# Contemporary Diabetes

**Series Editor**: Aristidis Veves, MD, DSc

For further volumes:
http://www.springer.com/series/7679

Alicia J. Jenkins • Peter P. Toth
Timothy J. Lyons
Editors

# Lipoproteins in Diabetes Mellitus

Humana Press

*Editors*
Alicia J. Jenkins, MD, FRACP
Health Sciences Center
Section of Endocrinology and Diabetes
University of Oklahoma
Oklahoma City, OK, USA

NHMRC Clinical Trials Centre
University of Sydney
Sydney, NSW, Australia

Timothy J. Lyons, MD, FRCP
Health Sciences Center
Section of Endocrinology and Diabetes
Harold Hamm Diabetes Center
University of Oklahoma
Oklahoma City, OK, USA

Peter P. Toth, MD, PhD
College of Medicine
University of Illinois
Peoria, IL, USA

ISBN 978-1-4614-7553-8 ISBN 978-1-4614-7554-5 (eBook)
DOI 10.1007/978-1-4614-7554-5
Springer New York Heidelberg Dordrecht London

Library of Congress Control Number: 2013944894



Printed on acid-free paper

Humana Press is a brand of Springer
Springer is part of Springer Science+Business Media (www.springer.com)

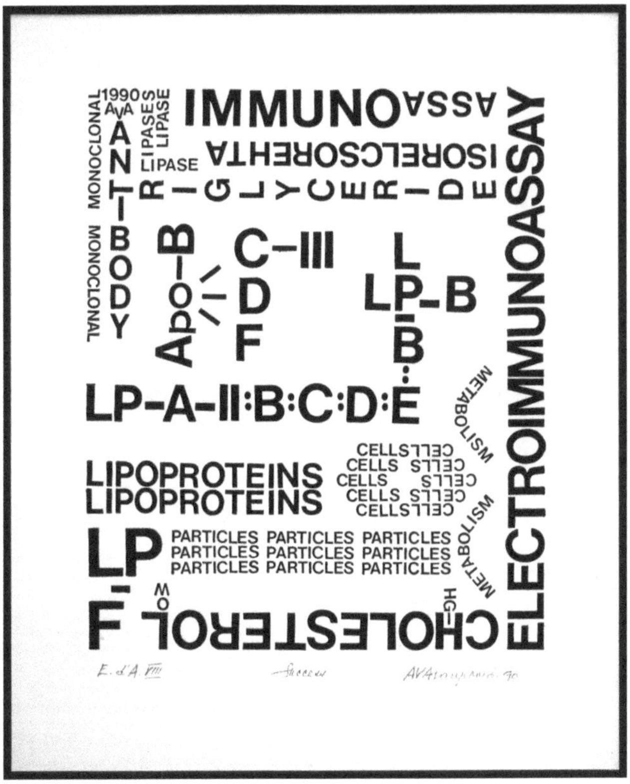


*"Success" by Alexandra Alaupovic (nee Vrbanic—born December 21, 1921, Podravska Slatina, Croatia—died January 2, 2013, Oklahoma City, OK, USA).*
*The artist created this work in recognition of the lipoprotein-related research by her husband Petar Alaupovic. Alexandra Alaupovic trained at the Academy of Visual Arts in Zagreb, University of Illinois and the University of Oklahoma, and was a Professor of Sculpture at the Oklahoma City University. Her work is exhibited in many public and private collections around the world. She is survived by her husband, daughter Betsy and grandsons Robert and Homer Clark.*

# Preface

Diabetes mellitus (DM) is becoming increasingly epidemic globally. The World Health Organization (WHO) estimates that the prevalence of DM varies between 8 and 10 % in all regions of the globe. Millions of new cases are diagnosed every year, and a substantial percentage of people with DM are undiagnosed either because they are not screened for the condition or because of inadequate access to healthcare. The epidemics of obesity, increased mechanization and reduced physical activity, cigarette smoking, and the fact that people are living longer have all contributed to the rise in Type 2 DM incidence. The incidence and prevalence of Type 1 DM is also increasing, perhaps also related to changes in the environment. Obesity, sedentary lifestyle, and cigarette smoking potentiate insulin resistance, which also promote atherosclerosis and the vascular complications of DM, as well as of Type 2 DM itself. Longer lifespan is associated with increased weight, lower levels of physical activity, and progressive loss of pancreatic islet cell mass. The US Centers for Disease Control estimates that 26.5 % of Americans 65 years of age or older have DM. According to the American Heart Association, in 2008, 18 million Americans had diagnosed DM, with another 7.1 million having undiagnosed DM; it is estimated that the prevalence of pre-diabetes in the US is 81.5 million. These staggering numbers are not unique to the United States. The worldwide rate of rise in DM is just as alarming. It is estimated that by the year 2030, 340 million people around the world will have DM and the figure is likely to be higher.

The risk for DM is strongly influenced by genetic and environmental factors. Risk for new onset DM is strongly influenced by race and ethnicity. Insulin resistance (IR) is the hallmark of pre-diabetes and Type 2 DM and is characterized by impaired transduction of insulin signaling pathways. Insulin resistance, which also occurs in Type 1 DM, results in hyperglycemia and is also associated with visceral organ steatosis, endothelial dysfunction, hypertension, increased systemic inflammatory and oxidative tone, a prothrombotic state, intracellular accumulation of toxic lipid intermediates (diacylglycerol, ceramide), as well as atherogenic dyslipidemia, among other changes. These metabolic disturbances greatly augment risk for the development of microvascular and macrovascular disease. The epidemic of DM is expected to result in one of the steepest rises in human morbidity and mortality ever observed outside of wartime. DM is the leading cause of proliferative retinopathy and adult onset blindness in working age adults, peripheral vascular disease and lower extremity amputation, end-stage renal disease and need for dialysis and renal transplantation, peripheral and autonomic neuropathy, and it magnifies the risk of myocardial infarction, stroke, and sudden death at least two- to four-fold. In addition to the human cost of this disease, there is an enormous economic burden associated with the clinical management and treatment of complications associated with DM.

*Lipoprotein in Diabetes Mellitus* is meant to be an authoritative and comprehensive reference on the many changes wrought by IR and DM on lipid and lipoprotein metabolism. Reducing the burden of atherogenic lipoproteins in serum is unequivocally associated with reductions in risk for cardiovascular events and may also ameliorate microvascular damage. The book begins by summarizing the various techniques to measure lipoproteins and their subclasses. In addition to delineating the molecular basis for how IR and DM alter lipid and lipoprotein handling in the gut, adipose tissue, liver, blood, and blood vessel wall, this volume explores how IR induces dyslipidemia, the glycation and oxidation of lipoproteins, and how alterations in immunity and cell surface receptor expression can impact lipoprotein metabolism. The mechanistic basis for why IR and DM increase risk for atherosclerosis as well as diabetic retinopathy and nephropathy are explored in detail. The design of clinical trials and the impact of lifestyle modification and of specific approved and investigational drug classes on diabetic dyslipidemia and risk for diabetes-related complications comprise the latter third of this volume. We thank our international panel of contributors for their clinical and basic scientific expertise and many insights. It is our sincerest hope that the clinicians who care for patients with IR and DM and the basic science researchers who explore mechanisms of vascular damage and protection will find this treatment of the issues covered herein timely and relevant and that it will significantly impact patient care in a positive and lasting way.

Oklahoma City, OK, USA — Alicia J. Jenkins, MD, FRACP
Peoria, IL, USA — Peter P. Toth, MD, PhD
Oklahoma City, OK, USA — Timothy J. Lyons, MD, FRCP

# Contents

# Contributors

**Jean Claude Ansquer** ClinSciences, Dijon, France

**Michael Aviram** The Lipid Research Laboratory, Technion Faculty of Medicine, Rappaport Family Institute for Research in the Medical Sciences and Rambam Medical Center, Haifa, Israel

**Harold Bays** Louisville Metabolic and Atherosclerosis Research Center, Louisville, KY, USA

**Alex Bobik** Vascular Biology and Atherosclerosis, BakerIDI Heart and Diabetes Insitute, Melbourne, VIC, Australia

**Eliot A. Brinton** Utah Foundation for Biomedical Research, Salt Lake City, UT, USA

Utah Lipid Center, Salt Lake City, UT, USA

**Alberico L. Catapano** Department of Pharmacological and Biomolecular Sciences, University of Milan, Milan, Italy

Center for the Study of Atherosclerosis, E. Bassini Hospital, Cinisello Balsamo, and IRCCS Multimedica, Milan, Italy

**Alan Chait** Division of Metabolism, Endocrinology and Nutrition, University of Washington School of Medicine, Seattle, WA, USA

**Peter Clifton** Sansom Institute University of South Australia, Adelaide, SA, Australia

**Michael Cobble** CMO Atherotech Diagnostics Lab, Birmingham, AL, USA

Canyons Medical Center, Sandy, UT, USA

**Thomas D. Dayspring** Foundation for Health Improvement and Technology, Richmond, VA, USA

**Christelle Foucher** ClinSciences, Dijon, France

**Val Gebski** NHMRC Clinical Trials Centre, University of Sydney, Sydney, NSW, Australia

**Per-Henrik Groop** Folkhälsan Research Center, Folkhälsan Institute of Genetics, Biomedicum Helsinki, Finland

Department of Medicine, Division of Nephrology, Helsinki University Central Hospital, Helsinki, Finland

Baker IDI Heart & Diabetes Institute, Melbourne, VIC, Australia

**Sandra J. Hamilton** Combined Universities Centre for Rural Health, University of Western Australia, Geraldton, WA, Australia

**Tony Hayek** The Lipid Research Laboratory, Technion Faculty of Medicine, Rappaport Family Institute for Research in the Medical Sciences and Rambam Medical Center, Haifa, Israel

**Andrzej S. Januszewski** Department of Medicine, The University of Melbourne, St. Vincent's Hospital, Melbourne, VIC, Australia

NHMRC Clinical Trials Centre, University of Sydney, Sydney, NSW, Australia

**Alicia J. Jenkins** Section of Endocrinology and Diabetes, University of Oklahoma Health Sciences Center, Oklahoma City, OK, USA

NHMRC Clinical Trials Centre, University of Sydney, Sydney, NSW, Australia

**Steven R. Jones** Department of Medicine, Cardiology Division, The Johns Hopkins University, Baltimore, MD, USA

**Parag H. Joshi** Johns Hopkins University, Baltimore, MD, USA

**Marielle Kaplan** The Laboratory of Clinical Biochemistry, Rappaport Family Institute for Research in the Medical Sciences, Rambam Medical Center, Haifa, Israel

**Anthony Keech** NHMRC Clinical Trials Centre, University of Sydney, Sydney, NSW, Australia

**Richard L. Klein** Division of Endocrinology, Diabetes, and Medical Genetics, Medical University of South Carolina, Charleston, SC, USA

**Gerhard M. Kostner** Medical University of Graz, Graz, Austria

**Karam M. Kostner** University of Queensland, Mater Hospital, Brisbane, Australia

**Barry Lewis** University of Sydney, Sydney, NSW, Australia

**Peter J. Little** Department of Pharmacy, RMIT University, Bundoora, VIC, Australia

Monash University, Melbourne, VIC, Australia

**Maria F. Lopes-Virella** Department of Medicine, Medical University of South Carolina, Charleston, SC, USA

Ralph A. Johnson VA Medical Center, Charleston, SC, USA

**Timothy J. Lyons** Section of Endocrinology & Diabetes, Harold Hamm Oklahoma Diabetes Center, University of Oklahoma Health Sciences Center, Oklahoma City, OK, USA

**Ville-Petteri Mäkinen** Folkhälsan Research Center, Folkhälsan Institute of Genetics, Biomedicum Helsinki, Finland

Department of Medicine, Division of Nephrology, Helsinki University Central Hospital, Helsinki, Finland

**Seth S. Martin** Johns Hopkins University, Baltimore, MD, USA

**Patrick D. Mize** Atherotech Diagnostics Lab, Birmingham, AL, USA

**Giuseppe D. Norata** Department of Pharmacological and Biomolecular Sciences, University of Milan and Center for the Study of Atherosclerosis, E. Bassini Hospital, Cinisello Balsamo, Italy

**David O'Neal** University of Melbourne, Department of Medicine, St. Vincent's Hospital, Fitzroy, Melbourne, VIC, Australia

**Narin Osman** RMIT University, Melbourne, VIC, Australia

**Daphne Owens** Diabetes Institute of Ireland, Beacon Hospital, Sandyford, Dublin, Ireland

Trinity College Dublin, Dublin, Ireland

**Angela Pirillo** Center for the Study of Atherosclerosis, E. Bassini Hospital, Cinisello Balsamo, and IRCCS Multimedica, Milan, Italy

**Vasudevan A. Raghavan** Cardiometabolic, Lipid Clinic & Medical Weight Management Services, Division of Endocrinology, Scott and White Center of Diagnostic Medicine, Temple, TX, USA

Texas A&M Health Sciences Center and College of Medicine, Temple, TX, USA

**Arthur Z. Schwartzbard** Leon H. Charney Division of Cardiology, Department of Medicine, Center for Prevention of Cardiovascular Disease, NYU School of Medicine, New York, NY, USA

University Langone School of Medicine, New York, NY, USA

**Kamalpreet Singh** Texas A&M Health Sciences Center and College of Medicine, Temple, TX, USA

**David R. Sullivan** Department of Clinical Biochemistry, Royal Prince Alfred Hospital, Camperdown, Sydney, NSW, Australia

**Nina Tolonen** Folkhälsan Research Center, Folkhälsan Institute of Genetics, Biomedicum Helsinki, Helsinki, Finland

Department of Medicine, Division of Nephrology, Helsinki University Central Hospital, Helsinki, Finland

**Gerald H. Tomkin** Diabetes Institute of Ireland, Beacon Hospital, Sandyford, Dublin, Ireland

Trinity College Dublin, Dublin, Ireland

**Peter P. Toth** University of Illinois School of Medicine, Peoria, IL, USA

**Henry A. Tran** Greenberg Division of Cardiology, Weill Cornell Medical College, New York, NY, USA

New York University Langone School of Medicine, New York City, NY, USA

**James A. Underberg** Division of General Internal Medicine, Center for Prevention of Cardiovascular, NYU School of Medicine, New York, NY, USA

**Gabriel Virella** Department of Microbiology and Immunology, Medical University of South Carolina, Charleston, SC, USA

**Gerald F. Watts** Cardiometabolic Research Centre, School of Medicine and Pharmacology, Royal Perth Hospital Unit, University of Western Australia, Perth, WA, Australia

**Mingyuan Wu** Section of Endocrinology & Diabetes, Harold Hamm Oklahoma Diabetes Center, University of Oklahoma Health Sciences Center, Oklahoma City, OK, USA

# Laboratory Assessment of Lipoproteins in Diabetes

1

David R. Sullivan and Barry Lewis

## Abbreviations

| | |
|---|---|
| Apo B | Apolipoprotein B |
| CETP | Cholesteryl ester transfer protein |
| CVD | Cardiovascular disease |
| HDL-C | High-density lipoprotein cholesterol |
| LDL-C | Low-density lipoprotein cholesterol |
| NHDL-C | Non-high-density lipoprotein cholesterol |
| TC | Total cholesterol |
| TG | Triglycerides |
| TRL | Triglyceride-rich lipoproteins |

## Introduction

### Lipids, Lipoproteins and Other Analytes in Diabetes

Type 1 and Type 2 diabetes mellitus are often regarded as abnormalities of insulin and glucose metabolism, but it is more appropriate to recognise that they disrupt the pathophysiology of macronutrient metabolism as a whole. Accordingly, it is essential to recognize the effects of diabetes on another major class of macronutrients, namely, lipids. The fundamental differences in the pathophysiology and treatment of Type 1 and Type 2 diabetes are manifest in the changes in lipoprotein metabolism that accompany these two common forms of diabetes. Consequently, the role of altered lipoprotein metabolism in the atherosclerotic process that underlies macrovascular complications may differ. Fully treated Type 1 diabetes often causes minimal disturbance to the lipoprotein profile, in fact the level of HDL-C may be slightly increased in insulin-treated patients [1, 2]. Nevertheless, glycation of the protein component of lipoproteins [3], as well as other modifications such as oxidation and immune complex formation (discussed in other chapters), may render lipoproteins dysfunctional in Type 1 diabetes. Consequently, the atherogenicity of the diabetic state in Type 1 diabetes, combined with the early age of onset, results in an increased lifelong risk of CVD that demands efforts to maintain lipoproteins at target levels or better [4]. This may be difficult to achieve in the face of complications of Type 1 diabetes such as renal impairment or the need for immune-suppressive therapy subsequent to renal, pancreas or islet cell transplantation. Hypercholesterolemia may occur in Type 1 diabetes in association with severe chronic hyperglycemia. Furthermore, insulin is required for the action of lipoprotein lipase, so early use of insulin therapy may be necessary in the massive hypertriglyceridemia associated with both forms of diabetes [5].

D.R. Sullivan (✉)
Department of Clinical Biochemistry, Royal Prince Alfred Hospital, Missenden Rd, Camperdown, Sydney, NSW 2050, Australia
e-mail: David.sullivan@sswahs.nsw.gov.au

B. Lewis
University of Sydney, Sydney, NSW, Australia

A.J. Jenkins et al. (eds.), *Lipoproteins in Diabetes Mellitus*, Contemporary Diabetes, DOI 10.1007/978-1-4614-7554-5_1, © Springer Science+Business Media New York 2014

**Table 1.1** Potential confounding factors that may affect lipoprotein assessment in Type 2 diabetes

| | |
|---|---|
| Intercurrent illness (with acute phase inflammation) | Increased VLDL (TG), reduced HDL-C, LDL-C |
| Hemoconcentration (dehydration, upright posture, prolonged tourniquet, squeezing to obtain fingerprick sample) | Proportionate increase in most analytes, including lipoproteins |
| Medications, menstrual cycle | Variable |
| Winter/summer | LDL-C lower in summer |
| Stress | Small unexplained increase is LDL-C reported |
| Food or caloric intake | Increased chylomicrons (TG) sufficient to undermine standardisation for purposes of classification and LDL-C calculation |
| Hemolysis or analytical delay | Predominantly affects other analytes (e.g. glucose and potassium levels) rather than lipids |
| Lipaemia | May require dilution<br>May interfere with turbidimetric analysis of Apolipoproteins |
| Presence and type of anticoagulant | Direct HDL-C now less likely to be affected |

On the other hand, Type 2 diabetes is associated with a well-characterized disturbance of the lipoprotein profile which features mild to moderate increase in triglyceride-rich lipoproteins (TRL), reduced HDL-C, smaller LDL size and modification of LDL particle composition, hence increased cardiovascular risk. Type 2 diabetes is by far the commoner variety and is becoming increasingly prevalent in the setting of increased dietary energy intakes and reduced activity levels both in affluent and developing societies; it will be the major focus of attention of this chapter.

Lipid abnormalities manifest as disturbances of the levels of the lipoproteins that transport lipids in the bloodstream. These disturbances contribute to the macrovascular complications of diabetes by influencing the processes that underlie atherosclerosis and thrombosis. Less frequently, they lead to massive increases in TG that greatly increase the risk of acute pancreatitis with associated loss of beta cell function. Recent evidence also suggests that disturbances in lipoprotein metabolism may contribute to some forms of microvascular complications of diabetes such as renal impairment, which is discussed in other chapters; however the relevant mechanisms are yet to be fully elucidated [6].

The laboratory assessment of lipoprotein status in diabetes relies on minimization of the effect of potential confounding factors which are summarised in Table 1.1. Sample collection procedures are designed to reduce preanalytical sources of error [7]. Sustained attention to standardisation and quality assurance has established a high level of reliability for routine lipid measurements which is maintained by a well-established system of internal and external quality assurance programmes [8, 9]. This process has been extended to include Apolipoproteins, most importantly Apo B [10] and Apo (a) [11].

One of the most clinically relevant sources of variability is the presence of intercurrent illness because the associated inflammatory response modifies the lipid and lipoprotein profile. It is important to note that the lipoprotein response to intercurrent illness shares some of the features of that associated with Type 2 diabetes, as will be described later. The magnitude of modifications associated with an inflammatory response is usually proportional to the severity of the underlying illness [12], but proportionately smaller responses should also be anticipated in association with minor intercurrent illnesses [13].

## Routine Lipoprotein Assessment

Clinical evaluation of lipoprotein metabolism in diabetes usually involves the measurement of total cholesterol, HDL-C and TG following a 12-h fast. LDL-C is derived from the fasting results by application of the Friedewald equation

[14] [LDL-C in mg/dl = TC−HDL-C−(TG/5), LDL-C in mmol/l = TC−HDL-C−(TG/2.2)], but this calculation becomes less reliable as TG levels increase beyond approximately 4 mmol/l (350 mg/dl). Non-fasting samples have been shown to be a more sensitive marker for the detection of individuals with increased risk of CVD [15], but the unstandardized nature of non-fasting samples [16] makes them unsuitable for the characterization or serial monitoring of lipid status in diabetes. Indeed, even fasting levels of TG and other lipids show considerable within-individual variability [17]. This has implications for the serial measurement of LDL-C and the fasting TG from which it was calculated. A change in a serial measurement can only be attributed to clinical factors if it is greater than would be expected due to other sources of variability [18]. The considerable biological variability of fasting TG will increase the proportion by which a serial measurement of fasting TG (and hence LDL-C) must differ in order to indicate a clinically significant alteration.

Increased levels of TRL may also cause variable interference with automated "direct" HDL-C measurements due to TRL cholesterol content. This may have resulted in a positive bias in the past. Method comparison studies prior to 2000 suggested good agreement between "separation" HDL-C methods and the reference method [19], even in the presence of Intralipid [20] or TRL [21]. Where positive bias occurred, it was attributed to incomplete precipitation with the comparator method [22–24] or the presence of Apolipoprotein E-containing HDL [25], but the sources of TG used in these studies had a relatively low cholesterol content. "Direct" HDL methods initially involved the use of α-cyclodextrin, and positive interference from TRL was described in some [26], but not all [23] studies. Since methods involving α-cyclodextrin have been superseded, several recent studies of "direct" HDL methods have reported positive biases which were attributed to TRL [27] or the presence of diabetes [28]. This is an important issue because any overestimation of HDL-C leads to a risk of under-diagnosis of the metabolic syndrome and insulin resistance, as well as under-calculation of LDL-C and NHDL-C. These combined effects would result in a substantial underestimation of absolute risk of CVD, leading to loss of opportunity to effectively identify and treat patients on the basis of their metabolic risk factors. It is possible that TRL may also interfere with "direct" LDL-C assays that utilize a similar strategy based on selective effect of detergents [29].

The accuracy of standard lipid measurements is extremely important because this quantitative information is applied directly to patient management. The atherogenic effect of LDL-C and other Apo B-containing lipoproteins and the probable anti-atherosclerotic effects of HDL-C represent independent risk factors for CVD. Whereas LDL-C (or TC) originally provided thresholds for initiation of treatment and targets for management, management decisions are now seen in a wider context that encompasses the overall (absolute) CVD risk of the patient. This incorporates the classic modifiable and non-modifiable risk factors to varying extents. The predominance of age is one of several inevitable limitations to the performance of the absolute risk calculation algorithms. Diabetes is no longer regarded as "coronary risk equivalent", but rather the presence or absence of diabetes is treated as a categorical variable, usually without adjustment for severity. Clinical uncertainty associated with intermediate levels of CVD risk has led to efforts to "reclassify" patients in this category by a variety of methods. Consequently, some algorithms allow adjustment for factors such as ethnicity, duration of diabetes, HbA1C level and the presence or absence of microalbuminuria (e.g. www.yourheartforecast.co.nz/). Whilst the additional CVD risk posed by the presence of diabetes often justifies active management of the lipid profile, clinicians need to remember that the presence of massive hypertriglyceridemia poses the more immediate risk of acute pancreatitis.

## LDL Composition and Particle Number

Clinical decision-making based purely on quantitative assessment of LDL-C and HDL-C is no longer appropriate, particularly in the presence of elevated TG, which is often the case in Type 2 diabetes. Increased levels of TRL promote the action of cholesteryl ester transfer protein (CETP), which leads to a reduction in HDL-C levels and a depletion in the amount of cholesterol carried per LDL particle. The extent of this process may depend on the severity of postprandial lipemia [30] such that these changes in HDL-C and LDL composition [31] are not completely reflected by the accompanying fasting TG level. Furthermore, the relationship between LDL-C and CVD risk becomes confounded [32] because the formation of "small dense LDL" results in an LDL-C concentration that is low relative to the number of LDL particles. This is illustrated by the superiority of other risk markers [33] such as NHDL-C (calculated as the difference between TC and HDL-C levels) which reflects the full range of potentially atherogenic lipoproteins. This superiority is thought to reflect the greater atherogenicity of the "small dense LDL" and hence the pre-eminence of particle number as the main determinant of the pro-atherogenic effect on non-HDL lipoproteins [34]. This conclusion is based on quantitative ultracentrifuge studies which are usually too tedious to perform for clinical purposes. Electrophoresis based on sizing gel techniques has attempted to circumvent this problem, leading to designation of so-called "pattern A" and "pattern B" profiles or estimations of LDL diameter. These methods are non-quantitative with respect to the number of atherogenic lipoprotein particles, so their clinical value may be marginal.

A more promising approach is based on the measurement of serum Apo B level [35]. All particles that contain Apo B (including chylomicrons, which contain Apo B48, and VLDL, LDL IDL and Lp(a), which contain Apo B 100) are capable of transporting lipid to peripheral sites and, as such, might be considered potentially atherogenic. All such particles contain a single molecule of Apo B, so Apo B provides a direct measurement of the number of particles. Human Apo B derived from the intestine is the product of post-translational modification (m-RNA editing) that yields a product that consists of the N-terminal fragment that represents 48 % of the complete Apo B protein. These two products are designated Apo B 48 and Apo B 100, respectively. Polyclonal antibodies, or monoclonals targeting the first half of the molecule, can be used to quantify both forms. Apo B levels do not change very much after a meal because the transport of dietary fat is largely accommodated by an increase in TG content, rather than an increase in total Apo B. This also reflects the fact that the number of Apo B 100 particles is large relative to the number of Apo B 48 particles. Hence Apo B measurement need not depend on fasting [36] or the ability to differentiate the Apo B 100 isoform.

The degree to which large TG-rich Apo B-containing particles can directly damage the artery wall is debateable, but all apo B 100-contaiining particles (with the exception of Lp(a)) are potential precursors of LDL. As a result, Apo B 100, which is largely reflected by total Apo B levels, quantitatively represents the pro-atherogenic potential of the lipoprotein profile. Furthermore, the predominance of LDL particles means that Apo B largely reflects LDL particle number. Evidence suggests that Apo B measurement is superior to LDL-C or NHDL-C for CVD risk assessment [37]. When combined with LDL-C measurement, the LDL-C:Apo B ratio can reflect the degree to which cholesterol depletion of LDL has led to the formation of "small, dense LDL".

Nuclear magnetic resonance (NMR) spectroscopy is a non-destructive analytical technique applied to plasma or serum that may be used to reflect the physical composition of lipoprotein particles, particularly their size and number. Consequently, NMR spectroscopy has been used to provide a more detailed picture of lipoprotein size distributions, including HDL species. The technique is unable to distinguish between LDL and Lp(a). Nevertheless studies suggest that NMR spectroscopy may provide additional benefit in terms of the clinical assessment of lipoprotein-associated CVD risk [38].

Tables 1.2, 1.3, and 1.4 are provided as a means of extending the benefits of Apo B measurement to include diagnosis.

**Table 1.2** An algorithm for the prediction of the likely class of lipoproteins responsible for dyslipidemia in approximate order of prevalence in Type 2 diabetes (adapted from de Graaf et al.) [23]

| Apolipoprotein B level | TG > 1.5 mg/dl (Y/N) | TG:ApoB ≥10 (Y/N) | TC (mg/dl): ApoB ≥6.2 (Y/N) | Lipoprotein |
|---|---|---|---|---|
| Apo B < 1.2 g/l | N | N | N | Normal |
| Apo B < 1.2 g/l | Y | N | N | VLDL[a] |
| Apo B ≥ 1.2 g/l | Y | N/A | N/A | LDL and VLDL[a, b] |
| Apo B ≥ 1.2 g/l | N | N/A | N/A | LDL[b] |
| Apo B = 0.75–1.2 g/l | Y | Y | N | Chylomicron and VLDL[a] |
| Apo B < 1.2 g/l | Y | N | Y | IDL or "remnants" |
| Apo B < 0.75 g/l | Y | Y | N | Chylomicrons alone[a] |

[a]LDL particle size (diameter) may be reduced, as in "small, dense LDL"
[b]LDL particle number may be increased, as in increased Apo B level

## Etiological Assessment

The clinical implications of dyslipidemia depend on the type of lipoprotein responsible for the alteration in lipid levels and the etiological reason for its accumulation. The atherogenic effect of various lipoproteins may differ depending on the etiological context in which they arise, and it should not be assumed that the lipoprotein profile in Type 1 or Type 2 diabetes is solely and necessarily based on that condition alone. Other secondary causes may modify the lipoprotein abnormality, whilst intercurrent primary lipoprotein disorders may influence or even dictate the lipoprotein profile. Tables 1.2, 1.3, and 1.4 provide a framework for diagnostic considerations that may modify clinical management. The first step in this process is the consideration of which lipoprotein class is responsible for any dyslipidemia in a person with diabetes. Though this may be inferred from the results of the automated laboratory tests, it cannot be relied upon. Traditionally, identification of the excess lipoproteins was achieved by lipid electrophoresis, but this non-quantitative method does little to enhance prognostic information. Tables 1.2, 1.3, and 1.4 present an extension of the use of Apo B levels to provide this information in an alternative and potentially more useful format [35]. The different lipoprotein patterns are presented in approximate order of their prevalence in Type 2 diabetes, but as will be explained, the first four are somewhat interchangeable. The last two are substantially less common.

## Predominant Hypertriglyceridemia and Hyperbetalipoproteinemia

Predominant hypertriglyceridemia due to increased VLDL (accompanied by low HDL-C) is the most common form of dyslipidaemia in people with Type 2 diabetes, but it is by no means universal. It may occur with or without an associated increase in cholesterol due to increased LDL. As a result, the first four profiles listed in Table 1.2 are relatively common in people with Type 2 diabetes. This is supported by the observation that Type 2 diabetes is a common secondary cause of the first three lipoprotein patterns in Table 1.3. Nevertheless, it is also important to note that other diseases may cause or contribute to such patterns of dyslipidaemia, and indeed several, such as renal impairment and medications, are common accompaniments of Type 2 diabetes, whilst others, such as obesity and corticosteroid use, represent secondary causes of Type 2 diabetes itself. Furthermore, the mere presence of diabetes does not exclude the possibility of intercurrent primary causes of dyslipidaemia. It has been argued that LDL-C levels in western society are pathologically high due to gene/environment interactions (referred to as "polygenic hypercholesterolemia"), and hence this pattern, the fourth in Table 1.4, may frequently accompany Type 2 diabetes.

Indeed, the first four patterns in Tables 1.2, 1.3, and 1.4 must be regarded as potentially interchangeable. This is highlighted by the condition

**Table 1.3** Causes of secondary dyslipidemia, including diabetes

| Excess lipoprotein accumulation | Causes |
|---|---|
| VLDL | Type 2 diabetes<br>Obesity/insulin resistance<br>Chronic renal impairment<br>Hemodialysis<br>Alcohol excess<br>Estrogen use<br>Glucocorticoid use<br>Retinol analogues<br>Other |
| LDL and VLDL | Type 2 diabetes<br>Obesity/insulin resistance<br>Cholestasis<br>Nephrotic syndrome<br>Peritoneal dialysis<br>Systemic lupus erythematosus<br>Polycystic ovary syndrome<br>Glucocorticoid use<br>HIV and highly active antiretroviral therapy<br>Antipsychotic drug use<br>Pregnancy<br>Other |
| LDL | Nephrotic syndrome<br>Hypothyroidism<br>Anabolic steroids<br>Other |
| Chylomicron and VLDL | Type 2 diabetes<br>Obesity/insulin resistance<br>Chronic renal impairment<br>Alcohol excess<br>Oestrogen use<br>Glucocorticoid use<br>Pregnancy<br>Other |
| IDL or "remnants" | Triggered or exacerbated by<br>Type 2 diabetes<br>Obesity/insulin resistance<br>Chronic renal impairment<br>Alcohol excess<br>Oestrogen use<br>Glucocorticoid use<br>Other |
| Chylomicrons alone | Acquired Apo C2 deficiency in systemic lupus erythematosus |

hyperbetalipoproteinemia, which is listed as a primary dyslipidaemia in Table 1.4. Hyperbetalipoproteinemia was previously referred to as familial combined hyperlipidaemia. It featured a variable lipoprotein picture that ranged from normal levels of LDL-C and TG to elevated levels of either or both. This variability was manifest within individuals and between individuals of affected families. It was regarded as a dominant monogenic condition and was more reliably identified by the overproduction of Apo B-containing particles, manifest as increased Apo B levels, even in normolipidemic cases. Whilst strong genetic predisposition remains evident, it is now clear that expression of the abnormality is highly dependent on other factors, most notably age and central adiposity [39]. As such, it has come to be regarded as one form of the spectrum of insulin resistance [40]. This implies that many subjects with Type 2 diabetes may have a genetic predisposition towards overproduction of Apo B-containing lipoproteins which might manifest as normolipemia, isolated elevation of LDL-C or TG levels or combined elevation of both. As explained previously, any tendency towards increased TG levels would trigger a decline in HDL-C due to the action of CETP. At the other end of the scale, if Type 2 diabetes is the result of non-genetic factors, those factors may also be sufficient to lead to hyperbetalipoproteinemia. It will be appreciated that even polygenic hypercholesterolemia can be regarded as a form of hyperbetalipoproteinemia.

## Saturation of Catabolic Pathways

Type 2 diabetes implies a tendency towards positive energy balance that favours excess serum levels of markers of macronutrient metabolism, most notably glucose, free fatty acids and TG. Furthermore, the previous sections highlight the association between Type 2 diabetes and the overproduction of serum lipoproteins. Consequently, Type 2 diabetes places increased demands on the catabolic pathways for TG and Apo B-containing lipoproteins, respectively. Most Apo B-containing particles undergo final catabolism via the LDL receptor. Competition for this receptor will increase LDL-C levels, and this is thought to contribute to increases in LDL-C and Apo B that are commonly associated with Type 2 diabetes. The LDL receptor also mediates the hepatic removal of catabolised TRL, known as "remnant particles"; in this case the receptor

**Table 1.4** Causes of primary dyslipidemia which may coexist with diabetes

| Excess lipoprotein accumulation | Primary causes |
|---|---|
| VLDL | Polygenic gene/environment interactions<br>Familial hypertriglyceridemia |
| LDL and VLDL | Polygenic gene/environment interactions<br>HyperApobetalipoproteinaemia preferred instead of "familial combined hyperlipidemia" |
| LDL | Polygenic gene/environment interactions<br>Familial hypercholesterolaemia |
| Chylomicron and VLDL | Polygenic gene/environment interactions<br>Exacerbation of familial hypertriglyceridemia or familial hyperchylomicronaemia |
| IDL or "remnants" | Dysbetalipoproteinaemia |
| Chylomicron | Familial hyperchylomicronaemia |

interacts with the Apolipoprotein E of these lipoproteins. The affinity of Apo E for the LDL receptor varies according to a genetically determined polymorphism: the E2:E2 genotype has the least affinity which causes mild impairment of remnant clearance, mild increase in TG and a mildly reduced LDL-C [41]. This polymorphism has a prevalence of about 1 %. If any cause of lipoprotein overproduction is also present, this "second hit" may saturate Apo E-mediated catabolism of "remnants" [42]. Massive accumulation of remnant particles, as reflected by an increase in TG and TC that is out of proportion to any increase in Apo B, is strongly atherogenic, and the severity may even be sufficient to saturate the removal of TG, as discussed below.

The catabolism of TG takes place on the endothelial surface of peripheral tissues due to the action of lipoprotein lipase. There are a number of genetic influences that affect the activity of lipoprotein lipase [43]. The rarest and severest impairments result in lipoprotein lipase deficiency, the last condition in Table 1.4. Nevertheless, individuals with Type 2 diabetes and less severely limited lipoprotein lipase activity may accumulate enough TG to fully saturate their lipolytic activity, particularly if they adopt a high-fat diet or deteriorates if their glycemic control (second last condition in Table 1.3). This may rapidly exacerbate TG levels, causing massive hypertriglyceridemia with attendant risk of acute pancreatitis. As mentioned above, the hypertriglyceridemia associated with accumulation of remnant particles may also saturate the activity of lipoprotein lipase.

## Apolipoprotein Measurement

Data supporting the use of Apo B measurement in appropriate circumstances has already been presented. Relatively inexpensive light-scattering methods are suitable for routine samples, but immuno-enzymatic or immuno-radiometric methods should be considered when lipemia is present because this may confound light-scattering techniques. The same considerations apply to the measurement of other Apolipoproteins.

Results of Apo A1 measurement carry the same implications as HDL-C, but evidence of clear-cut superiority is lacking [44]. Apo A1 cannot be incorporated in risk algorithms, and its widespread adoption is unlikely unless practical considerations lead to utilization in combination with Apo B. Apo E and Apo C3 are associated with both HDL and VLDL, but the VLDL fraction predominates, so the levels of these Apolipoproteins largely reflect the concentration of VLDL and TG. Apo C3 has demonstrated independent prognostic value in some studies [45], but its use is limited and standardisation of its measurement is at an early stage. Apo C2 plays a reciprocal role to Apo C3, but it is not measured as frequently. Apo A5 activity in the liver is a major determinant of plasma TG levels, but it is difficult to measure in the circulation [46]. Measurements of Apo A4, A2 and other minor apolipoproteins have yet to find major clinical applications.

Apolipoprotein (a) is an enigmatic Apolipoprotein that is covalently linked to LDL to form lipoprotein (a). Its homology with plasminogen makes it a putative inhibitor of thrombolysis, whilst its high degree of glycosylation renders it adherent to vessel wall matrix. Epidemiological studies supported by genome-wide association evidence conclude that it is an independent risk factor for cardiovascular disease [47]. It is largely under genetic control, but it may increase in the presence of renal impairment [48]. It can be measured by the methods mentioned above, but care must be taken with the standardization of the assay because the molecular size of the protein, which has a strong inverse relationship to its plasma level, shows remarkable variation between individuals [49].

## Other Laboratory Markers

One must not assume that abnormal lipoprotein status in people with Type 2 diabetes is solely due to the diabetic state. Consideration of additional primary and secondary causes provides additional prognostic information [50]. It is difficult, but plausible, to factor these considerations into clinical management decisions that are largely based on quantification and assessment of the absolute CVD (or other) risk of the individual patient. The greatest problem is the need to reclassify patients with intermediate levels of risk, so it is in this category that lipoprotein pattern and underlying etiology can be most helpful. Other forms of laboratory assessment also play a role in this regard. Detection, quantification and monitoring of pro-atherogenic diabetic complications, particularly renal impairment, warrant the measurement of urinary microalbumin, eGFR via creatinine and possibly, in future, cystatin C and/or N-gelatinase-associated lipocalin. The severity of hyperglycemia in diabetes, as quantified by serum glucose and glycated hemoglobin (usually as HbA1c) levels, also requires consideration. Biochemical modification of lipoproteins is not necessarily proportional to the severity of diabetes, so independent measurement of parameters such as oxidised LDL may eventually become relevant, but the evidence for their routine use has yet to accumulate [51]. Markers of other potentially atherosclerotic processes, such as inflammation, may also be relevant. It needs to be remembered that excess central adipose tissue, commonly associated with Type 2 diabetes, may be a source of adipokines, that include inflammatory markers such as C-reactive protein (measurable with a high-sensitivity assay) or lipoprotein-associated phospholipase A2. In this sense, raised levels of inflammatory markers may represent surrogate markers of Type 2 diabetes and pre-diabetes. Nevertheless, some guidelines do envisage a role for hs-CRP measurement in the reclassification of intermediate-risk patients [52]. Genome-wide association studies infer the existence of other independent mechanisms, some of which may pertain to both diabetes and its complications [53]. The capabilities of next-generation sequencing may permit the use of genetic techniques for the assessment of complex disorders such as diabetes and its complications [54].

## Summary

Clinical management of diabetes mellitus requires effective laboratory assessment of lipoprotein abnormalities. Diabetes may cause or exacerbate quantitative and/or qualitative changes in lipoproteins. Furthermore, diabetic complications may cause secondary dyslipidemia, whilst important forms of primary dyslipidemia may coexist with diabetes. The risk of macrovascular complications of diabetes can be anticipated by consideration of major cardiovascular risk factors including total cholesterol (TC), fasting triglyceride (TG) and high-density lipoprotein cholesterol (HDL-C), from which additional indicators such as low-density lipoprotein cholesterol (LDL-C) and non-HDL cholesterol (NHDL-C) may be derived. Like diabetes, dyslipidemia is a complex chronic condition that requires ongoing assessment and long-term surveillance.

## References


1. Taskinen MR, Kahri J, Koivisto V, Shepherd J, Packard CJ. Metabolism of HDL Apolipoprotein A-I and A-II in type 1 (insulin-dependent) diabetes mellitus. Diabetologia. 1992;35:347–56.
2. Dullaart RP. Plasma lipoprotein abnormalities in type 1 (insulin-dependent) diabetes mellitus. Neth J Med. 1995;46:44–54.
3. Nobecourt E, Tabet F, Lambert G, et al. Nonenzymatic glycation impairs the antiinflammatory properties of Apolipoprotein A-I. Arterioscler Thromb Vasc Biol. 2010;30:766–72.
4. Toth PP. An urgent matter-identifying your patients' cardiovascular risk and improving their outcomes. Commentary. J Fam Pract. 2009;58:S41–3.
5. Robinson DS, Speake BK. Role of insulin and other hormones in the control of lipoprotein lipase activity. Biochem Soc Trans. 1989;17:40–2.
6. Davis TME, Ting R, Best JD, et al. Effects of fenofibrate on renal function in patients with type 2 diabetes mellitus: the fenofibrate intervention and event lowering in diabetes (FIELD) study. Diabetologia. 2011;54:280–90.
7. Cooper GR, Myers GL. Clinical issues in cholesterol testing. J Med Assoc Ga. 1991;80:301–3.
8. Bachorik PS, Ross JW. National Cholesterol Education Program recommendations for measurement of low-density lipoprotein cholesterol: executive summary. The National Cholesterol Education Program Working Group on Lipoprotein Measurement. Clin Chem. 1995;41:1414–20.
9. Warnick GR, Wood PD. National Cholesterol Education Program recommendations for measurement of high-density lipoprotein cholesterol: executive summary. The National Cholesterol Education Program Working Group on Lipoprotein Measurement. Clin Chem. 1995;41:1427–33.
10. Contois JH, Warnick GR, Sniderman AD. Reliability of low-density lipoprotein cholesterol, non-high-density lipoprotein cholesterol, and Apolipoprotein B measurement. J Clin Lipidol. 2011;5:264–72.
11. Marcovina SM, Albers JJ, Scanu AM, et al. Use of a reference material proposed by the International Federation of Clinical Chemistry and Laboratory Medicine to evaluate analytical methods for the determination of plasma lipoprotein(a). Clin Chem. 2000;46:1956–67.
12. Dunham CM, Fealk MH, Sever 3rd WE. Following severe injury, hypocholesterolemia improves with convalescence but persists with organ failure or onset of infection. Crit Care. 2003;7:R145–53.
13. Gidding SS, Stone NJ, Bookstein LC, Laskarzewski PM, Stein EA. Month-to-month variability of lipids, lipoproteins, and Apolipoproteins and the impact of acute infection in adolescents. J Pediatr. 1998;133:242–6.
14. Friedewald WT, Levy RI, Fredrickson DS. Estimation of the concentration of low-density lipoprotein cholesterol in plasma, without use of the preparative ultracentrifuge. Clin Chem. 1972;18:499–502.
15. Nordestgaard BG, Benn M, Schnohr P, Tybjaerg-Hansen A. Nonfasting triglycerides and risk of myocardial infarction, ischemic heart disease, and death in men and women. [Reprint in Ugeskr Laeger. 2007 Nov 5;169(45):3865–8; PMID: 18031660]. JAMA. 2007;298:299–308.
16. Wilder LB, Bachorik PS, Finney CA, Moy TF, Becker DM. The effect of fasting status on the determination of low-density and high-density lipoprotein cholesterol. Am J Med. 1995;99:374–7.
17. Tolfrey K. Intraindividual variability of children's blood lipid and lipoprotein concentrations: a review. Prev Cardiol. 2002;5:145–51.
18. Dimitri G. "Critical difference" and biological variation of serum triglycerides. Clin Chem. 1994;40:501.
19. Rifai N, Cole TG, Iannotti E, et al. Assessment of interlaboratory performance in external proficiency testing programs with a direct HDL-cholesterol assay. Clin Chem. 1998;44:1452–8.
20. Nauck M, Marz W, Haas B, Wieland H. Homogeneous assay for direct determination of high-density lipoprotein cholesterol evaluated. Clin Chem. 1996;42:424–9.
21. Harris N, Galpchian V, Rifai N. Three routine methods for measuring high-density lipoprotein cholesterol compared with the Reference Method. Clin Chem. 1996;42:738–43.
22. de Keijzer MH, Elbers D, Baadenhuijsen H, Demacker PN. Evaluation of five different high-density lipoprotein cholesterol assays: the most precise are not the most accurate. Ann Clin Biochem. 1999;36:168–75.
23. Hubbard RS, Hirany SV, Devaraj S, Martin L, Parupia J, Jialal I. Evaluation of a rapid homogeneous method for direct measurement of high-density lipoprotein cholesterol. Am J Clin Pathol. 1998;110:495–502.
24. Okazaki M, Sasamoto K, Muramatsu T, Hosaki S. Evaluation of precipitation and direct methods for HDL-cholesterol assay by HPLC. Clin Chem. 1997;43:1885–90.
25. Okada M, Matsui H, Ito Y, Fujiwara A. Direct measurement of HDL cholesterol: method eliminating Apolipoprotein E-rich particles. J Clin Lab Anal. 2001;15:223–9.
26. Egloff M, Leglise D, Duvillard L, et al. Multicenter evaluation on different analyzers of three methods for direct HDL-cholesterol assay. Ann Biol Clin. 1999;57:561–72.
27. Perera NJ, Burns JC, Perera RS, Lewis B, Sullivan DR. Adjustment of direct high-density lipoprotein cholesterol measurements according to intercurrent triglyceride corrects for interference by triglyceride-rich lipoproteins. J Clin Lipidol. 2010;4:305–9.
28. Saeed BO, Smart P, Keeka G, Handley GH, Weaver JU. Comparison of two direct methods for HDL cholesterol measurement with an indirect precipitation method in diabetic patients. Diabetes Nutr Metabol Clin Exp. 2002;15:169–72.
29. Jun KR, Park H-I, Chun S, Park H, Min W-K. Effects of total cholesterol and triglyceride on the percentage

difference between the low-density lipoprotein cholesterol concentration measured directly and calculated using the Friedewald formula. Clin Chem Lab Med. 2008;46:371–5.
30. Sullivan DRCD, Le Couter DG, Lam CWK. The vascular implications of post-prandial lipoprotein metabolism. Clin Biochem Rev. 2004;25: 19–30.
31. Tsimihodimos V, Gazi I, Kostara C, Tselepis AD, Elisaf M. Plasma lipoproteins and triacylglycerol are predictors of small, dense LDL particles. Lipids. 2007;42:403–9.
32. Sniderman AD. Applying ApoB to the diagnosis and therapy of the atherogenic dyslipoproteinemias: a clinical diagnostic algorithm. Curr Opin Lipidol. 2004;15:433–8.
33. Sniderman A, Couture P, de Graaf J. Diagnosis and treatment of Apolipoprotein B dyslipoproteinemias. Nat Rev Endocrinol. 2010;6:335–46.
34. Jungner I, Sniderman AD, Furberg C, Aastveit AH, Holme I, Walldius G. Does low-density lipoprotein size add to atherogenic particle number in predicting the risk of fatal myocardial infarction? Am J Cardiol. 2006;97:943–6.
35. de Graaf J, Couture P, Sniderman A. A diagnostic algorithm for the atherogenic Apolipoprotein B dyslipoproteinemias. Nat Clin Pract Endocrinol Metab. 2008;4:608–18.
36. Langsted A, Freiberg JJ, Nordestgaard BG. Fasting and nonfasting lipid levels: influence of normal food intake on lipids, lipoproteins, Apolipoproteins, and cardiovascular risk prediction. Circulation. 2008;118: 2047–56.
37. Walldius G. Apolipoprotein B, (ApoB) more closely related to subclinical atherosclerosis than non-HDL cholesterol and LDL cholesterol. J Intern Med. 2010;268:549–51.
38. Cromwell WC, Otvos JD. Low-density lipoprotein particle number and risk for cardiovascular disease. Curr Atheroscler Rep. 2004;6:381–7.
39. Shamir R, Tershakovec AM, Gallagher PR, Liacouras CA, Hayman LL, Cortner JA. The influence of age and relative weight on the presentation of familial combined hyperlipidemia in childhood. Atherosclerosis. 1996;121:85–91.
40. Ascaso JF, Sales J, Merchante A, et al. Influence of obesity on plasma lipoproteins, glycaemia and insulinaemia in patients with familial combined hyperlipidaemia. Int J Obes Relat Metab Disord. 1997;21: 360–6.
41. Eto M, Watanabe K, Ishii K. Reciprocal effects of Apolipoprotein E alleles (epsilon 2 and epsilon 4) on plasma lipid levels in normolipidemic subjects. Clin Genet. 1986;29:477–84.
42. Retnakaran R, Connelly PW, Goguen J. Unmasking of type III hyperlipoproteinemia by hypothyroidism: a dramatic illustration of altered lipoprotein metabolism in a postpartum woman. Endocr Pract. 2005;11:394–8.
43. Lichtenstein L, Kersten S. Modulation of plasma TG lipolysis by Angiopoietin-like proteins and GPIHBP1. Biochim Biophys Acta. 1801;2010:415–20.
44. Cromwell WC. High-density lipoprotein associations with coronary heart disease: does measurement of cholesterol content give the best result? J Clin Lipidol. 2007;1:57–64.
45. Olivieri O, Martinelli N, Girelli D, et al. Apolipoprotein C-III predicts cardiovascular mortality in severe coronary artery disease and is associated with an enhanced plasma thrombin generation. J Thromb Haemost. 2010;8:463–71.
46. Dallinga-Thie GM, van Tol A, Hattori H, et al. Plasma Apolipoprotein A5 and triglycerides in type 2 diabetes. Diabetologia. 2006;49:1505–11.
47. Enkhmaa B, Anuurad E, Zhang W, Tran T, Berglund L. Lipoprotein(a): genotype-phenotype relationship and impact on atherogenic risk. Metab Syndr Relat Disord. 2011;9:411–8.
48. Shishehbor MH, Oliveira LPJ, Lauer MS, et al. Emerging cardiovascular risk factors that account for a significant portion of attributable mortality risk in chronic kidney disease. Am J Cardiol. 2008;101: 1741–6.
49. Mackness M, Hughes E, Heart UKLS. Variability in the measurement of lipoprotein(a) in the British Isles. Ann Clin Biochem. 2009;46:311–5.
50. Sullivan DRLB. A classification of lipoprotein disorders: implications for clinical management. Clin Lipidol. 2011;6:327–38.
51. Lyons TJ, Jenkins AJ. Lipoprotein glycation and its metabolic consequences. Curr Opin Lipidol. 1997;8: 174–80.
52. Genest J, McPherson R, Frohlich J, et al. 2009 Canadian Cardiovascular Society/Canadian guidelines for the diagnosis and treatment of dyslipidemia and prevention of cardiovascular disease in the adult - 2009 recommendations. Can J Cardiol. 2009;25:567–79.
53. Frayling TM. Genome-wide association studies provide new insights into type 2 diabetes aetiology. Nat Rev Genet. 2007;8:657–62.
54. Schnabel RB, Baccarelli A, Lin H, Ellinor PT, Benjamin EJ. Next steps in cardiovascular disease genomic research–sequencing, epigenetics, and transcriptomics. Clin Chem. 2012;58:113–26.

# Lipoprotein Subclasses and Cardiovascular Disease Risk in Insulin-Resistant Diabetes

**2**

Michael Cobble, Patrick D. Mize, and Eliot A. Brinton

## Insulin Resistance and Type 2 Diabetes

The pathophysiology of type 2 diabetes mellitus (T2DM) is characterized by insulin resistance (IR) in many tissues, including the liver and muscle, accompanied by progressive failure of adequate insulin secretion by the pancreatic β-cells [28]. Prior to the emergence of overt T2DM (i.e., fasting hyperglycemia), patients with "pre-diabetes" are seemingly healthy in that they have normal or only slightly elevated fasting glucose (impaired fasting glucose or IFG), but they have significantly impaired glucose tolerance (IGT) and IR. In this state there is progressive loss of β-cell function manifested as a loss of insulin secretion. Once the β-cell function declines 50–80 %, glucose levels cannot be brought to normal, even after an overnight fast, and so fasting hyperglycemia occurs and T2DM begins. Additional factors contributing to the onset of the T2DM phenotype are accelerated intracellular lipolysis in adipose tissue, defective incretin secretion by the gastrointestinal tract, inappropriate elevation (or lack of appropriate suppression) of glucagon secretion by pancreatic α-cells, increased glucose reabsorption in renal tubules, and IR in portions of the central nervous system responsible for regulating glucose homeostasis.

In both T2DM and in the prediabetes/IR state, a characteristic dyslipidemia occurs. The standard lipid profile often shows elevated plasma TG and non-HDL-C (defined as total cholesterol minus HDL-C) levels and reduced HDL-C [13, 15, 32, 88, 123]. In these cases, comprehensive lipid testing is likely to reveal additional abnormalities, including increased levels of remnant particles and a shift towards LDL particles which are smaller and denser on average. The shift towards small, dense LDL-C, called "Pattern B," is generally due primarily to an absolute increase in small, dense LDL and so is related to increased plasma concentrations of LDL particles and apoprotein B (apo B). This change can be assessed by measurement of (1) average or peak LDL size, (2) LDL particle concentrations, and (3) total plasma apo B levels.

The mechanisms by which insulin resistance could cause these changes may largely start with a lack of suppression of hormone-sensitive lipase by insulin in visceral adipocytes. This causes increased mobilization of free fatty acids from adipose tissue, which in turn leads to hepatic TG overload. Excess hepatic fatty acids and TG leads to increased hepatic secretion of VLDL particles, which results in elevated plasma TG levels.

M. Cobble, MD, AAFP, FNLA (✉)
CMO Atherotech Diagnostics Lab, Birmingham, AL, USA

Canyons Medical Center, 9355 S 1300 E, Sandy, UT 84094, USA
e-mail: MCobble@atherotech.com

P.D. Mize
Atherotech Diagnostics Lab, Birmingham, AL, USA

E.A. Brinton
Atherometabolic Research, Murray, UT, USA

A.J. Jenkins et al. (eds.), *Lipoproteins in Diabetes Mellitus*, Contemporary Diabetes,
DOI 10.1007/978-1-4614-7554-5_2, 

Further, insulin resistance is associated with reduced activity of lipoprotein lipase, which, by decreasing clearance of TG-rich lipoproteins from plasma, exacerbates the increase in plasma TG due to oversecretion of VLDL. Since TG-rich lipoproteins are the substrate which drives activity of cholesteryl ester transfer protein (CETP), high plasma TG levels result in a net increase in the core-lipid exchange between lipoproteins catalyzed by this enzyme. This results in TG loading of LDL and HDL particles, which in turn leads to relatively rapid TG lipolysis by hepatic lipase and reduced overall core-lipid content, which finally results in decreased particle size and increased particle density. Small, dense LDL appears to be more atherogenic than larger LDL for several reasons: (1) impaired binding to the LDL receptor resulting in impaired LDL clearance and prolonged plasma half-life; (2) greater entry past the endothelium into the subendothelial space; (3) greater adhesion to the subendothelial matrix, increasing dwell time in the space where lipoprotein modification and ingestion by macrophages principally occurs; and (4) a greater susceptibility to oxidation and other types of modification, increasing the likelihood of scavenging by macrophages. Since ingestion of modified LDL by macrophages in the artery wall appears to be the one of the principal driving forces in atherogenesis, excess production of small, dense LDL in the presence of elevated plasma TG levels may be a major mechanism of increased atherosclerosis and CVD in patients with high TG.

TG loading of the core of HDL also leads to relatively rapid TG lipolysis and net loss of core volume, similar to LDL. In contrast, however, it is not clear that increased production of small, dense HDL increases atherosclerosis or CVD. Instead, the loss of HDL core triglyceride results in the release of apo A-I from HDL. Once shed from HDL, apo A-I undergoes rapid glomerular filtration and catabolic loss. Since a large percentage of the anti-atherosclerotic effects of HDL are attributable to apo A-I, reductions in apo A-I levels appear to increase atherosclerosis and CVD. Finally, the enhanced action of CETP in the presence of high plasma TG levels results in excess transfer of cholesterol back to VLDL and IDL, which makes those particles more atherogenic. Thus, the constellation of dyslipidemic changes related to high TG dramatically increases the risk of CVD.

DeFronzo and colleagues [28] have reported a series of studies demonstrating severe impairment of insulin signal transduction pathways (e.g., insulin resistance substrate (IRS)-1 mediated) in lean T2DM patients and obese individuals with normal glucose tolerance. These insulin-signaling defects lead to abnormalities in intramyocellular glucose metabolism and decreased glucose by muscle, where it is less readily oxidized as fuel. This results in hyperglycemia, which appears to be pro-atherogenic via several mechanisms including adverse effects on lipoproteins and the artery wall. The latter includes impaired release of nitric oxide as a sign of endothelial dysfunction. In contrast, despite these insulin-resistant changes, the MAP kinase pathway retains its sensitivity to insulin, resulting in excessive stimulation and activation of downstream pathways involved in inflammation and atherogenesis. Thiazolidinediones (TZDs) comprise a class of antidiabetic drugs that simultaneously augment insulin signaling through IRS-1 and inhibit the MAP kinase pathways. In two prominent clinical trials of T2DM patients, CHICAGO and the TZD pioglitazone halted the progression of carotid and coronary atherosclerosis, respectively [82, 90]. Interestingly, these anti-atherosclerotic effects were related to increases in HDL-C levels. Of greater importance, pioglitazone also decreased a core composite of CVD events (myocardial infarction, stroke, and total or CVD mortality) in T2DM in the larger, longer PROactive (the Prospective Pioglitazone Clinical Trial in Macrovascular Events) study. Thus, effective interventions to inhibit the pathophysiological damage associated with the IR/DM phenotype are possible, underscoring the need for better utilization of diagnostic tools able to identify "at-risk" populations and their specific lipid disorders.

Restoration of glycemic control and alleviation of IR both promote plasma TG reduction, primarily by reducing the excess uptake of glucose and free fatty acids by the liver, which fuel excess hepatic TG production [28]. However, direct treatment of hyperglycemia may fail to normalize metabolism or the composition of LDL and HDL. Further complicating therapeutic intervention in T2DM is the deceptively normal lipid profile that frequently occurs with, or even without, initial treatment on dyslipidemia medications [13, 15, 88]. Further, reducing LDL-C levels, which are the primary target of dyslipidemia therapy, with statin monotherapy often fail to address the abovementioned lipoprotein abnormalities which contribute to excess atherosclerosis and CVD events in T2DM and IR [123]. It is critical, therefore, to understand how current lipid treatment options can be employed to more favorably impact the complex dyslipidemia often seen in IR/DM patient and to incorporate this knowledge into routine clinical practice. To address this therapeutic gap, it first may be necessary to address the diagnostic gap. That is, a standard lipid panel often provides little or no evidence of these abnormalities.

Direct measurement of total plasma apo B has been proposed, because it counts all potentially atherogenic lipoproteins [24, 115]. In addition, assessment of LDL particle concentration and direct measurement of subclasses of VLDL, LDL, and HDL also may help diagnose and quantify these derangements in lipoprotein metabolism [32, 56, 63].

## The Case for Evaluating Lipoprotein Subclasses

Standard lipid panels (e.g., total cholesterol, TG, LDL-C, and HDL-C) are performed using automated chemistry analyzers, with LDL-C being calculated using the Friedewald equation [36]. Elevated levels of LDL-C and non-HDL-C, and reduced HDL-C, have been identified as primary CVD risk factors in official lipid guidelines [88]. By reporting single values for lipoprotein cholesterol concentrations, the traditional lipid panel implies that lipoproteins, such as LDL-C and HDL-C, are single entities. Instead, lipoprotein particles span a continuum of size, density, cholesterol content, and TG content, with an especially large gradient for the TG-rich IDL and VLDL lipoproteins, and chylomicrons [60], as summarized schematically in Fig. 2.1. Further, over the past two decades, evidence has emerged to demonstrate that the standard lipid panel fails to identify many lipoprotein abnormalities which may contribute to elevated risk of CVD events [123].

Methods which sort lipoproteins by particle size (e.g., gradient gel electrophoresis (GGE) and nuclear magnetic resonance spectroscopy (NMR)) cannot separate IDL and Lp(a) from LDL as these subclasses have overlapping sizes. In contrast, differential particle density between LDL and Lp(a) allows separation of these related, but very different, lipoproteins by density gradient centrifugation (DGU) [60, 63].

Within each lipoprotein class, there is a wide range of lipoprotein sizes, related to considerable variability in the total cholesterol content of the particle [60, 88]. The fact that LDL-related lipoproteins vary substantially in size, density, and content of cholesterol and TG appears to explain much of the lack of precision in CVD risk estimation by the standard lipid panel, since it only provides the LDL-C concentration, and this is only as a rough calculation [63].

A key strategy to better estimate CVD risk is to focus on all atherogenic (apo B) particles. One parameter of this is non-HDL-C, which represents the total cholesterol content of VLDL, IDL, LDL, and Lp(a), and is a powerful predictor of CVD risk. Because there is one copy of apo B in each non-HDL particle, measurement of total plasma apo B, generally by immunoassay, directly reflects the total number of atherogenic particles. A third method is LDL particle number which can be calculated by NMR.

In a meta-analysis of clinical reports using LDL-C, non-HDL-C, and apo B as CVD markers, apo B was found to be the most reliable predictor of fatal or non-fatal ischemic cardiovascular events [115]. The mean relative risk ratio for apo B was 12 % greater than for LDL-C and 6 % higher than for non-HDL-C. Thus, over a 10-year period, an apo B-based strategy for evaluating and treating excess CVD risk might be estimated to prevent 500,000 more CVD events than a non-HDL-C

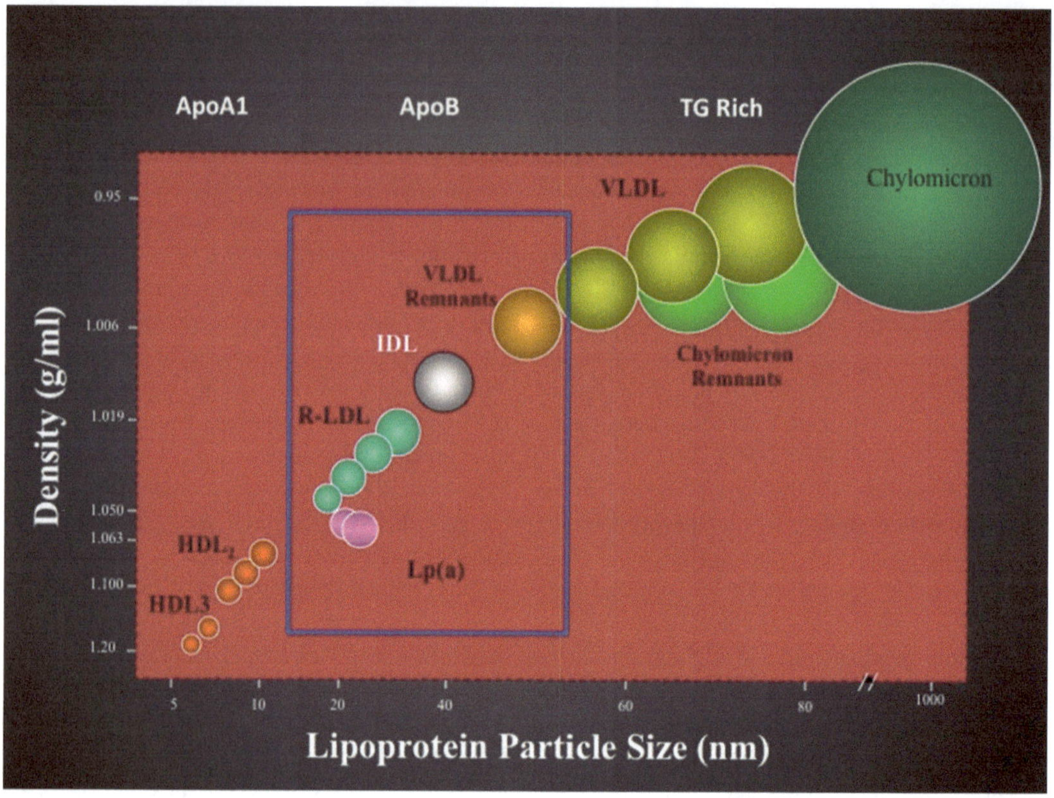


**Fig. 2.1** Lipoprotein size-density relationship. Lipid subclasses are present in a continuum of size and density, with an especially large gradient for the TG-rich lipoproteins IDL, VLDL, and chylomicrons. Technologies that sort by size (NMR and GGE) cannot separate IDL and Lp(a) from LDL-R, as these lipoproteins have overlapping sizes. IDL and Lp(a) differ by density; therefore, DGU is the best way to separate total LDL into its three components. Total LDL is made up of Lp(a), IDL, and real LDL or R-LDL. R-LDL is defined as total LDL-C minus Lp(a)-C minus IDL-C. Both Lp(a) and IDL are more atherogenic than LDL itself. Atherogenic remnant lipoproteins include IDL and VLDL3 (small/dense). These are elevated in MetSyn and T2DM and respond to low-carbohydrate diets. HDL2 is the more mature HDL subclass. HDL3 is less lipidated and smaller. The density range for IDL is 1.006–1.019 g/ml. Lp(a) and R-LDL are typically located in the density range of 1.019–1.063 g/ml. Lp(a) and small/dense LDL overlap in the density range of 1.050–1.063 g/ml. In addition, Lp(a) overlaps with IDL and large R-LDL when PAGGE is used, because of differences in electrophoretic mobility; however, Lp(a) size is actually 21–25 nm. Figure courtesy of Atherotech Labs, Inc., Birmingham, AL

strategy, while a non-HDL-C-based strategy might prevent 300,000 more CVD events than one based on calculated LDL-C alone.

In some clinical studies, the LDL particle number calculated as above by NMR has demonstrated a stronger correlation with CVD risk than has LDL-C. For example, in the Multi-Ethnic Study of Atherosclerosis (MESA), a lipoprotein subclass analysis in over 5,500 apparently healthy adults found a significant correlation between higher numbers of total or small LDL particles and increased carotid intima-media thickness (CIMT), a CVD risk factor [86]. By contrast, higher concentrations of total or large HDL particles were inversely correlated with CIMT. LDL particle subclasses remained significantly associated with CIMT after adjustment for both LDL-C and traditional lipids. LDL-C was also independently associated with worsened CIMT. However, there was no significant additional contribution of LDL-C to CIMT once the two LDL subclasses (large and small LDL particles) were included in the model. In the subgroup of participants with diabetes, both large and small LDL particle concentrations were significantly associated with CIMT.

The particle-size distribution of LDL varies significantly according to genetic factors and correlates inversely with CVD risk [60]. The predominance of larger, more buoyant LDL particles is termed Pattern A and suggests lower CVD risk. In contrast, Pattern B is typified by higher relative concentrations of small, dense LDL, which increases CVD risk by as much as fourfold, compared to Pattern A. Pattern A/B is the term for intermediate LDL particle size and it may roughly double CVD risk. In light of these differences in risk and the differing underlying pathophysiology of these patterns, it is suggested that each pattern warrants different therapeutic strategies [60].

In the process of lipolysis of TG from TG-rich lipoproteins, the core of the lipoproteins shrinks and the resulting smaller lipoproteins are called "remnants." Remnant lipoproteins tend to be more atherogenic than their parent lipoprotein. VLDL remnant particles include $VLDL_3$ and IDL. Levels of these VLDL remnant lipoproteins are elevated in patients with the metabolic syndrome (MetSyn) or IR/T2DM, and this elevation can be reduced with a diet low in total carbohydrate and especially in sugar content [50]. Interestingly, the IDL remnant particles may be more atherogenic, on a per particle basis, than is LDL, and it may be lowered less efficiently by statin treatment than are LDL levels. Lp(a) also seems especially atherogenic with a strong genetic influence and does not respond well to statin therapy [31, 107]. Elevated levels of IDL and Lp(a) usually can be lowered by niacin treatment [9], though whether this impacts risk for CVD events is as yet not established.

Lp(a) appears to consist of an LDL particle, to which has been added a large glycoprotein termed apo(a), attached to the apo B by a covalent bond. Apo(a) has a constant region and a variable region in which a peculiar secondary "loop" structure, termed a "kringle" due to its resemblance to a Dutch pastry by the same name, is repeated a variable number of times. Significant elevations of Lp(a) levels may double CVD risk in isolation [109], and when present concomitantly with elevated concentrations of small, dense LDL, CVD risk may jump by 25-fold [91]. Unfortunately, measurement of Lp(a) by the traditional protein assay may lack accuracy due to sensitivity of immunoassay kits to the number of kringle repeats in apo(a) [77]. Lp(a) can also be quantified by measurement of its cholesterol content by DGUC. Although this parameter of Lp(a) concentration is not the traditional one, there is evidence that it may be more reproducible than that of Lp(a) protein by immunoassay.

Among the major HDL subfractions, $HDL_2$, the larger subspecies, has been reported to be the more atheroprotective HDL subfraction [129], whereas $HDL_3$ has been reported to be less protective or even neutral in its relationship to CVD [8]. The opposite, however, has also been reported. Curiously, there appears to be heterogeneity in HDL subfraction effects among interventions which raise total HDL levels. For example, exercise [14] and niacin may raise $HDL_2$ more than $HDL_3$, whereas some but not all studies [128] [83] have suggested the opposite pattern of size-specific increase with ethanol and fibrates.

## LDL Subclasses

Quantification of LDL particle subclasses by NMR indicates a significantly stronger predictive value for the incidence of CVD events or disease progression than LDL-C [10, 65, 75, 95, 104, 107]. This association appeared to be independent of the standard lipid panel values. In one representative study, determination of LDL particle concentration and size by NMR found that particle concentration was a predictor of future CVD events in overtly healthy middle-aged women [10]. In general, the magnitude of LDL-particle predictive value was similar to that associated with standard lipid measurements, but less than the predictive value of measuring the inflammatory biomarker C-reactive protein (CRP).

In the Women's Health Study of middle-aged women with no history of CVD or cancer, LDL particle concentration was the best lipoprotein predictor of incident CVD events and stroke and was more strongly related to these outcomes than was apo B [10]. The Quebec Cardiovascular Study found that the combination of IR/diabetes, elevated small dense LDL-C, and elevated apo B synergistically confers a 20-fold increased risk for CVD events [122]. Tempering this viewpoint are studies where adjustment for the number of LDL particles (apo B or LDL particle concentration) attenuated the relationship between a predominance of small, dense LDL and atherosclerotic CVD [10, 49, 55, 65, 95, 105, 123]. Thus, the question of whether or not apo B-containing lipoproteins can develop a steep-enough gradient of atherogenicity across subtypes to achieve clinical relevance remains controversial. However, epidemiologic and clinical intervention trials have clearly demonstrated a stronger correlation with apo B concentration and subsequent CVD events than for LDL-C values and CVD events [114].

Small, dense LDL particles comprise an important component of the Pattern B pathophysiology associated with obesity, the MetSyn, and IR/DM (characterized by high TG, low HDL-C, and increased LDL particle number) [4, 12, 58, 84, 102]. Individuals with smaller average LDL size (18–21 nm) are more likely to present with IR and the metabolic syndrome and are at an increased risk for developing T2DM [33, 39, 40, 58].

Other predictive variables, such as higher concentrations of TG-rich lipoproteins or reduced HDL-C, might need to be considered. For example, Maki et al. [76] reported a significant association between progressive increases in carotid intima-media thickness (CIMT), a surrogate marker of early-stage atherosclerosis, and increased cholesterol in TG-rich lipoproteins and denser LDL lipoprotein subclasses, coupled with lower HDL-C concentrations, in normoglycemic adults at moderate risk for coronary heart disease (CHD). Further, epidemiology studies have consistently supported a stronger role for non-HDL-C in predicting subsequent CVD events than for LDL-C, independent of elevated TG concentrations [12, 26, 52, 72, 99].

## Triglyceride-Rich Lipoproteins

Increased cholesterol carried by TG-rich lipoproteins (VLDL, IDL, chylomicrons) is highly atherogenic and a prominent component of the IR/DM dyslipidemia phenotype linked to increased CVD risk [88]. Metabolic syndrome (MetSyn) or IR/T2DM dyslipidemia is characterized not only by high TG and low HDL-C concentrations but also by increases in the size of VLDL particles and decreases in the size of LDL and HDL [39, 125]. Larger VLDL lipoproteins/particles are strongly associated with TG, IR, and the MetSyn [39, 58]. High concentrations are defined as more than 5 nmol/L (>75th percentile in MESA) and confer an increased risk for developing T2DM [88]. In addition, VLDL-C correlates strongly with concentrations of TG-rich remnant particles [88]. An alternate view suggests that the superiority of non-HDL-C as a CVD predictor results from the association between non-HDL-C and LDL particle number, rather than from the atherogenicity of TG-rich lipoprotein remnants [25, 96]. This theory is based on the finding of elevated levels of small, dense LDL particles in individuals with hypertriglyceridemia, resulting in higher-than-expected LDL particle concentrations than predicted from LDL-C concentrations.

## HDL Subclasses

High concentrations of HDL-C are now firmly established as a beneficial condition that lowers CVD risk, and most published reports attribute the cardioprotective properties of HDL to HDL2 [88, 129]. Reduced concentrations of HDL lipoprotein subclasses are a prominent component of the IR/diabetic/MetSyn dyslipidemia phenotype linked to increased CVD risk [39, 58]. Among subjects in the MESA trial not treated with lipid-lowering medication, total HDL particle number was more strongly associated with carotid atherosclerosis than was HDL-C [86]. In the Pravastatin Limitation of Atherosclerosis in the Coronary Arteries (PLAC-I) statin intervention trial, a key finding was the negative association between progression of coronary artery disease and high levels of smaller HDL particle subclasses [104]. This correlation was independent of total HDL-C concentrations. In contrast, in the Veterans Affairs HDL Intervention Trial VAHIT total and small HDL particle numbers were independent predictors of recurrent CVD events [95].

In a representative group of prospective studies examining the relationship of HDL-C subclasses to CHD events, risk was significantly associated with both HDL2-C and HDL3-C in five studies [38, 68, 106, 111, 118], with HDL2-C but not HDL3-C in one study [67] and with HDL3-C but not HDL2-C in one study [124]. In another study, HDL-C, HDL2-C, and HDL3-C concentrations were all inversely associated with CIMT progression, which agreed with results reported previously for traditional HDL-C measurements [76]. The results were similar however for total HDL-C, HDL2-C, and HDL3-C. All three values correlated with CIMT progression; however, HDL-C, HDL2, and HDL3 were not superior in their prediction of CIMT progression.

In one of the longest prospective studies to examine the relationship between lipoprotein subclasses and coronary heart disease (CHD), 1,905 men from the Livermore Radiation Laboratory were followed for 29 [130] and 53 years [129]. Between 1954 and 1957, lipoprotein mass concentrations were determined using an analytic ultracentrifugation technique [43]. At the 10-year follow-up, the 38 men who developed clinical ischemic heart disease had significantly lower HDL2 (32 %), lower HDL3 (8 %), higher LDL (13 %), higher IDL (23 %), and higher small VLDL (21 %) mass compared to the total sample population. At the 29-year follow-up, 179 CHD deaths, 182 nonfatal myocardial infarctions, and 93 revascularization procedures were confirmed in 97 % of the cohort [130]. Total incident CHD was inversely related to HDL2 and HDL3 mass and concordantly related to LDL mass, IDL mass, and small and large VLDL mass concentrations, after adjustment for age. The lowest quartiles of both HDL2 mass and HDL3 mass independently predicted total incident CHD. Risk for premature CHD ($\leq$65 years old) was significantly greater in men within the lowest HDL2 and HDL3 quartiles plus high LDL mass concentrations. At the 53-year follow-up, the risk associated with the lowest HDL2 quartile increased significantly by 22 % for all-cause mortality, 63 % for total CHD, and 117 % for premature CHD mortality, when adjusted for age [129]. When adjusted for standard risk factors (age, total cholesterol, blood pressure, BMI, smoking) and the lowest HDL3-quartile, the corresponding risk increases were 14, 38, and 62 %, respectively. Men with HDL3 less than or equal to the 25th percentile had 28 % greater total CHD risk and 71 % greater risk of premature CHD risk. Higher LDL mass concentrations significantly increased total CHD risk by 3.8 % and premature CHD risk by 6.1 % for each 10 mg/dL rise in concentration. Thus, data from the first study to demonstrate an association between HDL subclasses and CVD risk support the conclusion that lower concentrations of the more buoyant HDL2 particle, and to a lesser extent HDL3, are associated with increased CVD risk. LDL mass as expected predicted risk; however, TG-rich lipoproteins and subclasses also were powerful predictors. Although still controversial, some investigations suggest that HDL2 particles may offer greater cardioprotective effects than HDL3 [34], though this is now questioned and being actively re-evaluated.

## Techniques for Measuring Lipoprotein Subclasses

There are several methods available to measure apolipoproteins and lipoprotein subclasses, including chemical analysis and immunoassays, gel electrophoresis (polyacrylamide gradient gel electrophoresis (PAGGE) or GGE), nuclear magnetic resonance (NMR), and density gradient ultracentrifugation (DGU) [11, 29, 41, 42, 56, 63]. The most common method is the standard lipid panel performed using automated chemistry analyzers. This method involves independent measurements of total cholesterol, HDL-C, and TG. LDL is estimated using the Friedewald equation [36].

$$[\text{FLDL-C}] = [\text{Total Cholesterol}] - [\text{HDL-C}] - [\text{TG}/5]$$

In the Friedewald relationship, the IDL and Lp(a) components of LDL are assumed to be 20 % of the TG concentration. This underscores the importance of obtaining a fasting TG measurement, because the elevated TG levels found postprandially can cause false-low estimation of Friedewald-calculated LDL (FLDL-C). For patients with TG >400 mg/dL, a direct LDL measurement should be performed to avoid this problem [78]. In reality, directly measuring LDL levels eliminates Friedewald equation inaccuracies caused by higher levels of TG and

TG-rich lipoproteins. FLDL-C levels do not correlate well with direct LDL levels in patients with diabetes or coronary or other atherosclerotic diseases [110], because many of these patients have high levels of TG-rich lipoproteins even with near-normal TG concentrations, the classic hallmark of an atherogenic lipoprotein profile.

Lipoprotein subclasses can be measured in many cases by direct measurement on chemistry analyzers, but measurements of multiple subclasses by this method is expensive and all subclasses are not captured. Techniques that can measure multiple lipoprotein subclasses simultaneously have been reviewed and compared [123]. PAGGE/GGE, NMR, and DGU represent widely used, practical options that simultaneously measure all lipoprotein subclasses.

## Gradient and Modified Nongradient Gel Electrophoresis

Because of the laborious nature of the original DGU technique (*described below*), other methods were developed to separate and measure lipoproteins and their subclasses based on physical properties, such as size. One of these techniques is nondenaturing gradient gel electrophoresis (PAGGE or GGE). Size separation of lipoproteins is accomplished by using polyacrylamide gradient gels (2–16 % cross-linking) in which the gel layers have decreasing pore size due to the increasing cross-linking of the polyacrylamide gel. Smaller size lipoprotein particles travel farther in the gel matrix while movement of larger lipoprotein particles is inhibited. Migration distance under these conditions is inversely related to particle diameter. Also, increasing electrophoresis time from 24 to 30 h does not significantly affect the relative mobility (separation) of the LDL peaks. The standard deviation of results typically range from 0.2 to 0.28 nm (CV < 1.0 %).

After the electrophoresis step is completed, the gels are removed from the holder and stained with one of a number of dyes (Coomassie Brilliant blue R-250 for protein detection, Sudan Black or Oil Red O for lipid detection) to reveal the shape and size of the separated lipoprotein fractions. Lipoprotein particle size is roughly inversely proportional to the particle density. The amount of the lipoprotein in each stained fraction is determined through the use of a densitometer, and a computer deconvolution program is used to convert the color density of each peak into a lipid concentration (mg/dL). Typical LDL profiles for Pattern A and B individuals are shown in Fig. 2.2.

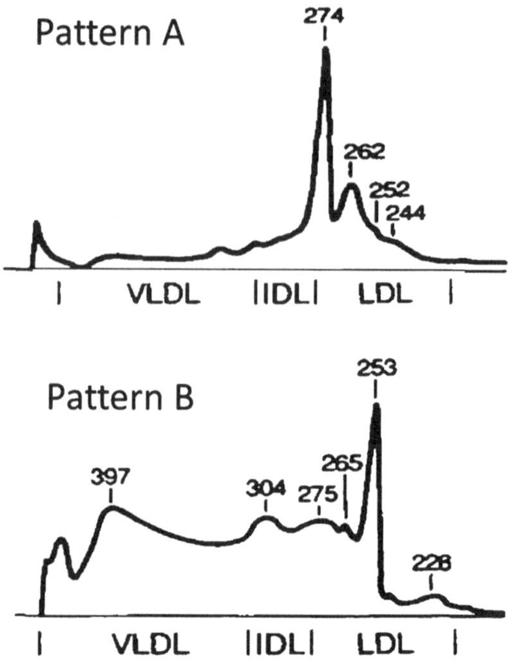


**Fig. 2.2** Representative LDL subclass analyses generated using PAGGE/GGE. The *black profile lines* are representative of the optical density of the gels containing the stained lipoproteins. These profiles are deconvoluted to yield the concentration of the individual LDL lipid subclasses. The Pattern A profile shows a predominance of large buoyant LDl particles skewing to the right with an absence of IDL or VLDL particles. The Pattern B profile with peak particle diameters less than 255 Å and the pattern skewed to the left with large amounts of IDl and VLDL particles. This lipid profile is for a patient with an atherogenic phenotype. Two gradient gels are necessary to size separate all lipoproteins (HDL and non-HDL). Reprinted with permission from Austin [4]

Application of this technique reveals multiple bands within the total LDL fraction of different subjects. The range of particle diameters comprised by LDL separated by this method is 21.8–27.8 nm, corresponding closely to the ranges determined by negative-staining electron microscopy [112]. Sodium dodecyl sulfate (SDS) polyacrylamide gel electrophoresis of the above fractions reveals only apo B. Importantly, similar-size lipoproteins separated by PAGGE/GGE have heterogeneous densities, while similar-density lipoproteins separated by DGU display multiple-size heterogeneity. Therefore, the output from these two techniques is complementary, but not necessarily identical [17]. One example of the use of PAGGE/GGE to characterize lipoprotein subclasses within a large population was reported for the Quebec Heart Study [121, 122]. Cholesterol in small, dense LDL (<25.5 nm) conferred a risk of four- to six-fold greater risk of ischemic heart disease than did cholesterol located within larger, more buoyant LDL particles.

## Nuclear Magnetic Resonance Spectroscopy

Both the PAGGE/GGE and DGU techniques rely on a physical separation of the lipoproteins, either by density or by size, before cholesterol analysis. Another method has been developed using nuclear magnetic resonance spectroscopy (NMR) to estimate lipoprotein particle number, size, and concentration without a separation step [92, 93]. This technique provides quantitative measurement of size fractions throughout the lipoprotein particle spectrum.

Lipoprotein particles are composed of an apoprotein and a mixture of cholesterol, phospholipids, cholesteryl esters, and triglycerides [56, 94]. The aggregate number of terminal methyl groups of these lipids yields a set of characteristic resonance signals over a defined part of the NMR spectrum. NMR uses these characteristic signals broadcast by lipoprotein subclasses of different sizes. Each subclass of VLDL, LDL, and HDL has a distinct spectral pattern, or a bulk particle signal, that is slightly shifted due to the different sizes of the VLDL, LDL, and HDL particles. This signal envelope contains the signals emitted by the terminal methyl group protons of the four types of lipid in the lipoprotein particles: phospholipid, unesterified cholesterol, cholesteryl ester, and triglyceride [56]. Each lipoprotein subclass signal emanates from the aggregate number of terminal methyl groups on the lipids contained within the particle, with the cholesteryl esters and triglycerides in the particle core each contributing three methyl groups, and the phospholipids and unesterified cholesterol in the surface shell each contributing two methyl groups. Because the methyl signals from these lipids are indistinguishable from each other, they overlap to produce a bulk lipid particle signal. The amplitude of each lipoprotein subclass signal serves as a measure of the particle concentration of that subclass. The measured amplitudes of lipoprotein subclass NMR signals are directly proportional to the number of particles emitting the signal, even when the amount of lipid or protein per particle varies from person to person. As a result, NMR-derived lipoprotein concentrations may differ from those measured by traditional methods. That said, studies of split samples have demonstrated good agreement between LDL and HDL particle sizes measured by NMR and GGE [47].

NMR spectra are recorded using a dedicated spectrometer over approximately 1 min and then computer deconvolution of the magnetic resonance signal generates a profile of the component lipoprotein particles corresponding to various sizes and concentrations [56]. The only specimens for which freezing may adversely affect NMR results are postprandial samples or samples with fasting triglyceride values greater than approximately 300 mg/dL. Freezing these samples may alter (lower) chylomicron and VLDL subclass concentrations. A representative spectral profile is shown in Fig. 2.3.

The use of NMR to quantify lipoprotein subclasses has some limitations [2]. When the proton-NMR spectra of 11 lipoprotein subclasses were recorded at physiological temperature, the methyl resonance region commonly used for lipoprotein analyses showed considerable overlap for all lipoprotein subclasses, with an intense distorted triplet-like signal at approximately 0.85 ppm and some cholesterol backbone-related resonances. The average relative errors of the quantifications denote noteworthy differences in the capability of the partial least squares analyses of the spectra to uncover the subclass-specific signal areas. The VLDL and HDL3 subclasses give the most accurate results, with considerably

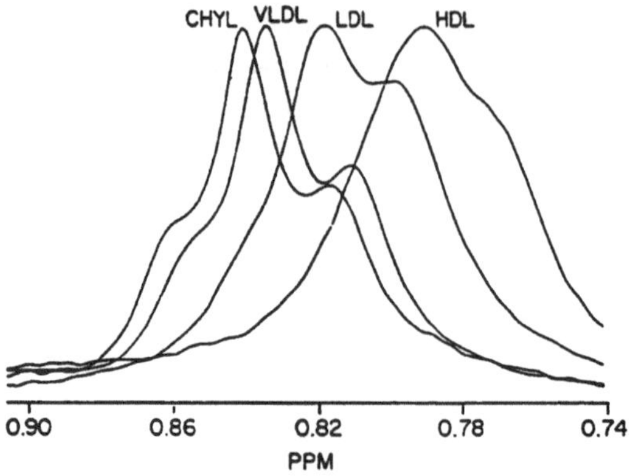


**Fig. 2.3** Lipoprotein components separated by nuclear magnetic resonance spectroscopy (NMR). Represented are the magnetic resonances of the methyl groups of cholesterol, phospholipids, cholesteryl esters, and triglycerides contained in the different classes of lipoproteins. The terminal methyl groups of the lipids yield a set of characteristic resonance signals over a defined part of the NMR spectrum. Because the methyl signals from these lipids are indistinguishable from each other, they overlap to produce a bulk lipid particle signal. Each subclass of VLDL, LDL, and HDL has a distinct spectral pattern that is slightly shifted due to the different sizes of the VLDL, LDL, and HDL particles. These signals are deconvoluted to yield both the size and concentration of lipoprotein subclass particle. Reprinted with permission from Otvos [93]

less accurate results for the HDL2, IDL, and the smaller LDL particles. At all noise levels there is an approximately ten-fold difference in the quantification accuracy between the most and least accurate (LDLl) values.

The similarity of the methyl signals, particularly for the LDL and HDL2 subclasses, and the small-sized differences within the LDL subclasses make the decreased quantification accuracy for the IDL, LDL, and HDL2 subclasses understandable. No explanation is apparent for why the accuracy for the LDL2 and LDL3 quantification appears to be three times better than that for the LDLl.

Exemplifying the use of NMR spectroscopy was a report by Freedman et al. [35] based on the Framingham Study, a large community-based epidemiology study spanning decades. There is a gender differential in CHD risk that narrows with advancing age. Freedman et al. [35] investigated the possible influence of lipoprotein subclasses on this phenomenon by measuring lipoprotein particle sizes and concentrations using NMR. They analyzed plasma samples from 1,692 female and 1,574 male participants in the Framingham Offspring Study. When adjusted for age and lipid concentration, women had a lipoprotein subclass profile suggestive of lower CVD risk, consisting of significantly lower concentrations of small LDL particles (median 209 vs. 367 nmol/L) and higher concentrations of large HDL particles (median 8 vs. 3 μmol/L). In addition, women had fewer small LDL particles ≤20.5 nm (11 % vs. 34 % nm) and larger HDL particles (mean 9.4 vs. 8.9 nm). This sex difference is similar to that observed for a GGE-measured LDL peak particle diameter of <25.5 nm (Pattern B) [35]. The female/male difference in HDL particle size decreased with age. There is no proffered evidence that this supports the change in CVD risk as a function of age. Surprisingly, the increased LDL-C concentration found in older women was attributable to higher concentrations of intermediate and large LDL particles, rather than small LDL particles. Despite the gender advantage in CVD risk at younger ages for women in the general population, women with diabetes have slightly greater CVD risk and mortality from myocardial infarctions than do men with diabetes [103], highlighting the dysregulation diabetes introduces into lipid metabolism.

From an analytical perspective, the NMR method used in the Freedman et al. [35] study had several advantages over classical electrophoresis or ultracentrifugation. By avoiding the need for physical fractionation of lipoprotein subclasses, which traditionally required hours-to-days and achieved only partial resolution of lipoprotein subclasses, NMR reduced fractionation to minutes and was completely automated. It also eliminated sources of analytical variability inherent in older separation procedures. In addition, NMR provides a direct measure of lipoprotein subclass particle concentrations, rather than basing quantification on the amount of cholesterol contained within lipoprotein particles or the relative degree of lipid-to-protein staining of separated particles. Counterbalancing these advantages were the measurement variability inherent in NMR determinations and the requirement for expensive equipment and a high level of technical expertise to perform this technique.

## Density Gradient Centrifugation

Some of the earliest reports on quantitation of plasma lipoproteins were based on the techniques of analytical and preparative ultracentrifugation [70]. Analytic ultracentrifugation was applied in the 1950s to the separations of lipoproteins by their rates of migration in an intense centrifugal field and remained in use through the end of the twentieth century [130]. It was the gold standard against which other techniques were calibrated [54, 71]. Differences in the density of lipoprotein class and subclasses in salt solutions (1.063 g/mL) cause different rates of separation, termed Svedberg flotation ($S_f$) rates, for VLDL, IDL, LDL, and HDL lipoproteins subclasses [29, 41–43, 62]. DGU flotation rates are controlled by the size, shape, and hydrated density of the particles. Major subclasses within LDL were defined as $S_f$ 12–20 (IDL) and $S_f$ 0–12; these are the components of total cholesterol that contribute to the standard LDL-C measurement. The HDL fraction is composed of three major subclasses: $F_{1.2}$ 0–3.5 (HDL3), $F_{1.2}$ 3.5–9 (HDL2), and $F_{1.2}$ 9–20 (HDL1). Analytical ultracentrifugation data from small healthy populations could be grouped into subpopulations with common characteristics. One subgroup had levels of small, dense LDL ($S_f$ 0–7) that were positively correlated with VLDL and inversely correlated with HDL2. Other subgroups had larger, more buoyant LDL ($S_f$ 7–12) and showed the opposite relationships with VLDL and HDL2. The gold standard method for LDL-C and HDL-C quantitation (beta quantitation) recommended by the US Centers for Disease Control (CDC) and the National Cholesterol Education Program (NCEP) is based on DGU [7].

The original DGU technique was used to demonstrate a predictive relationship between lipoproteins and their subclasses and the subsequent development of cardiovascular and coronary heart disease in large population studies, such as the Framingham Heart Study and the Lawrence Livermore Study [57, 129]. The Framingham Study was the first to show the relationship of total cholesterol and LDL to heart disease. Further, in a 53-year follow-up of the Lawrence Livermore Study, the protective effect of high concentrations of HDL2 was demonstrated.

More recently, the DGU technique has been refined by applying vertical spin ultracentrifugation (Vertical Auto Profile® [VAP] Atherotech Inc, Birmingham, AL) [63]. The original DGU technique is extremely time consuming (days) and required a laborious manual separation of the lipoprotein subclass fractions, followed by an enzymatic cholesterol assay. The VAP technique uses a salt density gradient to separate the lipids in a diluted serum sample. The gradient is subjected to a single, vertical spin, density gradient ultracentrifugation. Unlike most preparative ultracentrifugation methods, the vertical spin method separates all lipoproteins in less than 1 h. The separated lipoprotein classes are then continuously drained from the bottom of the centrifuge tube into the VAP continuous flow analyzer where they sequentially react with a cholesterol-specific enzymatic reagent producing a cholesterol concentration-dependent lipoprotein absorbance profile monitored by a spectrophotometer. The digital output from the spectrophotometer is collected electronically, and the resulting absorbance curve is deconvoluted to quantify individual lipoprotein classes and their respective subclasses using in-house developed software. This technique simultaneously measures cholesterol concentrations of all five lipoprotein classes: HDL, LDL1-4 (LDL without Lp(a) and IDL), IDL, Lp(a), and VLDL and their respective lipoprotein subclasses (HDL2, HDL3; LDL1, LDL2, LDL3, LDL4; VLDL1+2, VLDL3) [21, 22]. LDL is directly measured, not calculated as in the standard lipid panel, therefore non-fasting samples can be used for LDL determinations. Lipid subfractionation reveals the direct underlying pathophysiology of the dyslipidemia and may better suggest targeted treatment strategies or response to treatment.

A normal (Pattern A) cholesterol lipoprotein profile from the DGU VAP technique shows the relatively dense HDL separated from the lighter LDL fraction and the very light VLDL fraction (Fig. 2.4a). In sharp contrast, Fig. 2.4b shows the atherogenic phenotype typical of Pattern B in a T2DM patient with poor glycemic control. The LDL level is high and the peak is shifted to the left (more small, dense LDL). The amount of remnant lipoproteins (IDL and VLDL3) is highly

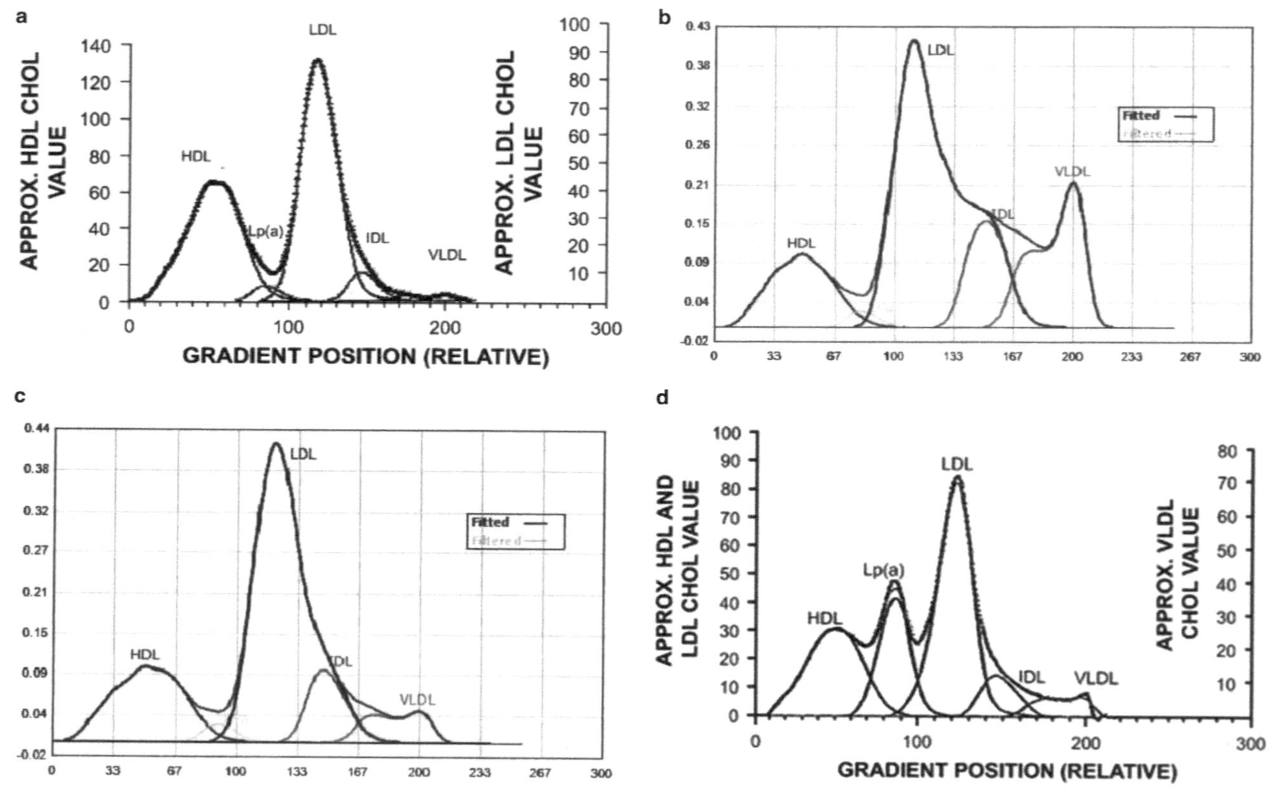


**Fig. 2.4** Representative lipoprotein subclass spectrum generated using the DGU VAP technique. (**a**) Pattern A profile from a healthy adult with no insulin resistance. The *x*-axis represents decreasing density. The lipoproteins separate from denser (HDL) to lighter (VLDL). The cholesterol profile (*dashed line*) is deconvoluted to yield the individual lipoprotein classes and subclasses (*solid lines*). The relative amounts of HDL, Lp(a), LDL, IDL, and VLDL and position of the LDL peak indicate that this is a normal lipid profile (Pattern A). (**b**) Pattern B profile from a T2DM patient with poor glycemic control ($HbA_{1c}$ 11.0 %; fasting plasma glucose 302 mg/dL). Note the elevated levels of TG, IDL, VLDL, and VLDL3. The HDL, LDL, IDL, and VLDL levels are 40, 145, 36, and 68 mg/dL, respectively; TG 443 mg/dL. The relative shift of the LDL peak compared to the LDL peak indicates small, dense LDL Pattern B. The large IDL and VLDL peaks indicate large amounts of remnant atherogenic lipoproteins. (**c**) Profile from a T2DM patient with excellent glycemic control ($HbA_{1c}$ 5.8 %; fasting plasma glucose 121 mg/dL). Lipoprotein abnormalities remain even after amelioration of hyperglycemia. The LDL peak is shifted towards the HDL peak and indicates that small, dense LDL is still present. The IDL and VLDL peaks are smaller, but indicate remnant atherogenic lipoproteins are present. The HDL, LDL, IDL, and VLDL levels are 45, 121, 22, and 25 mg/dL, respectively. (**d**) Profile from a T2DM patient with a normal standard lipid panel, but high levels of Lp(a) when analyzed by DGU ($HbA_{1c}$ 7.2 %; fasting plasma glucose 110 mg/dL). The large peak between the HDL and LDL peaks is the small dense Lp(a) peak. Figures courtesy of Atherotech Labs, Inc., Birmingham, AL

elevated as well as that whole VLDL level. Further, as shown in Fig. 2.4c, lipoprotein abnormalities remain in T2DM patients even after restoration of glycemic control. An example of a patient (Fig. 2.4d) with high Lp(a) and normal LDL levels is illustrative of lipoprotein abnormalities that can be missed with the standard lipid panel.

In summary, the great majority of patients with MetSyn/IR and T2DM show the classic atherogenic lipoprotein profile that is distinguished by a relatively small HDL peak, an LDL peak which may be of relatively normal size, and the presence of elevated levels of TG-rich IDL and VLDL.

## Clinical Evaluation of Lipoprotein Subclasses in the Insulin-Resistant/ Diabetic Population

### Correlation with IR/DM or MetSyn

Table 2.1 summarizes key findings from clinical investigations correlating specific changes in lipoprotein subclasses with the MetSyn and IR/DM. Higher LDL particle concentration and small, dense LDL particles, but not LDL-C, were strongly associated with MetSyn in the Framingham Heart Study [58]. Similar results were found in individuals with a wide range of insulin sensitivity/resistance and overt T2DM in the report from Garvey et al. [39]. The strongest relationships with IR/DM were found for large HDL particles (negative), large VLDL particles (positive), total LDL particles (positive), and small LDL particles (positive). Of note, no correlation was found between LDL-C concentration and the degree of insulin sensitivity or resistance. Similar strong subclass associations were found in IR/T2DM subjects in the Insulin Resistance Atherosclerosis Study (IRAS) [33, 40]. Of special interest, high concentrations of large VLDL particles and small HDL particle size predicted diabetes, independent of lipid values and insulin sensitivity. Echoing this finding, a preponderance of large VLDL particles and small HDL particles was selected in stepwise regression as predictors of T2DM in the Melbourne Collaborative Cohort Study [51]. TG concentrations were the only conventional lipid measure that predicted T2DM in a stepwise model that included total cholesterol, HDL-C, LDL-C, and TG. Thus, atherogenic lipoprotein abnormalities are a hallmark of adults who subsequently develop T2DM.

T2DM is often a consequence of overweight/obesity later in life, whereas type 1 diabetes is caused by autoimmune destruction of pancreatic β-cells and typically presents in young children. Therefore, the report from Alabakavoska et al. [1] raises interesting questions about the etiology of dyslipidemia in the setting of hyperglycemia. In this study, 89 % of healthy control children had Pattern A compared with Pattern B in 87 % of T1DM children, despite no significant differences in standard lipid panel between the two groups. Further, the T1DM group had a preponderance of LDL3 and LDL4, the small, dense, more atherogenic LDL lipoproteins.

### Correlation with CVD

Table 2.2 summarizes key findings from clinical investigations correlating specific changes in lipoprotein subclasses in patients with IR/DM or MetSyn with cardiac events or CVD risk biomarkers. Many clinical studies have found that adults with a preponderance of small, dense LDL particles and reduced HDL particles are more likely to develop the MetSyn and IR/DM [33, 39, 40, 58, 117] and subsequently experience CVD events [23, 74]. Other studies have found no predictive value for CVD risk [46, 58]. Thus, the current state of affairs remains in flux. However, there is no doubt that residual lipoprotein disease and CVD risk currently exists in both treated and untreated patients.

### Intervention Studies

Table 2.3 summarizes key findings from clinical investigations examining specific therapeutic interventions in patients with IR/DM or MetSyn

**Table 2.1** Overview of epidemiology investigations examining lipoprotein subclasses in patients with IR/DM or the metabolic syndrome (MetSyn)

| Publication | Trial name | *N* | Pop studied | Race (country) | Major findings | Subclass technique |
|---|---|---|---|---|---|---|
| Alabakovska [1] | NA | 30 vs. 100 | T1DM vs. NoHG children | NG (Macedonia) | T1DM children had lower HDL-C; 88.5 % had Pattern B dyslipidemia vs. 11 % in healthy children ($P<0.0001$). Mean LDL lipoprotein size was 24.6 vs. 26.4 nm, respectively ($P<0.0001$). LDL size in T1DM inversely correlated with TG ($P<0.05$); positively correlated with HDL-C ($P<0.05$) | PAGGE |
| Austin [6] | NA | 204 | IR, elderly adults | Finish (Finland) | At 3.5-year follow-up, this study was first to demonstrate that a predominance of small LDL is a risk factor for the future development of T2DM (twofold greater risk), independent of age, gender, IR, and BMI; not independent of fasting insulin or TG concentrations. An increase of 5 Å in LDL diameter was associated with a 16 % decrease in risk of T2DM | PAGGE |
| Chu [20] | NA | 21 vs. 23 | IR vs. NoHG adults | NG (US) | IR was associated with lower concentrations of HDL2 ($P<0.001$) and HDL3 ($P<0.001$); higher TG concentrations ($P<0.01$); higher concentrations of all TG-rich lipoprotein classes, including IDL ($P<0.02$); large, buoyant TG-rich VLDL1+2 ($P<0.01$); and small, dense cholesterol-rich VLDL3a+3b ($P<0.001$). Although LDL-C appeared to be higher in the IR individuals (3.44 vs. 3.24 mmol/L; $P<0.39$), this effect was partially attributable to the effects of a significantly higher IDL (0.49 vs. 0.39 mmol/L; $P<0.02$) in the setting of almost identical Lp(a) (0.19 vs. 0.18 mmol/L; $P<0.85$). IR was associated with a small, dense LDL lipoprotein ($P<0.001$). A higher proportion of IR individuals had LDL Pattern B ($P<0.001$) | DGU |
| Feingold [32] | NA | 29 vs. 87 | T2DM vs. NoHG male adults | NG (US) | T2DM associated with increased prevalence of LDL lipoprotein subclass Pattern B: 52 % vs. 24 % in NoHG ($P<0.025$). Clearance of TG-rich lipoproteins delayed in Pattern B vs. A in T2DM patients (mean 25 vs. 14 min; $P<0.01$) | PAGGE |
| Festa [33] | Insulin Resistance Atherosclerosis Study (IRAS) | 513 vs. 830 | IR/T2DM vs. NoHG adults | Caucasian, Black, Hispanic (US) | VLDL particle size and small HDL particle number predicted diabetes, independent of lipids and insulin sensitivity or resistance. The relation of both VLDL size and small HDL to incident diabetes was largely independent of glucose tolerance status at baseline, waist circumference, TG, and HDL-C. There was a linear increase in the incidence of diabetes across quartiles of VLDL size and to a lesser extent across quartiles of small HDL particle concentrations. Insulin sensitivity attenuated the relation to incident diabetes of VLDL size, but not of small HDL particles | NMR |

| | | | | | | |
|---|---|---|---|---|---|---|
| Friedlander [37] | Jerusalem Diabetes Prevalence Study | 390 | IR/T2DM vs. NoHG adults | Mixed (Israel) | Confirmed high TG, low HDL-C, fasting and postprandial insulin levels significantly associated with LDL lipoprotein subclass phenotypes. LDL-C, HDL-C, and TG were independently associated with LDL lipoprotein size. The addition of IR (insulinemia) and glucose concentration had no independent effects on LDL size. However, on a background of elevated LDL-C and IR, mean LDL size was lower. The association of IR and LDL size is not mediated directly through the level of insulinemia, but via alterations in lipid metabolism | PAGGE |
| Garvey [39] | NA | 46/46 vs. 56 | IR, T2DM vs. NoHG adults | 66 % Caucasian (US) | Lipid panel: IS vs. IR, only TG difference achieved statistical significance, elevated in IR ($P<0.03$); IS vs. DM, total cholesterol, LDL-C, and TG elevated in DM (all $P<0.05$). Subclass masses by NMR: IS vs. IR, total and large VLDL, total and small LDL elevated in IR (all $P<0.05$), large HDL lower in IR ($P<0.05$); IS vs. DM, total and large VLDL, total, intermediate, and small LDL, small HDL elevated in DM (all $P<0.05$); large LDL, total and large HDL lower in DM (all $P<0.05$) | NMR |
| Goff [40] | Insulin Resistance Atherosclerosis Study (IRAS) | 1,371 | IR/T2DM vs. NoHG adults | Black, Hispanic, non-Hispanic Caucasian (US) | Progressively elevated across categories of increasing glucose intolerance (all $P<0.05$): TG concentration, large and intermediate VLDL concentrations; total VLDL particle number and size; small LDL concentration; total LDL particle number. Progressively reduced across categories of increasing glucose intolerance (all $P<0.05$): Large and intermediate LDL concentration, LDL particle size, total and large HDL concentration, HDL particle size. Greater concentrations of small, dense LDL particles and lower concentrations of large LDL particles were associated with IR or greater adiposity. IR and adiposity were associated with higher large VLDL particle concentration and a shift to larger VLDL size, low HDL particle concentration | NMR |
| Haffner [48] | San Antonio Heart Study | 466 | IR & NoHG male adults | Hispanic, non-Hispanic Caucasian (US) | Mexican Americans: higher BMI, more IR, higher fasting TG, lower LDL lipoprotein size (all $P<0.05$). Pattern B trended higher in Mexican Americans (40 % vs. 34 %). In univariate analysis, LDL size significantly associated with glucose, insulin, male gender, total cholesterol, HDL-C, and TG. In multivariate analyses, higher TG, insulin, and glucose concentrations, lower HDL-C, and male gender were independent correlates of small, dense LDL. Pattern B predicted by higher insulin, higher TG, and male gender, independent of ethnicity | PAGGE |

(continued)

**Table 2.1** (continued)

| Publication | Trial name | *N* | Pop studied | Race (country) | Major findings | Subclass technique |
|---|---|---|---|---|---|---|
| Hodge [51] | Melbourne Collaborative Cohort Study (MCCS) | 754 vs. 59 | NoHG vs. T2DM adults | Born in Australia, UK, Greece, or Italy (Australia) | DM onset at 4years more prevalent in adults with Southern European origin. DM: higher BMI, total cholesterol, TG; lower HDL-C (all $P<0.05$). DM NMR subclasses: *Higher* VLDL size and particle number; large and medium VLDL concentrations; IDL concentration; LDL particles; medium-small and very small LDL concentration; small HDL concentration (all $P<0.05$). DM NMR subclasses: *Lower* LDL size; HDL size; large LDL concentration; large HDL concentration (all $P<0.05$). Concentration of VLDL particles (positive) and HDL particle size (negative) was selected by stepwise regression as predictors of T2DM. These associations were independent of other non-lipid risk factors, but not plasma TG. Factor analysis identified a factor from NMR variables, explaining 47 % of their variation, and characterized by a positive correlation with VLDL, particularly large and medium sized; more low-density lipoprotein (LDL) that were smaller and relatively smaller, but not more HDL particles. This factor was positively associated with diabetes incidence, but not independently of TG | NMR |
| Kulkarni [64] | NA | 78 | IR vs. NoHG adults | Asian Indian, Caucasian (US) | Asian Indians: *Higher* VLDL-C; TG; small, dense LDL (44 % vs. 21 %) (all $P<0.05$). Asian Indians: *Lower* HDL-C, HDL3-C, HDL2-C (all $P<0.05$). Increased prevalence of small, dense LDL type due to increased TG, with fasting insulin being one of the important determinants of TG. Fasting insulin was significantly increased in Asian Indians with small, dense LDL type compared with other Asian Indians, suggesting a significant role of IR in increasing the prevalence of small, dense LDL type | DGU |
| Kuller [66] | Multiple Risk Factor Intervention Trial (MRFIT) | 428 | MetSyn male adults | Caucasian, Black (US) | At 25-year follow-up, compared men with MetSyn who died of CHD vs. did not die of CHD or CVD. Total HDL particles, medium HDL particles, and baseline LDL-C were significant predictors of CHD death. LDL particles and VLDL particles were not significantly related to CHD death. Size of VLDL, LDL, or HDL particles is not significantly related to CHD death. The long-term risk of CHD among men with MetSyn was not related to the levels of CRP, insulin, adiponectin, or to the number of small LDL particles | NMR |

| | | | | | | |
|---|---|---|---|---|---|---|
| Lee [69] | NA | 40 vs. 40 | T2DM vs. NoHG male adults | Asian (South Korea) | DM: *Higher* TG, total cholesterol, smaller LDL lipoproteins (all $P<0.05$). Higher concentrations of small LDL positively correlated with TG, $HbA_{1c}$, and oxidized LDL; negatively correlated with HDL-C (all $P<0.05$) | PAGGE |
| | | | | | Stepwise multiple regression: TG, $HbA_{1c}$, and oxidized LDL, in descending order, were independent correlation factors for small-sized LDL proportion (all $P<0.05$) | |
| Selby [108] | Kaiser Permanente Women Twins Study | 682 | IR, T2DM, vs. NoHG adult female twins | Majority Caucasian (US) | IR/DM: higher prevalence of Pattern B. Mixed IR and NoHG ($n=564$ twins): TG, HDL-C, and IR predicted Pattern B ($P<0.05$). In 25 non-DM monozygotic twin pairs and discordant LDL pattern (i.e., removal of all genetic variability) each component of the IR syndrome was more apparent in the twin with Pattern B: higher TG, lower HDL-C, higher BMI, higher waist-to-hip ratio, higher systolic blood pressure (all $P<0.05$); trends for higher fasting and postprandial insulin | PAGGE |
| Tan [126] | NA | 44 | T2DM adults | Asian (Singapore) | In the HDL fraction, the majority of particles were small HDL (59 %), followed by medium particles (25 %); large particles comprised the smallest proportion (16 %). Findings were similar in the LDL fraction, with 56 % of LDL particles belonging to the small subclass. Only the concentrations of total and medium-sized HDL particles and not HDL-C, HDL size, ApoA-I, large- or small-sized HDL particles showed significant correlations with cholesterol efflux from macrophages incubated with apo B-depleted plasmas | NMR |

*CHD* coronary heart disease; *CVD* cardiovascular disease; *DGU* density gradient ultracentrifugation, including Vertical Auto Profile® (Atherotech Inc, Birmingham, AL); *IR* insulin resistant, includes patients diagnosed with impaired fasting glucose; *IS* insulin sensitive when measured by hyperinsulinemic-euglycemic clamp technique; *MetSyn* metabolic syndrome; *N* number of individuals in study population; *NA* not applicable; *NG* not given; *NoHG* normoglycemic, includes individuals with healthy insulin sensitivity; *NMR* nuclear magnetic resonance spectroscopy, including NMR LipoProfile (LipoScience, Inc., Raleigh, NC); *PAGGE* polyacrylamide gradient gel electrophoresis; *Pop* characteristics of population studied; *T1DM* type 1 diabetes mellitus; *T2DM* type 2 diabetes mellitus; *TG* triglycerides; *Vs* versus

**Table 2.2** Overview of clinical trials examining the association between lipoprotein subclasses and the emergence of cardiovascular disease in patients with IR/DM or the metabolic syndrome (MetSyn)

| Publication | Trial name | *N* | Pop studied | Race (country) | Major findings | Subclass technique |
|---|---|---|---|---|---|---|
| Bakogianni [8] | NA | 28 vs. 24 vs. 25 | T2DM + CAD vs. NoHG ± CAD male adults | NG (Greece) | T2DM patients with coronary artery disease (CAD) had higher TG compared with either NoHG/no CAD or NoHG/CAD ($P<0.05$). T2DM/CAD vs. NoHG/no CAD: reduced HDL-C, HDL2-C, and HDL3-C (all $P<0.05$). T2DM/CAD vs. NoHG/CAD: reduced HDL-C and HDL2-C (all $P<0.05$); no change in HDL3-C. Greater percentage reduction of cholesterol in HDL2 vs. HDL3 for both comparisons | DGU |
| Colhoun [23] | NA | 194 vs. 195 | T1DM vs. NoHG adults | NG (UK) | *Male* T1DM vs. NoHG: *Higher* large HDL, HDL size (all $P<0.05$); *Lower* medium VLDL concentration, total VLDL particles, total LDL + IDL particles, small HDL (all $P<0.05$) | NMR |
| | | | | | *Female* T1DM vs. NoHG: *Higher* small LDL, VLDL size, large HDL, HDL size (all $P<0.05$); *Lower* medium VLDL, small LDL, small HDL, (all $P<0.05$). LDL size and subclass were similar in diabetic and nondiabetic men. In women, diabetes was associated with less large and more small LDL and a reduced LDL size (mean difference 0.2 nm). This gender difference was significant. T1DM was associated with more large and less small HDL and, to a similar degree in both sexes, a higher HDL size (difference of 0.4 nm in men and 0.3 nm in women). No definitive abnormalities in VLDL size. In nondiabetic subjects, lower average HDL particle size, lower LDL size, and higher VLDL size were significantly associated with coronary calcification. Thus the HDL size differences with diabetes would be expected to be anti-atherogenic and the LDL size differences pro-atherogenic. No clear relationship between particle size and calcification in diabetic subjects was observed | |
| Gray [46] | Strong Heart Study | 4,505 | IR/DM vs. NoHG adults | Native American (US) | LDL size: smaller in men than in women; smaller in DM than in non-DM. In multivariate analyses, LDL size significantly related to components of the IR, including TG (inversely) and HDL-C (positively). In this population with low LDL-C, LDL lipoprotein size was not related to CVD | PAGGE |

| | | | | | | |
|---|---|---|---|---|---|---|
| Kathiresan [58] | Framingham Heart Study | 2,993 | MetSyn vs. NoHG adults | Majority Caucasian (US) | Male MetSyn: *Higher* total LDL particles, small LDL, total VLDL particle number, large and intermediate VLDL, apo B (all $P<0.05$); *lower* large LDL, total HDL particle number, large and small HDL (all $P<0.05$) | NMR |
| | | | | | Female MetSyn: *Higher* total LDL particles, small LDL, total VLDL particle number, large and intermediate VLDL, small HDL, LDL-C, apo B (all $P<0.05$); *Lower* large LDL, total HDL particle number, large HDL (all $P<0.05$), LDL particle number and small LDL particle number, but not LDL-C, strongly associated with MetSyn. Small LDL particle number is elevated in the MetSyn, increases with the number of MetSyn components, and most prominently was correlated with TG and HDL-C. Higher rate of CVD events with MetSyn vs. NoHG. A higher small LDL particle number was *not* associated with greater CVD event rates in people with the MetSyn | |
| Laasko [67] | NA | 213 | T2DM adults | Majority Caucasian (Finland) | *Died of CHD* vs. did not: No differences in LDL-C. For HDL-C, 1.01±0.04 vs. 1.20±0.02 mmol/L ($P<0.001$). For HDL2-C, 0.62±0.04 vs. 0.78±0.02 mmol/L, ($P<0.001$). No differences in HDL3-C. For VLDL-C, 2.07±0.28 vs. 1.37+0.10 mmol/L ($P<0.01$). For TG, 4.16±0.72 vs. 2.72±0.22 mmol/L ($P<0.01$) | DGU |
| | | | | | *Serious CHD event* vs. none: No differences in LDL-C. For HDL-C, 1.06±0.03 vs. 1.20±0.02 mmol/L ($P<0.001$). For HDL2-C, 0.66±0.03 vs. 0.79±0.02 mmol/L ($P=0.02$). No differences in HDL3-C. For VLDL-C, 1.81±0.20 vs. 1.38±0.11 mmol/L ($P<0.05$). For TG, 3.69±0.52 vs. 2.72±0.24 mmol/L ($P<0.01$) | |
| | | | | | *Univariate logistic regression analysis*: VLDL-C, TG positively associated and HDL-C, HDL2-C negatively associated with CHD death and all CHD events. The risk T2DM patients with having low HDL-C (23 % of patients), whatever their TG level, to die from CHD was fourfold ($P<0.001$) and for all CHD events, twofold ($P=0.002$). High TG (45 % of patients) was associated with a twofold risk for CHD death ($P=0.001$) and all CHD events ($P=0.008$). High non-HDL-C (>5.3 mmol/L; 84 % of patients) not associated with increased risk of CHD events. Simultaneous presence of low HDL-C (<0.9 mmol/L), high TG (>2.3 mmol/L), and high LDL-C (>4.1 mmol/L) (7 % of patients) increased the risk of CHD death (OR=4.0 [1.7–9.5], $P<0.001$) and all CHD in T2DM patients. In the study population, low HDL-C was the most important single predictor of future CHD events | |

(continued)

**Table 2.2** (continued)

| Publication | Trial name | *N* | Pop studied | Race (country) | Major findings | Subclass technique |
|---|---|---|---|---|---|---|
| Lyons [74] | Diabetes Control and Complications Trial/ Epidemiology of Diabetes Interventions and Complications (DCCT/EDIC) | 1,325 | T1DM adults | NG (US) | CIMT associations with lipoproteins were stronger for the internal than the common carotid artery, predominantly involving LDL. Internal CIMT was positively associated with LDL subclasses and particle concentration and with conventional LDL-C and ApoB in both genders. Common CIMT was associated, in men only, with large VLDL, IDL, conventional LDL-C, and apo B | NMR |
| Marso [79] | Diabetes Genome Project (DGP) | 66 vs. 119 | T2DM vs. NoHG adults | NG (US) | Low adiponectin levels are associated with atherogenic lipoproteins (elevated TG, small dense LDL-C, and low HDL-C), increased plaque volume, lipid-rich plaque, and IVUS-derived pathological intimal thickening in the total cohort that was driven by the nondiabetic population, suggesting an anti-atherogenic role in the early stages of lesion development. Adiponectin levels did *not* correlate with DM | DGU |
| | | | | | Adiponectin levels correlated with TG ($r=-0.27$, $P=0.0002$) and HDL-C ($r=-0.4$, $P<0.003$), small dense LDL3 ($r=-0.27$, $P=0.003$) and LDL4 ($r=-0.25$, $P=0.0005$), and the large, more buoyant LDL2 ($r=0.18$, $P=0.015$) | |
| Soedamah-Muthu [117] | Pittsburgh Epidemiology of Diabetes Complications Study (EDC) | 118 | T1DM children at baseline | NG (US) | Ten-year follow-up: CAD vs. no CAD. CAD: *Higher* non-HDL-C, TG, apo B, apo A1/HDL-C, total small, medium, and large VLDL, total, small and medium LDL, medium HDL (all $P<0.05$); Trend for higher LDL-C and total cholesterol; *Lower* HDL-C, LDL size, total and large HDL, HDL size (all $P<0.05$) | NMR |
| | | | | | In T1DM both lipid mass and particle concentrations of all three VLDL subclasses, small LDL, medium LDL, and medium HDL were increased in CAD cases compared to no CAD controls, while large HDL was decreased | |

*Abbreviations*: *CIMT* carotid intima-media thickness; *DGU* density gradient ultracentrifugation, including Vertical Auto Profile® (Atherotech Inc, Birmingham, AL); *IR* insulin resistant, includes patients diagnosed with impaired fasting glucose; *MetSyn* metabolic syndrome; *N* number of individuals in study population; *NA* not applicable; *NG* not given; *NMR* nuclear magnetic resonance spectroscopy, including NMR LipoProfile (LipoScience, Inc., Raleigh, NC); *NoHG* normoglycemic, includes individuals with healthy insulin sensitivity; *PAGGE* polyacrylamide gradient gel electrophoresis; *Pop* characteristics of population studied; *TG* triglycerides; *Tx* treatment; *Vs* versus; *Wks* weeks

**Table 2.3** Overview of intervention clinical trials examining lipoprotein subclasses in patients with IR/DM or the metabolic syndrome (MetSyn)

| Publication | Trial name | *N* | Pop studied | Race (country) | Tx duration (wks) | Tx | Major findings | Subclass technique |
|---|---|---|---|---|---|---|---|---|
| Chainani-Wu [16] | Multisite cardiac lifestyle intervention program | 131 | T1 or T2DM vs. NoHG adults | NG (US) | 12 | Intensive lifestyle intervention | Comprehensive lifestyle intervention that included a low-fat, whole-foods, plant-based diet, exercise, stress management, and group support meetings. 131 participants (59 % women and 43 % with DM), 56 with CHD (38 % women and 27 % DM), and 75 at high risk with >3 CHD risk factors and/or DM (76 % women and 55 % DM)<br>In whole cohort, reduction in large and small VLDL particles; size of VLDL particles; total LDL particles; total, large, and small HDL particles (all $P<0.05$). In subgroup with diagnosed CHD, reduction in total and small LDL particles; total and small HDL particles (all $P \leq 0.05$); increased HDL size ($P<0.05$). In subgroup at high risk for CHD, reduction in large VLDL particles and size; total, large, medium, and small HDL particles (all $P \leq 0.05$) | NMR |
| Chilton [18] | Diabetes therapy Utilization: Researching changes in Hb$A_{1c}$, weight and other factors Through Intervention with exenatide once weekly (DURATION-1) | 211 | T2DM adults | Caucasian, Black, Hispanic, Asian (Canada, US) | 30 | Exenatide once weekly vs. twice daily | Once-weekly exenatide was associated with a clinically important shift in lipoprotein pattern away from small, dense LDL4-C, despite the appearance of a benign lipid profile at baseline. Exenatide significantly reduced hsCRP independent of restored glycemic control and weight loss | DGU |
| Deeg [27] | GLAI study | 369 vs. 366 | T2DM adults | Caucasian, Black, Hispanic, Asian, other (Colombia, Mexico, Puerto Rico, US) | 24 | Pioglitazone, rosiglitazone | First study to demonstrate that PIO and ROSI have significantly different effects on lipoprotein subclass particle concentrations and sizes despite similar effects on glycemic control and IR. PIO increased total VLDL particle concentration less than ROSI and decreased VLDL particle size more than ROSI. PIO treatment reduced total LDL particle concentration, whereas ROSI treatment increased it. Both treatments increased LDL particle size, with PIO treatment having a greater effect. Whereas PIO increased total HDL particle concentration and size, ROSI decreased them; both increased HDL-C. | NMR |

(continued)

**Table 2.3** (continued)

| Publication | Trial name | *N* | Pop studied | Race (country) | Tx duration (wks) | Tx | Major findings | Subclass technique |
|---|---|---|---|---|---|---|---|---|
| Gómez-Pérez [45] | NA | 106 | T2DM adults | NG (Mexico) | 24 | Troglitazone, placebo | Troglitazone significantly improved IS; higher HDL-C and lower TG; reduced lighter VLDL1. The change in HDL-C resulted from a combination of higher HDL3-C and lower HDL2-C. Troglitazone reduces TG by lowering the TG content of VLDL1 and increases HDL-C by increasing HDL3-C | DGU |
| Howard [53] | Stop atherosclerosis in native diabetics study (SANDS) | 418 | T2DM adults | Native American (US) | 156 | Statin plus other drugs as needed | First study to establish CIMT regression in T2DM with aggressive lipid and blood pressure interventions compared with standard therapy. Aggressive therapy (vs. standard) reduced total cholesterol; LDL-C; non-HDL-C; total and small VLDL particles; total, large, and small LDL particles; apo B (all $P \leq 0.05$) | NMR |
| May [81] | Diabetes and combined lipid therapy regimen (DIACOR) | 300 | T2DM adults | NG (US) | 12 | Simvastatin, fenofibrate, both | Combination therapy reduced dense VLDL-C compared with fenofibrate ($P<0.001$) or simvastatin ($P<0.0001$); simvastatin reduced IDL-C compared with fenofibrate ($P=0.003$) Combination therapy ameliorated Pattern B dyslipidemia; reduced TG, dense VLDL-C, and Lp(a); increased HDL3 and LDL particle size | DGU |
| Miller [85] | SILHOUETTE | | T2DM adults | NG (USA) | 6 | Simvastatin, placebo | Statin (simvastatin) reduced TG-rich lipoproteins (VLDL-C, VLDL3, IDL, LDL subclasses) | DGU |
| Nakano [87] | NA | 25 vs. 25 | T2DM adults | Asian (Japan) | 12 | Pioglitazone, metformin | PIO, but not MET, reduced large VLDL; increased in serum adiponectin levels (each $P<0.001$). In the PIO group, the change in large VLDL correlated positively with changes in $HbA_{1c}$ ($r=0.468$, $P=0.0174$), HOMA-IR ($r=0.593$, $P=0.0014$), very small LDL ($r=0.714$, $P<0.0001$) and net electronegative charged modified LDL ($r=0.412$, $P=0.0399$), and inversely with changes in adiponectin level ($r=-0.526$, $P=0.0061$) | Gel-permeation HPLC |
| Niemeijer-Kanters [89] | NA | 50 | T2DM adults | NG (The Nether-lands) | 30 | Treated to lipid targets, simvastatin, gemfibrozil, acipimox, combinations | At week 0, 24 patients (48 %) were characterized by small dense LDL Pattern B. After treatment, a shift towards normal LDL lipoprotein size was observed in 17 patients. HDL-C was significantly lower in these patients compared to those who had LDL subclass pattern A. Multivariate regression analysis revealed VLDL-C or TG and HDL3-C as independent predictors of LDL lipoprotein size. Change in HDL2-C was an independent determinant for change in LDL particle size | DGU |

| | | | | | | | | |
|---|---|---|---|---|---|---|---|---|
| Perez [98] | NA | 177 (81 vs. 96) | T2DM adults | Caucasian, Black, Hispanic, Asian (US) | 24 | Pioglitazone, background, metformin or sulfonylurea (2 separate studies) | PIO combination treatment: increased average and peak LDL lipoprotein size ($P<0.0001$; range 0.29–0.39 nm for average; 0.36–0.55 nm for peak lipoprotein size); decreased TG ($P<0.05$). Shifts in HDL and LDL distribution showed an increase in large lipoproteins and a decrease in small lipoproteins ($P<0.05$); increased HDL2, decreased HDL3. For PIO + MET: increased levels of Apo AI, Apo AI/AII-containing HDL, and Lp(a) ($P<0.05$) | PAGGE |
| Pontrelli [101] | NA | 20 | IR/T2DM adults | NG (Canada) | 9 | Atorvastatin, placebo | Statin decreased the density of LDL lipoproteins; shift from small, dense LDL to more buoyant and less atherogenic lipoproteins; reduction in total cholesterol (41 %), LDL-C (55 %), TG (32 %), and ApoB (40 %) (all $P<0.05$). Mean LDL lipoprotein diameter increased from small, dense LDL to intermediate LDL. At baseline, LDL lipoproteins were predominantly found in the small, dense subclass; statin resulted in a shift in the profile to the larger and more buoyant LDL subclass | PAGGE |
| Shimabukuro [113] | NA | 16 vs. 15 | T2DM adults | Asian (Japan) | 24 | Pitavastatin, atorvastatin | Statins (atorvastatin vs. pitavastatin): reduced total cholesterol, LDL-C, non-HDL-C and LDL-C/HDL-C ($P<0.05$). Pitavastatin increased HDL-C ($P<0.05$); reduced Apo AI and apo B ($P<0.01$). Atorvastatin reduced TG, apo B ($P<0.01$). Large, medium, and small VLDL; large, medium, small, and very small LDL decreased equally after treatment with either statin ($P<0.05$). TG decreased in most VLDL and LDL lipoprotein subclasses after atorvastatin treatment; TG was decreased only in medium HDL subclasses after pitavastatin | HPLC |
| Soedamah-Muthu [116] | Collaborative Atorvastatin Diabetes Study (CARDS) | 69 vs. 53 | T2DM adults | NG (UK) | 24 | Atorvastatin, Placebo | Statin decreased TG; LDL-C; Apo B; medium and small VLDL; large and medium LDL ($P<0.05$). Statin increased large HDL with little change in small HDL; as a result average HDL particle size increased ($P<0.05$) | NMR |
| Tomassini [127] | Vytorin vs. atorvastatin in patients with type 2 diabetes mellitus and hypercholesterol-anemia Study (VYTAL) | 1,013 | T2DM adults | Caucasian, Black, Asian, Hispanic, Native American, other (US) | 6 | Simvastatin plus ezetimibe vs. atorvastatin | Ezetimibe/simvastatin reduced LDL-C; LDL1-C; LDL2-C; LDL3-C; real LDL-C; IDL-C; IDL1-C; IDL2-C; VLDL-C; VLDL3-C; and remnant-like lipoprotein cholesterol (RLP-C) more than atorvastatin (all $P<0.05$). Ezetimibe/simvastatin increased HDL-C; HDL3-C; VLDL1 + 2-C (all $P<0.05$). Changes in LDL4-C and LDL-C subclass patterns (A, B, and I) were comparable for both treatments. Generally, similar results were observed for patients with TG levels <200 and ≥200 mg/dL. Frequency of Pattern B was also reduced more in patients with higher TGs for both treatments | DGU, PAGGE |

*Abbreviations*: *DGU* density gradient ultracentrifugation, including Vertical Auto Profile® (Atherotech Inc, Birmingham, AL); *IR* insulin resistant, includes patients diagnosed with impaired fasting glucose; *HPLC* high performance liquid chromatography; *MetSyn* metabolic syndrome; *N* number of individuals in study population; *NA* not applicable; *NG* not given; *NMR* nuclear magnetic resonance spectroscopy, including NMR LipoProfile (LipoScience, Inc., Raleigh, NC); *NoHG* normoglycemic, includes individuals with healthy insulin sensitivity; *PAGGE* polyacrylamide gradient gel electrophoresis; *Pop* characteristics of population studied; *TG* triglycerides; *Tx* treatment; *Vs* versus; *Wks* weeks with changes in lipoprotein subclasses and other biomarkers for CVD risk.

Carotid artery intima-media thickness (CIMT) is a surrogate measure of early-stage atherosclerosis correlated with risk factors for CVD [73, 76, 100, 119, 120]. Statin and fibrate treatments each inhibit the rate of carotid intima-media thickness (CIMT) progression [3, 80, 131]. In a direct-comparison study, fibrate therapy demonstrated a significantly greater CIMT and a steeper CIMT-to-time relationship than statin therapy [19]. These differences were not explained by differences in LDL-C concentrations. Similar outcomes have been reported for individuals with IR/T2DM or MetSyn. In a statin trial in T2DM patients with low HDL-C, active treatment reduced TG-rich lipoprotein subclasses and promoted a less atherogenic lipoprotein profile [85]. In a population of genetically similar T2DM adults with no prior history of cardiovascular events, statin therapy for 3 years reduced total cholesterol and LDL-C in parallel with reduced CIMT, i.e., regression of atherosclerosis [53]. In addition, aggressive therapy was more effective than standard therapy in decreasing apo B, LDL particle concentrations (both small and large particles), and VLDL size and particle number. There was a trend for an association between reduced LDL particle concentrations and CIMT regression.

Thiazolidinediones (TZDs) are insulin sensitizers and potent inhibitors of lipolysis in adipose tissue [28]. TZDs also mobilize lipid out of the muscle, liver, and pancreatic β-cells, thereby reducing the lipotoxicity that occurs with worsening IR/DM. For example, in T2DM patients the TZD pioglitazone reduced LDL particle number, despite significantly increasing LDL-C concentration; and this effect was attributed to a large increase in LDL size and cholesterol content [44].

Other antidiabetic therapies are also starting to demonstrate effects on lipoprotein subclasses and CVD risk reduction. For example, post hoc analysis of a clinical trial in T2DM patients administered the GLP-1 receptor agonist exenatide suggests significant improvements in the pro-atherogenic phenotype with exenatide treatment [18]. In T2DM patients participating in the exenatide DURATION-1 clinical trial [30], in which 80 % presented with a lipid Pattern B, i.e., the LDL-C distribution was skewed towards the smaller LDL3-C and LDL4-C. After treatment, a clinically important shift in lipoprotein pattern away from small, dense LDL4-C lipoproteins was observed, consistent with the corresponding reduction in serum TG. Reductions in TG rich remnant lipoproteins were also significant [18]. Exenatide therapy also significantly increased the more buoyant HDL2-C lipoprotein, even after adjustment for treatment reductions in $HbA_{1c}$ and body weight.

## Concluding Remarks

The physiological continuum of metabolic syndrome, IR, and diabetes is associated with elevations in TG-rich lipoproteins (VLDL and IDL) and redistribution of elevated cholesterol among LDL and HDL subclasses. The pro-atherogenic phenotype characterized by small, dense LDL lipoproteins is at least doubled in people with diabetes, attributable in part to dysregulation of TG-rich lipoprotein clearance. Standard lipid panels (e.g., TG, total cholesterol, calculated LDL-C, and HDL-C) fail to identify many lipoprotein abnormalities that contribute to CVD events. Clustering of subclass lipoprotein and particle changes are extremely common in diabetes. Technologies (e.g., PAGGE, NMR, DGU) have been developed that allow clinicians to integrate lipoprotein subclass measures into more comprehensive treatment strategies based on each patient's detailed dyslipidemic profile. Clinical investigations have validated the strengths and weaknesses of each methodology and provide an emerging confirmation of the use of lipoprotein subclass profiles in predicting CVD risk. Further work regarding such measures, response to treatment, and outcomes data is warranted.

## References

1. Alabakovska SB, Labudovic DD, Tosheska KN, Spiroski MZ, Todorova BB. Low density lipoprotein subclass distribution in children with diabetes mellitus. Bratisl Lek Listy. 2008;109:155–9.
2. Ala-Korpela M, Lankinen N, Salminen A, Suna T, Soininen P, Laatikainen R, Ingman P, Jauhiainen M,

Taskinen M, Héberger K, Kaski K. The inherent accuracy of [1]H NMR spectroscopy to quantify plasma lipoproteins is subclass dependent. Atherosclerosis. 2007;190:352–8.
3. Amarenco P, Labreuche J, Lavallée P, Touboul P-J. Statins in stroke prevention and carotid atherosclerosis: systematic review and up-to-date meta-analysis. Stroke. 2004;35:2902–9.
4. Austin MA, Brunzell JD, Fitch WL, Krauss RM. Inheritance of low density lipoprotein subclass patterns in familial combined hyperlipidemia. Arterioscler Thromb Vasc Biol. 1990;10:520–30.
5. Austin MA, King MC, Vranizan KM, Krauss RM. Atherogenic lipoprotein phenotype. A proposed genetic marker for coronary heart disease risk. Circulation. 1990;82:495–506.
6. Austin MA, Mykkänen L, Kuusisto J, Edwards KL, Nelson C, Haffner SM, Pyörälä K, Laakso M. Prospective study of small LDLs as a risk factor for non–insulin dependent diabetes mellitus in elderly men and women. Circulation. 1995;92:1770–8.
7. Bachorick PS, Ross JW. National Cholesterol Education Program recommendations for measurement of low-density lipoprotein cholesterol: executive summary. Clin Chem. 1995;41:1414–20.
8. Bakogianni MC, Kalofoutis CA, Skenderi KI, Kalofoutis AT. Clinical evaluation of plasma high-density lipoprotein subfractions (HDL2, HDL3) in non-insulin-dependent diabetics with coronary artery disease. J Diabetes Complications. 2001;15:265–9.
9. Ballantyne C, Gleim G, Liu N, et al. Effects of coadministered extended-release niacin/laropiprant and simvastatin on lipoprotein subclasses in patients with dyslipidemia. J Clin Lipidol. 2012;6(3):235–43.
10. Blake GJ, Otvos JD, Rifai N, Ridker PM. LDL particle concentration and size as determined by NMR spectroscopy as predictors of cardiovascular disease in women. Circulation. 2002;106:1930–7.
11. Blanche PJ, Gong EL, Forte TM, Nichols AV. Characterization of human high density lipoproteins by gradient gel electrophoresis. Biochim Biophys Acta. 1981;665:408–19.
12. Boumaiza I, Omezzine A, Rejeb J, et al. Apolipoprotein B and non-high-density lipoprotein cholesterol are better risk markers for coronary artery disease than low-density lipoprotein cholesterol in hypertriglyceridemic metabolic syndrome patients. Metab Syndr Relat Disord. 2010;8: 515–22.
13. Brunzell JD, Davidson M, Furberg CD, Goldberg RB, Howard BV, Stein JH, Witztum JL. Lipoprotein management in patients with cardiometabolic risk: consensus statement from the American Diabetes Association and the American College of Cardiology Foundation. Diabetes Care. 2008;31:811–22.
14. Campbell SC, Moffatt RJ, Kushnick MR. Continuous and intermittent walking alters HDL(2)-C and LCATa. Atherosclerosis. 2011;218:524–9.
15. Catapano AL, Reiner Z, De Backer G, Graham I, Taskinen M, Wiklund O, Agewall S, Alegria E, Chapman MJ, Durrington P, Erdine S, Halcox J, Hobbs R, Kjekshus J, Filardi PP, Riccardi G, Storey RF, Wood D. ESC/EAS guidelines for the management of dyslipidaemias: The Task Force for the management of dyslipidaemias of the European Society of Cardiology (ESC) and the European Atherosclerosis Society (EAS). Atherosclerosis. 2011;217S:S1–44.
16. Chainani-Wu N, Weidner G, Purnell DM, Frenda S, Merritt-Worden T, Pischke C, Campo R, Kemp C, Kersh ES, Ornish D. Changes in emerging cardiac biomarkers after an intensive lifestyle intervention. Am J Cardiol. 2011;108:498–507.
17. Chapman MJ, Laplaud PM, Luc G, Forgez P, Bruckert E, Goulinet S, Lagrange D. Further resolution of the low density lipoprotein spectrum in normal human plasma: physicochemical characteristics of discrete subspecies separated by density gradient ultracentrifugation. J Lipid Res. 1988;29:442–58.
18. Chilton R, Toth PP, Ramirez G, Cobble M, Walsh B, Chiquette E. Treatment with exenatide BID and QW for 30 weeks was associated with favorable lipid subclass changes. Diabetologia. 2011;54 Suppl 1:P799. Accessed Jan 26, 2012 at http://www.abstractsonline.com/Plan/ViewAbstract.aspx?sKey=04f097f3-144b-4788-a3ee-15f397f53c9f&cKey=053cc9fd-fe9b-4593-8746-594a8cf83802&mKey=%7bBAFB2746-B0DD-4110-8588-E385FAF957B7%7d.
19. Chironi G, Simon A, Gariepy J, Balice M, Del-Pino M, Levenson J. Differential associations of statin and fibrate treatment with carotid arterial remodeling. Am J Hypertens. 2005;18:1476–81.
20. Chu JW, Abbasi F, Kulkarni KR, Lamendola C, McLaughlin TL, Scalisi JN, Reaven GM. Multiple lipoprotein abnormalities associated with insulin resistance in healthy volunteers are Identified by the vertical auto profile-II methodology. Clin Chem. 2003;49:1014–7.
21. Chung BH, Wilkinson T, Geer JC, Segrest JP. Preparative and quantitative isolation of plasma lipoproteins: rapid, single discontinuous density gradient ultracentrifugation in a vertical rotor. J Lipid Res. 1980;21:284–91.
22. Chung BH, Segrest PJ, Cone JT, et al. High resolution plasma lipoprotein cholesterol profiles by a rapid, high volume semi-automated method. J Lipid Res. 1981;22:1003–14.
23. Colhoun HM, Otvos JD, Rubens MB, Taskinen MR, Underwood SR, Fuller JH. Lipoprotein subclasses and particle sizes and their relationship with coronary artery calcification in men and women with and without type 1 diabetes. Diabetes. 2002;51:1949–56.
24. Contois JH, McConnell JP, Sethi A, Csako G, Devarag S, Hoefner DM, Warnick GR. Apolipoprotein B and cardiovascular disease risk: position statement from the AACC lipoproteins and vascular diseases division working group on best practices. Clin Chem. 2009;55:407–19.
25. Cromwell WC, Otvos JD, Keyes MJ, et al. LDL particle number and risk of future cardiovascular disease in the Framingham Offspring Study - implications

for LDL management. J Clin Lipidol. 2007;1: 583–92.
26. Cui Y, Blumenthal RS, Flaws JA, et al. Non-high-density lipoprotein cholesterol level as a predictor of cardiovascular disease mortality. Arch Intern Med. 2001;161:1413–9.
27. Deeg MA, Buse JB, Goldberg RB, Kendall DM, Zagar AJ, Jacober SJ, Khan MA, Perez AT, Tan MH. on behalf of the GLAI study investigators. Pioglitazone and rosiglitazone have different effects on serum lipoprotein particle concentrations and sizes in patients with type 2 diabetes and dyslipidemia. Diabetes Care. 2007;30:2458–64.
28. DeFronzo RA. From the triumvirate to the ominous octet: a new paradigm for the treatment of type 2 diabetes mellitus. Diabetes. 2009;58:773–95.
29. DeLalla OF, Gofman JW. Ultracentrifugal analysis of serum lipoproteins. Methods Biochem Anal. 1954;1:459–78.
30. Drucker DJ, Buse JB, Taylor K, et al. for the DURATION-1 Study Group. Exenatide once weekly versus twice daily for the treatment of type 2 diabetes: a randomised, open-label, non-inferiority study. Lancet. 2008;372:1240–50.
31. Enkhmaa B, Anuurad E, Zhang W, Tran T, Berglund L. Lipoprotein(a): genotype-phenotype relationship and impact on atherogenic risk. Metab Syndr Relat Disord. 2011;9:411–8.
32. Feingold KR, Grunfeld C, Pang M, Doerrler W, Krauss RM. LDL subclass phenotypes and triglyceride metabolism in non-insulin-dependent diabetes. Arterioscler Thromb Vasc Biol. 1992;12:1496–502.
33. Festa A, Williams K, Hanley AJG, Otvos JD, Goff DC, Wagenknecht LE, Haffner SM. Nuclear magnetic resonance lipoprotein abnormalities in prediabetic subjects in the insulin resistance atherosclerosis study. Circulation. 2005;111:3465–72.
34. Franceschini G, Bondoli A, Granata D, Mercuri V, Negri M, Tosi C, Sirtori CR. Reduced HDL2 levels in myocardial infarction patients without risk factors for atherosclerosis. Atherosclerosis. 1987;68:213–9.
35. Freedman DS, Otvos JD, Jeyarajah EJ, Shalaurova I, Cupples LA, Parise H, D'Agostino RB, Wilson PWF, Schaefer EJ. Sex and age differences in lipoprotein subclasses measured by nuclear magnetic resonance spectroscopy: The Framingham Study. Clinical Chem. 2004;50:1189–200.
36. Friedewald W, Levy R, Fredrickson D. Estimation of concentration of low-density lipoprotein cholesterol in plasma, without use of the preparative ultracentrifuge. Clin Chem. 1972;18:499–502.
37. Friedlander Y, Kidron M, Caslake M, Lamb T, McConnell M, Bar-On H. Low density lipoprotein particle size and risk factors of insulin resistance syndrome. Atherosclerosis. 2000;148:141–9.
38. Fujimoto WY, Bergstrom RW, Boyko EJ, Chen KW, Leonetti DL, Newell-Morris L, Shofer JB, Wahl PW. Visceral adiposity and incident coronary heart disease in Japanese-American men: The 10-year follow-up results of the Seattle Japanese-American Community Diabetes Study. Diabetes Care. 1999;22: 1808–12.
39. Garvey WT, Kwon S, Zheng D, Shaughnessy S, Wallace P, Hutto A, Pugh K, Jenkins AJ, Klein RL, Liao Y. Effects of insulin resistance and type 2 diabetes on lipoprotein subclass particle size and concentration determined by nuclear magnetic resonance. Diabetes. 2003;52:453–62.
40. Goff Jr DC, D'Agostino Jr RB, Haffner SM, Otvos JD. Insulin resistance and adiposity influence lipoprotein size and subclass concentrations. Results from the insulin resistance atherosclerosis Study. Metabolism. 2005;54:264–70.
41. Gofman JW. Serum lipoproteins and the evaluation of atherosclerosis. Ann N Y Acad Sci. 1956;64:590–5.
42. Gofman JW, Lindgren F, Elliott H, et al. The role of lipids and lipoproteins in atherosclerosis. Science. 1950;111:166–71.
43. Gofman JW, Young W, Tandy R. Ischemic heart disease, atherosclerosis, and longevity. Circulation. 1966;34:679–97.
44. Goldberg RB, Kendall DM, Deeg MA, Buse JB, Zagar AJ, Pinaire JA, Tan MH, Khan MA, Perez AT, Jacober SJ. for the GLAI study investigators. A comparison of lipid and glycemic effects of pioglitazone and rosiglitazone in patients with type 2 diabetes and dyslipidemia. Diabetes Care. 2005;28:1547–54.
45. Gómez-Pérez FJ, Aguilar-Salinas CA, Vázquez-Chávez C, Fanghänel-Salmón G, Gallegos-Martínez J, Gómez-Diaz RA, Salinas-Orozco S, Chavira-López IJ, Sánchez-Reyes L, Torres-Acosta EM, Tamez R, López A, Guillén LE, Cesarman G. Further insight on the hypoglycemic and nonhypoglycemic effects of troglitazone 400 or 600 mg/d: effects on the very-low-density and high-density lipoprotein particle distribution. Metabolism. 2002;51:44–51.
46. Gray RS, Robbins DC, Wang W, Yeh JL, Fabsitz RR, Cowan LD, Welty TK, Lee ET, Krauss RM, Howard BV. Relation of LDL size to the insulin resistance syndrome and coronary heart disease in American Indians: The Strong Heart Study. Arterioscler Thromb Vasc Biol. 1997;17:2713–20.
47. Grundy SM, Vega GL, Otvos JD, Rainwater DL, Cohen JC. Hepatic lipase influences high density lipoprotein subclass distribution in normotriglyceridemic men: genetic and pharmacological evidence. J Lipid Res. 1999;40:229–34.
48. Haffner SM, Mykkanen L, Valdez RA, Paidi M, Stern MP, Howard BV. LDL size and subclass pattern in a biethnic population. Arterioscler Thromb Vasc Biol. 1993;13:1623–30.
49. Hallman DM, Brown SA, Ballantyne CM, Sharrett AR, Boerwinkle E. Relationship between low-density lipoprotein subclasses and asymptomatic atherosclerosis in subjects from the Atherosclerosis Risk in Communities (ARIC) Study. Biomarkers. 2004;9:190–202.
50. Hite AH, Berkowitz VG, Berkowitz K. Low-carbohydrate diet review: shifting the paradigm. Nutr Clin Pract. 2011;26:300–8.

51. Hodge AM, Jenkins AJ, English DR, O'Dea K, Giles GG. NMR-determined lipoprotein subclass profile predicts type 2 diabetes. Diabetes Res Clin Pract. 2009;83:132–9.
52. Holewijn S, den Heijer M, Swinkels DW, Stalenhoef AF, de Graaf J. Apolipoprotein B, non-HDL cholesterol and LDL cholesterol for identifying individuals at increased cardiovascular risk. J Intern Med. 2010;268:567–77.
53. Howard WJ, Russell M, Fleg JL, Mete M, Ali T, Devereux RB, Galloway JM, Otvos JD, Ratner RE, Roman MJ, Silverman A, Umans JG, Weissman NJ, Wilson C, Howard BV. Prevention of atherosclerosis with low-density lipoprotein cholesterol lowering-lipoprotein changes and interactions: the SANDS study. J Clin Lipidology. 2009;3:322–31.
54. Hulley SB, Cook SG, Wilson WS, Nichaman MZ, Hatch FT, Lindgren FT. Quantitation of serum lipoproteins by electrophoresis on agarose gel: standarization in lipoprotein concentration units (mg/100 mg) by comparison with analytical ultracentrifugation. J Lipid Res. 1971;12:420–33.
55. Ip S, Lichtenstein AH, Chung M, Lau J, Balk EM. Systematic review: association of low-density lipoprotein subfractions with cardiovascular outcomes. Ann Intern Med. 2009;150:474–84.
56. Jeyarajah EJ, Cromwell WC, Otvos JD. Lipoprotein particle analysis by nuclear magnetic resonance spectroscopy. Clin Lab Med. 2006;26:847–70.
57. Kannel WB, Dawber TR, Friedman GD. Risk factors in coronary heart disease. An evaluation of several serum lipids as predictors of coronary heart disease. The Framingham Study. Ann Intern Med. 1964;61:888–99.
58. Kathiresan S, Otvos JS, Sullivan LM, Keyes MJ, Schaefer EJ, Wilson PWF, D'Agostino RB, Vasan RS, Robins SJ. Increased small low-density lipoprotein particle number: a prominent feature of the metabolic syndrome in the Framingham Heart study. Circulation. 2006;113:20–9.
59. Krauss RM. Heterogeneity of plasma low-density lipoproteins and atherosclerosis risk. Curr Opin Lipidol. 1994;5:339–49.
60. Krauss RM, Blanche PJ. Detection and quantitation of LDL subfractions. Curr Opin Lipidol. 1992;3:377–83.
61. Krauss RM, Burke DJ. Identification of multiple subclasses of plasma low density lipoproteins in normal humans. J Lipid Res. 1982;23:97–104.
62. Krauss RM, Lindgren FT, Ray RM. Interrelationships among subgroups of serum lipoproteins in normal human subjects. Clin Chim Acta. 1980;104:275–90.
63. Kulkarni KR. Cholesterol profile measurement by vertical auto profile method. Clin Lab Med. 2006;26:787–802.
64. Kulkarni KR, Markovitz JH, Nanda NC, Segrest JP. Increased prevalence of smaller and denser LDL particles in Asian Indians. Arterioscler Throm Vasc Biol. 1999;19:2749–55.
65. Kuller L, Arnold A, Tracy R, et al. Nuclear magnetic resonance spectroscopy of lipoproteins and risk of coronary heart disease in the cardiovascular health study. Arterioscler Thromb Vasc Biol. 2002;22: 1175–80.
66. Kuller LH, Grandits G, Jerome D, Cohen JD, Neaton JD, Prineas R. for the Multiple Risk Factor Intervention Trial Research Group. Lipoprotein particles, insulin, adiponectin, C-reactive protein and risk of coronary heart disease among men with metabolic syndrome. Atherosclerosis. 2007;195:122–8.
67. Laakso M, Lehto S, Penttilä I, Pyörälä K. Lipids and lipoproteins predicting coronary heart disease mortality and morbidity in patients with non-insulin dependent diabetes. Circulation. 1993;88:1421–30.
68. Lamarche B, Moorjani S, Cantin B, et al. Associations of HDL2 and HDL3 subfractions with ischemic heart disease in men. Prospective results from the Québec Cardiovascular Study. Arterioscler Thromb Vasc Biol. 1997;17:1098–105.
69. Lee W, Min WK, Chun S, Jang S, Kim JQ, Lee DH, Park JY, Park H, Son JE. Low-density lipoprotein subclass and its correlating factors in diabetics. Clin Biochem. 2003;36:657–61.
70. Lindgren FT, Jensen LC, Wills RD, Freeman NK. Flotation rates, molecular weights and hydrated densities of the low-density lipoproteins. Lipids. 1969;4: 337–44.
71. Lindgren FT, Silvers A, Jutaglr R, Layshot L, Bradley DD. A comparison of simplified methods for lipoprotein quantification using the analytic ultracentrifuge as a standard. Lipids. 1977;12:278–82.
72. Liu J, Sempos CT, Donahue RP, Dorn J, Trevisan M, Grundy SM. Non-high-density lipoprotein and very-low-density lipoprotein cholesterol and their risk predictive values in coronary heart disease. Am J Cardiol. 2006;98:1363–8.
73. Lorenz MW, Markus HS, Bots ML, Rosvall M, Sitzer M. Prediction of clinical cardiovascular events with carotid intima-media thickness: a systematic review and meta-analysis. Circulation. 2007;115: 459–67.
74. Lyons TJ, Jenkins AJ, Zheng D, Klein RL, Otvos JD, Yu Y, Lackland DT, McGee D, McHenry MB, Lopes-Virella M, Garvey WT, DCCT/EDIC Research Group. Nuclear magnetic resonance-determined lipoprotein subclass profile in the DCCT/EDIC cohort: associations with carotid intima-media thickness. Diabet Med. 2006;23:955–66.
75. Mackey RH, Kuller LH, Sutton-Tyrrell K, Evans RW, Holubkov R, Matthews KA. Lipoprotein subclasses and coronary artery calcium in postmenopausal women from the healthy women study. Am J Cardiol. 2002;90:71–6.
76. Maki KC, Dicklin MR, Davidson MH, Mize PD, Kulkarni KR. Indicators of the atherogenic lipoprotein phenotype measured with density gradient ultracentrifugation predict changes in carotid intima-media thickness in men and women. Vasc Hlth Risk Manag. 2012;8:31–8.
77. Marcovina SM, Albers JJ, Gabel B, Koschinsky ML, Gaur VP. Effect of the number of apolipoprotein(a)

kringle 4 domains on immunochemical measurements of lipoprotein(a). Clin Chem. 1995;41:246–55.
78. Marniemi J, Maki J, Maatela J, Jarvisalo J, Impivaara O. Poor applicability of the Friedewald formula in the assessment of serum LDL cholesterol for clinical purposes. Clin Biochem. 1995;28:285–9.
79. Marso SP, Mehta SK, Frutkin A, House JA, McCrary JR, Kulkani KR. Low adiponectin levels are associated with atherogenic dyslipidemia and lipid-rich plaque in nondiabetic coronary arteries. Diabetes Care. 2008;31:989–94.
80. Masoura C, Pitsavos C, Aznaouridis K, Skoumas I, Vlachopoulos C, Stefanadis C. Arterial endothelial function and wall thickness in familial hypercholesterolemia and familial combined hyperlipidemia and the effect of statins. A systematic review and meta-analysis. Atherosclerosis. 2011;214:129–38.
81. May HT, Anderson JL, Pearson RR, Jensen JR, Horne BD, Lavasani F, Yannicelli HD, Muhlestein JB. Comparison of effects of simvastatin alone versus fenofibrate b alone versus simvastatin plus fenofibrate on lipoprotein subparticle profiles in diabetic patients with mixed dyslipidemia (from the Diabetes and Combined Lipid Therapy Regimen study). Am J Cardiol. 2008;101:486–9.
82. Mazzone T, Meyer PM, Feinstein SB, Davidson MH, Kondos GT, D'Agostino Sr RB, Perez A, Provost JC, Haffner SM. Effect of pioglitazone compared with glimepiride on carotid intima-media thickness in type 2 diabetes: a randomized trial. JAMA. 2006;296:2572–81.
83. McKenney JM, Jones PH, Bays HE, et al. Comparative effects on lipid levels of combination therapy with a statin and extended-release niacin or ezetimibe versus a statin alone (the COMPELL study). Atherosclerosis. 2007;192:432–7.
84. McNamara JR, Campos H, Ordovas JM, Peterson J, Wilson PW, Schaefer EJ. Effect of gender, age, and lipid status on low density lipoprotein subfraction distribution. Results from the Framingham Offspring Study. Arterioscler Thromb Vasc Biol. 1987;7:483–90.
85. Miller M, Dobs A, Yuan Z, Battisti WP, Palmisano J. The effect of simvastatin on triglyceride-rich lipoproteins in patients with type 2 diabetic dyslipidemia: a SILHOUETTE trial sub-study. Curr Med Res Opin. 2006;22:343–50.
86. Mora S, Szklo M, Otvos JD, Greenland P, Psaty BM, Goff DC, O'Leary DH, Saad MF, Tsai MY, Sharrett AR. LDL particle subclasses, LDL particle size, and carotid atherosclerosis in the Multi-Ethnic Study of Atherosclerosis (MESA). Atherosclerosis. 2007;192:211–7.
87. Nakano K, Hasegawa G, Fukui M, Yamasaki M, Ishihara K, Tooru Takashima T, Kitagawa Y, Fujinami A, Ohta M, Hara H, Adachi T, Masakazu Ogata M, Hiroshi Obayashi H, Naoto NN. Effect of pioglitazone on various parameters of insulin resistance including lipoprotein subclass according to particle size by a gel-permeation high-performance liquid chromatography in newly diagnosed patients with type 2 diabetes. Endocrine J. 2010;57:423–30.
88. NCEP Expert Panel. Third report of the National Cholesterol Education Program (NCEP) expert panel on detection, evaluation, and treatment of high blood cholesterol in adults (Adult Treatment Panel III) final report. Circulation. 2002;106:3143–421.
89. Niemeijer-Kanters SD, Dallinga-Thie GM, de Ruijter-Heijstek FC, Algra A, Erkelens DW, Banga JD, Jansen H. Effect of intensive lipid-lowering strategy on low-density lipoprotein particle size in patients with type 2 diabetes mellitus. Atherosclerosis. 2001;156:209–16.
90. Nissen SE, Nicholls SJ, Wolski K, Nesto R, Kupfer S, Perez A, Jure H, De Larochelliere R, Staniloae CS, Mavromatis K, Saw J, Hu B, Lincoff AM, Tuzcu EM, PERISCOPE Investigators. Comparison of pioglitazone versus glimepiride on progression of coronary atherosclerosis in patients with type 2 diabetes: the PERISCOPE randomized controlled trial. JAMA. 2008;299:1561–73.
91. Nordestgaard BG, Chapman MJ, Ray K, et al. European Atherosclerosis Society Consensus Panel. Lipoprotein(a) as a cardiovascular risk factor: current status. Eur Heart J. 2010;31:2844–53.
92. Otvos JD, Jeyarajah EJ, Bennett DW. Quantification of plasma lipoproteins by proton nuclear magnetic resonance spectroscopy. Clin Chem. 1991;37:377–86.
93. Otvos JD, Jeyarajah EJ, Bennett DW, Krauss RM. Development of a proton nuclear magnetic resonance spectroscopic method for determining plasma lipoprotein concentrations and subspecies distributions from a single, rapid measurement. Clin Chem. 1992;38:1632–8.
94. Otvos JD, Jeyarajah EJ, Cromwell WC. Measurement issues related to lipoprotein heterogeneity. Am J Cardiol. 2002;90(Suppl):22i–9.
95. Otvos JD, Collins D, Freedman DS, et al. Low-density lipoprotein and high-density lipoprotein particle subclasses predict coronary events and are favorably changed by gemfibrozil therapy in the Veterans Affairs High-Density Lipoprotein Intervention Trial. Circulation. 2006;113:1556–63.
96. Otvos JD, Mora S, Shalaurova I, Greenland P, Mackey RH, Goff DC. Clinical implications of discordance between low density lipoprotein cholesterol and particle number. J Clin Lipidol. 2011;5:105–13.
97. Packard CJ. Triacylglycerol-rich lipoproteins and the generation of small, dense low-density lipoprotein. Biochem Soc Trans. 2003;31(Pt 5):1066–9.
98. Perez A, Khan M, Johnson T, Karunaratne M. Pioglitazone plus a sulphonylurea or metformin is associated with increased lipoprotein particle size in patients with type 2 diabetes. Diabetes Vasc Dis Res. 2004;1:44–50.
99. Pischon T, Girman CJ, Sacks FM, Rifai N, Stampfer MJ, Rimm EB. Non-high-density lipoprotein cholesterol and apolipoprotein B in the prediction of

coronary heart disease in men. Circulation. 2005; 112:3375–83.
100. Polak JF, Pencina MJ, Pencina KM, O'Donnell CJ, Wolf PA, D'Agostino RB. Carotid-wall intima–media thickness and cardiovascular events. N Engl J Med. 2011;365:213–21.
101. Pontrelli L, Parris W, Adeli K, Cheung RC. Atorvastatin treatment beneficially alters the lipoprotein profile and increases low-density lipoprotein particle diameter in patients with combined dyslipidemia and impaired fasting glucose/type 2 diabetes. Metabolism. 2002;51:334–432.
102. Reaven GM, Chen YI Y, Jeppesen J, Maheux P, Krauss RM. Insulin resistance and hyperinsulinemia in individuals with small, dense, low density lipoprotein particles. J Clin Invest. 1993;92:141–6.
103. Roeters van Lennep JE, Westerveld HT, Erkelens DW, van der Wall EE. Risk factors for coronary heart disease: implications of gender. Cardiovasc Res. 2002;53:538–49.
104. Rosenson RS, Otvos JD, Freedman DS. Relations of lipoprotein subclass levels and low-density lipoprotein size to progression of coronary artery disease in the Pravastatin Limitation of Atherosclerosis in the Coronary Arteries (PLAC-I) trial. Am J Cardiol. 2002;90:89–94.
105. Sacks FM, Campos H. Low-density lipoprotein size and cardiovascular disease: a reappraisal. J Clin Endocrinol Metab. 2003;88:4525–32.
106. Salonen JT, Salonen R, Seppänen K, Rauramaa R, Tuomilehto J. HDL, HDL2, and HDL3 subfractions, and the risk of acute myocardial infarction. A prospective population study in eastern Finnish men. Circulation. 1991;84:129–39.
107. Schaefer EJ, McNamara JR, Tayler T, Daly JA, Gleason JL, Seman LJ, Ferrari A, Rubenstein JJ. Comparisons of effects of statins (atorvastatin, fluvastatin, lovastatin, pravastatin, and simvastatin) on fasting and postprandial lipoproteins in patients with coronary heart disease versus control subjects. Am J Cardiol. 2004;93:31–9.
108. Selby JV, Austin MA, Newman B, Zhang D, Quesenberry CP, Mayer EJ, Krauss RM. LDL subclass phenotypes and the insulin resistance syndrome in women. Circulation. 1993;88:381–7.
109. Seman LJ, DeLuca C, Jenner JL, et al. Lipoprotein(a)-cholesterol and coronary heart disease in the Framingham Heart study. Clin Chem. 1999;45:1039–46.
110. Senti M, Pedro-Botet J, Rubies-Prat J, Vidal-Barraquer F. Secondary prevention of coronary heart disease in patients with extracoronary atherosclerosis: a need for accuracy of low density lipoprotein determination. Angiology. 1996;47:241–6.
111. Sharrett AR, Ballantyne CM, Coady SA, et al. Coronary heart disease prediction from lipoprotein cholesterol levels, triglycerides, lipoprotein(a), apolipoproteins A–I and B, and HDL density subfractions: the Atherosclerosis Risk in Communities (ARIC) Study. Circulation. 2001;104:1108–13.
112. Shen MMS, Krauss RM, Lindgren FT, Forte TM. Heterogeneity of serum low density lipoproteins in normal human subjects. J Lipid Res. 1981;22:236–44.
113. Shimabukuro M, Higa M, Tanaka H, Shimabukuro T, Yamakawa K, Masuzaki H. Distinct effects of pitavastatin and atorvastatin on lipoprotein subclasses in patients with type 2 diabetes mellitus. Diabet Med. 2011;28:856–64.
114. Sniderman AD, Furberg CD, Keech A, et al. Apolipoproteins versus lipids as indices of coronary risk and as targets for statin treatment. Lancet. 2003;361:777–80.
115. Sniderman AJ, Williams K, Contois JH, Monroe HM, McQueen MJ, de Graaf J, Furberg CD. A meta-analysis of low-density lipoprotein cholesterol, non-high-density lipoprotein cholesterol, and apolipoprotein B as markers of cardiovascular risk. Circ Cardiovasc Qual Outcomes. 2011;4:337–45.
116. Soedamah-Muthu SS, Colhoun HM, Thomason MJ, Betteridge DJ, Durrington PN, Hitman GA, Fuller JH, Julier K, Mackness MI, Neil HA, CARDS Investigators. The effect of atorvastatin on serum lipids, lipoproteins and NMR spectroscopy defined lipoprotein subclasses in type 2 diabetic patients with ischaemic heart disease. Atherosclerosis. 2003;167:243–55.
117. Soedamah-Muthu SS, Chang Y-F, Otvos J, Evans RW, Orchard TJ. Lipoprotein subclass measurements by nuclear magnetic resonance spectroscopy improve the prediction of coronary artery disease in Type 1 diabetes. A prospective report from the Pittsburgh Epidemiology of Diabetes Complications Study. Diabetologia. 2003;46:674–82.
118. Stampfer MJ, Sacks FM, Salvini S, Willett WC, Hennekens CH. A prospective study of cholesterol, apolipoproteins, and the risk of myocardial infarction. N Engl J Med. 1991;325:373–81.
119. Stein JH, Johnson HM. Carotid intima-media thickness, plaques, and cardiovascular disease risk implications for preventive cardiology guidelines. J Amer Coll Cardiol. 2010;55:1608–10.
120. Stein JH, Korcarz CE, Hurst RT, Lonn E, Kendall CB, Mohler ER, Najjar SS, Rembold CM, Post WS, American Society of Echocardiography Carotid Intima-Media Thickness Task Force. Use of carotid ultrasound to identify subclinical vascular disease and evaluate cardiovascular disease risk: a consensus statement from the American Society of Echocardiography Carotid Intima-Media Thickness Task Force. Endorsed by the Society for Vascular Medicine. J Am Soc Echocardiogr. 2008;21:93–111.
121. St-Pierre AC, Ruel IL, Cantin B. Comparison of various electrophoretic characteristics of LDL particles and their relationship to the risk of ischemic heart disease. Circulation. 2001;104:2295–9.
122. St-Pierre AC, Cantin B, Dagenais GR, et al. Low-density lipoprotein subfractions and the long-term risk of ischemic heart disease in men: 13-year follow-up data from the Québec Cardiovascular Study. Arterioscler Thromb Vasc Biol. 2005;25:553–9.

123. Superko HR. Advanced lipoprotein testing and subfractionation are clinically useful. Circulation. 2009;119:2383–95.
124. Sweetnam PM, Bolton CH, Yarnell JW, et al. Associations of the HDL2 and HDL3 cholesterol subfractions with the development of ischemic heart disease in British men. The Caerphilly and Speedwell Collaborative Heart Disease Studies. Circulation. 1994;90:769–74.
125. Tan KCB, Shiu SWM, Chu BYM. Roles of hepatic lipase and cholesterol ester transfer protein in determining low density lipoprotein subfraction distribution in Chinese patients with noninsulin-dependent diabetes mellitus. Atherosclerosis. 1999;145:273–8.
126. Tan HC, Tai ES, Sviridov D, Nestel PJ, Ng C, Chan E, Teo Y, Wai DC. Relationships between cholesterol efflux and high-density lipoprotein particles in patients with type 2 diabetes mellitus. J Clin Lipidol. 2011;5:467–73.
127. Tomassini JE, Mazzone T, Goldberg RB, Guyton JR, Weinstock RS, Polis A, Jensen E, Tershakovec AM. Effect of ezetimibe/simvastatin compared with atorvastatin on lipoprotein subclasses in patients with type 2 diabetes and hypercholesterolaemia. Diabetes Obes Metab. 2009;11:855–64.
128. van Tol A, van der Gaag MS, Scheek LM, van Gent T, Hendriks HF. Changes in postprandial lipoproteins of low and high density caused by moderate alcohol consumption with dinner. Atherosclerosis. 1998;141 Suppl 1:S101–3.
129. Williams PT. Fifty-three year follow-up of coronary heart disease versus HDL2 and other lipoproteins in Gofman's Livermore Cohort. J Lipid Res. 2012;53: 266–72.
130. Williams PT, Feldman DE. Prospective study of coronary heart disease vs. HDL2, HDL3, and other lipoproteins in Gofman's Livermore Cohort. Atherosclerosis. 2011;214:196–202.
131. Zhu S, Su G, Meng QH. Inhibitory effects of micronized fenofibrate on carotid atherosclerosis in patients with essential hypertension. Clin Chem. 2006;52: 2036–42.

# Insulin Resistance and Atherosclerosis

# 3

Kamalpreet Singh and Vasudevan A. Raghavan

## Introduction

Easy and affordable availability of calorie-dense food substrates and increasing adoption of a sedentary lifestyle sans regular exercise have resulted in an increase in the incidence and prevalence of obesity worldwide. A major consequence is the increase in the number of those with diabetes mellitus (DM), which is projected to reach about 300 million people worldwide by 2020 [1]. Following the discovery of insulin by Banting, McLeod, and Best in 1922, it was widely thought that human diabetes mellitus was largely due to a deficiency in the secretion of the hormone. However, in 1936 Sir Harold Percival Himsworth [2] noted variations in the responses of diabetic patients to insulin and proposed the notion that insulin insensitivity, not insulin deficiency, was the defining biochemical defect in many diabetics. In the spring of 1939, he also delivered the Goulstonian Lectures at the Royal College of Physicians of London, highlighting this new paradigm. These lectures were eventually published in 1939 [3–6]. The discovery of the immunoassay method for quantification of human insulin by Yalow and Berson in 1960 [7] soon led to the realization that in many individuals with diabetes, insulin resistance was often characterized by "compensatory" hyperinsulinemia. This has implications as discussed in subsequent sections.

DM is a group of metabolic diseases characterized by hyperglycemia resulting from defects in insulin secretion, insulin action, or both. The vast majority of DM cases belong to two etiopathogenetic categories commonly referred to as type 1 diabetes mellitus (T1DM) and type 2 diabetes mellitus (T2DM). In T1DM, the cause is an absolute deficiency of insulin secretion, and "at-risk" individuals can often be identified by serological testing of autoimmune markers of pancreatic islet cell damage and also by genetic markers. In T2DM, by far the more prevalent variety, the cause is a combination of resistance to insulin action and an inadequate compensatory insulin secretory response. In the latter category, a clinically asymptomatic period where the patient experiences a degree of hyperglycemia sufficient to cause pathologic and functional changes in various target tissues may be present for a long period of time before DM is detected. During this asymptomatic period, it is possible to demonstrate an abnormality in carbohydrate metabolism by measurement of plasma fasting glucose or after a challenge with an oral glucose load [8].

K. Singh
Texas A&M Health Sciences Center and College of Medicine, Temple, TX, USA

V.A. Raghavan, MBBS, MD, MRCP(UK) (✉)
Cardiometabolic, Lipid Clinic & Medical Weight Management Services, Division of Endocrinology, Scott and White Center of Diagnostic Medicine, 1605 S 31st Street, Temple, TX 76508, USA

Texas A&M Health Sciences Center and College of Medicine, Temple, TX, USA
e-mail: abu_vasudevan@hotmail.com

A.J. Jenkins et al. (eds.), *Lipoproteins in Diabetes Mellitus*, Contemporary Diabetes,
DOI 10.1007/978-1-4614-7554-5_3, © Springer Science+Business Media New York 2014

## Insulin Resistance Pathways

Insulin resistance (IR) represents an altered and suboptimal biological response to normal insulin concentrations. While the definition encompasses several biological actions of insulin in the body, it typically refers to a state in which a given concentration of insulin is associated with a subnormal glucose response [9]. Through its highly integrated actions on carbohydrate, protein, and lipid metabolism, insulin exerts a significant effect on the regulation of glucose homeostasis, most apparent in its effects in three tissues: liver, muscle, and adipose tissue. Insulin's actions are initiated by interaction with a specific transmembrane protein receptor, encoded by a single gene composed of 22 exons located on chromosome 19 [10]. Detailed insulin effects, insulin receptor interaction, and mechanisms of IR are beyond the scope of this review and are discussed elsewhere in detail [9], but it appears that two major post-receptor signaling pathways convey the insulin signal downstream [11, 12]. One pathway involving the phosphorylation of insulin receptor substrate (IRS)-1 and (IRS)-2 and activation of phosphatidyl inositol 3-kinase (hereafter referred to as PI3K pathway) appears to be necessary for mediating metabolic effects of insulin [13, 14]. The second signaling pathway appears to involve the phosphorylation of Shc and activation of Ras, Raf, MEK, and mitogen-activated protein (MAP) kinases (Erk 1 and 2) (hereafter referred to as MAPK pathway). In contrast to the PI3K pathway, activation of the MAPK pathway contributes solely to the nuclear and mitogenic effects of insulin and plays no role in mediating the metabolic actions of insulin [15, 16].

Subsequent reports by Jiang and Cusi et al. [17, 18] have established the concept of "selective insulin resistance." Jiang et al. [17] compared insulin signaling via the PI3K and MAPK pathways in vascular tissue of lean and obese Zucker rats using both in vivo and ex vivo studies. They demonstrated a significant decrease in the ability of insulin to stimulate the phosphorylation of IRS-1, the association of the p85 regulatory subunit of PI3K with IRS-1, the activity of PI3K, and the phosphorylation of Akt (a downstream serine kinase of the PI3K pathway) in the vasculature of obese insulin-resistant rats. In contrast, the stimulatory effect of insulin on MAPK remained intact in these animals. Cusi et al. [18] studied the two pathways of insulin signaling in human muscle biopsy samples obtained from patients with T2DM, obese nondiabetic individuals, and lean control subjects before and after euglycemic-hyperinsulinemic clamp. Insulin stimulation of the PI3K pathway was dramatically reduced in obese nondiabetic individuals and virtually absent in T2DM patients. In contrast, insulin stimulation of the MAPK pathway was normal in obese and diabetic subjects. Subsequent studies [19, 20] have similarly established that insulin resistance has differential effects on these two pathways. As IR often is associated, especially earlier in the natural course of DM, with hyperinsulinemia, it follows that the mitogenic pathway effects of insulin are amplified in T2DM and indeed prediabetes/other insulin-resistant states (see Fig. 3.1).

## Atherosclerosis

Ross and Glomset [21] proposed more than three decades ago a proliferative model for atherosclerosis, where endothelial denuding injury led to platelet aggregation, release of platelet-derived growth factor, and proliferation of smooth muscle cells in the arterial intima, thereby forming the nidus of the atherosclerotic plaque and updating the centuries' old Virchow's concept of "response to injury" model (initially proposed in 1856) which envisaged atherosclerosis merely as a passive deposition of lipid debris in arterial walls. This simplistic concept has since evolved largely due to the advances in cell biology techniques, and current thinking is that atherosclerosis is indeed a complex process invoking endothelial dysfunction, vascular smooth muscle dysfunction, immune dysfunction, and inflammation [22, 23].

Atherosclerosis is an inflammatory process that selectively affects arteries and is highly prevalent in both genders. Thrombo-occlusive complications of atherosclerosis including stroke and

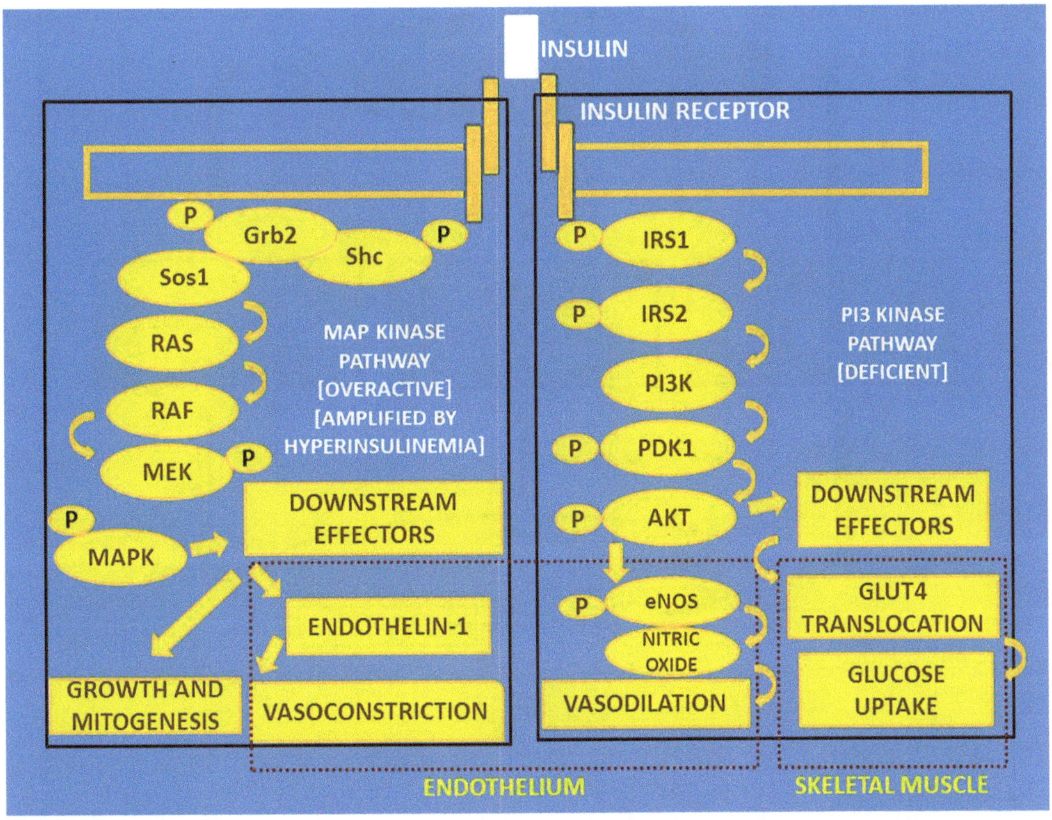


**Fig. 3.1** Insulin resistance (IR) is selective to the PI3K (predominantly metabolic) effects of insulin. Hyperinsulinemia, a common concomitant of IR, results in exaggerated MAPK (predominantly nuclear and mitogenic) effects of insulin

myocardial infarction are major causes of morbidity and mortality. Thrombo-occlusive complications of atherosclerosis including stroke and myocardial infarction are major causes of morbidity and mortality. Atherosclerosis is perhaps initiated by endothelial dysfunction and in the presence of structural alterations such as the absence of a confluent luminal elastin layer and the exposure of proteoglycans [2], in which apolipoprotein-B (apoB) enriched particles such as low-density lipoprotein (LDL) accumulate in the subendothelial space. Elevated levels of circulating LDL cholesterol (LDL-c) facilitate atherosclerosis and cardiovascular disease (CVD) [24]. ApoB100 binding to negatively charged extracellular matrix proteoglycans leads to intimal retention of LDL particles, where they are vulnerable to oxidative modification by reactive oxygen species and enzymes such as myeloperoxidase or lipoxygenases released from inflammatory cells. Oxidized LDL (oxLDL) promotes expression of adhesion molecules and the secretion of chemokines by endothelial cells, which in conjunction with platelet-derived chemokines drive immune cell infiltration into the intima. Early lesions ("fatty streaks") consist of T cells and monocyte-derived macrophage-like foam cells loaded with lipids. Accrual of dying cells and other cellular debris along with cholesterol crystals forms a necrotic core. Fibroatheromatous plaques are covered by a fibrous cap composed of collagen and smooth muscle cells (SMCs), which are replaced by macrophages in the thinning inflamed caps that are prone to rupture. The "shoulder" regions are heavily infiltrated by T cells and mast cells, which produce enzymes and proinflammatory mediators, contributing to adventitial inflammation of advanced plaques [25]. The pathogenesis of atherosclerosis is discussed in greater detail elsewhere [26].

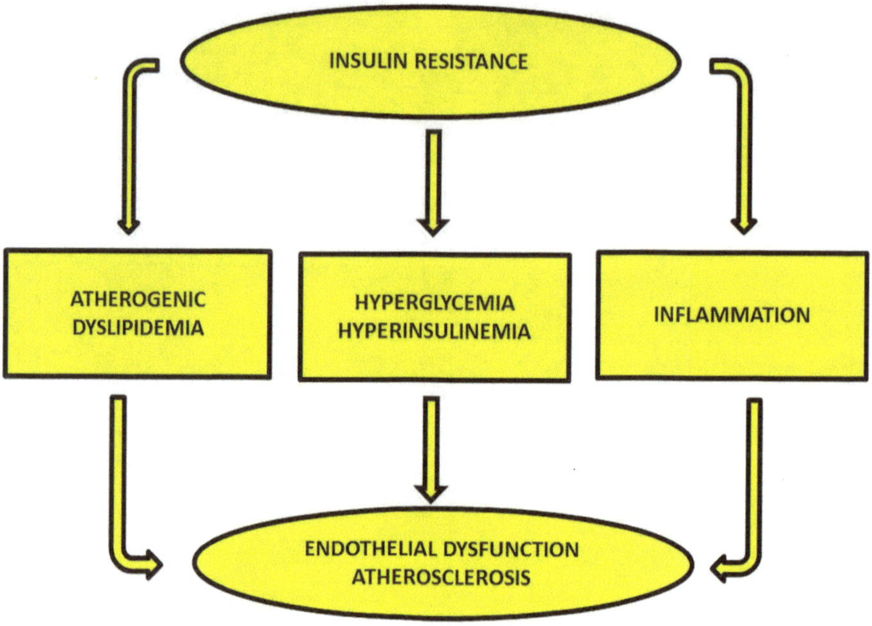


**Fig. 3.2** Insulin resistance-related processes are associated with endothelial dysfunction and promotion of atherosclerosis

IR is associated with processes that facilitate atherosclerosis (see Fig. 3.2). The pathophysiological processes involved in the initiation and progression of early atherosclerotic lesions are somewhat different from those associated with the formation of clinically dangerous plaques [27, 28], and distinguishing the effects of IR and hyperglycemia on these processes is important. As alluded to earlier, early-to-mid-stage atherogenesis involves the subendothelial retention of apoB-containing lipoproteins, activation of endothelial cells, recruitment of monocytes and other inflammatory cells, cholesterol loading of lesional cells, and migration of smooth muscle cells to the intima. In contrast, advanced plaque progression is influenced primarily by processes that promote plaque necrosis and thinning of a collagenous "scar" overlying the lesion, called the fibrous cap. The objective of this chapter is to describe how IR and hyperglycemia promote atherogenesis and plaque progression. It should be noted that IR and hyperglycemia are likely to have additive or synergistic pro-atherogenic effects in the setting of T2DM. For example, glucotoxicity may contribute to IR, and treatment of hyperglycemia in T2DM has been shown to improve IR in some tissues [29].

## Role of Atherogenic Dyslipidemia

Altered metabolism of triglyceride-rich lipoproteins (TGRLP) is an important part of the metabolic environment in insulin-resistant states. Figure 3.3 illustrates the lipid pathways that operate in IR states. Insulin promotes synthesis of nonesterified fatty acids (NEFA) or free fatty acid (FFA) and its assimilation into triacylglycerols. In obesity and other IR states, excessive adipose tissue breakdown leads to increased hepatic delivery of FFA. This leads to increased hepatic synthesis and secretion of triglyceride-laden very low-density lipoprotein (VLDL). Impaired clearance of VLDL and chylomicrons (intestinally derived) leads to prolonged plasma retention of these particles. These partially lipolyzed remnants, which include cholesterol-enriched intermediate-density lipoproteins (IDLs), are

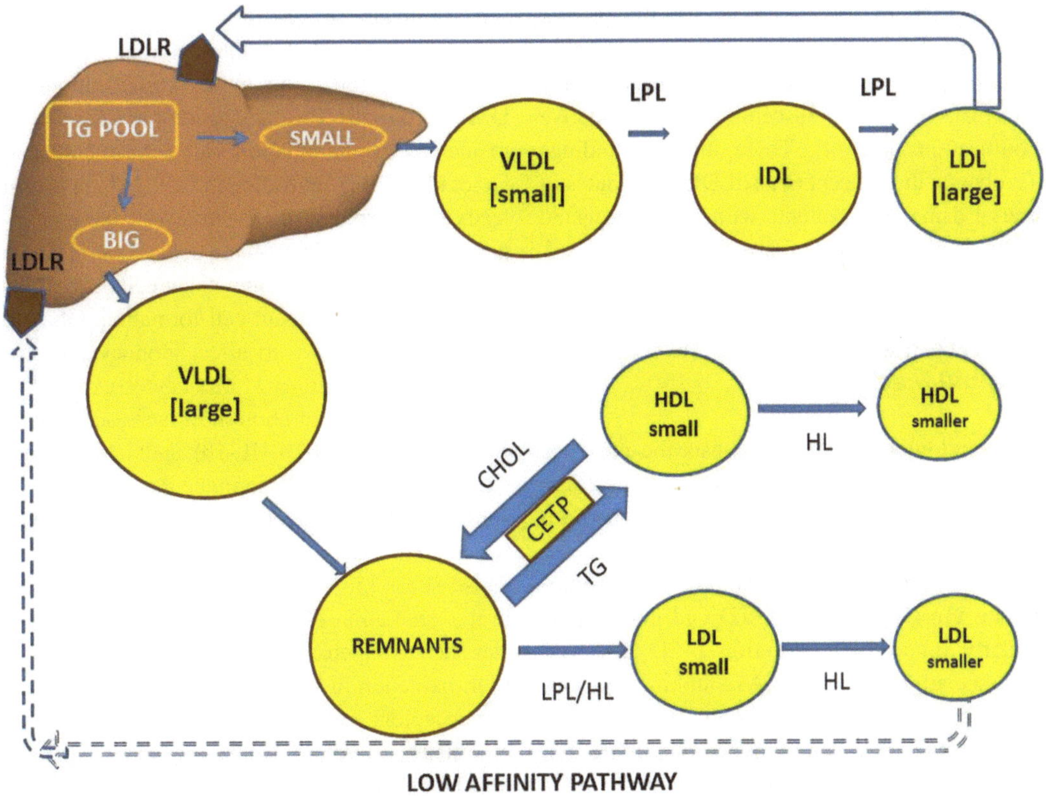


**Fig. 3.3** Insulin resistance: lipid pathways leading to atherogenic dyslipidemia

very atherogenic in humans and in a number of animal models [30, 31]. Increased hepatic production and/or slow plasma clearance of VLDL leads to increased production of precursors of small dense LDL (sdLDL) particles. As many as seven distinct LDL subspecies which differ in their metabolic behavior and pathological roles have been identified [32]. Plasma VLDL levels correlate with increased density and decreased size of LDL [33, 34]. In addition, LDL size and density are inversely related to plasma levels of high-density lipoprotein (HDL), especially the $HDL_2$ subclass [35]. sdLDL particles arise from the intravascular processing of specific larger VLDL precursors in multiple steps, including lipolysis [32]. TG enrichment of the lipolytic products occurs mainly through the action of cholesteryl ester transfer protein (CETP) and, together with hydrolysis of triglyceride and phospholipids by hepatic lipase, leads to increased production of sdLDL particles [30, 31]. Another reason for prolonged plasma retention time for these particles is the reduced affinity of the hepatic LDL receptors for these particles [32].

HDL particles are heterogeneous, and multiple subclasses differing in diameter and density have been identified, ranging from the small dense $HDL_{3c}$, $HDL_{3b}$, and $HDL_{3a}$ to the larger $HDL_{2a}$ and $HDL_{2b}$ [36]. The reasons for the reduction in plasma HDL concentration in IR states are multifactorial, but a major factor appears to be the increased transfer of cholesterol from HDL to TGRLP, with reciprocal transfer of triglyceride to HDL. Triglyceride-laden HDL particles are hydrolyzed by hepatic lipase and subsequently rapidly catabolized and cleared from plasma [37]. Typically, the reduced HDL levels in plasma of patients with T2DM are manifest as reductions in the $HDL_{2b}$ subspecies and relative or absolute increases in smaller denser $HDL_{3b}$ and $HDL_{3c}$.

Increased atherogenicity of sdLDL appears to be related to a number of properties, including reduced LDL receptor affinity [38, 39], greater propensity for transport into the subendothelial space [40], increased binding to arterial wall proteoglycans [41], and susceptibility to oxidative modifications [42–44]. These in vitro findings corroborate the concept that sdLDL contributes to arterial damage in patients with the atherogenic dyslipidemia seen in insulin-resistant states.

## Dysglycemia and Atherosclerosis: Possible Mechanisms

Epidemiological research suggests the presence of an association between glycemic control and CVD risk [45]. Data from the United Kingdom Prospective Diabetes Study (UKPDS) suggested more or less a linear relationship between hemoglobin A1c (HbA1c) and CVD end points, particularly myocardial infarction [46]. However, the association between HbA1c and microvascular complications is stronger than it is for macrovascular outcomes such as myocardial infarction, stroke, or cardiovascular death, raising the question if glucose plays a greater role in the pathogenesis of microvascular than macrovascular outcomes in DM. Similar relationships between hyperglycemia and CVD outcomes have been demonstrated in T1DM, but the association seems less pronounced [47].

It has been suggested that glucose might act directly or indirectly via the generation of advanced glycation end products (AGEs) or reactive oxygen species. AGEs are a class of chemical by-products that result from the combination of protein and sugar (usually glucose) and are increasingly recognized as a mediator of hyperglycemia-induced cytopathology. Hyperglycemia inside the cell increases diacylglycerol (DAG) levels, a critical activating cofactor for the classic isoforms of protein kinase C, kinase-β, kinase-δ, and kinase-α [48–51]. Protein kinase C (PKC) activation leads to a variety of gene effects. The vasodilator nitric oxide (NO) levels are low because nitric oxide synthase (eNOS) expression is reduced, while the vasoconstrictor endothelin-1 expression is increased. Levels of transforming growth factor-β (TGF-β) and plasminogen activator inhibitor-1 (PAI-1) are also increased [51–55]. Several studies have demonstrated that inhibition of PKC prevented early renal and retinal complications of DM [52, 55, 56]. PKC activation has been linked to increased inflammation via increased nuclear factor κB (NFκB) activation [57, 58], which in turn leads to the expression of several proinflammatory genes, including adhesion molecules that facilitate monocyte adhesion to endothelial cells [57]. This eventually leads to foam cell formation. Glucose has also been shown to affect monocyte/macrophage activation in vitro. Monocytes exposed to high glucose concentration show increased expression of interleukin-1β (IL-1β) and interleukin-6 (IL-6) [59]. This results in induction of PKC, activation of NFκB, and robust release of superoxide, which could play a role in glucose-mediated oxidative stress [59]. Glucose auto-oxidation results in the generation of several reactive oxygen species such as superoxide anion, which can facilitate LDL oxidation in vitro [60]. Cell-surface scavenger receptors on arterial macrophages take up modified lipoproteins including oxidized LDL (oxLDL) that have become oxidized as a result of glucose-mediated oxidative stress [60, 61] or modified by AGEs [61]. Moreover, AGE-modified albumin can inhibit scavenger receptor B1 (SR-B1)-mediated efflux of cholesterol to HDL [62]. AGE proteins in the circulation may also interfere with the functions of SR-B1 in reverse cholesterol transport by inhibiting the selective uptake of HDL-cholesteryl ester, as well as cholesterol efflux from peripheral cells to HDL. Thus, hyperglycemia affects alterations in the delivery and removal of lipid from macrophages by lipoproteins and other proteins.

## Endothelial Dysfunction in Insulin-Resistant States

Studies in human obesity and IR have revealed a clear association between the chronic activation of proinflammatory signaling pathways and decreased insulin sensitivity. For example, elevated levels of tumor necrosis factor-α (TNF-α), interleukin-6 (IL-6), and interleukin-8 (IL-8) have all been reported in various diabetic and insulin-resistant states [63–67]. The inflammatory marker C-reactive protein (CRP), a nonspecific acute-phase reactant synthesized predominantly in the liver, is commonly elevated in states characterized by IR [68]. Also, experiments in naturally occurring rodent models of obesity, knockout, and transgenic mice as well as detailed studies of insulin signaling at the molecular level have begun to elucidate the mechanistic links between obesity-induced inflammation and insulin-resistant states.

The precise pathways by which accrual of excess adipose tissue initiates systemic inflammation are unclear. One theory holds that adipose tissue expansion leads to adipocyte hypertrophy and hyperplasia, eventually outstripping the local oxygen supply leading to hypoxia and activation of cellular stress pathways [69]. This causes cell-autonomous inflammation and the release of cytokines and other proinflammatory signals. Adipokines such as resistin, leptin, and adiponectin perhaps also affect inflammation and insulin sensitivity. Locally secreted chemokines attract proinflammatory macrophages into the adipose tissue where they form crown-like structures around large dead or dying adipocytes. These tissue macrophages then release cytokines that further perpetuate inflammation involving neighboring adipocytes, thereby exacerbating inflammation and IR. Hepatic inflammation from steatosis occurs in obesity, whereby hepatocyte stress pathway responses may be triggered resulting in hepatocyte-autonomous inflammation. Activation of Kupffer cells (macrophage-like cells in the liver) releases locally acting cytokines and exacerbates inflammation and promotes hepatic insulin resistance. In addition, overnutrition is often accompanied by elevations in tissue and circulating FFA concentrations, and saturated FFAs can directly activate proinflammatory responses in vascular endothelial cells, adipocytes, and myeloid-derived cells [70]. A state of systemic inflammation then occurs.

TNF-α, a proinflammatory cytokine secreted predominantly by monocytes and macrophages, has varied biological effects on lipid metabolism, coagulation, and endothelial function. Activation of the TNF receptor results in the stimulation of NFκB signaling via inhibitor of nuclear factor kappa-B kinase subunit beta (IKKb). A landmark study by Hotamisligil [71] showed that adipose tissue isolated from different obese rodent models overexpressed TNF-α. His group also showed that neutralization of TNF-α in obese fa/fa rats ameliorated IR [71]. Similar correlations between TNF-α levels, obesity, and IR were soon demonstrated in humans [67]. Corresponding in vitro experiments demonstrated that by activating IKKb, TNF-α stimulation leads to serine phosphorylation of IRS, attenuating its ability to transduce insulin-mediated cellular events [72]. Mice genetically deficient in TNF-α or the TNF-α receptor 1 gene (TNFR1) do not develop IR caused by high-fat feeding or obesity [73].

TNF-α also affects insulin signaling independent of IRS1. TNF-α-treated cultured 3T3-L1 adipocytes show reduced expression of the insulin receptor, IRS1, and Glut4 genes, as well as a decrease in insulin-stimulated glucose uptake [74]. Ruan et al. also showed that TNF-α induced a decrease in many 3T3-L1 adipocyte genes, including GLUT4, hormone-sensitive lipase (HSL), long-chain fatty acyl CoA synthetase, adiponectin, the transcription factor CCAAT-/enhancer-binding protein-alpha (C/EBP), and the nuclear receptors peroxisome proliferator-activated receptor gamma (PPARɣ) and retinoic acid x receptor (RXR). As many of these genes have direct and indirect effects on glucose homeostasis, changes in adipocyte expression of these genes will likely contribute to IR [75].

c-Jun N-terminal kinase 1 (JNK1) (encoded by MAPK8) also contributes to the development of IR in obese and diabetic states. Hirosumi et al. [76] found elevated JNK activity in liver, adipose tissue, and skeletal muscle of obese insulin-resistant mice, and knockout of JNK1 ($JNK1^{-/-}$) resulted in the amelioration of IR in high-fat-diet-fed (HFDF) mice. At the cellular level, these workers also showed that JNK1 knockout led to decreased IRS1 phospho-Ser307 in the liver. Importantly, deletion of JNK1 also caused resistance to the development of obesity, so the improved insulin sensitivity in these animals could be a result of decreased adiposity and/or decreased JNK1 activity in insulin target cells. The role of JNK2 has also been assessed in studies and seems to play a significant role in the development of obesity-induced IR. Recent data suggest that JNK2 can be involved in metabolic regulation when JNK1 is absent, since $JNK1^{+/-}JNK2^{-/-}$ mice phenocopy $JNK1^{-/-}$ mice in their reduced adiposity and improved insulin sensitivity [77]. It appears that functional in vivo interactions between these isoforms may contribute to the regulation of insulin action.

Salicylate and its derivative acetyl salicylic acid (or aspirin) have been in use to treat symptoms of T2DM for a very long time. At higher doses, they are effective in reducing blood sugar levels, but adverse effects such as gastrointestinal bleeding and tinnitus have precluded their widespread use in this context [78]. These agents are weak inhibitors of IKKb, thus preventing IRS1 serine307 phosphorylation with some insulin-sensitizing effects [79]. Kim et al. [80] showed that lipid infusion causes acute IR in rodents and pretreatment of lipid-infused rats with salicylates improves glucose utilization in skeletal muscle, as measured during hyperinsulinemic-euglycemic clamp studies. They also performed lipid infusions in IKKb heterozygous knockout mice ($IKKb^{+/-}$) and reported similar improvements in insulin sensitivity when compared to wild-type controls [80]. Yuan et al. showed that TNF-α treatment of 3T3-L1 adipocytes induces IR, an effect that could be prevented by pretreatment of cells with aspirin. A parallel experiment was performed in adipocytes using okadaic acid to activate IKKb independent of TNF-α stimulation, and again, aspirin prevented okadaic acid-induced IR. In vivo studies of aspirin-treated obese rats and mice have shown that salicylate pretreatment protects them from IR [81]. Mice with a liver-specific constitutively active IKKb transgene (LIKK) developed hyperglycemia and decreased hepatic insulin sensitivity with mild secondary systemic IR in skeletal muscle. There was liver expression of the proinflammatory markers IL-6, IL-1β, and TNF-α similar to that found in the liver of obese mice. In rescue experiments, LIKK mice treated with sodium salicylate or IL-6-neutralizing antibodies had markedly improved insulin sensitivity. In addition, mice expressing the liver-specific IκBα super-repressor transgene (LISR), which prevents the activation of IKKb, protected both LIKK and obese mice from hepatic IR. Another important finding in this study was the elevated expression of the macrophage-specific markers, Emr1 (also known as F4/80) and Cd68, in the livers of LIKK and obese mice. Co-expression of LISR and LIKK in compound transgenic mice reduced both IR and the expression of these same macrophage markers. These data indicate that hepatic inflammation caused by a high-fat diet is mediated by both hepatocytes and Kupffer cells (liver macrophages) [82]. These studies highlight the role of IKKb in the development of obesity and inflammation-induced IR.

As alluded to before, nitric oxide (NO) is an endogenous signaling molecule produced by nitric oxide synthase and acts as a signal transduction molecule for a number of physiological processes such as vasodilation. It is also involved in many pathophysiologic states such as IR. Several IR inducers such as FFAs, proinflammatory cytokines, and oxidative stress activate the expression of Nos*2*, the gene that encodes iNOS [83]. NO reduces Akt activity by causing s-nitrosylation of a specific cysteine residue [84]. Increased iNOS activity also results in the degradation of IRS1 in cultured skeletal muscle cells [83]. *Nos2* knockout mice are protected from obesity-induced skeletal muscle IR, and this is associated with improved PI3K-Akt activity [85]. It appears that *Nos2* is also required for the development of sepsis-induced skeletal muscle IR, perhaps also mediated by the s-nitrosylation of the insulin receptor IRS1 and Akt [86, 87]. These studies suggest that increased iNOS activity may play a direct role in the pathogenesis of IR.

Macrophages and lymphocytes elaborate interleukin-10 (IL-10) which exerts anti-inflammatory activity by inhibiting TNF-α-induced NFκB expression, via reduction in IKK activity and inhibition of NFκB DNA-binding activity [88]. It has been shown in human subjects that IR is more prevalent in subjects with reduced serum levels of IL-10 [89]. Consistent with the concept that IL-10 may have insulin-sensitizing effects is the laboratory evidence that mice treated with IL-10 did not become insulin resistant when treated with either IL-6 or lipid infusions [89]. Lumeng et al. showed that IL-10-treated 3T3-L1 adipocytes are protected from TNF-α-induced cellular IR [90]. Recombinant IL-10 therapy of conditions such as psoriasis has raised hopes that immunomodulation of IL-10 activity can be a potential treatment of IR [91].

## Atherosclerosis in Insulin-Resistant States: Role of Macrophage

A key discovery in the arena of obesity-induced inflammation and IR was the finding that bone marrow-derived macrophages are present in adipose tissue of obese mice and humans [92, 93]. Weisberg et al. compared adipose tissue RNA profiles for various mouse models of obesity and found that a subset of genes, while not typically expressed in adipocytes, were confirmed through immunohistochemistry to be adipose tissue-resident macrophage-derived. The percentage of macrophages in a given adipose tissue depot positively correlated with adiposity and adipocyte size. They also found that adipose tissue macrophages were responsible for nearly all adipose tissue TNF-α expression and a significant portion of Nos2 and IL-6 expression. They quantified the infiltration of macrophages in subcutaneous adipose tissue from obese human subjects and reported that as high as 50 % of the total cell content consists of macrophages compared to 10 % in lean controls [92]. Xu et al. [93] reported similar findings and showed that thiazolidinedione (TZD) treatment could repress the expression of macrophage-specific genes, providing an additional mechanism by which TZD treatment improves insulin sensitivity.

A study by Arkan et al. [94] showed that inhibition of the macrophage inflammatory pathway protects mice from obesity-induced insulin resistance. In this study, the investigators generated both a myeloid-specific deletion of IKKb (IKKb$^{\Delta mye}$) and liver-specific deletion of IKKb (IKKb$^{\Delta hep}$). They found that IKKb$^{\Delta hep}$ mice are protected from high-fat-diet-induced hepatic IR but that this was a tissue-autonomous effect, since these mice still developed IR in the muscle and fat. There was a significant reduction in the expression of inflammatory markers in the liver suggesting that inactivation of inflammation can prevent HFD-induced insulin resistance. Also, tissue-specific deletion of IKKb in myeloid cells (IKKb$^{\Delta mye}$ mice) led to improvement in insulin sensitivity with globally improved insulin action in the muscle, liver, and fat. As such, these results showed that inactivation of myeloid-IKKb activity prevented systemic IR, most likely by blocking local paracrine interaction between resident macrophages and insulin target tissues.

Monocyte chemoattractant protein-1 (MCP-1), also known as chemokine ligand 2 (Ccl2), and its cognate receptor chemokine receptor 2 (Ccr2) are also major components of IR in obese mice. MCP-1 is a chemokine secreted primarily by macrophages and endothelial cells that promotes the recruitment of monocytes to inflamed tissues. Ccr2 is expressed in monocytes but also in the lung, spleen, and thymus [95]. Weisberg et al. found that obesity-matched *Ccr2*$^{-/-}$ mice displayed reduced adipose tissue macrophage infiltration, reduced hepatic steatosis, decreased inflammatory profiles, and improved systemic insulin sensitivity. *Ccr2* deficiency also attenuated high-fat-diet-induced weight gain by causing a reduction in caloric intake, highlighting the possible involvement of Ccr2 in the control of eating behavior. Also, treatment of obese mice with a pharmacological antagonist of Ccr2 led to decreased adipose tissue macrophage infiltration and improved insulin sensitivity [96]. Complementary studies on MCP-1 have shown that its expression is increased in obese mice, suggesting that changes in MCP-1 levels promote the recruitment of macrophages to adipose tissue which then causes inflammation and IR. Studies on transgenic mice that overexpress MCP-1 under the control of the adipose tissue-specific AP2 promoter found that MCP-1 overexpression is associated with macrophage infiltration and IR [97, 98]. Kanda et al. [98] also showed that the onset of these abnormalities in obese mice could be prevented by genetic deletion of MCP-1. MCP-1 may also have a role in energy metabolism. Unlike other studies, Inouye et al. [99]

showed that HFD-fed MCP-1 KO mice developed hyperinsulinemia and increased adiposity independent of adipose tissue macrophage levels, which were unchanged. Differences in experimental approaches as well as the complexity/redundancy of chemokine signaling may have accounted for these conflicting conclusions. In total, most evidence suggests that the MCP-1/Ccr2 axis could provide an important mechanistic link between obesity, adipose tissue inflammation, and IR.

## Endoplasmic Reticulum Stress

Yet another potential cause of inflammation in obesity is the so-called endoplasmic reticulum (ER) stress. This idea is based on the premise that nutrient excess causes mechanical stress, excess lipid accumulation and protein synthesis, and abnormal energy metabolism, all of which lead to an overburdened ER. This "hyper-synthetic" state in the ER interrupts the normal folding of proteins and activates the so-called unfolded protein response (UPR), thereby triggering stress response pathways. The role of the UPR is both to alleviate the ER stress and, paradoxically, to activate apoptosis depending on the nature and severity of the stressor [100]. Özcan et al. [101] showed that ER stress induction is associated with IR via JNK-mediated serine phosphorylation of IRS-1, in cultured liver cells. They also demonstrated that obese mice deficient for one allele of X-box-binding protein-1 (XBP1), a transcription factor that promotes the expression of molecular chaperones in response to ER stress, are more severely insulin resistant compared to obese controls. These mice exhibit ER stress, increased JNK activity, and IRS1 serine phosphorylation. This group also showed that reduction of ER stress by oral administration of active chemical chaperones improved glucose homeostasis in obese mice [102]. A recent study [103] found that fetuin-A levels were increased in those who suffered with DM and nonalcoholic fatty liver disease (NAFLD). In this study, a total of 180 age- and sex-matched subjects with normal glucose tolerance, NAFLD alone, newly diagnosed diabetes mellitus (NDDM) alone, and those with both NDDM and NAFLD were recruited. They found that the levels of fetuin-A were significantly increased in NDDM with NAFLD as compared with subjects who had NDDM alone or NAFLD alone. They further used HepG2 cells to investigate the regulation of fetuin-A. Treatment with ER stress activator, thapsigargin, increased the expression of fetuin-A mRNA and protein in a time- and dose-dependent manner. Pretreatment with the ER stress inhibitor, 4-phenylbutyrate reversed high glucose- or palmitate-induced fetuin-A expression. Furthermore, treating both streptozotocin induced and high-fat-diet-induced diabetic mice with 4-phenylbutyrate not only decreased hepatic fetuin-A levels, but also improved hyperglycemia. ER stress induced by hyperglycemia and palmitate increased the expression of fetuin-A and further contributed to the development of IR.

The authors of another study [104] sought to distinguish the adaptive and deleterious effects of lipid-induced ER stress on hepatic insulin action. Exposure of human hepatoma HepG2 cells or mouse primary hepatocytes to the saturated fatty acid palmitate enhanced ER stress in a dose-dependent manner. Exposure of HepG2 cells to prolonged mild ER stress activation induced by low levels of thapsigargin, tunicamycin, or palmitate augmented insulin-stimulated Akt phosphorylation, with subsequent attenuation of the acute stress response to high-level palmitate challenge. In contrast, exposure of HepG2 cells or hepatocytes to severe ER stress induced by high levels of palmitate was associated with reduced insulin-stimulated Akt phosphorylation and glycogen synthesis, as well as increased expression of glucose-6-phosphatase. Attenuation of ER stress using chemical chaperones (trimethylamine N-oxide or tauroursodeoxycholic acid) partially protected against the lipid-induced changes in insulin signaling. These findings in liver cells suggested that mild ER stress associated with chronic low-level palmitate exposure induced an adaptive UPR that enhances insulin signaling and protects against the effects of high-level palmitate. However, in the absence of chronic adaptation, severe ER stress induced by high-level palmitate exposure induces deleterious UPR signaling that contributes to IR and metabolic dysregulation.

## Conclusion

Insulin resistance is a complex metabolic defect that most likely has several etiologies dependent on the individual's genetic substrate and the underlying pathophysiologic state. Atherogenic dyslipidemia, hyperinsulinemia, dysglycemia, inflammation associated with obesity, and ectopic steatosis in liver and skeletal muscle all collude to facilitate endothelial dysfunction and predispose to the initiation and propagation of atherosclerosis. With regard to the relationship between insulin resistance and atherosclerosis, a fascinating array of cellular and metabolic defects have been demonstrated in elegantly done laboratory studies and human studies, yet more research is needed to define ways by which human intervention can fundamentally alter the metabolic and vascular milieu and slow the pace of atherosclerosis and favorably impact CVD outcomes. Underscoring the need is the fact that a majority of diabetic patients die from cardiovascular disease, and to date, aggressive management of the various risk factors does not seem to abrogate the so-called residual risk. Lifestyle methods leading to a reduction in body weight have salutatory effects on insulin resistance and CVD outcomes and remain a mainstay in the therapeutic armamentarium of a physician seeking to improve the overarching effects of the insulin-resistant state.

## References


1. Muoio DM, Newgard CB. Mechanisms of disease: molecular and metabolic mechanisms of insulin resistance and beta-cell failure in type 2 diabetes. Nat Rev Mol Cell Biol. 2008;9:193–205.
2. Himsworth HP. Diabetes mellitus. Lancet. 1936;227:127–30.
3. Himsworth HP. The mechanism of diabetes mellitus. Lancet. 1939;234:1–6.
4. Himsworth HP. The mechanism of diabetes mellitus. Lancet. 1939;234:65–8.
5. Himsworth HP. The mechanism of diabetes mellitus. Lancet. 1939;234:118–22.
6. Himsworth HP. The mechanism of diabetes mellitus. Lancet. 1939;234:171–6.
7. Yalow RS, Berson SA. Immunoassay of endogenous plasma insulin in man. J Clin Invest. 1960;39: 1157–75.
8. American Diabetes Association. Diagnosis and classification of diabetes mellitus. Diabetes Care. 2012;35 Suppl 1:S64–71.
9. Moller DE, Flier JS. Insulin resistance–mechanisms, syndromes, and implications. N Engl J Med. 1991;325:938–48.
10. Seino S, Seino M, Nishi S, Bell GI. Structure of the human insulin receptor gene and characterization of its promoter. Proc Natl Acad Sci USA. 1989;86:114–8.
11. Cheatham B, Kahn CR. Insulin action and the insulin signaling network. Endocr Rev. 1995;16: 117–42.
12. White MF. The IRS-signalling system: a network of docking proteins that mediate insulin action. Mol Cell Biochem. 1998;182:3–11.
13. Shepherd PR, Kahn BB. Glucose transporters and insulin action–implications for insulin resistance and diabetes mellitus. N Engl J Med. 1999;341:248–57.
14. Shulman GI. Cellular mechanisms of insulin resistance in humans. Am J Cardiol. 1999;84:3J–10.
15. Sasaoka T, Rose DW, Jhun BH, Saltiel AR, Draznin B, Olefsky JM. Evidence for a functional role of Shc proteins in mitogenic signaling induced by insulin, insulin-like growth factor-1, and epidermal growth factor. J Biol Chem. 1994;269:13689–94.
16. Sasaoka T, Ishiki M, Sawa T, et al. Comparison of the insulin and insulin-like growth factor 1 mitogenic intracellular signaling pathways. Endocrinology. 1996;137:4427–34.
17. Jiang ZY, Lin YW, Clemont A, et al. Characterization of selective resistance to insulin signaling in the vasculature of obese Zucker (fa/fa) rats. J Clin Invest. 1999;104:447–57.
18. Cusi K, Maezono K, Osman A, et al. Insulin resistance differentially affects the PI 3-kinase- and MAP kinase-mediated signaling in human muscle. J Clin Invest. 2000;105:311–20.
19. Zecchin HG, Bezerra RM, Carvalheira JB, et al. Insulin signalling pathways in aorta and muscle from two animal models of insulin resistance–the obese middle-aged and the spontaneously hypertensive rats. Diabetologia. 2003;46:479–91.
20. Law RE, Meehan WP, Xi XP, et al. Troglitazone inhibits vascular smooth muscle cell growth and intimal hyperplasia. J Clin Invest. 1996;98:1897–905.
21. Ross R, Glomset JA. The pathogenesis of atherosclerosis (first of two parts). N Engl J Med. 1976;295: 369–77.
22. Libby P, Hansson GK. Involvement of the immune system in human atherogenesis: current knowledge and unanswered questions. Lab Invest. 1991;64: 5–15.
23. Hansson GK, Libby P. The immune response in atherosclerosis: a double-edged sword. Nat Rev Immunol. 2006;6:508–19.
24. Hansson GK, Hermansson A. The immune system in atherosclerosis. Nat Immunol. 2011;12:204–12.
25. Yla-Herttuala S, Bentzon JF, Daemen M, et al. Stabilisation of atherosclerotic plaques. Position paper of the European Society of Cardiology (ESC)

Working Group on atherosclerosis and vascular biology. Thromb Haemost. 2011;106:1–19.
26. Weber C, Noels H. Atherosclerosis: current pathogenesis and therapeutic options. Nat Med. 2011;17:1410–22.
27. Lusis AJ. Atherosclerosis. Nature. 2000;407:233–41.
28. Tabas I. Macrophage death and defective inflammation resolution in atherosclerosis. Nat Rev Immunol. 2010;10:36–46.
29. Henry RR. Glucose control and insulin resistance in non-insulin-dependent diabetes mellitus. Ann Intern Med. 1996;124:97–103.
30. Krauss RM. Triglycerides and atherogenic lipoproteins: rationale for lipid management. Am J Med. 1998;105:58S–62.
31. Krauss RM. Atherogenicity of triglyceride-rich lipoproteins. Am J Cardiol. 1998;81:13B–7.
32. Berneis KK, Krauss RM. Metabolic origins and clinical significance of LDL heterogeneity. J Lipid Res. 2002;43:1363–79.
33. McNamara JR, Jenner JL, Li Z, Wilson PW, Schaefer EJ. Change in LDL particle size is associated with change in plasma triglyceride concentration. Arterioscler Thromb. 1992;12:1284–90.
34. McNamara JR, Campos H, Ordovas JM, Peterson J, Wilson PW, Schaefer EJ. Effect of gender, age, and lipid status on low density lipoprotein subfraction distribution. Results from the Framingham Offspring Study. Arteriosclerosis. 1987;7:483–90.
35. Krauss RM, Williams PT, Lindgren FT, Wood PD. Coordinate changes in levels of human serum low and high density lipoprotein subclasses in healthy men. Arteriosclerosis. 1988;8:155–62.
36. Blanche PJ, Gong EL, Forte TM, Nichols AV. Characterization of human high-density lipoproteins by gradient gel electrophoresis. Biochim Biophys Acta. 1981;665:408–19.
37. Hopkins GJ, Barter PJ. Role of triglyceride-rich lipoproteins and hepatic lipase in determining the particle size and composition of high density lipoproteins. J Lipid Res. 1986;27:1265–77.
38. Campos H, Arnold KS, Balestra ME, Innerarity TL, Krauss RM. Differences in receptor binding of LDL subfractions. Arterioscler Thromb Vasc Biol. 1996;16:794–801.
39. Pascot A, Lemieux I, Prud'homme D, et al. Reduced HDL particle size as an additional feature of the atherogenic dyslipidemia of abdominal obesity. J Lipid Res. 2001;42:2007–14.
40. Bjornheden T, Babyi A, Bondjers G, Wiklund O. Accumulation of lipoprotein fractions and subfractions in the arterial wall, determined in an in vitro perfusion system. Atherosclerosis. 1996;123:43–56.
41. Anber V, Griffin BA, McConnell M, Packard CJ, Shepherd J. Influence of plasma lipid and LDL-subfraction profile on the interaction between low density lipoprotein with human arterial wall proteoglycans. Atherosclerosis. 1996;124:261–71.
42. Chait A, Brazg RL, Tribble DL, Krauss RM. Susceptibility of small, dense, low-density lipoproteins to oxidative modification in subjects with the atherogenic lipoprotein phenotype, pattern B. Am J Med. 1993;94:350–6.
43. de Graaf J, Hak-Lemmers HL, Hectors MP, Demacker PN, Hendriks JC, Stalenhoef AF. Enhanced susceptibility to in vitro oxidation of the dense low density lipoprotein subfraction in healthy subjects. Arterioscler Thromb. 1991;11:298–306.
44. Tribble DL, Holl LG, Wood PD, Krauss RM. Variations in oxidative susceptibility among six low density lipoprotein subfractions of differing density and particle size. Atherosclerosis. 1992;93:189–99.
45. Kannel WB, McGee DL. Diabetes and glucose tolerance as risk factors for cardiovascular disease: the Framingham study. Diabetes Care. 1979;2:120–6.
46. Turner RC, Millns H, Neil HA, et al. Risk factors for coronary artery disease in non-insulin dependent diabetes mellitus: United Kingdom Prospective Diabetes Study (UKPDS: 23). BMJ. 1998;316: 823–8.
47. Prince CT, Becker DJ, Costacou T, Miller RG, Orchard TJ. Changes in glycaemic control and risk of coronary artery disease in type 1 diabetes mellitus: findings from the Pittsburgh Epidemiology of Diabetes Complications Study (EDC). Diabetologia. 2007;50:2280–8.
48. Koya D, King GL. Protein kinase C activation and the development of diabetic complications. Diabetes. 1998;47:859–66.
49. Derubertis FR, Craven PA. Activation of protein kinase C in glomerular cells in diabetes. Mechanisms and potential links to the pathogenesis of diabetic glomerulopathy. Diabetes. 1994;43:1–8.
50. Xia P, Inoguchi T, Kern TS, Engerman RL, Oates PJ, King GL. Characterization of the mechanism for the chronic activation of diacylglycerol-protein kinase C pathway in diabetes and hypergalactosemia. Diabetes. 1994;43:1122–9.
51. Koya D, Jirousek MR, Lin YW, Ishii H, Kuboki K, King GL. Characterization of protein kinase C beta isoform activation on the gene expression of transforming growth factor-beta, extracellular matrix components, and prostanoids in the glomeruli of diabetic rats. J Clin Invest. 1997;100:115–26.
52. Ishii H, Jirousek MR, Koya D, et al. Amelioration of vascular dysfunctions in diabetic rats by an oral PKC beta inhibitor. Science. 1996;272:728–31.
53. Kuboki K, Jiang ZY, Takahara N, et al. Regulation of endothelial constitutive nitric oxide synthase gene expression in endothelial cells and in vivo : a specific vascular action of insulin. Circulation. 2000;101: 676–81.
54. Studer RK, Craven PA, DeRubertis FR. Role for protein kinase C in the mediation of increased fibronectin accumulation by mesangial cells grown in high-glucose medium. Diabetes. 1993;42:118–26.
55. Feener EP, Xia P, Inoguchi T, Shiba T, Kunisaki M, King GL. Role of protein kinase C in glucose- and angiotensin II-induced plasminogen activator inhibitor expression. Contrib Nephrol. 1996;118:180–7.
56. Koya D, Haneda M, Nakagawa H, et al. Amelioration of accelerated diabetic mesangial expansion by

treatment with a PKC beta inhibitor in diabetic db/db mice, a rodent model for type 2 diabetes. FASEB J. 2000;14:439–47.
57. Piga R, Naito Y, Kokura S, Handa O, Yoshikawa T. Short-term high glucose exposure induces monocyte-endothelial cells adhesion and transmigration by increasing VCAM-1 and MCP-1 expression in human aortic endothelial cells. Atherosclerosis. 2007;193:328–34.
58. Yan SD, Schmidt AM, Anderson GM, et al. Enhanced cellular oxidant stress by the interaction of advanced glycation end products with their receptors/binding proteins. J Biol Chem. 1994;269:9889–97.
59. Dasu MR, Devaraj S, Jialal I. High glucose induces IL-1beta expression in human monocytes: mechanistic insights. Am J Physiol Endocrinol Metab. 2007;293:E337–46.
60. Kawamura M, Heinecke JW, Chait A. Pathophysiological concentrations of glucose promote oxidative modification of low density lipoprotein by a superoxide-dependent pathway. J Clin Invest. 1994;94:771–8.
61. Miyazaki A, Nakayama H, Horiuchi S. Scavenger receptors that recognize advanced glycation end products. Trends Cardiovasc Med. 2002;12:258–62.
62. Ohgami N, Miyazaki A, Sakai M, Kuniyasu A, Nakayama H, Horiuchi S. Advanced glycation end products (AGE) inhibit scavenger receptor class B type I-mediated reverse cholesterol transport: a new crossroad of AGE to cholesterol metabolism. J Atheroscler Thromb. 2003;10:1–6.
63. Roytblat L, Rachinsky M, Fisher A, et al. Raised interleukin-6 levels in obese patients. Obes Res. 2000;8:673–5.
64. Straczkowski M, Dzienis-Straczkowska S, Stepien A, Kowalska I, Szelachowska M, Kinalska I. Plasma interleukin-8 concentrations are increased in obese subjects and related to fat mass and tumor necrosis factor-alpha system. J Clin Endocrinol Metab. 2002;87:4602–6.
65. Hotamisligil GS, Spiegelman BM. Tumor necrosis factor alpha: a key component of the obesity-diabetes link. Diabetes. 1994;43:1271–8.
66. Sartipy P, Loskutoff DJ. Monocyte chemoattractant protein 1 in obesity and insulin resistance. . 2003;100:7265–70.
67. Hotamisligil GS, Arner P, Caro JF, Atkinson RL, Spiegelman BM. Increased adipose tissue expression of tumor necrosis factor-alpha in human obesity and insulin resistance. J Clin Invest. 1995;95:2409–15.
68. Visser M, Bouter LM, McQuillan GM, Wener MH, Harris TB. Elevated C-reactive protein levels in overweight and obese adults. JAMA. 1999;282:2131–5.
69. de Luca C, Olefsky JM. Inflammation and insulin resistance. FEBS Lett. 2008;582:97–105.
70. Kim F, Tysseling KA, Rice J, et al. Free fatty acid impairment of nitric oxide production in endothelial cells is mediated by IKKbeta. Arterioscler Thromb Vasc Biol. 2005;25:989–94.
71. Hotamisligil GS, Shargill NS, Spiegelman BM. Adipose expression of tumor necrosis factor-alpha: direct role in obesity-linked insulin resistance. Science. 1993;259:87–91.
72. Hotamisligil GS, Peraldi P, Budavari A, Ellis R, White MF, Spiegelman BM. IRS-1-mediated inhibition of insulin receptor tyrosine kinase activity in TNF-alpha- and obesity-induced insulin resistance. Science. 1996;271:665–8.
73. Uysal KT, Wiesbrock SM, Marino MW, Hotamisligil GS. Protection from obesity-induced insulin resistance in mice lacking TNF-alpha function. Nature. 1997;389:610–4.
74. Stephens JM, Lee J, Pilch PF. Tumor necrosis factor-alpha-induced insulin resistance in 3T3-L1 adipocytes is accompanied by a loss of insulin receptor substrate-1 and GLUT4 expression without a loss of insulin receptor-mediated signal transduction. J Biol Chem. 1997;272:971–6.
75. Ruan H, Hacohen N, Golub TR, Van Parijs L, Lodish HF. Tumor necrosis factor-alpha suppresses adipocyte-specific genes and activates expression of preadipocyte genes in 3T3-L1 adipocytes: nuclear factor-kappaB activation by TNF-alpha is obligatory. Diabetes. 2002;51:1319–36.
76. Hirosumi J, Tuncman G, Chang L, et al. A central role for JNK in obesity and insulin resistance. Nature. 2002;420:333–6.
77. Tuncman G, Hirosumi J, Solinas G, Chang L, Karin M, Hotamisligil GS. Functional in vivo interactions between JNK1 and JNK2 isoforms in obesity and insulin resistance. . 2006;103:10741–6.
78. Williamson RT. On the treatment of glycosuria and diabetes mellitus with sodium salicylate. Br Med J. 1901;1:760–2.
79. Yin MJ, Yamamoto Y, Gaynor RB. The anti-inflammatory agents aspirin and salicylate inhibit the activity of I(kappa)B kinase-beta. Nature. 1998;396:77–80.
80. Kim JK, Kim YJ, Fillmore JJ, et al. Prevention of fat-induced insulin resistance by salicylate. J Clin Invest. 2001;108:437–46.
81. Yuan M, Konstantopoulos N, Lee J, et al. Reversal of obesity- and diet-induced insulin resistance with salicylates or targeted disruption of Ikkbeta. Science. 2001;293:1673–7.
82. Cai D, Yuan M, Frantz DF, et al. Local and systemic insulin resistance resulting from hepatic activation of IKK-beta and NF-kappaB. Nat Med. 2005;11:183–90.
83. Sugita H, Fujimoto M, Yasukawa T, et al. Inducible nitric-oxide synthase and NO donor induce insulin receptor substrate-1 degradation in skeletal muscle cells. J Biol Chem. 2005;280:14203–11.
84. Yasukawa T, Tokunaga E, Ota H, Sugita H, Martyn JA, Kaneki M. S-nitrosylation-dependent inactivation of Akt/protein kinase B in insulin resistance. J Biol Chem. 2005;280:7511–8.
85. Perreault M, Marette A. Targeted disruption of inducible nitric oxide synthase protects against obesity-linked insulin resistance in muscle. Nat Med. 2001;7:1138–43.
86. Carvalho-Filho MA, Ueno M, Carvalheira JB, Velloso LA, Saad MJ. Targeted disruption of iNOS

prevents LPS-induced S-nitrosation of IRbeta/IRS-1 and Akt and insulin resistance in muscle of mice. Am J Physiol Endocrinol Metab. 2006;291:E476–82.
87. Carvalho-Filho MA, Ueno M, Hirabara SM, et al. S-nitrosation of the insulin receptor, insulin receptor substrate 1, and protein kinase B/Akt: a novel mechanism of insulin resistance. Diabetes. 2005;54: 959–67.
88. Schottelius AJ, Mayo MW, Sartor RB, Baldwin Jr AS. Interleukin-10 signaling blocks inhibitor of kappaB kinase activity and nuclear factor kappaB DNA binding. J Biol Chem. 1999;274:31868–74.
89. van Exel E, Gussekloo J, de Craen AJ, et al. Low production capacity of interleukin-10 associates with the metabolic syndrome and type 2 diabetes : the Leiden 85-plus study. Diabetes. 2002;51: 1088–92.
90. Lumeng CN, Bodzin JL, Saltiel AR. Obesity induces a phenotypic switch in adipose tissue macrophage polarization. J Clin Invest. 2007;117:175–84.
91. Asadullah K, Sterry W, Volk HD. Interleukin-10 therapy–review of a new approach. Pharmacol Rev. 2003;55:241–69.
92. Weisberg SP, McCann D, Desai M, Rosenbaum M, Leibel RL, Ferrante Jr AW. Obesity is associated with macrophage accumulation in adipose tissue. J Clin Invest. 2003;112:1796–808.
93. Xu H, Barnes GT, Yang Q, et al. Chronic inflammation in fat plays a crucial role in the development of obesity-related insulin resistance. J Clin Invest. 2003;112:1821–30.
94. Arkan MC, Hevener AL, Greten FR, et al. IKK-beta links inflammation to obesity-induced insulin resistance. Nat Med. 2005;11:191–8.
95. Kurihara T, Bravo R. Cloning and functional expression of mCCR2, a murine receptor for the C-C chemokines JE and FIC. J Biol Chem. 1996;271: 11603–7.
96. Weisberg SP, Hunter D, Huber R, et al. CCR2 modulates inflammatory and metabolic effects of high-fat feeding. J Clin Invest. 2006;116:115–24.
97. Kamei N, Tobe K, Suzuki R, et al. Overexpression of monocyte chemoattractant protein-1 in adipose tissues causes macrophage recruitment and insulin resistance. J Biol Chem. 2006;281:26602–14.
98. Kanda H, Tateya S, Tamori Y, et al. MCP-1 contributes to macrophage infiltration into adipose tissue, insulin resistance, and hepatic steatosis in obesity. J Clin Invest. 2006;116:1494–505.
99. Inouye KE, Shi H, Howard JK, et al. Absence of CC chemokine ligand 2 does not limit obesity-associated infiltration of macrophages into adipose tissue. Diabetes. 2007;56:2242–50.
100. Rutkowski DT, Kaufman RJ. That which does not kill me makes me stronger: adapting to chronic ER stress. Trends Biochem Sci. 2007;32:469–76.
101. Ozcan U, Cao Q, Yilmaz E, et al. Endoplasmic reticulum stress links obesity, insulin action, and type 2 diabetes. Science. 2004;306:457–61.
102. Ozcan U, Yilmaz E, Ozcan L, et al. Chemical chaperones reduce ER stress and restore glucose homeostasis in a mouse model of type 2 diabetes. Science. 2006;313:1137–40.
103. Ou HY, Wu HT, Hung HC, Yang YC, Wu JS, Chang CJ. Endoplasmic reticulum stress induces the expression of Fetuin-A to develop insulin resistance. Endocrinology. 2012;153(7):2974–84.
104. Achard CS, Laybutt DR. Lipid-induced endoplasmic reticulum stress in liver cells results in two distinct outcomes: adaptation with enhanced insulin signaling or insulin resistance. Endocrinology. 2012; 153(5):2164–77.

# Apoproteins and Cell Surface Receptors Regulating Lipoprotein Metabolism in the Setting of Type 2 Diabetes

4

Thomas D. Dayspring

## Introduction

The epidemic of diabetes mellitus that is occurring throughout the world portends a drastic increase in the incidence of macrovascular atherosclerotic disease, the leading cause of death, in addition to all of its other morbidities. There are an estimated 18.3 million Americans >20 years of age who have physician-diagnosed diabetes, an additional 7.1 million adults with undiagnosed DM, and ~81.5 million adults with prediabetes (e.g., fasting blood glucose of 100 to >126 mg/dL). The prevalence of prediabetes in the US adult population is nearly 37 % [1]. Diabetes, especially type 2 diabetes mellitus (T2DM), is a lipidosis which has classically been described as a secondary lipid disorder.

Lipids are broadly defined as nonpolar molecules that are not soluble in water but are soluble in nonpolar solvents. Physiologically lipids contribute to numerous biologic processes including energy supply, membrane structure, membrane function, cellular signal transduction, mediation of inflammation, and steroid and bile acid synthesis. Some lipids are amphipathic molecules having unique molecular structures where one end of the molecule is polar and the other is not: with the polar end having some water solubility and the other end not. Such molecules are critically important for structure of lipid monolayers (lipoproteins and micelles) and lipid bilayers (cell membranes). Within membranes are specific areas of "functional" lipids termed lipid rafts where protein expression and other actions such as caveolae formation occurs.

Although there are multiple risk factors, many of which are treatable and are associated with or result in atherosclerotic plaques, there is only one sine qua non for the disease, namely, an accumulation of sterols within arterial wall macrophages (foam cells) [2]. It is crucial to recognize that hydrophobic sterols, noncholesterol sterols, and glycerolipids are trafficked in plasma and potentially into the arterial wall as components of protein-enwrapped particles called lipoproteins, in effect making atherogenesis a lipoprotein-mediated disease [3, 4]. Lipid and lipoprotein biology and physiology are immensely complex and the purpose of this chapter is to first, review basic sterol and glycerolipid biochemistry and lipid homeostasis including synthesis, absorption, and incorporation into and transportation within lipoproteins, and second, examine what changes occur and the consequences of those changes in the T2DM patient. Lipid homeostasis is regulated by (1) several nuclear transcription factors which mediate lipogenesis, (2) cellular membrane proteins involved with lipoprotein lipidation and delipidation, (3) catabolic receptors, (4) lipolytic enzymes, and (5) lipid transfer proteins. These will all be discussed in this chapter.

T.D. Dayspring (✉)
Foundation for Health Improvement and Technology,
737 North Fifth Street, Suite 200, Richmond,
VA 23219, USA
e-mail: tdayspring@aol.com

A.J. Jenkins et al. (eds.), *Lipoproteins in Diabetes Mellitus*, Contemporary Diabetes,
DOI 10.1007/978-1-4614-7554-5_4, © Springer Science+Business Media New York 2014

## Lipoprotein Structure and Nomenclature

Understanding lipoproteins requires a realization that there is a constant, continually ongoing, dynamic remodeling of the lipoprotein particles where lipid molecules and surface apoproteins are gained and lost and reacquired through complex pathways involving neutral lipid interchange between particles, hydrolysis of lipids (lipolysis), as well as particle catabolism [5]. Simply stated, lipoproteins and their lipid content are in a continuous state of constant dynamic flux and such behavior is often not reflected in standard lipid concentration measurements. Lipoproteins were originally separated by their density and were named from most to least buoyant as chylomicrons, very-low-density (VLDL), intermediate-density (IDL), low-density (LDL), and high-density lipoproteins (HDL). The lipoprotein particles can be further separated into subparticles of incremental buoyancies and sizes ranging from large (more buoyant) to smaller (less buoyant or dense). Buoyancy and density are determined by the molecular weight of the lipid and protein molecules in a given particle, and, in general, proteins have much higher molecular weights than lipids. Thus, the large, lipid-rich lipoproteins are the most buoyant and the smaller lipid-poor, protein-rich lipoproteins are denser. Within a specific family of lipoproteins, the smaller subspecies are always more dense than the larger ones and the term small and dense or large (fluffy) and buoyant is therefore redundant, i.e., a small LDL is by definition a dense LDL.

The glycerolipids, triglycerides or triacylglycerols (TG), and phospholipids (PL) are molecules in which three and two fatty acids (FA), respectively, are esterified to glycerol, a three-carbon carbohydrate. TG serve as a carrier of energy (9 kcal/g) which can be oxidized in muscles or stored in adipocytes. Typically PL consist of a saturated and a long-chain polyunsaturated FA including the omega-6 and omega-3 FA. Plasma PL not present on lipoproteins are bound to phospholipid transfer protein (PLTP) [6] and plasma FA not found in PL or TG are bound to albumin and referred to as free fatty acid or nonesterified fatty acids. Sterols are divided into zoosterols which include free or unesterified cholesterol (UC) and its precursors such as lathosterol and phytosterols (several exist, with sitosterol and campesterol being the most common). Molecules that have a structure that is very similar to cholesterol are termed noncholesterol sterols. A saturated sterol is called a stanol and is characterized by the absence of the double bond at the Δ5 position in the B ring. For example, sitosterol (a sterol) when reduced becomes sitostanol (a stanol). One cholesterol metabolite is cholestanol which is the stanol form of cholesterol. UC has a –OH (hydroxy) group at the #3 carbon position of the A ring, whereas cholesteryl ester (CE) has the –OH group replaced via the action of the enzyme acyl-cholesterol acyltransferase (ACAT) of which two isoforms exist ACTA1 and ACAT2, with a long-chain fatty acid (typically palmitic or oleic acid) forming cholesteryl palmitate or cholesteryl oleate. Unlike cholesterol, phytosterols are not a good substrate for ACAT and are not readily esterified in enterocytes or hepatocytes.

Lipoproteins are polymolecular assemblies of apoproteins and lipids including UC, CE, noncholesterol sterols, TG, and PL whose collective function is to traffic lipids to and from various tissues. All lipoproteins consist of a surface monolayer of amphipathic PL and UC molecules which surrounds the particle core consisting of a variable mixture of the hydrophobic TG and CE molecules (Fig. 4.1). Hydrophobic CE is relegated to the core of the particles away from the water in plasma, and this biochemical property is the reason that as lipoproteins lipidate, they become spherical, which, because the volume of a sphere is a function of the third power of the radius, vastly expand the number of TG lipid molecules and their 9 kcal/g of energy that can be trafficked. Providing structure, stability and aqueous solubility in plasma to the lipids are apoproteins, which assemble with the surface and core lipids. Once an apoprotein is lipidated it is called an apolipoprotein. Apart from structural functions, they also serve as ligands for various receptors and enzymes involved with particle formation and catabolism. Specific lipoproteins have very different core lipid concentrations

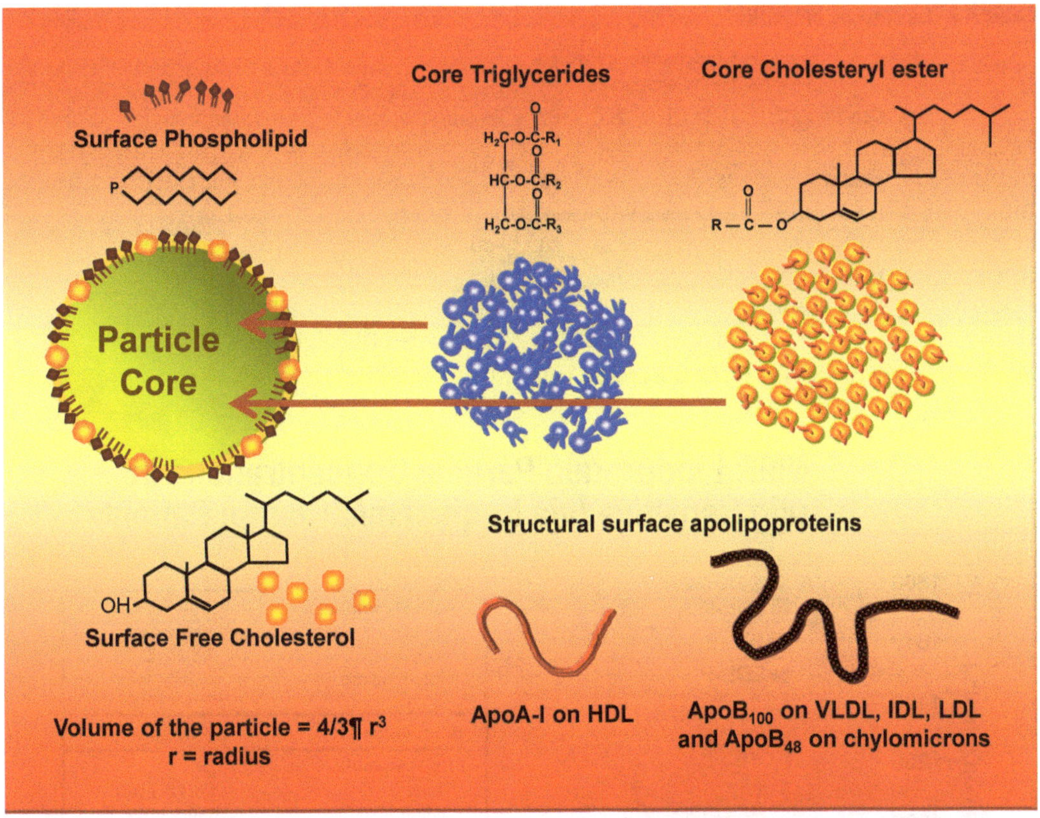


**Fig. 4.1** Lipoprotein structure involves amphipathic surface molecules PL and UC and the core consists of a variable mixture of nonpolar CE and TG. Providing structure and solubility are surface apolipoproteins. Because the volume of a sphere is related to the third power of the radius, even small lipoproteins can traffic significant numbers of lipid molecules per particle

**Table 4.1** Human apolipoproteins

| Apolipoprotein | Molecular weight | Lipoprotein association | Function |
|---|---|---|---|
| ApoA-I | 28,331 | HDL, chylomicrons | Activates ACAT, ABCA1 |
| ApoA-II | 17,380 | HDL, VLDL, Chylos | FFA metabolism, RCT, antiox |
| ApoA-IV | 44,000 | Chylomicrons, HDL | Chylo production, RCT, LCAT |
| ApoA-V | 39,000 | Chylos, VLDLs, HDLs | TG metabolism |
| ApoB-48 | 240,000 | Chylomicrons | Structural protein |
| ApoB-100 | 513,000 | VLDL, IDL, LDL | Binds to LDL receptor |
| ApoC-I | 7,000 | VLDL, HDL | Inhibits C-11, CETP |
| ApoC-II | 8,837 | Chylos, VLDL, HDL | Activates lipoprotein lipase |
| ApoC-III | 8,751 | Chylos, VLDL, HDL | Inhibits lipoprotein lipase |
| ApoD | 32,500 | HDL | CETP |
| ApoE | 34,145 | Chylos, VLDL, IDL, HDL | Binds to LDLr and LRP |

which can dynamically vary from particle to particle in the same and different individuals [7]. Phospholipids are amphipathic molecules and that unique property allows their polar end to interact with the water in plasma, enhancing lipoprotein plasma solubility. Although there are many known apolipoproteins with multiple functions (Tables 4.1 and 4.2), the main structural peptides are apolipoprotein B (apoB) and apolipoprotein A-I [8]. ApoB, the only non-exchangeable

**Table 4.2** Lipoprotein properties

| | | Composition by weight (% by weight) | | | | Relative | |
|---|---|---|---|---|---|---|---|
| | Density kg/L | UC+CE | TG | PL | Protein | volume[a] | Apolipoproteins |
| Chylomicron | < 0.95 | -5 | –90 | –4 | –1 | 700,000 | 8-48, A-1, C-1, C-11, C-111, E |
| VLDL | <1.006 | 25 | 55 | 18 | 8 | 360 | 8-100, A-ll, C-1, C-11, C-111, E |
| IDL | 1.006–1.019 | Between a VLDL and LDL | | | | | 8-100, E |
| LDL | 1.019–1.063 | 55 | 6 | 20 | –20 | 32 | 8-100 |
| HDL2 | 1.063–1.125 | 22 | 5 | 33 | 40 | 3 | A-1, A-ll, C-1, C-11, C-111, E |
| HDL3 | 1.125–1.210 | 17 | 3 | 25 | 55 | 1 | A-1, A-ll |
| Lp(a) | 1.04–1.13 | 48 | 9 | 21 | 22 | - LDL | B-100, a |

[a]For the purpose of comparison, HDL3 is assigned a value of 1

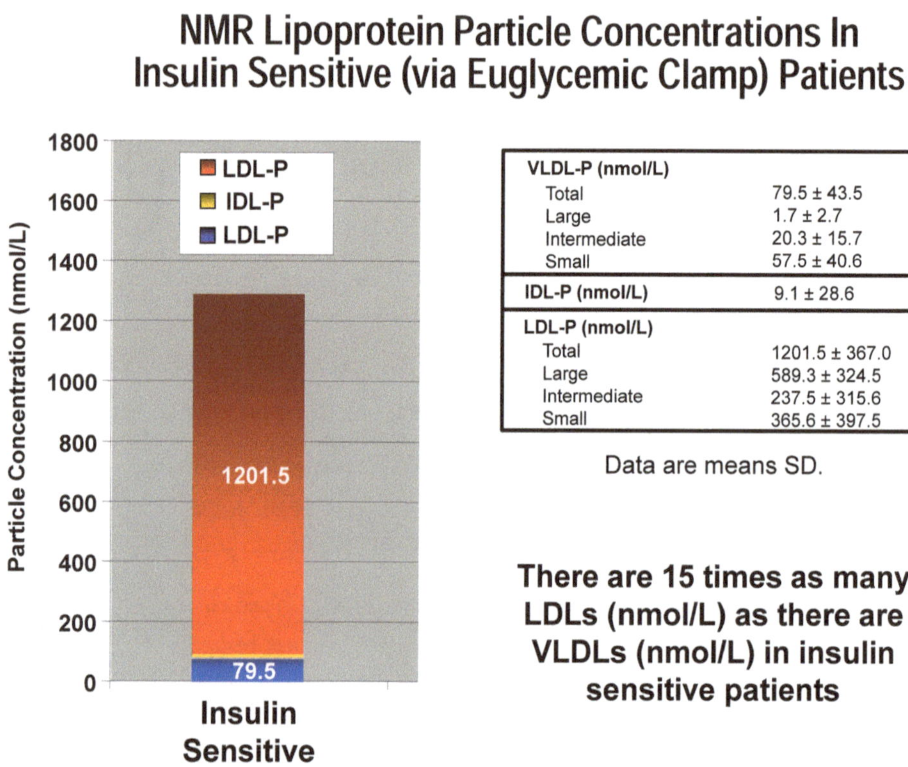


**Fig. 4.2** NMR lipoprotein particle concentrations in insulin sensitive (via euglycemic clamp) patients. Adapted from Garvey et al. Diabetes 2003;52(2):453-462. Reference [110] in chapter

apolipoprotein, exists in two isoforms: the hepatic synthesized apo$B_{100}$ and an intestinally produced truncated apo$B_{48}$, so named as it has 48 % of the molecular weight of apo$B_{100}$. Apo$B_{48}$ is missing the LDL receptor-binding domain [9]. VLDL, IDL, and LDL contain a single molecule of apolipoprotein $B_{100}$ [10]. Under normal physiologic conditions the plasma residence time of VLDL is approximately 2–6 h, IDL ~ 1 h, and LDL 1.5–3 days [11]. Therefore, approximately >90 % of apoB actually represents LDL particle concentration (LDL-P), and apoB is thus not particularly informative in quantifying VLDL particle concentration (VLDL-P) [12, 13] (Fig. 4.2).

The apoA-I family of lipoproteins are the HDL class and they remain the most complex

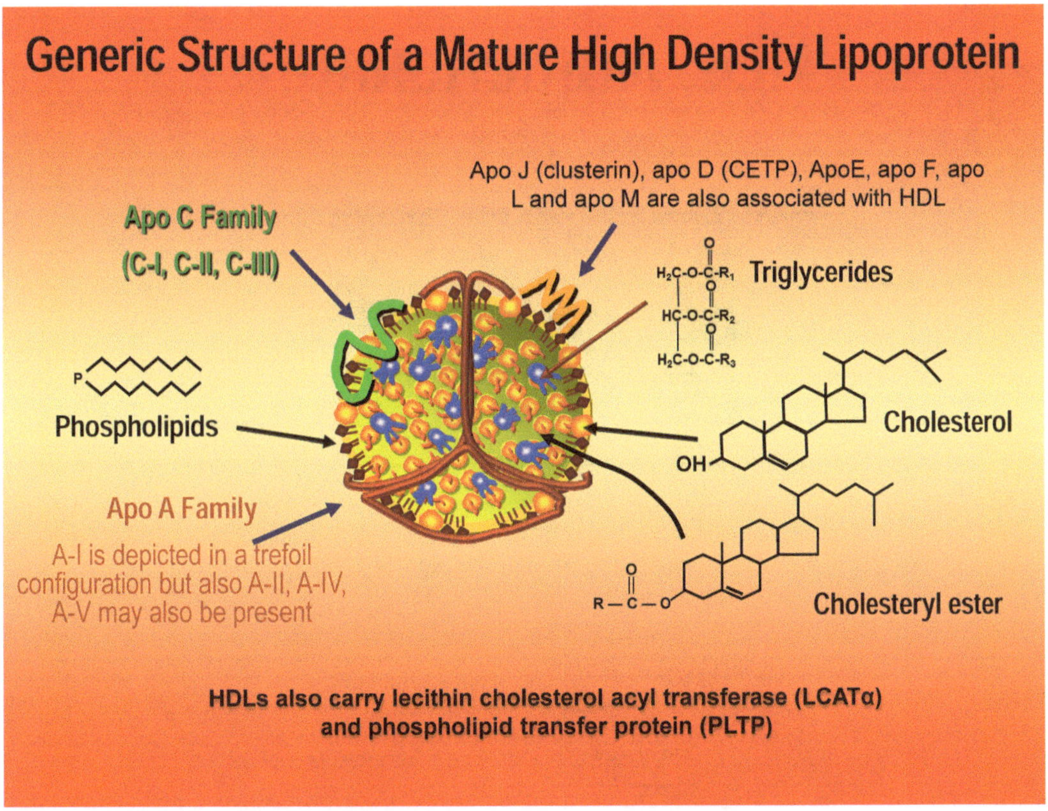


**Fig. 4.3** HDL particles are very small lipoproteins with a core of TG and cholesterol ester. The major surface apoproteins are A-I, A-II, or A-IV and ApoC family and ApoE family. HDL-C refers to the cholesterol mass

and enigmatic of all lipoproteins. HDLs not only traffic cholesterol and TG, but a large variety of other lipids including fat-soluble vitamins, phospholipids (e.g., phosphatidylcholine), and sphingolipids (sphingosin-1-phosphate, sphingomyelin, and ceramide), all of which are associated with many biological functions [14]. Collectively these are referred to as its lipidome. The protein cargo (proteome) of HDL is comprised of over 100 proteins, and these play defining roles in determining the functionality of HDL. HDLs acquire sterols from cells as they efflux UC, esterify the acquired UC using lecithin–cholesterol acyltransferase (LCAT), and then deliver the UC and CE elsewhere. HDLs are in a constant and dynamic state of lipidation and delipidation or remodeling and utilize a variety of cell membrane sterol transporters, lipid transfer proteins, and lipolytic enzymes to accomplish such [15]. There are many genetic, lifestyle, hormonal, metabolic, and inflammatory influences on HDL's makeup and function, and many of these may be manipulated by pharmacologic and lifestyle interventions. Structurally HDLs are similar to all lipoproteins with a one-molecule thick surface of PL and UC and a core of mostly CE but also a small amount of TG. The main structural protein of HDL is one to five copies of apolipoprotein A-I arranged in a "trefoil" configuration [10] (Fig. 4.3).

HDL nomenclature can be very confusing and some terms are technology dependent. There is a numerical ultracentrifuge classification where super large HDLs (not always present) are called HDL1. As the particles shrink in size, the names change to HDL2b, HDL2a (both large with b being larger than a) and HDL3a, HDL3b and HDL3c (with 3a being the largest and 3c the smallest). These terms are also used by labs utilizing ultracentrifugation or gradient gel electrophoretic fractionation. NMR spectroscopic

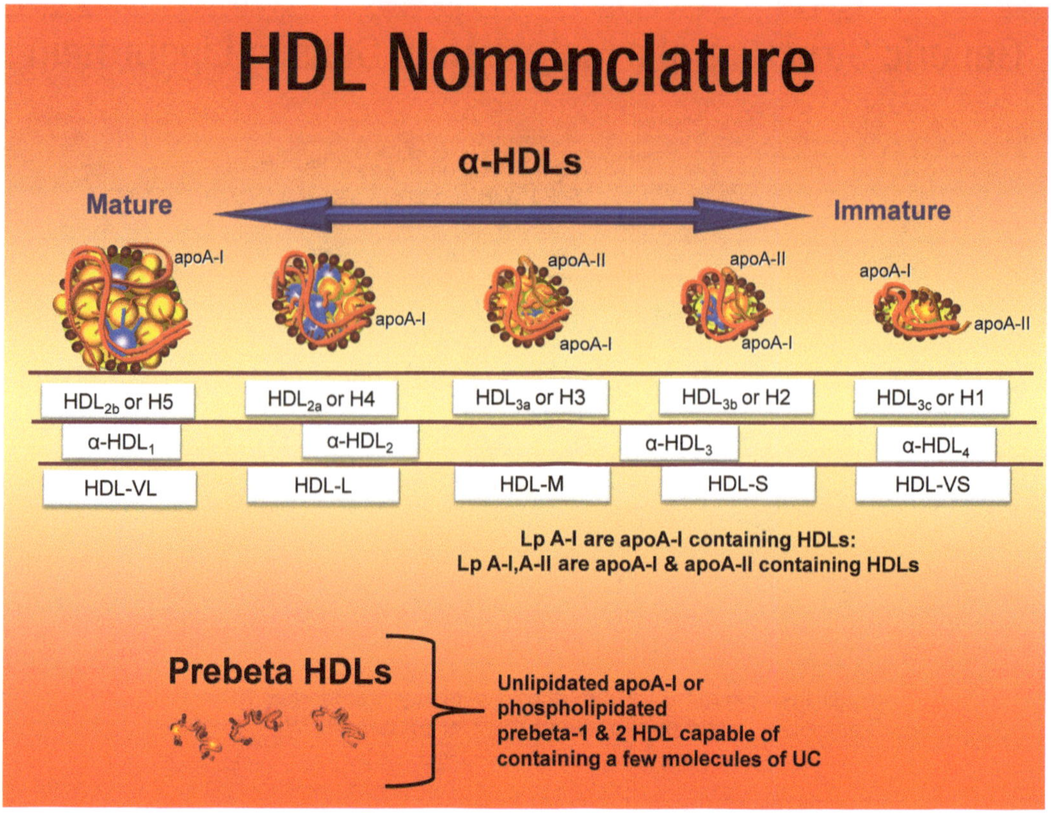


**Fig. 4.4** HDL particles can be separated two-dimensional electrophoresis and apoA-I staining into prebeta and alpha lipoproteins. The former are unlipidated apoA-I or phospholipidated A-I. Each HDL can have from 1 to 5 molecules of apoA-I. The α-HDLs range in size from small and dense to larger and more buoyant. There can be from one to five molecules of apoA-I per HDL particle; thus, apoA-I is only an approximation of the number (concentration) of HDL particles. ApoA-II is present, predominantly on the smaller species. *Dayspring original artwork*

classification of HDLs uses the terms H1 through 5 (with 5 being largest). Labs using 2D electrophoresis with apoA-I staining report apoA-I, prebeta-HDL, and the α-HDL subspecies. Some laboratories report how much cholesterol is in various HDL subspecies (i.e., $HDL_2$-C). The newest attempt from a group of experts to simplify HDL naming to simply refer to the particles as very small, small, medium, large, and very large. Classically those species have been called HDL1 (very large); HDL2a and HDL2b (large); HDL3a, HDL3b, and HDL3c (medium or small); and unlipidated apoA-I or prebeta (discoidal). Another system differentiates unlipidated apoA-I and prebeta HDLs (1 and 2) from large alpha HDLs (1, 2, 3, and 4 ranging from very large to small). NMR cannot measure unlipidated apoA-I or prebeta HDLs, but because of their transient existence, they only represent about 5 % of total HDL particles (HDL-P) [16] (Fig. 4.4).

## Measurement of Lipids and Lipoproteins

There are many ways of measuring lipoproteins in the laboratory including analyzing their density, their surface apolipoproteins, their core lipid content (expressed as TG or cholesterol mass per deciliter of plasma), or by NMR spectroscopy which determines the number of terminal methyl groups on CE, TG, and PL and translates that to particle numbers [17]. In clinical practice the majority of clinicians evaluate lipoproteins using lipid concentrations such as total particle cholesterol or TG or subparticle cholesterol mass per unit of plasma volume [18]. With respect to lab nomenclature and lipoprotein particle concentrations, (P) is added to the particle abbreviation and the value is expressed as nanomoles (nm) or micromoles (μmols) per liter. Lipoprotein particle concentrations can be determined using apolipoproteins, nuclear NMR [19], ion mobility transfer technologies [20], or ultracentrifugation with LDL staining.

$$\text{Total VLDL-P} = \text{chylomicron-P} + \text{large VLDL-P} + \text{medium VLDL-P} + \text{small VLDL-P}$$

Total IDL-P (not typically separated into subparticles)

$$\text{Total LDL-P} = \text{Large LDL-P} + \text{medium LDL-P} + \text{small LDL-P}$$

$$\text{Total HDL-P} = \text{Large HDL-P} + \text{medium HDL-P} + \text{small HDL-P}$$

With respect to cholesterol mass measurements, (-C) is added to the particle abbreviation and the value is expressed as mg per deciliter (dL) or millimoles per liter (mmol/L).

$$\text{Total cholesterol} = \text{VLDL-C} + \text{IDL-C} + \text{LDL-C} + \text{HDL-C} + \text{Lp(a)-C}$$

Calculated VLDL-C = TG/5 using the Friedewald formula [21].

Calculated

$$\text{LDL-C} = \text{IDL-C} + \text{LDL-C} + \text{Lp(a)-C}$$

using the formula

$$\text{LDL-C} = \text{TC-}[\text{HDL-C} + \text{VLDL-C}].$$

$$\text{Non-HDL-C} = \text{TC-HDL-C} = \text{apoB-C}$$

One should never confuse specific lipoprotein lipid and lipoprotein concentrations such as LDL-C with LDL-P or apoB or HDL-C with HDL-P. Each is a valid way of measuring LDL or HDL and when they correlate highly (*r* values) with each other as they often do, they are said to be concordant. However, when cholesterol and lipoprotein particle concentrations do not correlate, they are said to be discordant. With respect to LDLs and HDLs, it is not uncommon to have high or low LDL-C and HDL-C with respective low or high LDL-P and HDL-P values. Lipoproteins that are CE-poor will require larger numbers of particles to traffic a given amount of core cholesterol and, conversely, cholesterol-rich LDL or HDL will require fewer particles to traffic the cholesterol mass. The cholesterol mass or number of cholesterol molecules per particle is a function of both the particle volume and core lipid makeup. Since the volume of a sphere is $4/3\pi(r^2)$, even subtle changes in particle diameter can cause tremendous changes in the number of particles required for lipid trafficking. The same is true of the particle core ratio of TG to CE [22, 23]. Adding to potential discordance between cholesterol mass and particle concentrations is the fact that both calculated and directly assayed cholesterol concentrations often fail to meet accuracy standards [24, 25].

## Cellular Lipid Homeostasis

Because cholesterol can crystallize and cause cytotoxicity, cells maintain tight cholesterol homeostasis. All cells can synthesize UC as well as acquire it and FA through a variety of methods including cell membrane receptors which act as sterol or FA influx transporters or lipoprotein delipidation or internalization receptors (Table 4.3).

**Table 4.3** Synthesis, remodeling, and catabolism of circulating HDL particles

| Cell surface membrane receptors | |
|---|---|
| Lipoprotein endocytosis | LDL receptor (LDLr) |
| | LDL receptor-related protein (LRP) |
| | ApoA-1 beta-chain synthase or holoparticle receptor |
| Influx transporters | |
| | Niemann–Pick C1 like-1 protein (NPC1L1) |
| | Scavenger receptor 81 (SR-81) |
| Fatty acid transport proteins (FATP) efflux transporters | |
| | ATP-binding cassette transporters; A8CA1, A8CG1, A8CG, A8CG8 |
| | Scavenger receptor 81 |
| | Putative transintestinal cholesterol efflux transporter |

Cells can also efflux sterols via free diffusion down their concentration gradient, a family of sterol efflux proteins called ATP-binding cassette transporters (ABC) [26], and UC, CE, TG, and PL can be exported by lipoprotein synthesis and secretion. Specialized cells such as enterocytes and hepatocytes can acquire UC through a sterol influx protein called the Niemann–Pick C1 like-1 protein (NPC1L1) which is expressed at both the jejunal lumen/enterocyte and the hepatobiliary interfaces [27]. Many cells express the scavenger receptor B1 (SR-B1) a bidirectional transporter which can participate in the efflux or influx of CE [28]. Sterols can also be effluxed from enterocytes and hepatocytes into the gut lumen or bile, respectively, using heterodimers of the sterol efflux transporters ABCG5 and ABCG8 [29]. Cells can also acquire UC and CE via receptors that internalize lipoproteins such as LDL receptors (LDLr) [30], LDL receptor-related proteins (LRP) [31], or ectopic β-chain of ATP synthase [32]. There are also putative receptors yet to be classified that perform these functions including an enterocyte protein involved with transintestinal cholesterol efflux (TICE) [33]. Cellular sterol homeostasis is regulated through synchronized action of all of the above mechanisms.

With respect to lipids, the human diet includes TG, FA, UC, CE, and phytosterols and to a lesser degree some stanols. Intestinal esterolases and lipases convert some of the ingested CE into UC and TG to FA and monoacylglycerols. However, after a meal the majority of the UC in the jejunum is of biliary origin. All of the lipids in the gut lumen are collectively organized and emulsified by lecithin (e.g., phosphatidylcholine) which is a phospholipid in biliary secretions. The lipids are then surrounded and organized by amphipathic bile acids into mixed biliary micelles which consist of mixtures of UC, phytosterols, stanols, phospholipids, monoacylglycerols, and FA. The micelles "ferry" these lipids to the epithelium of the intestinal microvilli. Once there, FA are absorbed into enterocytes by passive diffusion or fatty acid transport proteins [34]. The unesterified sterols, but not stanols, in the micelles are taken up by enterocytes via a sterol permease NPC1L1 protein, which utilizes other proteins (AP2-clathrin) to facilitate sterol absorption [35]. NPC1L1 is not involved with FA absorption and in part is regulated by PPAR-α and PPAR-Δ and is expressed at both the brush border of the intestinal epithelium and at the hepatobiliary cell junction [36]. Most humans absorb about 50 % of the sterols in the gut, but some people are hyperabsorbers (60–80 %) and some are hypoabsorbers (~20–40 %) [37]. NPC1L1 is also expressed at the hepatobiliary interface where it facilitates reentry of biliary UC back into the liver. Only UC, not esterified sterols, can be absorbed by NPC1L1. Once UC enters an enterocyte or hepatocyte, it is subject to esterification catalyzed by ACAT2 (acetyl-coenzyme A acetyltransferase 2) or within lipoproteins catalyzed by LCAT (lecithin–cholesteryl acyltransferase). Unlike UC, phytosterols are poor substrates for human ACAT and LCAT. Thus, ACAT2 in the enterocyte is a major regulator of sterol absorption [38]. Upon esterification of UC (the active and amphipathic form of cholesterol) becomes CE (the storage or transportation, hydrophobic form of cholesterol). In hepatocytes UC can upon exposure to 7α-hydroxylase be converted into the primary bile acids (cholate or chenodeoxycholate) which are effluxed into the biliary system via the bile salt export protein (ABCB11) [39].

## The Apolipoprotein B Family of Lipoproteins

In the endoplasmic reticulum of enterocytes and hepatocytes, CE via the action of microsomal TG transfer protein joins with TG and apolipoprotein $B_{48}$ (enterocyte) or $B_{100}$ (hepatocyte) to form primordial chylomicrons or VLDL, respectively. Phospholipidation and additional TG lipidation of the particle occurs at the Golgi apparatus resulting in mature TG-rich lipoproteins. Evidence suggests apolipoprotein A-V (apoA-V) may have an inhibitory effect on this process as apoA-V modulates VLDL TG mobilization as well as secretion [40]. Also involved as a regulator of chylomicron synthesis and lipid absorption is apolipoprotein A-IV (apoA-IV), which, because of its large size, functions as a

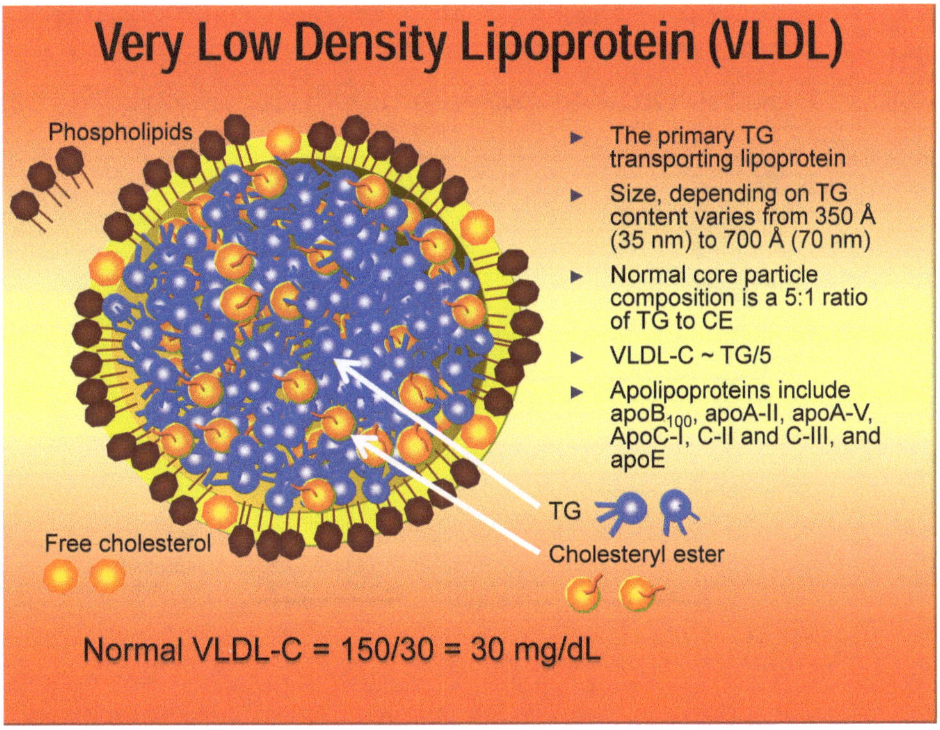


**Fig. 4.5** Very-low-density lipoprotein is a large TG-rich particle that carries several apoproteins: $ApoB_{100}$, ApoA-II, apoA-V, ApoC-I, apoC-II and apoC-III, and apoE. The primary function of VLDL is to traffic TG to myocytes and adipocytes and PL to the periphery. *Dayspring artwork*

stabilizing, expandable lipid interface, enhancing particle formation. Interestingly, through effects on the hypothalamus and vagus nerve (gastric), apoA-IV also serves as a mediator of satiety and appetite [41].

Under physiologic conditions the largest lipoproteins, chylomicrons and VLDLs, traffic large amounts of TG and PL, which are released during TG-hydrolysis (de-esterification) or lipolysis. Under fasting conditions Friedewald noted almost all of the plasma TG are trafficked within VLDL particles and a typical VLDL carries five times more TG than cholesterol and thus VLDL-C can be estimated by dividing TG/5 [21] (Fig. 4.5). That calculation changed the practice of clinical lipidology as it allowed clinicians to calculate LDL-C using the formula LDL-C = TC − [HDL-C + VLDL-C]. If one assumes a normal TG value is < 150 mg/dL, then a desirable VLDL-C is ≤ 30 mg/dL [42]. An American Heart Association expert panel recently defined an optimal TG to be < 100 mg/dL [43]. As hydrolysis of TG occurs during lipase-mediated lipolysis, the TG-rich lipoproteins shrink and shed much of their surface PL which are picked up by PLTP (phospholipid transfer protein) and delivered to cells or maturing HDL particles. As the large TG-rich VLDL loses its core and surface lipids, it becomes smaller and denser. An LDL is basically a VLDL that has lost its TG and is therefore a cholesterol-enriched lipoprotein with a core of four or more times CE than TG. Any LDL, independent of its size, that has an excess core TG will be necessarily CE-poor [44]. Normally HDLs traffic very little TG and their core is 90–95 % CE; hence, TG-rich HDLs will be cholesterol-poor which can cause a low HDL-C value. The apoB-containing lipoproteins acquire their core lipids during their genesis in enterocytes or hepatocytes, whereas the apoA-I particles are sterol lipidated via a variety of cell membrane efflux transporters.

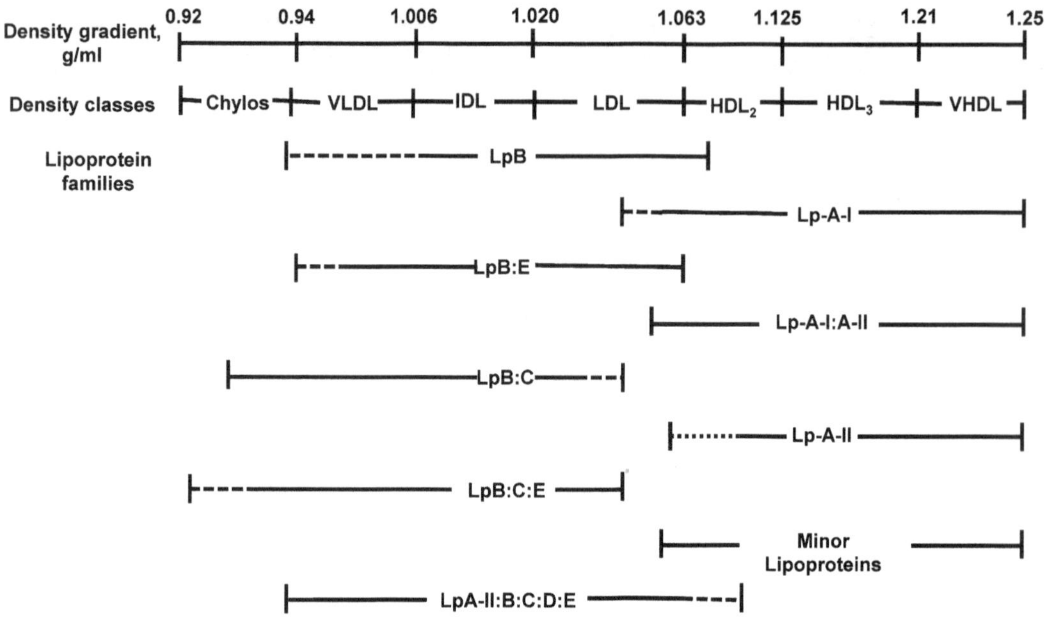


**Fig. 4.6** The relationship of individual apolipoprotein A (apoA)- and apoB-containing lipoprotein (Lp) families defined by their unique apolipoprotein composition to major lipoprotein density classes against the density (d) gradient background ($d$=0.92–1.25 g/mL). The lines under lipoprotein families designate the approximate density boundaries, with *solid lines* depicting the actual localization of each lipoprotein family and *dotted lines* the possible localization of each lipoprotein family. Lipoprotein families represent polydisperse systems of particles, each of which has a different lipid/protein ratio, but the same qualitative apolipoprotein composition. The polydisperse character of lipoprotein families is the main reason for their overlap within certain density segments (*Chylos* chylomicron, *HDL* high-density lipoprotein, *IDL* intermediate-density lipoprotein, *LDL* low-density lipoprotein, *VHDL* very high-density lipoprotein, *VLDL* very low density lipoprotein.) From Current Atherosclerosis Reports 2003, 5:459-467

Lipoproteins can also undergo additional lipidation or delipidation using a lipid transfer protein called apolipoprotein D (apoD) or cholesteryl ester transfer protein (CETP), which can exchange or swap one molecule of CE for CE, TG for TG, or CE for TG (often referred to as neutral lipids as they do not carry any charged group) [45]. The transfer of lipids between members of the apoB family themselves or the apoA-I family themselves is called a homotypic exchange, whereas the swapping of lipids between apoB and apoA-I particles is termed heterotypic. This lipid exchange is crucial to efficient lipid trafficking and dynamic remodeling of lipoproteins. Any lipoprotein acquiring TG will be subject to the lipolytic action of numerous lipases and, thus, TG-rich LDLs and HDLs would tend to become smaller and denser.

Other than apoB and apoA-I, there are numerous other apolipoproteins present on lipoproteins which perform multiple functions [46] (Fig. 4.6). All apoproteins but apoB are exchangeable, meaning they can transfer between lipoprotein species. Some act as ligands that direct and bind the lipoproteins to various cell membrane receptors or endothelial surface molecules, some are involved with activation or inactivation of various lipolytic enzymes such as lipoprotein lipase and other enzymes, and some serve as lipid acceptor proteins. Many of the apoproteins exist as genetically determined isoforms, which create individual and population differences in lipoprotein metabolism. Apart from apoproteins related to lipoprotein modulation, HDLs also transport numerous other proteins (over 50 have been identified), many of which are immunomodulatory

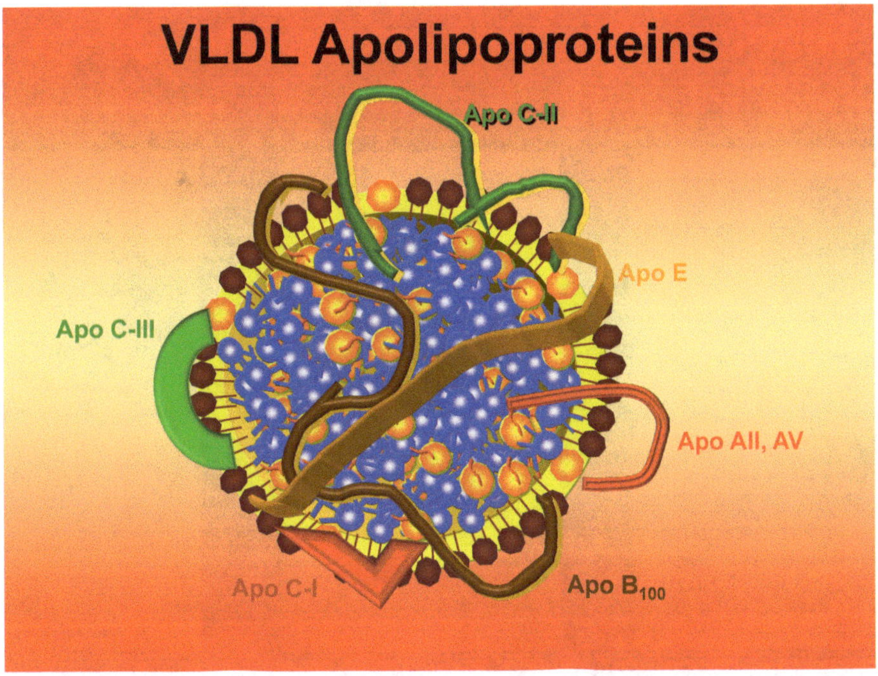


**Fig. 4.7** Very-low-density lipoprotein is a large TG-rich particle that carries several apolipoproteins. C-II is a ligand for lipoprotein lipase. ApoC-I blocks LPL, HL, CETP, LCAT, VLDLr, and LDLr. ApoC-II binds to and activates LPL. ApoC-III interferes with apoC-II/LPL binding and apoE binding to receptors. ApoB is a ligand for LDL receptor. ApoE is a ligand for the LDL, VLDL receptor, and the LDL receptor-related protein (LRP). C-III inhibits the action of LPL and the ability of apoE to act with receptors. ApoA-II inhibits VLDL lipolysis and apoA-V helps bind TG-rich lipoproteins to HSPG in areas of LPL expression. *Dayspring artwork*

in function. Collectively they are referred to as the HDL proteome [47].

Under normal physiologic conditions when lipoproteins have the proper core ratios of lipids, the following lipid trafficking pathways are operative. TG-rich chylomicrons are secreted into the lymphatic circulation (chylomicrons) where they make their way into plasma and join hepatically excreted TG-rich VLDLs. ApoA-V is part of TG-rich lipoprotein formation [48] and traffics with the particle as do multiple copies of apolipoprotein C-II (apoC-II), a ligand for LPL, and apolipoprotein C-I (apoC-I) and C-III (apoC-III) [49–51] (Fig. 4.7). ApoA-I is synthesized in hepatocytes and jejunal enterocytes and is secreted into plasma where it is rapidly lipidated but some apoA-I is also initially carried into plasma on chylomicron surfaces [52]. Delipidation of TG-rich particles or lipolysis occurs as TGs are hydrolyzed by lipoprotein lipase (LPL), a potent triglyceridase upregulated in large part by insulin in muscle and adipocyte vascular beds [53]. ApoA-V is important in the docking of TG-rich lipoproteins to heparan sulfate proteoglycans (HSPGs) in endothelial cell lipid rafts in the area of LPL expression and thus enhances lipolysis. ApoA-V is also involved with docking to the LDLr and LRP [54]. Chylomicron lipolysis is normally quite rapid due to the large size of these particles which contain multiple copies of apoC-II (an activator of LPL) resulting in smaller, TG-poorer particles called "chylomicron remnants." Two proteins, lipase maturation factor 1 (LMF1) and glycosylphosphatidylinositol-anchored high-density lipoprotein-binding protein 1 (GPIHBP1), regulate LPL maturation and binding and thus are important mediators of TG-rich lipoprotein lipolysis [55]. LPL is synthesized in the endoplasmic reticulum of myocytes and adipocytes where LMF 1 plays an essential role in the formation of catalytically active LPL, a process called lipase maturation, which then

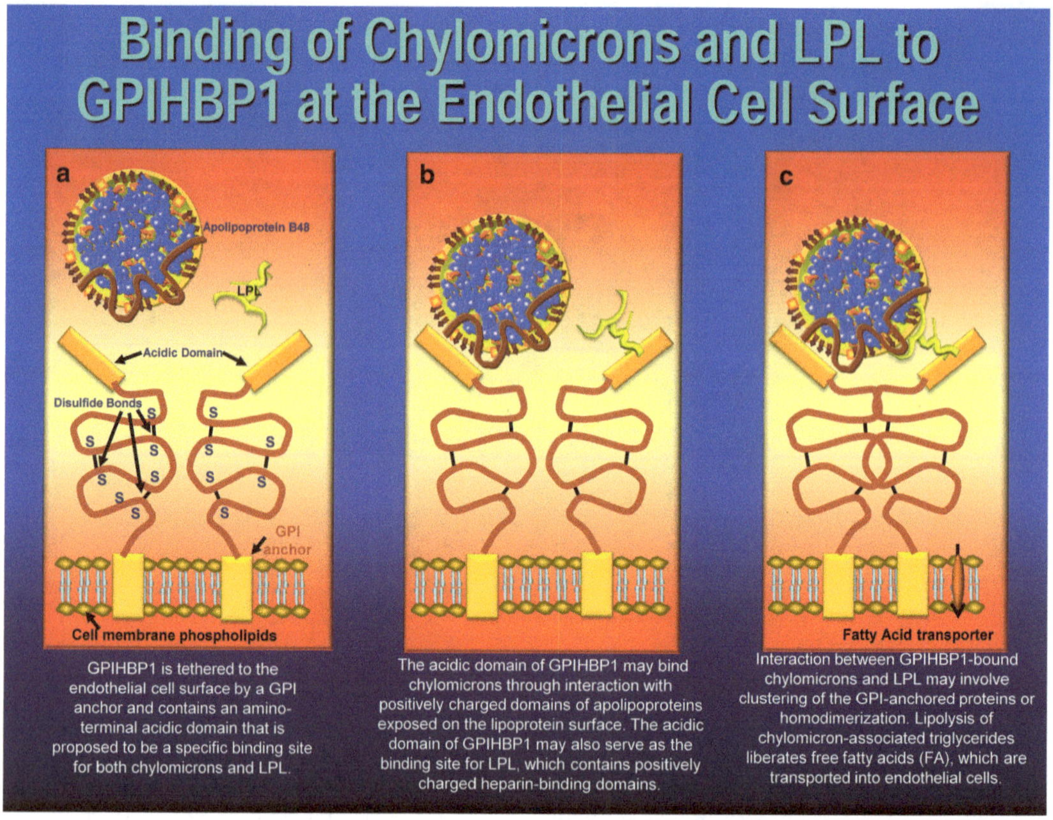


**Fig. 4.8** Adapted from Ory DS. Chylomicrons and lipoprotein lipase at the endothelial surface (reference [56] in the chapter). Model for binding of chylomicrons and LpL to GPIHBP1 at the endothelial cell surface. (**a**) GPIHBP1 is tethered to the endothelial cell surface by a GPI anchor and contains an amino-terminal acidic domain that is proposed to be a specific binding site for both chylomicrons and LpL. (**b**) The acidic domain of GPIHBP1 may bind chylomicrons through interaction with positively charged domains of apolipoproteins exposed on the lipoprotein surface. The acidic domain of GPIHBP1 may also serve as the binding site for LpL, which contains positively charged heparin-binding domains. (**c**) Interaction between GPIHBP1-bound chylomicrons and LpL may involve clustering of the GPI-anchored proteins or homodimerization. Lipolysis of chylomicron-associated triglycerides liberates free fatty acids (FA), which are transported into endothelial cells

translocates to the luminal surface of endothelial cells where it binds to HSPGs. GPIHBP1 provides a platform for apoC-II binding to LPL. In vascular endothelial cells where GPIHBP1 is expressed, lipid rafts also express syndecan1 and fatty acid transporters such as CD-36 [56] (Fig. 4.8). ApoA-V also facilitates interactions between the TG-rich lipoproteins and GPIHBP1 [57].

ApoA-IV contributes to lipolysis by facilitating efficient release of apoC-II from either HDL or VLDL, and once apoC-II is anchored by GPIHBP1, it binds to and activates LPL [53], resulting in hydrolysis of TG in chylomicrons or VLDL [58]. The resultant remnants are ultimately internalized by VLDL receptors in extrahepatic tissues [59] and by hepatic LDLr and LRP using apolipoprotein E (apoE) as a ligand. Another important regulator of TG-rich lipoprotein lipolysis is apoC-I which inhibits the binding of VLDL by LDLr, LRP or the VLDL receptor [60]. Such inhibition of TG-rich lipoprotein binding to lipoprotein receptors is thought to be due to the ability of apoC-I to alter or camouflage the conformation of apoE on TG-rich lipoprotein or to displace apoE from these particles. ApoC-I is also known to inhibit LPL, hepatic lipase (HL), phospholipase A2, as well as CETP [61], where it accounts for most of the CETP-inhibitory activity that is associated with human plasma HDL [62]. A chylomicron half-life is normally less than an hour, whereas VLDL lipolysis ranges from 2 to 6 h.

ApoC-III is synthesized in hepatocytes and enterocytes and is also a potent regulator of lipolysis [63]. It is present in three isoforms related to the number of sialic acid molecules (0, 1, or 2) terminating the oligosaccharidic portions of the protein, apoC-$III_0$, apoC-$III_1$, and apoC-$III_2$. In plasma the isoform makeup is ~10, 55, and 35 % of the total apoC-III levels. ApoC-$III_1$ and apoC-III2 correlate more with TG levels than apoC-$III_0$ and apoC-$III_2$ is associated with generation of small LDL. Collectively apoC-III stimulates VLDL assembly and secretion, inhibits LPL, in part by affecting binding of TG-rich lipoproteins to HSPG, and interferes with VLDLr, LRP, and LDLr uptake of lipoproteins [64, 65].

As the TG molecules are hydrolyzed by lipoprotein lipase to FA and monoacylglycerols, the TG-rich lipoproteins shrink, resulting in the loss of large amounts of their surface PL as well as some surface apolipoproteins. ApoC-III redistributes from VLDL to HDL and becomes ready for reuse and subsequent retransfer back to newly synthesized VLDL particles [66]. The now smaller particles carrying much less TG and PL still have their CE core: such particles are called VLDL and chylomicron remnants. The particles which were formerly TG-rich are now much less TG-rich and are trafficking primarily CE. The FA released from the TG can enter myocytes to be oxidized for energy, enter adipocytes and be reconverted to and stored as TG, or bind to albumin and be trafficked for use elsewhere. The PL can be taken up by the cell membranes or bind to phospholipid transfer proteins (PLTP) and carried to other cells or to maturing (lipidating) HDL particles. Ultimately, VLDL size decreases and density increases to the point where they become IDLs which under normal circumstances are rapidly removed by hepatic LDLr to which they dock via their $apoB_{100}$ and apoE. This receptor attachment is aided by HL, which has both triglyceridase and phospholipase properties resulting in additional particle lipolysis creating apoB-containing LDL particles. LDL is a predominantly cholesterol-rich lipoprotein with a core TG/CE ratio of ≥4:1 [67]. The LDLs typically circulate for 1.5 to 3 days before most (90 %) are cleared by hepatic LDLr [68]. During their plasma residence time, LDLs are subject to homotypic exchange via CETP of their core CE for TG with VLDLs or heterotypic exchange with HDLs. CETP-mediated exchange of neutral lipids can be inhibited by apoC-I and apolipoprotein F (apoF) [69]. Since every cell in humans can synthesize cholesterol de novo, very little LDL-mediated delivery of cholesterol is necessary. Persons with hypobetalipoproteinemia have very low levels of LDL-C and suffer no cholesterol deficiency consequences [70]. Normally LDLs are cleared by LDLr binding to apoB and the process of LDLs returning their core CE to the liver, much of which originated in HDLs, is termed "indirect reverse cholesterol transport."

## The Apolipoprotein A-I Family of Lipoproteins

Aside from the apoB particles whose main mission is to traffic TG and phospholipids is the HDL family of apoA-I lipoproteins. Unlike chylomicrons and VLDLs, HDLs are created not in enterocytes or hepatocytes, but rather in plasma by the lipidation of secreted apoA-I and apolipoprotein A-II (apoA-II). Regulated primarily by peroxisomal proliferator-activated receptor-α (PPAR-α), apoA-I is produced and released by hepatocytes and enterocytes. The unique helical structure of apoA-I gives it an affinity for cholesterol binding. Lipidation occurs along cell membrane surfaces with excess UC; activation of the liver X receptor (LXR) in turn upregulates cell membrane cholesterol efflux proteins including ABCA1. Unlipidated apoA-I accepts effluxed UC and PL, creating pre-beta HDL species. ApoA-I lipidation activates lecithin–cholesteryl acyltransferase-α (LCAT-α) which catalyzes the transfer of fatty acids from the sn2 position of PL to the 3-hydroxy group on UC, changing the amphipathic UC into the hydrophobic CE. The molecular polarity change drives the CE away from the apoA-I particle surface of the

HDL to its core explaining why, as the HDL matures, it converts from a discoidal to a spherical particle. ApoA-IV in HDL can activate LCAT and in free form in both lymph and plasma may also play critical roles in mediating ABCA1 cholesterol efflux. Additional HDL lipidation occurs via attachment of larger, more mature HDL species to ABCG1 sterol efflux transporters, SR-B1, or even by free diffusion from cells into larger HDL species [66]. As the HDL matures, it picks up, transfers, and reacquires numerous proteins (its proteome), including several apoproteins involved with lipoprotein catabolism and clearance including CETP, the apoC family, apoE, apolipoprotein A-II (apoA-II), apolipoprotein L (apoL), and apolipoprotein M (apoM), and others involved in a multitude of functions [71].

With respect to trafficking UC and CE, the vast majority (> 90 %) of HDL lipidation occurs via ABCA1 expression at the liver, small intestine, and adipocyte tissue [72].

In effect a serum HDL-C represents cholesterol derived from the gut and the liver and is not a reflection of peripheral cholesterol efflux. This suggests that HDLs evolved not solely to perform RCT but also delivery of hepatic- and enterocytic-derived UC elsewhere, primarily to steroidogenic tissues and adipocytes [73]. The likely reason HDLs have a 5-day half-life is to serve as a rapidly available supply of CE for the adrenal cortex under stressful hypercorticoid conditions like inflammation and infection [74] and as a repository for urgently needed immunoproteins. Because of those functions, many refer to HDLs as an innate part of the immune system [75]. A major part of HDL's antiatherogenic potential is the ability to efflux both CE and UC from sterol-laden macrophages (foam cells) in atherosclerotic plaque referred to as macrophage reverse cholesterol transport (ΩRCT). Compared to total body cholesterol, the amount of cholesterol in plaque is very small, and ΩRCT, although cardioprotective, does not contribute significantly to a serum HDL-C value [76]. Other than trafficking cholesterol to the tissues mentioned above, HDLs through numerous pathways can facilitate fecal excretion of cholesterol. HDLs can return UC and CE to the liver where it is delipidated by SR-B1, or endocytosed by LDLr (using apoE as a ligand), or the ectopic β chain of ATP synthase (holoparticle) receptor [77]. HDLs can also be delipidated by a putative enterocyte receptor and the UC exported to the gut lumen via ABCG5 and ABCG8 transporters in a process now termed transintestinal cholesterol efflux or TICE [33]. HDLs returning cholesterol to the liver or gut is called direct RCT. However, a major part of RCT is HDLs heterotypically exchanging its CE for TG with apoB particles (chylomicrons, VLDLs, IDLs, and primarily LDLs). The apoB particles now carrying a CE load acquired from HDLs are cleared by the liver, in essence returning substantial cholesterol in what is now called indirect RCT. Total RCT is the sum of direct and indirect RCT and it should be clear that a serum HDL-C by itself has no relationship with this complex and dynamic HDL-mediated trafficking of cholesterol system [78]. The TG-rich HDLs undergo additional lipolysis utilizing HL and endothelial lipase [79]. During this process some apoA-I is shed and is cleared via cubilin and megalin in renal tubules [80]. In effect, apoA-I is constantly being synthesized, secreted, lipidated, delipidated, and ultimately cleared by the liver, gut, or kidney.

In summary, lipid homeostasis, fatty acids, and cholesterol, derived mostly from the liver and gut, but also peripheral cells, are trafficked as components of lipoproteins: FA for energy and cell membranes, and cholesterol for cell membranes and steroidogenesis. Excess cholesterol in the form of UC and CE is returned to the gut for fecal elimination or to the liver where UC is secreted into bile or converted to a bile acid for potential fecal excretion or become part of a newly formed VLDL or effluxed to a prebeta HDL. The system obviously is complex and mediated by dozens of genes, enzymes, proteins, and receptors, and pathology in any of those will negatively affect lipid (energy and sterol) homeostasis.

## Insulin Resistance and Type 2 Diabetes

For the remainder of this chapter, lipoprotein pathophysiology related to insulin resistance (IR) and/or T2DM will be reviewed. A normal person is sensitive to the hormone insulin which regulates carbohydrate and fatty acid metabolism, lipogenesis, lipolysis, and, hence, energy homeostasis. Insulin mediates the uptake of glucose into cells where in muscles and liver it can be converted to and stored as glycogen. In IR there is impaired signaling via the phosphoinositol-3 kinase pathway allowing the buildup of toxic lipid metabolites, such as FA acyl CoA, diacylglycerol, and ceramide in numerous tissues including the liver, pancreatic beta cells, and adipocytes [81]. It is the IR-related lipid-mediated macrovascular complications, in large part related to atherothrombotic events, that result in the high morbidity and mortality risk seen in T2DM.

*Cholesterol Synthesis and Absorption*: Major epidemiological trials like Framingham Offspring [82], PROCAM [please define acronym 83], and Cardiovascular Risk in Young Finns Study [84] have related increased CV risk in patients with increased levels of phytosterols which are measurable markers of sterol absorption. Miettinen showed that in the Scandinavian Simvastatin Survival Study (4S), a high-risk secondary prevention trial of statin-/placebo-treated patients with high LDL-C, hypoabsorbers did and hyperabsorbers did not have a beneficial effect of simvastatin, theoretically because hyperabsorbers are typically hyposynthesizers of cholesterol and therefore less likely to be responsive to a statin [85]. In the DEBATE [Drugs and Evidence-Based Medicine in the Elderly] study, low-cholesterol absorption was associated with fewer recurrent cardiovascular events and with better survival in elderly patients despite frequent abnormalities of glucose metabolism [86]. Intestinal function is abnormal in diabetics and several enterocytic sterol homeostatic regulatory changes occur in IR patients. Conflicting studies have described T2DM as having either reduced [87] or increased cholesterol absorption [88]. A recent study demonstrated cholesterol absorption was highest in the lean insulin-sensitive participants, whereas cholesterol synthesis was highest in the lean IR and obese IR participants [89]. In another experiment 3-hydroxy-3-methylglutaryl coenzyme A (HMGCoA) reductase, the rate-limiting enzyme for cholesterol synthesis, is increased in animal models of diabetes in both the liver and small intestine [90].

Rats made diabetic by injection of streptozotocin are hyperabsorbers of cholesterol which was explained by changes in intestinal absorption-regulating proteins, namely, an upregulation of NPC1L1, ACAT2, and microsomal triglyceride transfer protein (MTP) and a reduced expression of ABCG5 and ABCG8 [91]. Lally et al. showed that diabetic patients had more NPC1L1 mRNA than the control subjects ($p<0.02$) and expression of ABCG5 and ABCG8 mRNA was lower in the diabetic patients ($p<0.05$) and MTP expression was increased ($p<0.05$). There was a positive correlation between NPLC1L1 and MTP mRNA ($p<0.01$) and a negative correlation between NPC1L1 and ABCG5 mRNA ($p<0.001$) [92]. In addition, an increase in apolipoprotein $B_{48}$ synthesis has been demonstrated in animal models of diabetes and insulin resistance. Generally, apoB synthesis and utilization is driven by increased lipid substrate availability. Hyperabsorption is a manifestation of intestinal dysfunction and leads to abnormal chylomicron composition which, via the action of CETP, will directly influence the composition of other circulating lipoproteins [93].

Experts have speculated on whether knowing one is or is not a hyperabsorber or hypersynthesizer of cholesterol would be useful in deciding on lifestyle and drug therapies, and there are both null and supporting data on this. Certainly, statins and statins plus cholesterol absorption inhibitors such as ezetimibe improve lipid and lipoprotein abnormalities in T2DM [94]. Of interest is that potent statin monotherapy can significantly increase cholesterol and noncholesterol sterol absorption, which has the potential to offset some of the benefit of inhibiting synthesis [95].

## The TG/HDL Axis: ApoB-Containing Lipoproteins

The major lipid abnormality in T2DM has been called a TG/HDL axis disorder and is characterized by variable TC and LDL-C but elevations of fasting and often postprandial TG and reductions in HDL-C [96]. Underlying these lipid concentration abnormalities are significant changes in the number, size, core lipid composition, and proteome of lipoproteins. It then becomes crucial to understand what happens to previously described lipoprotein genesis and trafficking of lipids in the IR patient with TG/HDL abnormalities. Clinicians are going to have to respect the pathology related to TG-rich lipoproteins and TG levels which heretofore were not deemed to be of concern (<150 mg/dL). Typically the liver in IR patients has increased pools of retained lipids, especially that of TG which results from an imbalance between the uptake and synthesis of fatty acids and their oxidation and export [97]. Both hyperinsulinemia and hyperglycemia induce the expression of the lipogenic gene-activating hepatic sterol regulatory element-binding protein 1c (SREBP1c) and the carbohydrate-responsive element-binding protein (ChREBP) [98].

The more lipid substrate (especially triglycerides) available in the hepatocyte or enterocyte cytosol, the more apoB will be lipidated rather than catabolized (Fig. 4.9). Insulin reduces MTP expression via activation of the mitogen-activated protein kinase (MAPK) pathway [99]. Normally, lipidation of apoB creates a primordial VLDL that evolves into a normally composed, sized, and secretable VLDL2 [100]. Secretion of VLDL2 is the same in IR and insulin-sensitive subjects. When there is a lack of lipid pool, there is improper folding and rapid degradation of apoB and less VLDL is produced [101]. The major cause of hypertriglyceridemia in the HOMA-IR person is the increased availability of free FA substrate causing hepatic overproduction and secretion of larger TG-rich VLDL1, resulting in increased plasma concentrations of apoB and TG [102] (Figs. 4.9 and 4.10). A recent nutritional study demonstrated apoB production had a strong relation with dietary fructose and especially fructose corn syrup and not glucose [103]. In a kinetic study, plasma glucose, insulin, and free fatty acids together explained 55 % of the variation in VLDL1 TG production rate [104]. The large VLDL1 seen in T2DM are normally suppressed by insulin, but not when IR is present. The apoB100-containing VLDL2 are converted to VLDL1 by the addition of a major load of triglycerides in the endoplasmic reticulum (the same is true of enterocyte $apoB_{48}$ and chylomicron formation). VLDL1 creation also is dependent upon ADP ribosylation factor 1 (a small GTP-binding protein) which is involved with translocation from ER to the Golgi apparatus where final synthesis including much of the TG acquisition and phospholipidation occurs [105, 106]. The time between $apoB_{100}$ production and lipidation to create large VLDL1 is approximately 15 min [105]. Insulin resistance results in diminished phosphatidylinositol-3-kinase that may add to the increased VLDL secretion [107]. In humans, the mean residence time of VLDL1 apoB is the main determinant of apoB pool size and of plasma TG concentration [108]. There is an increased production of VLDL1, as well as a reduction in the catabolic rate of apoB-containing lipoproteins, in particular IDL and LDL.

**Fig. 4.9** (**a**) Adapted from Arterioscler Thromb Vasc Biol. 2008;28:1225-1236 [reference 109 in chapter]. The assembly process starts in the rough endoplasmic reticulum (ER) by the biosynthesis and concomitant (cotranslational) translocation of apolipoprotein B100 (apoB100) to the lumen of this organelle. ApoB100 interacts cotranslationally with the microsomal triglyceride transfer protein (MTP) and is thereby lipidated to form a primordial particle (pre-VLDL). Alternatively, apoB100 fails to be lipidated and misfolds. This results in a sorting to degradation. Thus, the protein is unfolded and retracted to cytosol, ubiquitinated, and sorted to proteasomal degradation. Pre-VLDL is converted to VLDL2 late in the ER compartment. VLDL2 exits the ER at specific exit sites of this organelle by Sar1/Cop II vesicles, which fuse to become the ER–Golgi intermediate compartment (ERGIC) (7). ERGIC fuses with Cis-Golgi. In the Golgi apparatus, VLDL2 is converted to VLDL1 by the addition of a bulk load of triglycerides. This lipidation process differs from that which gives rise to pre-VLDL and VLDL2. The formation of VLDL1 may involve the formation of a lipid droplet in the lumen of the secretory pathway. The mechanism behind the formation of lipid droplets in the secretory pathway may follow that of cytosolic lipid droplets. Such droplets are formed from the microsomal membranes under the influence of the enzymes phospholipase D1 and ERK2 as well as of adipocyte differentiation-related protein (also known as adipophilin and caveolin). The formation of the cytosolic droplets also involves a fusion step that is dependent on microtubules and the motor protein dynein. (**b**) Triglycerides, VLDL, and apolipoprotein B. Adapted from Adiels M et al. Arterioscler Thromb Vasc Biol. 2005;25:1697-1703 [Reference 104 in chapter]

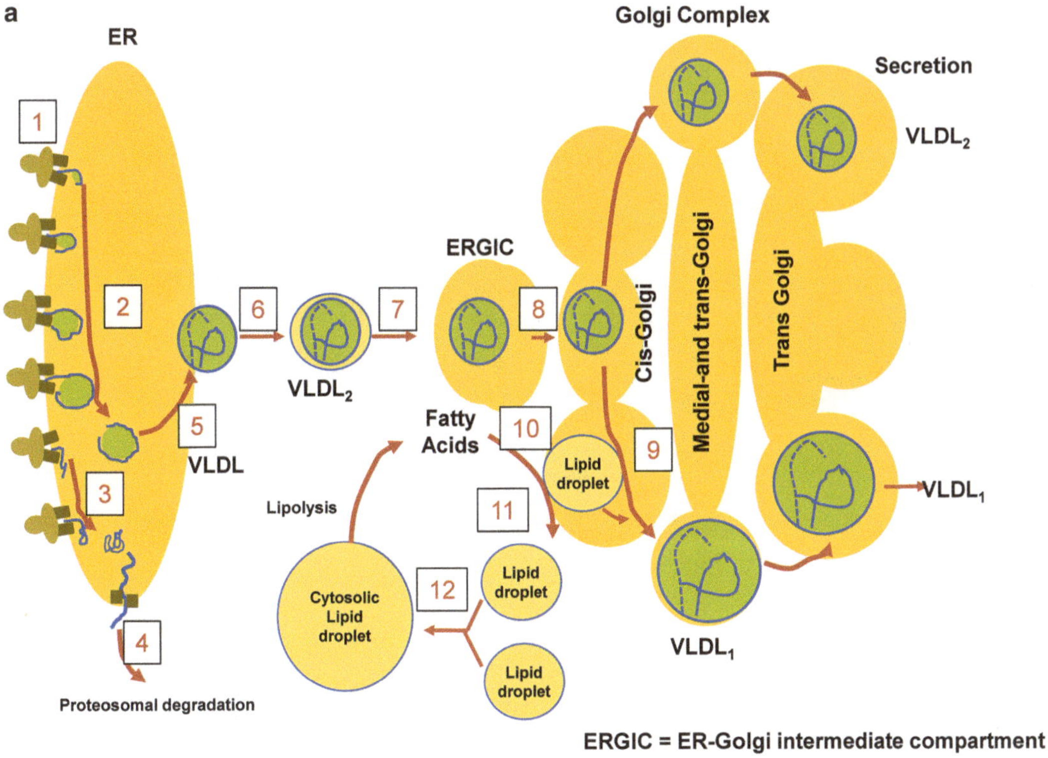


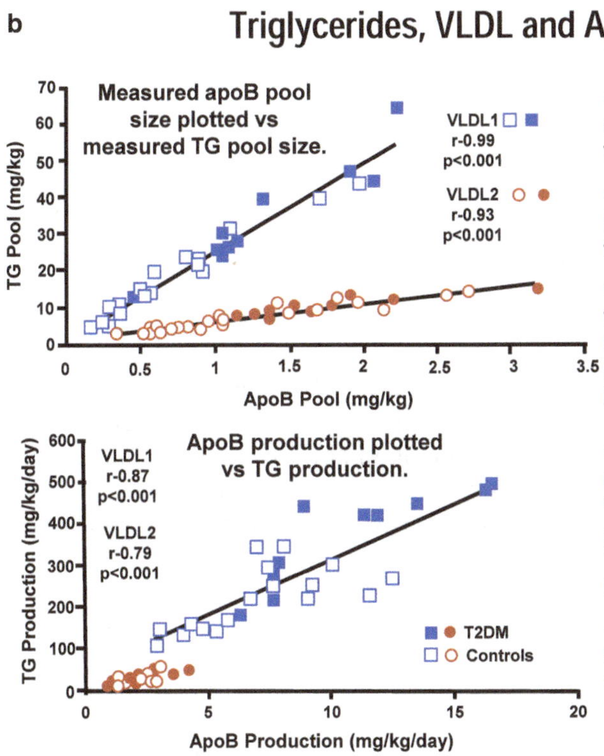


- There was a strong, linear correlation between the apoB and TG pools in both VLDL1 and VLDL2.
- The VLDL1 pools were significantly larger in DM2 than in controls (P<0.01), although data for all subjects plot on the same line.
- The same strong correlation was observed in the subgroups VLDL1 (controls, r=0.97, P<0.001; DM2, r=0.97, P<0.001) and VLDL2 (controls, r0.95, P0.001; DM2, r=0.92, P<0.001)

- There was a strong, linear correlation between apoB and TG production in both VLDL1 and VLDL2 and a significantly higher production of both VLDL1 apoB and VLDL1 TG in DM2 than in control subjects (apoB, P<0.01; TG, P<0.001).
- The TG-apoB ratio of VLDL1 and VLDL2 (ie, the slope of the lines) showed no significant differenced between DM2 and control subjects

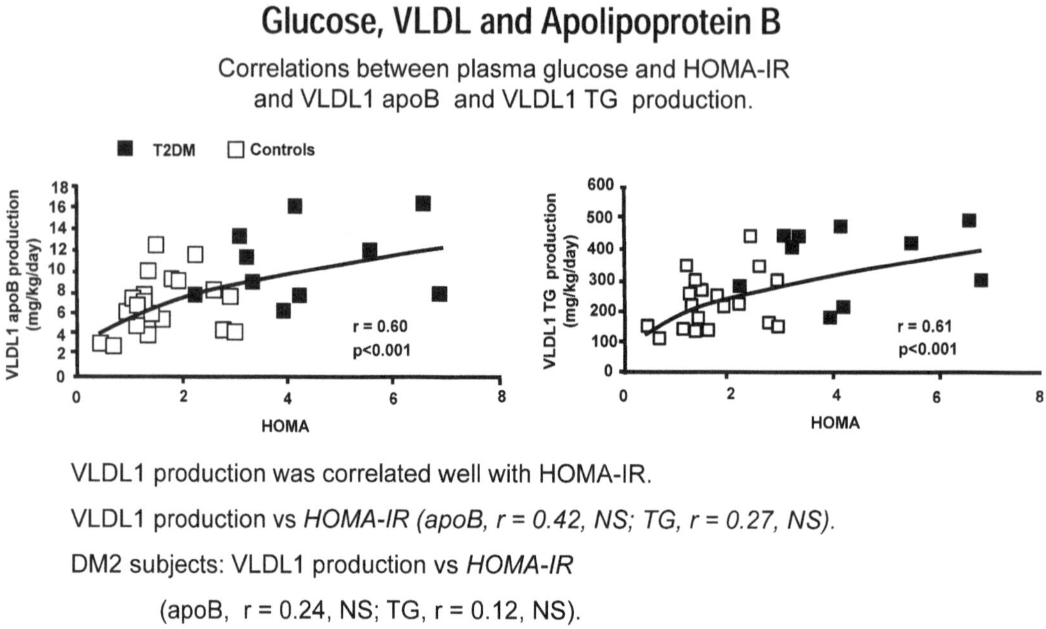


**Fig. 4.10** Glucose, VLDL, and apolipoprotein B. Adapted from Adiels M et al. Arterioscler Thromb Vasc Biol. 2005;25:1697-1703 [Reference 104 in chapter]

Collectively this leads to increased levels of apoB related to large VLDL-P and LDL-P. The catabolism of apoA-I, the main apolipoprotein of HDL, is increased by 48 %, but apoA-I production is increased by 25 %, probably because of some compensatory effect. This production/clearance imbalance results in a 16 % reduction in the concentration of HDL apoA-I [109] (Fig. 4.11). Garvey et al. in an elegant insulin clamp study analyzing NMR-derived particle concentrations showed that as the patients' status progressed from insulin sensitive to insulin resistance to T2DM, there are increases of VLDL-P, IDL-P, and most especially LDL-P [110].

VLDL lipolysis is delayed in T2DM due to several mechanisms. As previously mentioned several apolipoproteins are involved with efficient VLDL catabolism including apoE, apoA-II, apoA-IV, apoA-V, ApoC-I, apoC-II, apoC-III, apoD, and apoF. Many of those apolipoproteins have altered function in IR persons and T2DM. Ultimately lipolysis of TG-rich lipoproteins requires apoC-II to activate LPL and thus release of apoC-II from either HDL or VLDL allows for LPL-mediated hydrolysis of TG in nascent chylomicrons and VLDLs [111]. In a small study of diabetic patients vs. normolipemic controls who had TG-tolerance tests, the diabetics displayed typical postprandial hypertriglyceridemia, but although apoA-V levels were similar in the two groups, paradoxically the diabetics had increased postprandial apoA-V in non-HDL particles which is suggestive that apoA-V is not involved in the regulation of TG in the postprandial state [112]. In another study, the postprandial (after an oral fat load) increase of apoA-V was confirmed and was related to plasma TG and VLDL1-TG but also to apoC-III. It was thought the increase of apoA-V simply reflected the increase of VLDL particles related to apoC-III overproduction [113]. *ApoA-V* genotypes do not appear to have an impact on risk of development of T2DM [114].

ApoC family members are crucial to the synthesis of TG-rich lipoproteins as well as their lipolysis and catabolism. High concentrations of ApoC-I and ApoC-III are associated with increased triglycerides in men with the metabolic syndrome. These findings in humans were first seen in Hyplip2 congenic mouse strain studies which

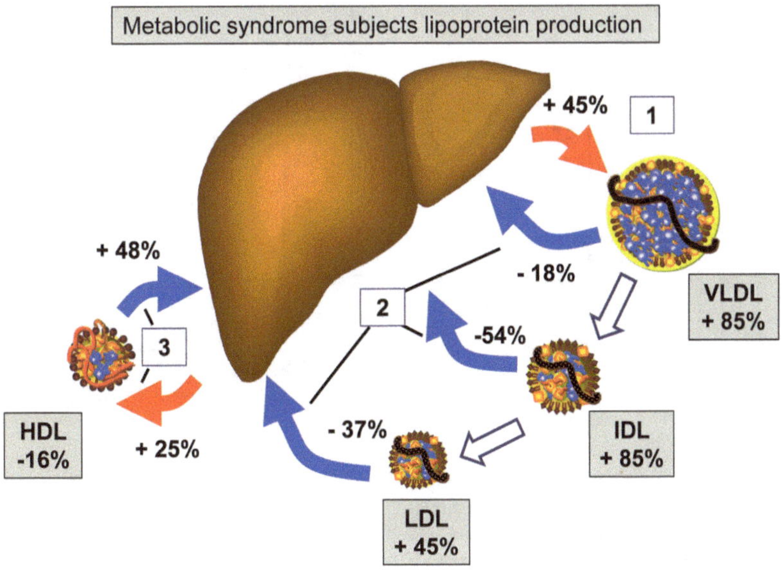


**Fig. 4.11** Adapted from Arterioscler Thromb Vasc Biol. 2008;28:1225-1236 [reference 109 in chapter]. Changes in lipoprotein metabolism in T2DM and the metabolic syndrome. Subjects diagnosed with the metabolic syndrome display, most noticeably, an increased production of VLDL (1), and there is a reduction in the catabolic rate of apoB-containing lipoproteins, in particular IDL and LDL (2). Together, these result in increased concentrations of apoB-containing lipoproteins. The catabolism of apoA-I, the main apolipoprotein of HDL, is increased by 48 %, but apoA-I production is increased by 25 %, probably because of some compensatory effect (3). This results in a 16 % reduction in the concentration of HDL apoA-I

related the elevated TG to delayed catabolism of VLDL, which in turn led to decreased FA delivery to visceral adipose tissue [115]. In obese males with the metabolic syndrome, apoC-I and ApoC-III levels were mainly related to the visceral adipose tissue (VAT) compartment (measured using nuclear magnetic resonance). This was related to a higher expression of LPL in VAT versus subcutaneous adipose tissue (SAT). The ApoC-I and ApoC-III inhibition of LPL therefore contributed to both higher TG and lower VAT area in human subjects. The difference in effect of ApoC-I and ApoC-III on TG concentrations in this study underlines the stronger inhibition of LPL by ApoC-III compared with ApoC-I [116] (Figs. 4.12 and 4.13).

All apoCs are distributed in a cycling process between TG-rich apoB lipoproteins and HDL. In the fasting state, apoC-II and apoC-III are equally distributed between HDL and VLDL, whereas apoC-I is mostly trafficked with HDL (>90 %). Thus, in the exchange of apolipoproteins after a meal, more apoC-I is transferred than other apoCs. The apoC-I enrichment of TRLs after a meal affects particle catabolism and is involved with the formation of VLDL and chylomicron CE-rich atherogenic remnants. A paradox is that apoC-I is not known to interfere with TG hydrolysis as studies have shown that apoC-I-enriched TRLs undergo normal hydrolysis forming smaller TRLs and remnants. Because apoC-I is a potent inhibitor of apoE-mediated uptake of TG-rich lipoproteins by LDLr, VLDLr, and LRP, particle clearance is impaired. ApoC-I-enriched particles which have compositional abnormalities (TG-rich) have increased plasma residence time allowing CETP-mediated exchange of core TG for CE utilizing heterotypic and homotypic pathways which over time make the remnants even more CE-rich. Numerous studies have demonstrated that CE-rich remnants are atherogenic, and delayed remnant clearance during the postprandial state is a well-established feature of patients with coronary artery disease (CAD) [117]. Interestingly ApoC-I is a more potent inhibitor of CETP when it is on HDL but not the apoB

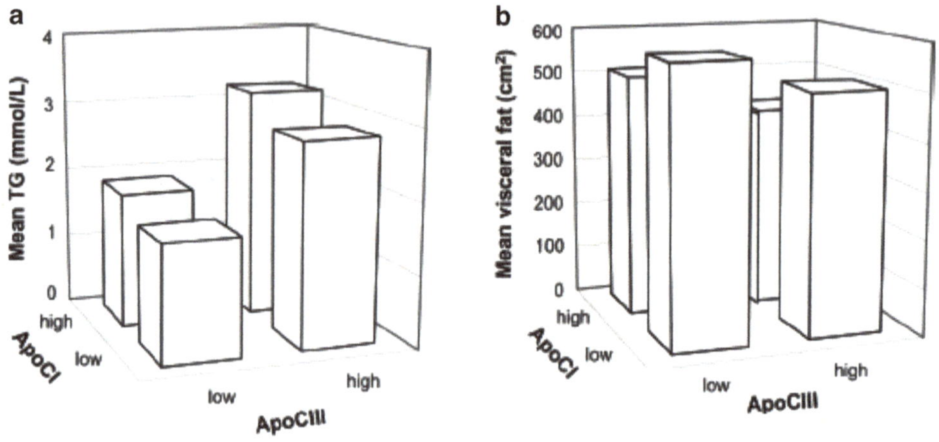


**Fig. 4.12** Illustration of the inverse relationship of ApoC-I and ApoC-III concentrations with plasma triglyceride concentration (*positive*, **a**) and with visceral adipose tissue area (*negative*, **b**). ApoC-I/ApoC-III median/mean low, ApoC-I/ApoC-III median/mean high. Groups: (1) low ApoC-I and ApoC-III ($n=35$), (2) high ApoC-I/low ApoC-III ($n=21$), (3) low ApoC-I/high ApoC-III ($n=14$), and (4) high ApoC-I and ApoC-III ($n=28$). Triglyceride concentration: 1 vs. 3, 1 vs. 4, and 2 vs. 4: $p<0.001$. 2 vs. 3: $p<0.01$. Visceral adipose tissue area: low ApoC-I and apoC-III vs. high ApoC-I and ApoC-III: $p<0.001$. From van der Ham RL, Alizadeh Dehnavi R, Berbée JF, Putter H, de Roos A, Romijn JA, Rensen PC, Tamsma JT. Diabetes Care. 2009;32:184-6 [Reference 116 in chapter]

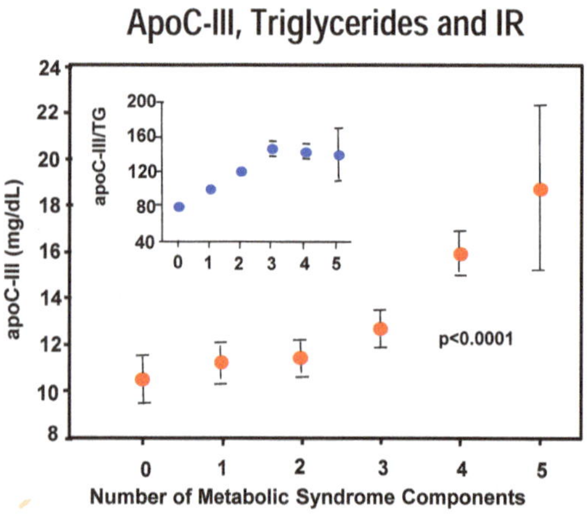


**Fig. 4.13** Mean of apoC-III concentration according to the number of metabolic syndrome components. Data normalized for TG values (*figure inset*) show statistically significant trends for the apoC-III/TG ratio ($p<0.0001$). Hermes Florez et al. Atherosclerosis 2006;188:134-141

particles. Thus, the transfer of apoC-I from HDL to TG-rich lipoproteins facilitate atherogenic remnant formation, suggesting a dual role of apoC-I: (1) preventing remnant formation and premature atherosclerosis if attached to HDL and (2) promoting remnant formation and atherosclerosis if transferred to TG-rich lipoproteins [118]. ApoC-I content of postprandial TG-rich lipoproteins has been shown to be a risk factor for early atherosclerosis in normolipidemic healthy middle-aged men, supporting the conclusion that the enrichment of remnant lipoproteins with cholesterol is not favorable. ApoC-I on TG-rich lipoproteins has been linked to increased CIMT [119] (Fig. 4.14). There are not a lot of published studies evaluating apoC-I, per se, in diabetes. In an evaluation of women with PCOS, those with IR were characterized by statistically significantly elevated levels of apoC-I compared with those of non-IR patients. ApoC-I correlated with BMI, TG, HDL-C, apoA-I, and HOMA-IR [120].

ApoC-III is perhaps the most complex and enigmatic apolipoprotein. For some time, it has been known that apoC-III-enriched particles were a significant CHD risk factor. ApoC-III levels are associated with hypertriglyceridemia, increases in VLDL-P and VLDL-TG, and inversely related to the size of LDL particles [121]. In the Cholesterol and Recurrent Events (CARE) trial, both the plasma concentrations of VLDL particles and apoC-III in VLDL and LDL were better predictors of coronary heart disease

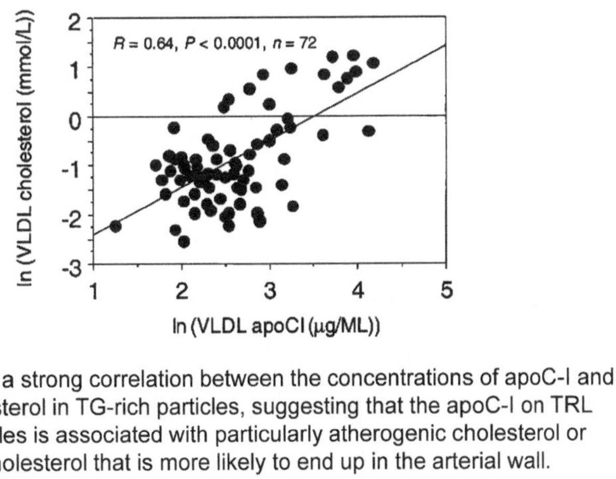


**Fig. 4.14** From Hamsten A, Silveira A, Boquist S, Tang R, Bond G, de Faire U, Björkegren J. The apolipoprotein CI content of triglyceride-rich lipoproteins independently predicts early atherosclerosis in healthy middle-aged men. J Am Coll Cardiol 2005;45:1013-7 [Reference 119 in chapter]

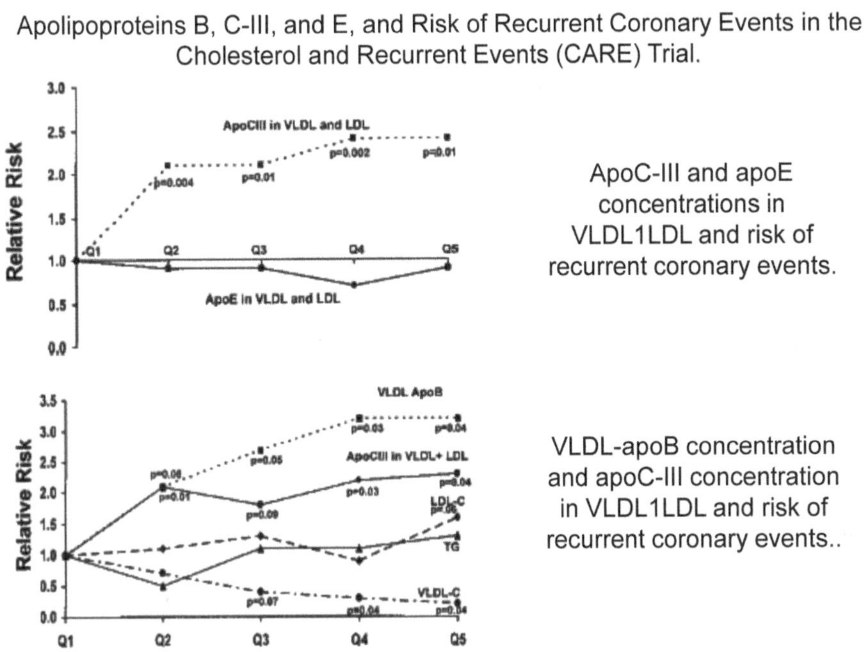


**Fig. 4.15** Sacks FM, Alaupovic P, Moye LA, Cole TG, Sussex B, Stampfer MJ, Pfeffer MA, Braunwald E. VLDL, Circulation. 2000;102:1886-1892 [Reference 122 in chapter]

risk than was plasma TG [122] (Fig. 4.15). In CARE diabetic status compared to nondiabetic status per se was not associated with high concentrations of apoC-III-containing TG-rich lipoprotein particles, if their plasma TG levels were similar [123]. Because the *apoC-III* location on chromosome 11 is near insulin response elements, a link to diabetes has been surmised [124]. Several nuclear transcription factors (NTF) influence apoC-III. One is Foxo1 which provides a molecular link between insulin resistance and the pathogenesis of diabetic hypertriglyceridemia. Foxo1 is a substrate of Akt/protein kinase B and glucocorticoid inducible kinase, which is involved with insulin signaling and in modulating both hepatic and intestinal apoC-III expression. Under both insulin-deficient and insulin-resistant conditions, Foxo1 expression is deregulated, contributing

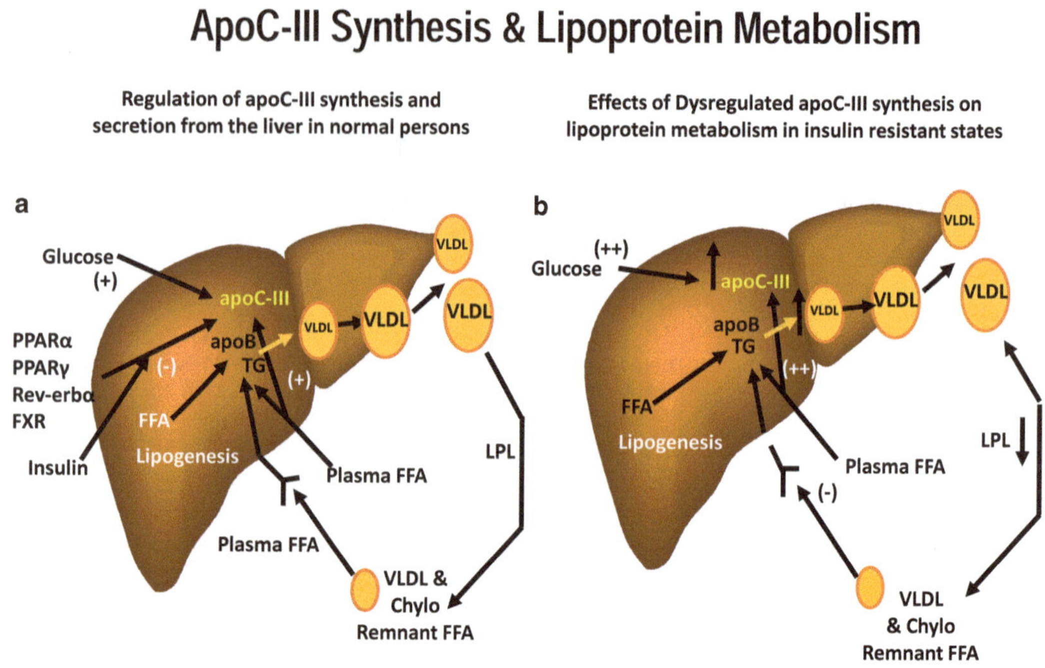


**Fig. 4.16** From Ginsburg and Brown. Arterioscler Thromb Vasc Biol 2011;31;471-473 [Reference 127 in chapter]. (**a**) Under normal conditions, apoC-III gene expression and synthesis are regulated by several factors, including nuclear transcription factors PPAR-α, PPARγ, Rev-erb, farnesoid X receptor, as well as insulin and glucose. All are inhibitory except for glucose, which stimulates apoC-III expression. Plasma free fatty acids (FFA) stimulate apoC-III secretion, but it is not known whether this occurs at the transcriptional or posttranslational level. ApoC-III in plasma inhibits lipoprotein lipase-mediated catabolism of VLDL (and chylomicrons) and inhibits the uptake of VLDL (and chylomicron) remnants by the liver. In addition, apoC-III may increase VLDL assembly and secretion. (**b**) In states of insulin resistance, any inhibitory role of insulin on apoC-III expression may be lost, whereas higher glucose levels, particularly in patients T2DM, would further stimulate apoC-III expression. Increased plasma FFA delivery to the liver would exacerbate this problem. The results of dysregulated apoC-III synthesis and secretion would be defective LPL-mediated lipolysis of TG-rich lipoproteins and reduced remnant lipoprotein clearance. Thus, dysregulated apoC-III synthesis and secretion could play a major role in the genesis of the diabetic, insulin-resistant dyslipidemia. In addition, accumulation of apoC-III-rich apoB-containing lipoproteins might have direct atherogenic consequences

to the increased apoC-III production and impaired plasma TG metabolism [125]. Hepatic nuclear factor 4-alpha (HNF-4α) which regulates LPL is also a strong positive regulator of apoC-III expression [126]. HNF-4α is stimulated by glucose and the carbohydrate-responsive element-binding protein (ChREBP). In individuals with IR and diabetes, there is a loss of insulin-mediated suppression of apoC-III that, coupled with glucose-stimulated apoC-III expression, leads to hypertriglyceridemia [127, 128] (Fig. 4.16). New findings demonstrate that apoC-III can play an additional "feedback" role in PPAR-α -mediated metabolic and inflammatory functions by controlling lipolytic generation of PPAR-α ligands. Because apoC-III expression is suppressed and LPL activity is stimulated by PPAR-α, a positive feedback system may exist. Individuals with high apoC-III levels may have impaired generation of endogenous PPAR-α ligands. Such a scenario is likely is patients with IR [129].

Accelerated conversion of buoyant LDL with apoC-III to dense LDL raises the possibility that apoC-III positively modulates the action of hepatic lipase, contributing to an increase in concentration of plasma dense LDL [130]. ApoC-III also interacts with SR-B1 and ABCA1, which will affect lipidation and delipidation of HDL.

HDL particle size shifted toward smaller sizes with increases of plasma apoC-III levels, especially when the elevations of apoC-III and apoC-II were simultaneous. The higher apoA-I concentrations also modified the effect of apoC-III on HDL subclass distribution profile. Dynamic remodeling of HDL is impaired when large-sized HDL2b particles decreased greatly in hypertriglyceridemic subjects, characterized by elevated apoC-III and C-II and lower apoA-I [131].

Like apoC-I the majority of apoC-III is found in the HDL fraction in normolipidemic individuals and on TG-rich lipoproteins in patients with elevated levels of plasma triglyceride. In plasma, different lipoproteins (whether apoB- or apoA-I-containing) have different numbers of apoC-III molecules, which may be determined by both the structure and the composition of the lipoproteins. Whether all of the apoC-III is exchangeable or not, it significantly affects the fate of the particle on which it resides, affecting potentially atherogenic VLDL, IDL, and small LDL [132] (Fig. 4.17). ApoC-III also interacts with apoE and thus VLDL metabolism is influenced by both their content of apoE and apoC-III. VLDL E+ and IDL E+ had lower fractional catabolic rates and much higher apolipoprotein C-III (apoC-III) content than did the corresponding E- particles [133]. Reanalysis of data suggests that some VLDLs, IDLs, and LDLs contain several molecules of apoC-III, whereas others contain none [134]. Less than half of HDLs contain apoC-III [135]. There are several mechanisms at play with respect to how apoC-III influences lipoproteins. Overproduction of apoC-III and apoB lipoproteins that contain apoC-III is a common feature of patients with hypertriglyceridemia. ApoC-III inhibits receptor-mediated uptake of these lipoproteins by the liver and thus VLDL containing apoC-III are channeled down the lipolytic cascade to LDL, particularly to smaller LDL that have a slower clearance rate from plasma leading to elevations of both small and total LDL-P. Indeed, increases of LDL particles containing apoC-III (LpB:C-III) were significantly associated with increases in small, dense LDL levels in healthy males independent of TG levels [136]. Many reports indicate that increased apoC-III content may contribute to inflammatory factors related to atherogenesis [137]. ApoC-III stimulates monocytes and endothelial cells to produce cytokines such as tumor necrosis factor-α and adhesion molecules, and it activates insulin-resistance pathways in endothelial cells causing endothelial dysfunction [138]. ApoC-III also stimulates adipocytes to produce cytokines and suppresses their production of adiponectin [139, 140] (Fig. 4.18).

Although not commonly appreciated, apoA-II is not solely an HDL apoprotein but also traffics with TG-rich lipoproteins and induces postprandial hypertriglyceridemia. In mice several features of the metabolic syndrome were associated with moderate to high expression of human apolipoprotein A-II. Overexpression of human apoA-II in mice led to postprandial accumulation of intestinal TRL for several hours, in a manner that one expects in IR patients [141]. Brewer suggests increased levels of apoC-III, apoC-I, or apoA-II on the apoB-containing lipoproteins may alter lipoprotein metabolism causing increased levels of atherogenic remnants. In some patients with hypertriglyceridemia, apoA-II is associated with the apoB-containing lipoproteins suggesting that the lipoproteins containing apoA-II were not effectively metabolized by LPL, and the increased plasma levels of these triglyceride-rich remnants were due to defective lipolysis [142] (Fig. 4.19). ApoA-II transfers from HDL to VLDL in vitro, resulting in VLDL that was a poorer substrate for LPL suggesting one function of apoA-II is to regulate the metabolism of TG-rich lipoproteins, with HDL serving as a plasma reservoir of apoA-II. Mice which overexpress mouse apoA-II, exhibit a marked hypertriglyceridemia, hypercholesterolemia, and increased plasma FFA, as well as insulin resistance, increased adiposity, and increased atherosclerosis [143]. ApoA-II prematurely released from poorly maturing HDL particles in persons with certain hypoalphalipoproteinemias may contribute to the elevated TG levels seen in such patients.

ApoE has multiple effects on lipogenesis, lipid absorption and lipoprotein formation, and catabolism and receptor-mediated clearance. TG-rich lipoproteins typically carry several copies

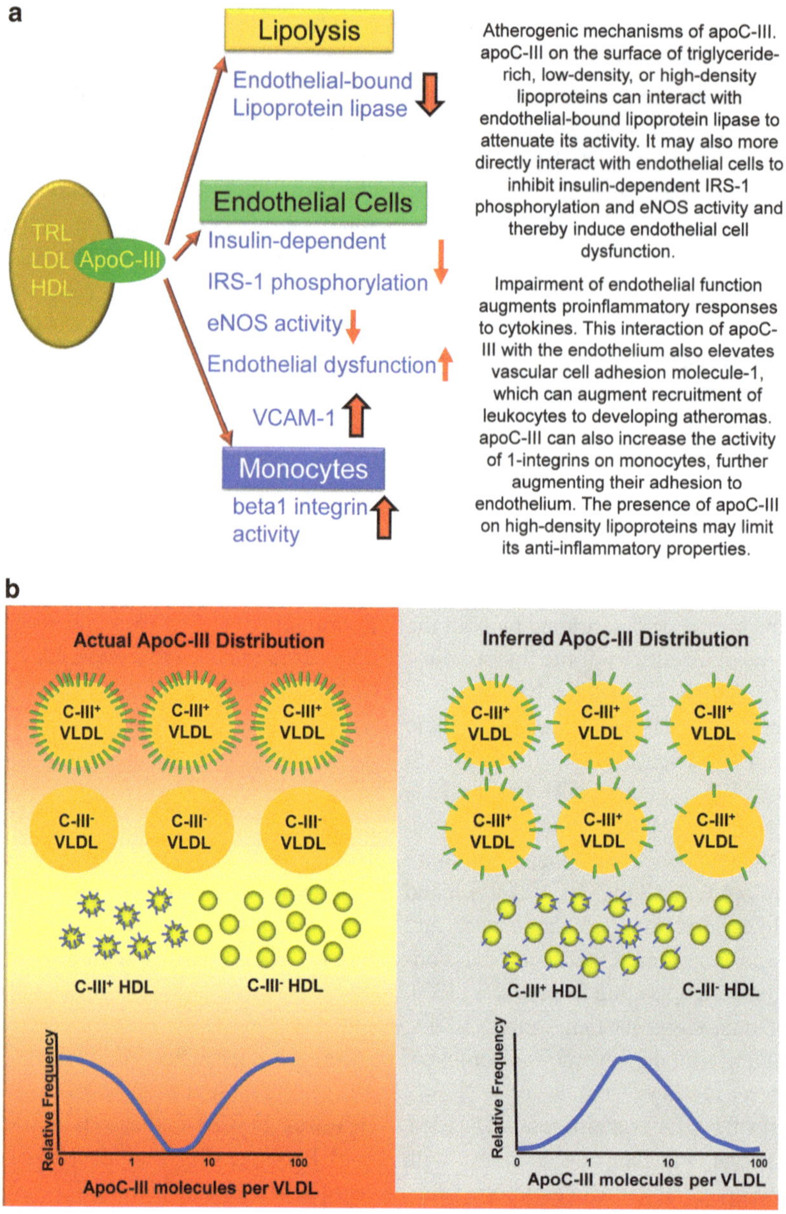


**Fig. 4.17** (**a**) Atherogenic mechanisms of apoC-III. apoC-III on the surface of triglyceride-rich, low-density, or high-density lipoproteins can interact with endothelial-bound lipoprotein lipase to attenuate its activity. It may also more directly interact with endothelial cells to inhibit insulin-dependent IRS-1 phosphorylation and eNOS activity and thereby induce endothelial cell dysfunction. Impairment of endothelial function augments proinflammatory responses to cytokines. This interaction of apoC-III with the endothelium also elevates vascular cell adhesion molecule-1, which can augment recruitment of leukocytes to developing atheromas. apoC-III can also increase the activity of 1-integrins on monocytes, further augmenting their adhesion to endothelium. The presence of apoC-III on high-density lipoproteins may limit its anti-inflammatory properties. Adapted from Bobik A. Apolipoprotein C-III and atherosclerosis: beyond effects on lipid metabolism. Circulation. 2008;118:702-4 [Reference 137 in chapter]. (**b**) Adapted from Sachs F et al. J Lip Res 2011;52:1067-70 [Reference 131 in chapter]. Comparison between the actual lipoprotein distribution of apoC-III and the distribution inferred from the one-pool concept of plasma apoC-III metabolism. There are on average ~20–50 apoC-III molecules on each VLDL particle. About 50 % of VLDL contain apoC-III (C-III+), and the other half of VLDL do not contain apoC-III at all (C-III–). The apoC-III distribution pattern within VLDL has an inverse bell shape (*left panel*). On the other hand, the one-pool concept of plasma apoC-III metabolism suggests that apoC-III exchanges freely and randomly within VLDL and HDL and also between VLDL and HDL. In this scenario, the vast majority of VLDL and HDL would contain some apoC-III molecules and would have a normal distribution pattern (*right panel*). There would be few VLDL or HDL containing large numbers of apoC-III molecules and one would be unlikely to find lipoproteins without apoC-III

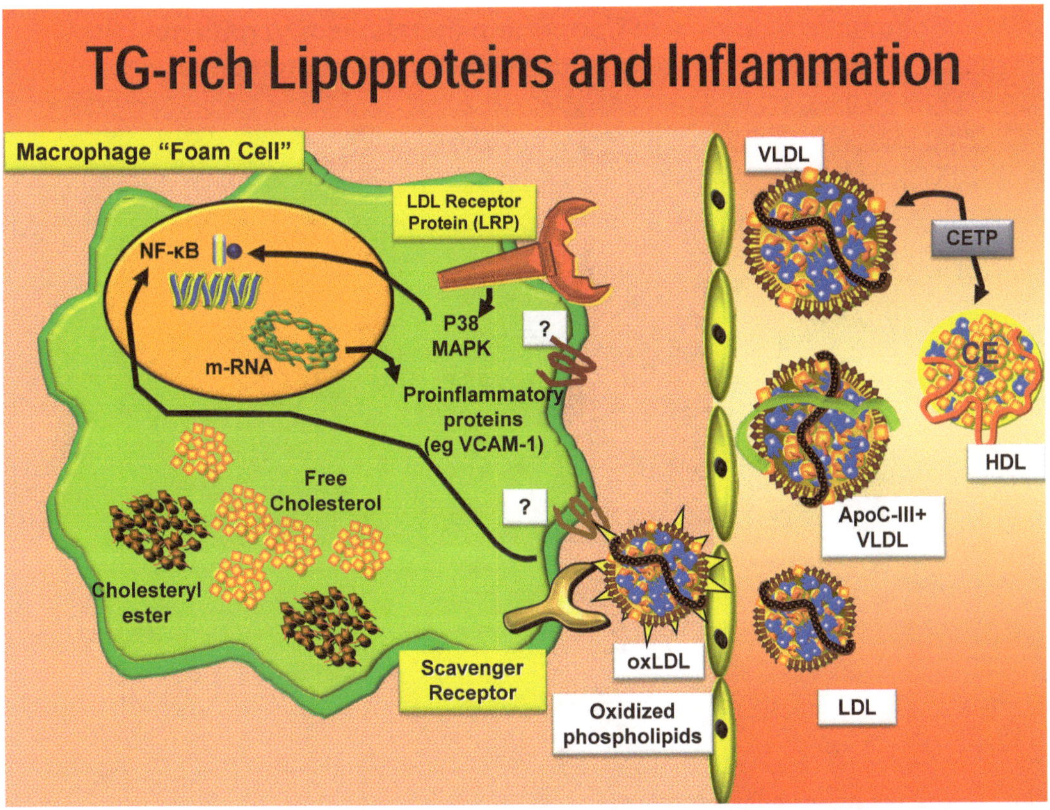


**Fig. 4.18** Adapted from Peter Libby Circulation Research 2007;100:299-3011 [Reference 104 in text]. Oxidation of LDL releases bioactive lipids that incite inflammation in vascular tissues through scavenger receptors and putative (?) receptors. Binding and internalization of TG-rich lipoproteins activates P38 MAP kinase and NFκB. ApoC-III+VLDL and LDL also activate proinflammatory functions of endothelial cells via a pertussis-sensitive, proteins kinase C (PKC)-mediated pathway that can stimulate via NFκB recruitment of leukocytes

of apoE, which exist in several genotypes (*E3/*E3, *E3/*E4, *E2/*E3, *E4/*E4, *E2/*E4, and *E2/*E2), some of which are associated with lipid/lipoprotein disorders. With respect to mice with STZ-induced diabetes, investigation reveals ApoE4 causes severe dyslipidemia and atherosclerosis independent of its interaction with LDLr. ApoE4-expressing livers have reduced fatty acid oxidation, which contributes to the accumulation of tissue and plasma lipids [144]. Southern European ethnicity does not confer an independent survival advantage in community-based Australian type 2 diabetic patients, but the APOE4 carriers were at higher risk of cardiac death [145].

ApoE polymorphisms have been implicated in predisposition to diabetes but the results of the individual studies have been inconclusive. A meta-analysis of population-based case–control genetic-association studies relating apoE polymorphisms and T2DM which included 30 studies reported data of apoE genotypes in 5,423 T2DM patients and 8,197 healthy unrelated controls and revealed a significant role played by the E2 allele carriers, who were at elevated risk for T2DM (odds ratio = 1.18, 95 % CI: 1.02, 1.35). Meta-regression analysis provided some weak evidence that the risk conferred by E2 allele is mediated through altering serum lipid levels [146]. The relationship between *APOE* and fatal and nonfatal CHD was examined among 10,035 men and 12,134 women, aged 44–79 years, from the Norfolk, England, arm of the European Prospective Into Nutrition and Cancer Study (1993–2007). During an average of 11 years of follow-up, 2,712 CHD events were documented.

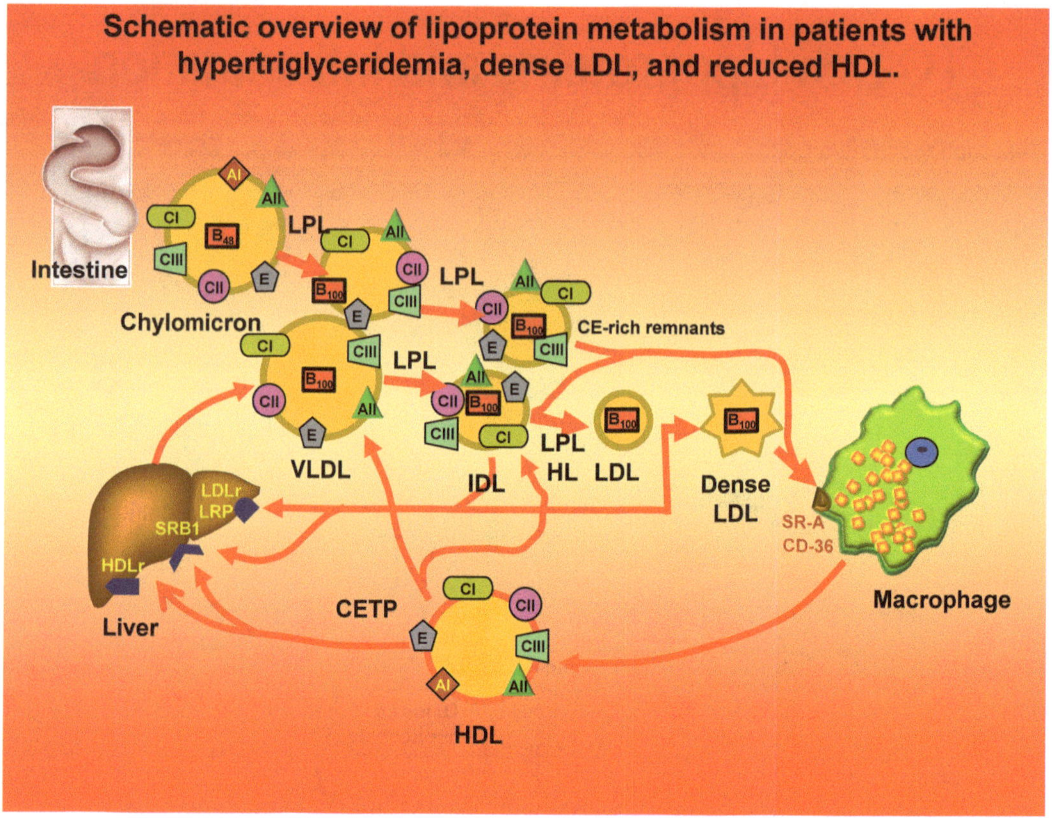


**Fig. 4.19** Schematic overview of lipoprotein metabolism in patients with hypertriglyceridemia, dense LDL, and reduced HDL. Adapted from Am J Cardiol. 1999;83:3F-12F [Reference 142 in chapter]

In the largest prospective cohort study to date, CHD risk was not associated with *APOE* genotype after controlling for a variety of cardiovascular risk factors, particularly the ratio of low- to high-density lipoprotein cholesterol [147]. A Turkish group assessed the apoE polymorphism in 295 patients with atherosclerotic disease (124 of them had diabetes). Findings suggested that apoE polymorphism was not related to the development of atherosclerosis in patients and was not associated with the lipid levels in patients with type 2 diabetes [148]. In the CARE trial, apoE concentrations in plasma or in VLDL+LDL were associated with CHD but were linked to apoC-III retarding their clearance. Also, apoE in HDL was an independent predictor of recurrent coronary events and explains the weaker relation between plasma triglycerides and coronary events [122].

Another apolipoprotein involved with TG-rich lipoproteins is apoL-I which was discovered in 1997 and has been found in human atherosclerotic vascular tissue. Typically, apoL-I associates with HDL particles [149] but in the HDL Atherosclerosis Treatment Study (HATS), there were significant associations between apoL-I and VLDL-TG and elevated glucose. VLDL-TG was the specific TG component associated with apoL-I and ~50 % of patients with high apoL-I levels had an elevated glucose phenotype compared with <15 % of those in the low apoL-I cluster. This supports the hypothesis that high apoL-I levels may be a novel marker of an atherogenic phenotype [150]. PCSK9, an LDLr peptidase, has emerged as a major regulator of the LDLr, but it also limits visceral adipogenesis likely via adipose VLDLr regulation. In vivo, endogenous hepatic PCSK9 has been shown to regulate VLDLr protein levels in adipose tissue. This regulation is achieved by circulating PCSK9 and thus helps regulate fat metabolism [151].

## The TG/HDL Axis: The HDL- and apoA-I-Containing Lipoproteins

The very large HDL lipidome is an area ripe for research. Ceramide, an HDL component, has been implicated in the pathogenesis of insulin resistance and has many proinflammatory properties such as impaired Huh7 cell (a well-differentiated hepatocyte) viability, mitochondrial function, and insulin signaling [152]. A kinetic study revealed that increased HDL apoA-I catabolism, a significant effector of low apoA-I in the metabolic syndrome, may be largely associated with dysregulation of VLDL-apoB metabolism (i.e., elevated plasma triglyceride and VLDL-apoB concentration and overproduction of VLDL-apoB), insulin resistance, and, to a lesser extent, low adiponectin concentration [153]. Compared with lean individuals, overweight–obese individuals had significantly higher HDL apoA-I fractional catabolic rate ($0.21 \pm 0.01$ vs. $0.33 \pm 0.01$ pools/day; $p < 0.001$) and production rate (PR; $11.3 \pm 4.4$ vs. $15.8 \pm 2.77$ mg/kg per day; $p = 0.001$). In the lean group, HDL apoA-I PR was significantly associated with apoA-I concentration ($r = 0.455$, $p = 0.004$), whereas in the overweight–obese group, both HDL apoA-I fractional catabolic rate ($r = -0.396$, $p = 0.050$) and HDL apoA-I PR ($r = 0.399$, $p = 0.048$) were significantly associated with apoA-I concentration. After adjustment for fasting insulin or Homeostasis Model Assessment (HOMA) score, HDL apoA-I PR was an independent predictor of apoA-I concentration [154]. In part the catabolic rate is related to heterotypic exchange of TG for CE between apoB and apoA-I particles, resulting in TG-rich HDLs which are subject to lipolytic catabolism and release of apoA-I making it available for renal excretion.

SR-B1 is involved with lipidation and delipidation of mature HDL particles. In a study of 16 men, postprandial lipemia caused structural changes to HDL so there was enhanced SR-BI and ABCG1-dependent efflux to large HDL2 particles. Although that is seemingly beneficial, postprandial lipemia was equally associated with enhancing formation of CE-enriched, TG-rich lipoprotein particles through the action of CETP and by inducing structural changes in HDL particles that reduce the direct return of HDL-CE to the liver [155]. Also affecting SR-B1 and ABCA1 efflux in vivo in transgenic mice in a reciprocal manner was modulation of HDL PL content. The type of lipase acting on HDL in vivo may also determine which FC efflux pathway the HDL serves. Efflux was examined by overexpressing either endothelial lipase (EL) or phosphatidylserine phospholipase (PS-PLA1) in human apoA-I transgenic mice. Overexpression of EL led to large reductions in the serum PL/apoA-I ratio (−60 %), total cholesterol (TC; −9 %), and HDL cholesterol (−91 %). Relative to the serum before overexpression of EL, the efflux potential of the serum via SR-BI decreased by 90 % and ABCA1-mediated efflux increased by 63 %. In contrast to overexpression of EL, overexpression of PS-PLA1 led to increases in the PL/apoA-I ratio (88 %), TC (78 %), HDL cholesterol (57 %), and HDL size. The efflux potential of the serum increased by 60 % via SR-BI and decreased by 57 % via ABCA1 [156].

## The TG/HDL Axis: Relating apoB- and apoA-I-Containing Lipoproteins

It has been known for decades the dyslipidemia or more aptly named dyslipoproteinemia associated with IR and T2DM was characterized by normal or abnormal levels of TC and LDL-C but also elevated TG and reduced HDL-C. Szapary and Rader coined the term the TG/HDL axis and noted its high association with CV risk [96]. NCEP declared that low HDL-C is a major and independent risk factor for CV risk [42]. It continues to be debated whether TG levels have such independent predictive powers on CV risk although a large meta-analysis showed TG had moderate and highly significant associations and, even though TG lost some predictive power when adjusted for HDL-C, it remained an independent predictor [157]. Major new insight as to the risk associated with elevated TG comes from the Metabolic, Lifestyle, and Nutrition Assessment in Young Adults (MELANY) study that followed 13,953 apparently healthy, untreated, young men (age 26–45 years) with TG levels less than <300 mg/dL over 5.5 years. The risk for CHD in men with high-tertile TG levels at baseline changed depending on the tertile at time of follow-up (hazard ratios, 8.23 [95 % CI, 2.50–27.13] for high (>131 mg/dL)/high (≥148 mg/dL), 6.84 [CI, 1.95–23.98] for high (131 mg/dL)/intermediate (94–147 mg/dL), and 4.90 [CI, 1.01–24.55] for high (>131 mg/dL)/low (≤93 mg/dL), compared with the stable low/low group). The risk for CHD in men with low-tertile levels at baseline also changed depending on the tertile at follow-up (hazard ratios, 3.81 [CI, 0.96–15.31] for low/intermediate and 6.76 [CI, 1.34–33.92] for low (≤81 mg/dL)/high (≥148 mg/dL), compared with the stable low/low group). The conclusion was that TG measurements over time can help CV risk assessment in young men (Fig. 4.19). A decrease in initially elevated TG levels was associated with a decrease in CHD risk compared with stable high TG levels. However, this risk remains higher than in those with persistently low TG levels [158]. Additional analysis showed two TG levels 5 years apart also identified young men at increased risk for diabetes, independent of traditional risk factors and of associated changes in BMI and lifestyle parameters. Two measurements of fasting triglyceride levels obtained 5 years apart can assist in identifying apparently healthy young men at increased risk for diabetes, independent of traditional risk factors and of associated changes in BMI and lifestyle parameters. Men in the lowest tertile of triglyceride levels (≤81 mg/dL) who progressed to the highest tertile (≥148 mg/dL) over follow-up (low-high) exhibited a hazard ratio (HR) of 12.62 (95 % CI, 3.52–31.34) compared with those remaining in the lowest tertile at both time points (reference group: low-low). Whereas men who were at the top triglyceride level tertile throughout follow-up [high (≥131 mg/dL)-high (≥148 mg/dL)] had a HR for diabetes of 7.08 (2.52–14.45), those whose triglyceride level decreased to the lowest tertile [high (≥131 mg/dL) to low(≤81 mg/dL)] exhibited a HR of 1.97 (0.67–6.13). Alterations in triglyceride levels during follow-up were associated with changes in BMI, physical activity, and eating breakfast habit ($p<0.05$), but remained an independent modifier of diabetes risk even after adjustment for such changes [159] (Fig. 4.20).

The answer to understanding TG and its relationship to CV risk is to study its relationship to atherogenic lipoproteins especially a change in the core TG of lipoproteins has a significant influence on how those particles are trafficked and catabolized. The lipoprotein hallmark of IR is the synthesis and secretion of the large VLDL1 particles. As noted normolipemic patients do not create significant amounts of VLDL1. A normal VLDL particle has a core TG/CE ratio of 5 to 1 [21]. Normally the TG-rich VLDL particles and chylomicrons undergo rapid lipolysis and vanish within 2–6 h but such is not the case when IR is at play where delayed catabolism and increased plasma residence time is the rule, leading to increased fasting and postprandial TG levels [160] (Fig. 4.21). The elevated TG by itself leads to endothelial dysfunction, elevation of inflammatory markers, hypercoagulability, and increased blood viscosity. The delayed catabolism is due to several factors already discussed, including imbalance of apoA-II, apoC-I, apoC-III, CETP activity, and impaired LPL function. The longer the residence times of TG-rich lipoproteins, the greater the chance that both homotypic and heterotypic exchange of neutral lipids occurs between lipoproteins utilizing CETP. The TG-rich VLDLs and chylomicrons send their core TG to IDLs and LDLs or to HDLs in exchange for CE. In the process the VLDLs and chylomicrons become TG-poorer and CE-rich. LPL-mediated hydrolysis of core TG occurs the particles reduce in size and shed surface phospholipids, creating atherogenic remnant lipoproteins [1H]. In essence the remnants are very large formerly TG-rich but converted to CE-enriched particles. One must keep in perspective that despite the risk associated with remnants, that risk is not solely due to VLDL-P per se but rather marked elevation of LDL-P [110, 161] (Fig. 4.22). In a Japanese study it was $apoB_{100}$-carrying lipoproteins (VLDL remnants), not $apoB_{48}$ lipoproteins, that were the major subset of remnants associated with sudden cardiac death in the

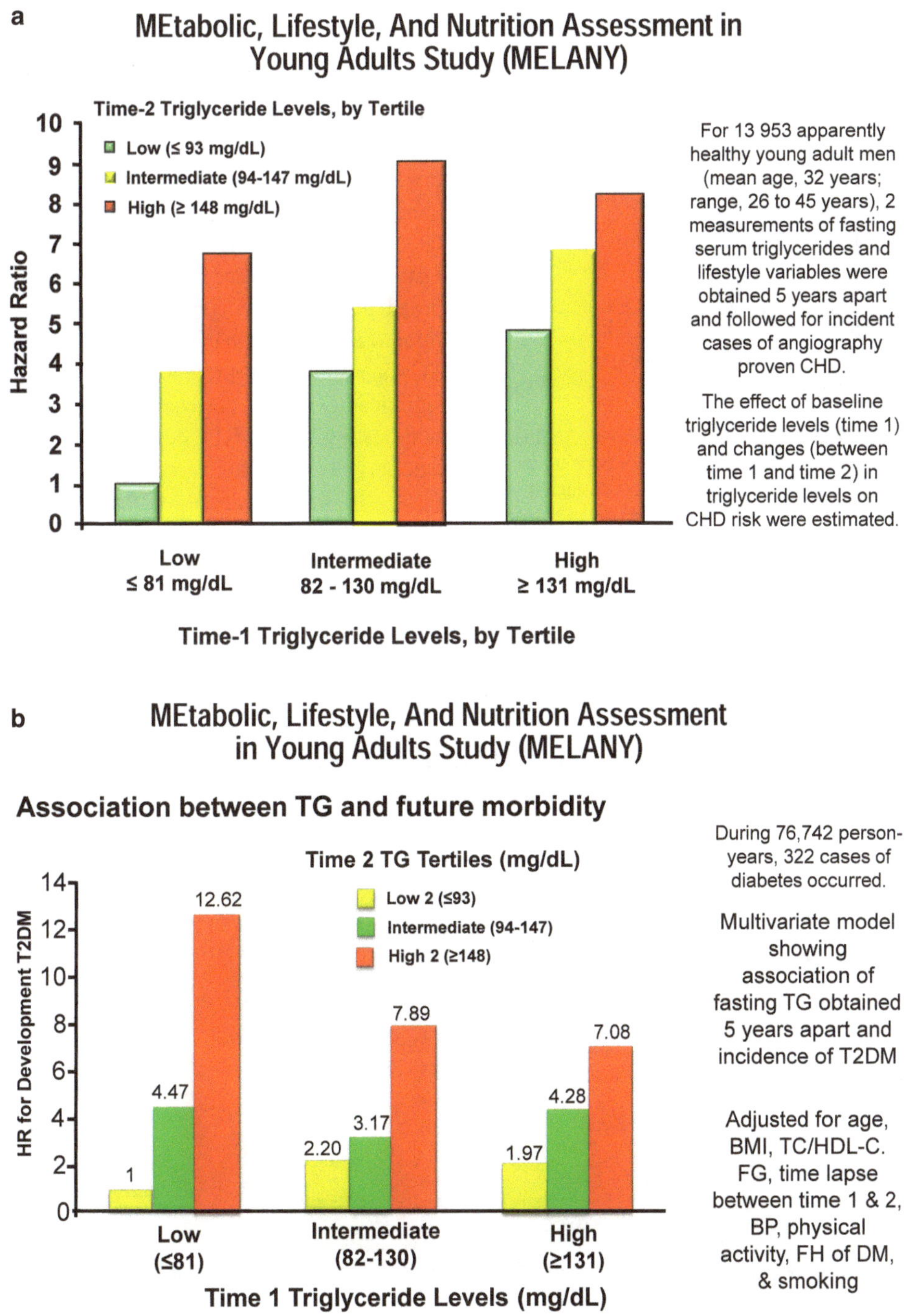


**Fig. 4.20** (**a**) Metabolic, Lifestyle, and Nutrition Assessment in Young Adults (MELANY) study. Adapted from Tirosh A et al. Ann Intern Med. 2007;147:377-385 [Reference 158 in chapter]. (**b**) Metabolic, Lifestyle, and Nutrition Assessment in Young Adults (MELANY) study. Adapted from Tirosh A et al. Diabetes Care 2008;31:2032-2037 [Reference 159 in chapter]

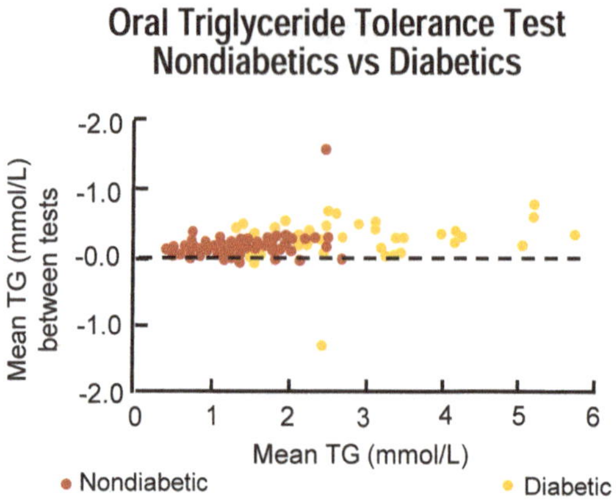


**Fig. 4.21** Mean difference plot comparing triglyceride concentrations at the 6-h time point for patients with no diabetes and diabetes. Adapted from Mohanlal N & Holman R. Diabet Care 2004;27:89-94 [Reference 160 in chapter]

postprandial state, regardless of the severity of coronary atherosclerosis [162]. Using newer analytical methods, data suggested the major part (approximately 80 % or more) of remnants are VLDL remnants, not chylomicron remnants. It was also found that plasma TG vs. remnant-TG concentrations in the postprandial state correlated significantly higher with risk than in the fasting state [163]. The increased TG in the postprandial state mainly consisted of TG in remnant lipoproteins. In normal volunteers, postprandial TG vs. remnant lipoprotein concentrations were significantly more correlated when compared with fasting TG vs. RLP concentrations, and the authors concluded increased sensitivity of non-fasting TG in predicting the CV risk (events) may be directly explained by the increase of remnant lipoproteins in the postprandial state [164]. However, in the Copenhagen General Population

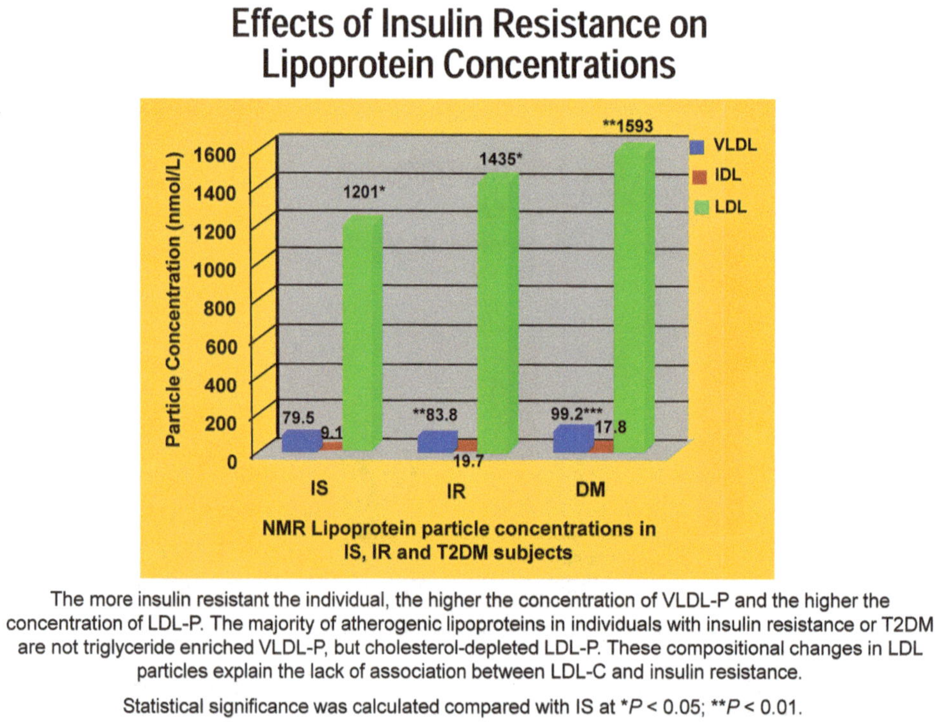


**Fig. 4.22** Data is from Garvey et al. Diabetes 2003;52(2):453-462. Reference [110] in chapter. Actual graph is from Rosenson R, et al. Atherosclerosis 213 (2010) 1-7. Reference [161] in chapter. Dyslipidemia was evaluated using both NMR lipoprotein subclass analysis and conventional lipid panel, and insulin sensitivity as the maximal glucose disposal rate (GDR) during hyperinsulinemic clamps in 56 insulin-sensitive, 46 insulin-resistant, and 46 untreated subjects with type 2 diabetes

Study, lipid and apolipoprotein concentrations, as a function of time since the last meal, were evaluated in 58,434 individuals (participation rate 45 %) from the general population, 2,270 of who had diabetes. TG increased up to 17.7 mg/dL after normal food intake in individuals with and without diabetes. No statistically significant differences in postprandial apoB were seen although apoB fluctuate to higher levels more in diabetics [165]. Nakajima has also suggested that remnant-like lipoprotein particles, not LDL particles, are the major oxidized lipoproteins in plasma [166]. Lipolysis of TG-rich LP will be delayed with an excess of C-III and the apoC-II/apoC-III ratio has been used as a predictor of lipolytic rate with high ratios associated with decreased plasma residence time.

The increased CETP-mediated exchange of core lipids inT2DM results in TG-rich and CE-poor LDLs and HDLs. The size of the LDL or HDL does not affect the lipid transfer, and small or large LDLs and HDLs can be TG acceptors or CE donors as can large TG-rich and CE-poor LDLs and HDLs. TG-rich LDLs are an underappreciated part of dyslipoproteinemia. Patients with elevations of LDL-TG (defined as > 54 mg/dL) may have low, normal, or elevated LDL-C levels but because these LDLs are CE depleted, they are almost always associated with elevated LDL-P or apoB. This was studied in 1,309 patients not taking lipid-lowering drugs in the Ludwigshafen Risk and Cardiovascular Health (LURIC) study. Among these, 739 individuals had angiographic CAD (>20 % stenosis) and 570 subjects served as control subjects. The association of LDL-TG (odds ratio [OR], 1.30; 95 % CI, 1.19–1.43; $p < 0.001$) with CAD was stronger than that of LDL-C (OR, 1.10; 95 % CI, 1.00–1.21; $p = 0.047$). The predictive value of LDL-TG for CAD was independent of LDL-C. High-sensitivity C-reactive protein (hs-CRP), serum amyloid A, fibrinogen, interleukin 6, intercellular adhesion molecule-1 (ICAM-1), and vascular adhesion molecule-1 (VCAM-1) increased in parallel to LDL-TG. CRP, ICAM-1, and VCAM-1 were inversely related to LDL-C. The authors speculate that since HL is subject to modulation by inflammatory cytokines, low-grade systemic inflammation might be the cause rather than the consequence of high LDL-TG. In 114 individuals with impaired fasting glucose, impaired glucose tolerance, or type 2 diabetes mellitus subjects with high LDL-TG, LDLs were depleted of CE, and VLDLs, IDLs, and dense LDLs were significantly elevated, i.e., apoB was elevated. The authors concluded that LDL-TG is a better indicator for atherogenic alterations of LDL metabolism than is LDL-C as at any given concentration of LDL particles, LDL-C would be low once LDL-TGs were high [167] (Figs. 4.23 and 4.24).

Of additional interest is the actual molecular structure and shape of TG-rich LDLs. LDL particles vary in their receptor-binding affinity and susceptibility to oxidative modifications. LDLs must be thought of as dynamically remodeling particles, and changes in particle composition, shape, and size, as well as apoB conformation will affect LDL function and receptor binding. Small LDL shows lower affinity to the LDL receptor, but increased unspecific binding to cell surfaces [168]. LDLs also may undergo a structural transition at body temperature and which may affect LDLr recognition. Below the transition temperature, the core-located lipids are arranged in an ordered liquid-crystalline phase whereas above the temperature, the neutral lipids are organized in a fluid, oil-like, randomly distributed state. If the LDLs are TG rich, the core lipids remain in their fluid phase, independent of temperature, and such LDLs have less affinity from LDLr compared to normolipidemic LDL. When LDL core TG is normal, the core CE is immobilized, causing a higher core viscosity. Under these conditions, the activity of CETP is lower [169]. It has also been speculated that when core lipids are in the liquid-crystalline state, surface phospholipids can be altered which could change the LDL shape from spherical to elliptical [170]. If the TG-rich LDs and HDL particles undergo additional lipolysis with HL, they can transform into small LDL or HDL with the latter being subject to break up and renal excretion of surface apoA-I. Atherogenesis is related to the accumulation and retention (binding to proteoglycans) of LDL in the arterial subendothelium [171].

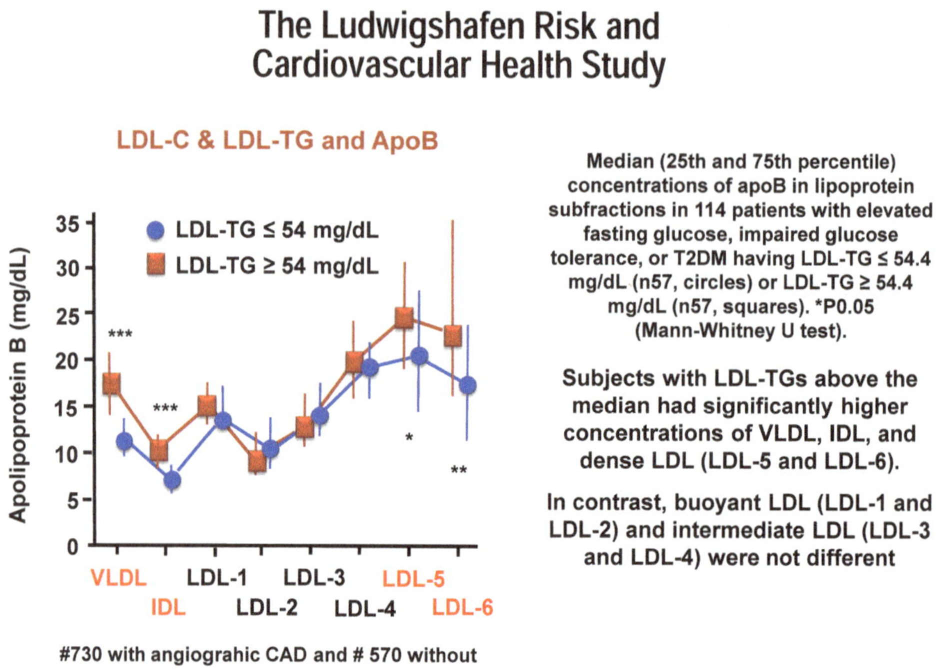


**Fig. 4.23** The Ludwigshafen Risk and Cardiovascular Health study. Adapted from Marz W et al. Circulation. 2004;110:3068-3074 [Reference 167 in chapter]

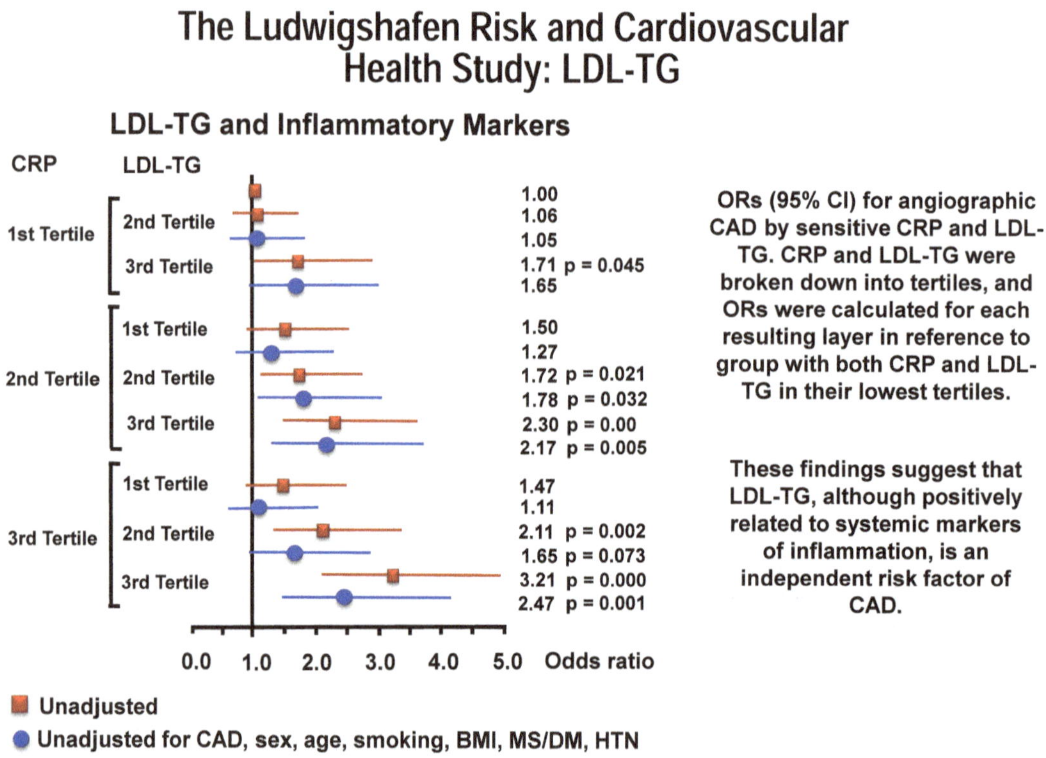


**Fig. 4.24** The Ludwigshafen Risk and Cardiovascular Health study: LDL-TG. Adapted from Marz W et al. Circulation. 2004;110:3068-3074 [Reference 167 in chapter]

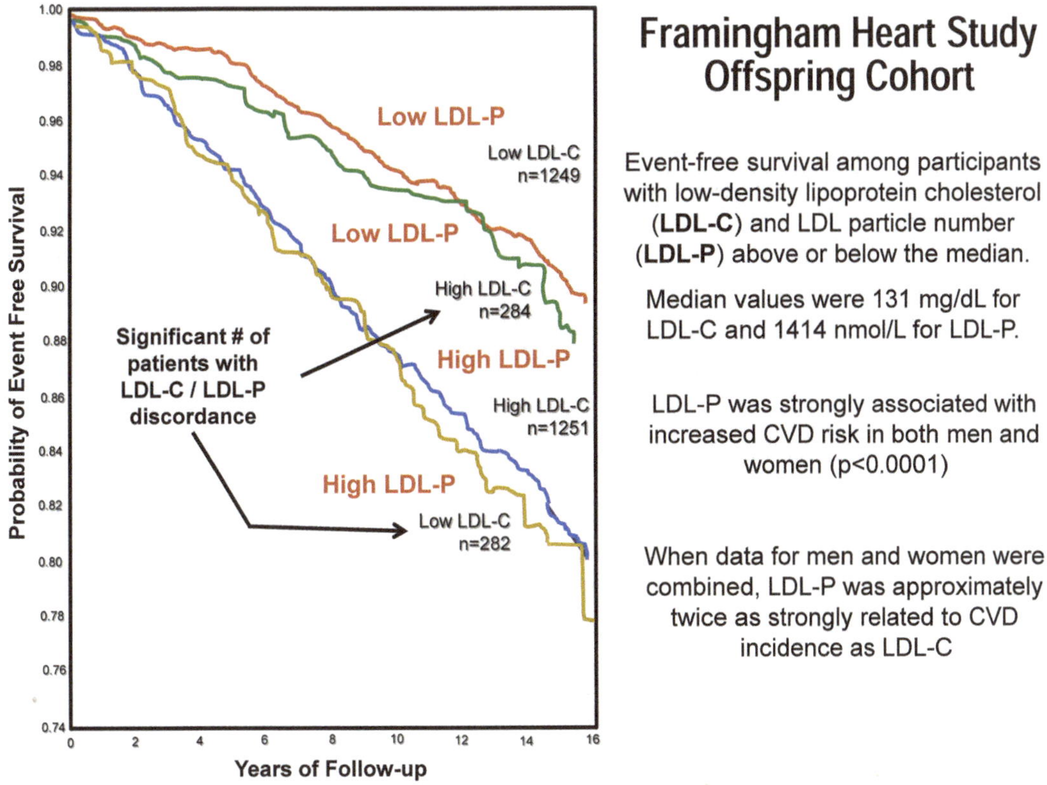


**Fig. 4.25** Framingham Heart Study Offspring cohort. Adapted from Cromwell W et al. J Clin Lipidol 2007;1:583-592 [Reference 175 in chapter]

Several studies have suggested that the small LDL is quite prone to oxidation and binding to HSPG. Subintimal oxidation of LDL is an initial process in atherogenesis. Lp-PLA2 is known to have high affinity for and traffic with the small LDL species [172, 173].

Despite the discussion of LDL core composition and size, the major factor driving the particle into the arterial wall is particle number. Older studies have related atherogenesis to the smaller, higher density LDL but several newer studies which adjusted for LDL-P reveal the LDL size does not maintain statistically significant independence as a CV risk factor [174]. A major area of lipid/lipoprotein clinical importance in IR and T2DM is the significant discordance between three measurements that typically have excellent correlation, specifically LDL-C and apoB and LDL-P. As discussed in the Garvey study, although VLDLs contribute to apoB, the vast majority of apoB particles are LDLs [110] and apoB measurement should be regarded as an assay of LDL-P. The American Association of Clinical Chemistry (AACC) in a position statement [13] reiterated that apoB is a measure of LDL-P and not a measure of VLDL or VLDL remnants. Cromwell in an evaluation of CV death over 16 years in the Framingham Offspring trial (4th examination cycle 1987–1991) showed that CV risk was related not per se to high or low LDL-C but rather elevated or not elevated LDL-P. Adding VLDL-P to the equation added little to risk prediction. There were far less events in those in the lowest quartile of LDL-P than the equivalent quartile of LDL-C [175] (Fig. 4.25). Recent data from MESA also highlighted the fact that when LDL-C and LDL-P are discordant, abnormal changes in CIMT follow LDL-P better than LDL-C [176]. In another study of T2DM patients, 84 % of patients who had an

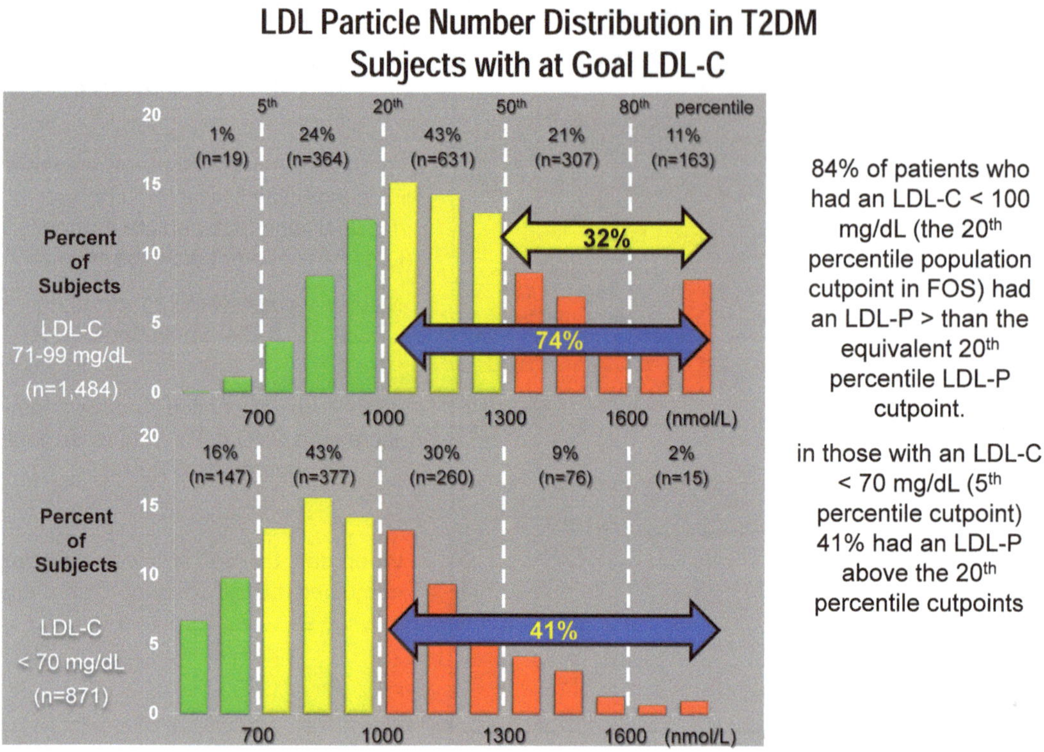


**Fig. 4.26** LDL particle number distribution in T2DM subjects with at goal LDL-C. Adapted from Cromwell W & Otvos J (Am J Cardiol 2006;98:1599-1602) [Reference 177 in chapter]

LDL-C < 100 mg/dL (the 20th percentile population cut point in FOS) had an LDL-P > than the equivalent 20th percentile LDL-P cut point. Of more concern was that in those with an LDL-C < 70 mg/dL (5th percentile cut point), 41 % had an LDL-P above the 20th percentile cut points [177] (Fig. 4.26). Sniderman has demonstrated this discordance in multiple trials comparing CV risk to LDL-C versus apoB [178]. The level of TG in metabolic syndrome patients that is associated with at-risk levels of LDL-P is far lower than previously inferred. In FOS as triglyceride levels increased from 80 to 250 mg/dL, the number of total LDL particles rose dramatically beginning with TG > 130 mg/dL while the levels of LDL-C remained low [179] (Fig. 4.27).

Low HDL-C is of course the other component of the TG/HDL axis. Often underappreciated is that triglycerides also have a profound influence on HDLs affecting HDL-P, HDL-TG, HDL-C, and HDL functionality. As discussed, due to heterotypic CETP exchange of neutral lipids, HDL particles become TG-rich and CE-poor. It is one reason that low HDL-C (<40 mg/dL) is associated with abnormal, at-risk levels of LDL-P (Fig. 4.28). Rader suggests TG-enrichment of HDL, and its subsequent hydrolysis by HL, impacts on HDL function [180, 181]. Such HDLs are subject to further lipolysis by HL and endothelial lipase resulting in smaller, denser HDL species, and apoA-I dissociates from the smallest of those particles [182]. EL and HL are upregulated in IR and may act in tandem with HL being more of a triglyceridase and EL a phospholipase. Most lipoproteins cannot pass into the glomerulus, but lipids bound to filtered apolipoproteins can be excreted via the renal tubule proteins megalin and cubilin. Dissociation of apoA-I from HDL or failure of apoA-I to incorporate into HDL enhances renal apoA-I catabolism via cubilin-mediated tubular excretion [183, 184] (Fig. 4.29).

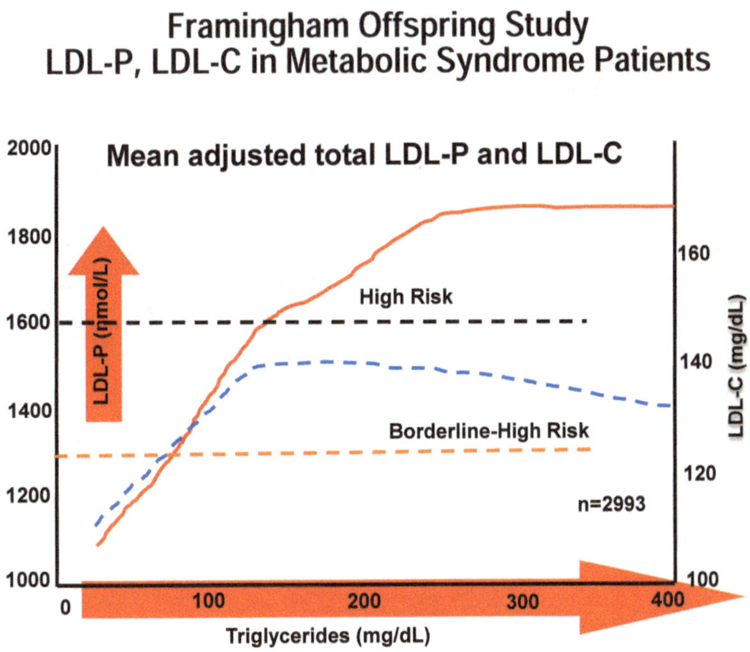


**Fig. 4.27** Framingham Offspring study LDL-P, LDL-C in metabolic syndrome patients. Adapted from Kathiresan S, Otvos JD, Sullivan LM et al. Circulation. 2006;113:20-29. [Reference 179 in chapter]

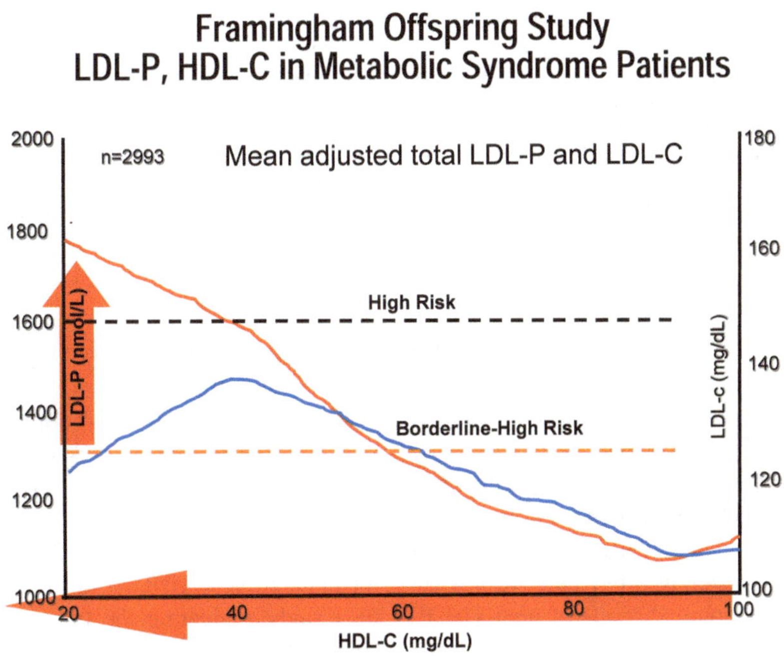


**Fig. 4.28** Framingham Offspring study LDL-P, HDL-C in metabolic syndrome patients. Adapted from Kathiresan S, Otvos JD, Sullivan LM et al. Circulation. 2006;113:20-29. [Reference 179 in chapter]

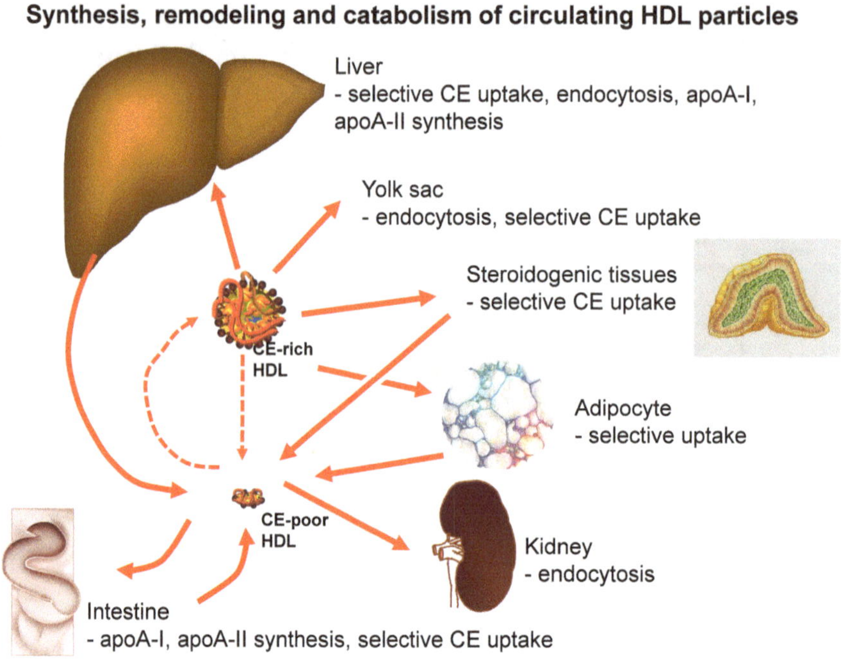


**Fig. 4.29** (1) Formation of small (discoidal) HDL particles from apolipoprotein A-I and A-II synthesized in the intestine and complexed with phospholipid and free cholesterol transferred from other lipoprotein particles and tissues. (2) Formation of spherical HDL of increased size promoted by further lipid loading and lecithin–cholesterol acyltransferase-catalyzed esterification of cholesterol. (3) Selective CE uptake (mediated by scavenger receptor BI; SR-BI) and endocytosis (unknown receptor) in the liver. (4) Selective CE uptake (mediated by SR-BI) in steroidogenic tissue, e.g., adrenals, testis, and ovary. (5) Formation of small cholesterol-poor HDL particles originating from HDL particles subjected to selective uptake in the steroidogenic tissues. (6) Formation of small cholesterol-poor HDL particles originating from (a) HDL particles subjected to selective uptake in the liver or (b) apolipoprotein A-I and A-II synthesized in the liver. (7) Reduction of HDL size as a result of lipolysis (effect of hepatic lipase, lipoprotein lipase, and endothelial lipase) and transfer of CE and phospholipid to other lipoproteins as promoted by CE transfer protein and the phospholipid transfer protein. (8) Renal filtration and subsequent endocytosis (mediated by cubilin) of lipid-poor apolipoprotein A-I and probably also some small filterable HDL particles (smaller than 8 nm). (9) Endocytosis (mediated by cubilin) of HDL and selective CE uptake in the yolk sac/early placenta of the pregnant organism. Adapted & modified from Moestrup SK and Kozyraki R. Cubilin, Curr Opin Lipidol. 2000;11:133-140. [Reference 184 in chapter]

The preβ-1 HDL particles are poorly lipidated HDL particles composed of one or two molecules of apoA-I and small amounts of PL and UC. Hypertriglyceridemic patients including those with metabolic syndrome exhibit significantly higher plasma preβ-1 HDL concentrations compared to healthy individuals. CETP and HL-/EL-induced remodeling of HDLs results in increased production and levels of preβ-1 HDL particles. The increased HL activity that has been observed in patients with high TG generates preβ-1 HDL. The net result of these changes is the elevation of preβ-1 HDL levels and the reduction in the concentrations of large α-migrating HDL [185]. It has been shown that increases in preβ-1 HDL concentrations reflect an impairment in HDL maturation and in dynamic remodeling of HDL and are a sign of impaired RCT [186–188]. PLTP activity is also increased in patients with high triglyceride values [189], and LCAT activity, required for maturation of HDL, is also decreased [190]. In a study evaluating the functional effects of HDL with respect to endothelial nitric oxide and superoxide production, endothelium-dependent vasodilation, and early endothelial progenitor cell-mediated endothelial repair, HDL from healthy persons promoted each of these functions. These endothelial effects of HDL were impaired in HDL from T2DM patients [191].

## Conclusions

In summary, examination of lipoprotein changes present in drug naive IR and T2DM patients with or without TG/HDL axis abnormalities reveals elevations of apoB particles (specifically increased remnants), significantly increased numbers of LDL particles, and decreased apoA-I and total HDL-P characterized by decreases in the larger alpha HDL species and increases in the prebeta-1 species. Many of these abnormalities are related to abnormal cholesterol absorption, synthesis, cellular efflux, and its trafficking in lipoproteins whose function is modulated by numerous apolipoproteins and cell surface receptors. Such patients therefore have high apoB/apoA-I ratios and high LDL-P/HDL-P ratios which were identified as the best predictors of CV risk in INTERHEART and VA-HIT and Women's Health Study, respectively [192–194]. More readily available to practicing clinicians is the TG/HDL-C ratio of which there are several studies linking high ratios>3.0 with insulin resistance [195], small LDL size [196], CV outcomes and all-cause mortality in women [197], as a predictor of residual risk in those treated to LDL-C goal [198], as a predictor of first coronary event in men [199], and with microvascular complications of diabetes [200]. In children with a TG-to-HDL-C ratio ≥2.0, there was a two- to threefold higher risk of elevated ALT levels and concentric LV hypertrophy than those with a TG-to-HDL-C ratio<2.0, independent of confounding factors [201].

There are other factors influencing HDL-C concentrations in diabetes. ABCA1 expression and protein concentrations in leukocytes, as well as function in cultured skin fibroblasts, were evaluated in drug naive T2DM men with variable degrees of hyperglycemia. All were abnormal and associated with low HDL-C. There are other conflicting studies with some showing ABCA1 directly influences glycemia via its action on β-cell insulin secretion, but other data suggest that it is glucose which modifies ABCA1 [202, 203].

A review of the NMR-measured lipoprotein changes typical of patients with TG/HDL axis abnormalities reveals increased total LDL-P and reduced total HDL-P and high LDL-P/HDL-P ratios. Subparticle examination identifies increased large VLDL-P, increased VLDL size, increased small LDL-P, decreased LDL size, decreased large HDL-P, and decreased HDL size. These parameters have been examined in the large ($n$=28,345) Women's Health Study of whom over 13.3 years 1,687 cases of T2DM occurred. Lipoproteins subfractions differed substantially by size in T2DM patients compared to normal patients. Small LDL and small HDL were positively associated with diabetes (quintile 5 vs. 1 [adjusted hazard ratios and 95 % CIs], 4.04 [3.21–5.09] and 1.84 [1.54–2.19], respectively). By contrast, large LDL and large HDL were inversely associated with diabetes (quintile 1 vs. 5, 2.50 [2.12–2.95] and 4.51 [3.68–5.52], respectively). For VLDL, large particles imparted higher risk than small particles (quintile 5 vs. 1, 3.11 [2.35–4.11] and 1.31 [1.10–1.55], respectively). Lipoprotein particle size remained significant after adjusting for standard lipids (HDL-C and TG) and nonlipid factors [204].

## References

1. Roger VL, Go AS, Lloyd-Jones DM, Benjamin EJ, Berry JD, Borden WB, et al. Heart disease and stroke statistics–2012 update: a report from the American Heart Association. Circulation. 2012;125:e12–230.
2. Roberts WC. It's the cholesterol, stupid! Am J Cardiol. 2010;106:1364–6.
3. Williams KJ, Tabas I. Lipoprotein retention- and clues for atheroma regression. Arterioscler Thromb Vasc Biol. 2005;25:1536–40.
4. Fredrickson DS, Levy RI, Lees RS. Fat transport in lipoproteins—an integrated approach to mechanisms and disorders. N Engl J Med. 1967;276:34–44.
5. Biggerstaff KD, Wooten JS. Understanding lipoproteins as transporters of cholesterol and other lipids. Adv Physiol Educ. 2004;28:105–6.
6. Tzotzas T, Desrumaux C, Lagrost L. Plasma phospholipid transfer protein (PLTP): review of an emerging cardiometabolic risk factor. Obes Rev. 2009;10:403–11.

7. Alaupovic P. The concept of apolipoprotein-defined lipoprotein families and its clinical significance. Curr Atheroscler Rep. 2003;5:459–67.
8. Kwitterovich PO. The Johns Hopkins textbook of dyslipidemia. Philadelphia: Wolters Kluwer/ Lippincott Williams and Wilkens; 2010.
9. Glickman RM, Rogers M, Glickman JN. Apolipoprotein B synthesis by human liver and intestine in vitro. Proc Natl Acad Sci. 1986;83:5296–300.
10. Huang R, Silva RA, Jerome WG, Kontush A, Chapman MJ, Curtiss LK, et al. Apolipoprotein A-I structural organization in high-density lipoproteins isolated from human plasma. Nat Struct Mol Biol. 2011;18:416–22.
11. Packard CJ, Demant T, Stewart JP, Bedford D, Caslake MJ, Schwertfeger G, et al. Apolipoprotein B metabolism and the distribution of VLDL and LDL subfractions. J Lipid Res. 2000;41:305–18.
12. Sniderman AD, Scantlebury T, Cianflone K. Hypertriglyceridemic hyperapob: the unappreciated atherogenic dyslipoproteinemia in type 2 diabetes mellitus. Ann Intern Med. 2001;135:447–59.
13. Contois JH, McConnell JP, Sethi AA, Csako G, Devaraj S, Hoefner DM, et al. Apolipoprotein B and cardiovascular disease risk: position statement from the AACC Lipoproteins and Vascular Diseases Division Working Group on Best Practices. Clin Chem. 2009;55:407–19.
14. Hoofnagle AN, Vaisar T, Mitra P, Chait A. HDL lipids and insulin resistance. Curr Diab Rep. 2010;10:78–86.
15. Tsompanidi EM, Brinkmeier MS, Fotiadou EH, Giakoumi SM, Kypreos K. HDL biogenesis and functions: role of HDL quality in atherosclerosis. Atherosclerosis. 2010;208:3–9.
16. Rosenson RS, Brewer Jr HB, Chapman MJ, Fazio S, Hussain MM, Kontush A, et al. HDL measures, particle heterogeneity, proposed nomenclature, and relation to atherosclerotic cardiovascular events. Clin Chem. 2011;57:392–410.
17. Lau JF, Smith DA. Advanced lipoprotein testing: recommendations based on current evidence. Endocrinol Metab Clin North Am. 2009;38:1–31.
18. Rifai N, Warnick GR, Dominiczak MH. Handbook of lipoprotein testing. 2nd ed. Washington DC:AACC Press; 2000.
19. Freedman DS, Otvos JD, Jeyarajah EJ, Barboriak JJ, Anderson AJ, Walker JA. Relation of lipoprotein subclasses as measured by proton nuclear magnetic resonance spectroscopy to coronary artery disease. Arterioscler Thromb Vasc Biol. 1998;18:1046–53.
20. Musunuru K, Orho-Melander M, Caulfield MP, Li S, Salameh WA, Reitz RE, et al. Ion mobility analysis of lipoprotein subfractions identifies three independent axes of cardiovascular risk. Arterioscler Thromb Vasc Biol. 2009;29:1975–80.
21. Friedewald WT, Levy RI, Fredrickson DS. Estimation of the concentration of low-density lipoprotein cholesterol in plasma, without use of the preparative ultracentrifuge. Clin Chem. 1972;18:499–502.
22. Sniderman AD. Can conclusions that seem discordant be concordant after all? J Clin Lipidol. 2011;5:261–3.
23. Dayspring T, Dall T, Abuhajir M. Moving beyond LDL-C: incorporating lipoprotein particle numbers and geometric parameters to improve clinical outcomes. Res Rep Clin Cardiol. 2010;1:1–10.
24. Marniemi J, Maki J, Maatela J, Jorma J, Jarvisalo J, Impivarra O. Poor applicability of the Friedewald formula in the assessment of serum LDL cholesterol for clinical purposes. Clin Biochem. 1995;28:285–9.
25. Contois JH, Warnick GR, Sniderman AD. Reliability of low-density lipoprotein cholesterol, non-high-density lipoprotein cholesterol, and apolipoprotein B measurement. J Clin Lipidol. 2011;5:264–72.
26. Voloshyna I, Reiss AB. The ABC transporters in lipid flux and atherosclerosis. Prog Lipid Res. 2011;50:213–24.
27. Yu L, Bharadwaj S, Brown JM, Ma Y, Du W, Davis MA, et al. Cholesterol-regulated translocation of NPC1L1 to the cell surface facilitates free cholesterol uptake. J Biol Chem. 2006;10(281):6616–24.
28. Rigotti A, Miettinen HE, Krieger M. The role of the high-density lipoprotein receptor SR-BI in the lipid metabolism of endocrine and other tissues. Endocr Rev. 2003;24:357–87.
29. Brewer Jr HB, Santamarina-Fojo S. New insights into the role of the adenosine triphosphate-binding cassette transporters in high-density lipoprotein metabolism and reverse cholesterol transport. Am J Cardiol. 2003;91(7A):3E–11.
30. Goldstein JL, Brown MS. Molecular medicine. The cholesterol quartet. Science. 2001;292:1310–2.
31. Williams SE, Ashcom JD, Argraves WS, Strickland DK. A novel mechanism for controlling the activity of alpha 2-macroglobulin receptor/low density lipoprotein receptor-related protein. Multiple regulatory sites for 39-kDa receptor-associated protein. J Biol Chem. 1992;5(267):9035–40.
32. Martinez LO, Jacquet S, Esteve JP, Rolland C, Cabezón E, Champagne E, et al. Ectopic beta-chain of ATP synthase is an apolipoprotein A-I receptor in hepatic HDL endocytosis. Nature. 2003;421:75–9.
33. van der Velde AE, Brufau G, Groen AK. Transintestinal cholesterol efflux. Curr Opin Lipidol. 2010;21:167–71.
34. Ballantyne CM. Clinical lipidology: a companion to Braunwald's heart disease. 1st ed. Philadelphia: Saunders/Elsevier; 2009. Chapter 3.
35. Ge L, Wang J, Qi W, Miao HH, Cao J, Qu YX, et al. The cholesterol absorption inhibitor ezetimibe acts by blocking the sterol-induced internalization of NPC1L1. Cell Metab. 2008;7:508–19.
36. Mathur SN, Watt KR, Field FJ. Regulation of intestinal NPC1L1 expression by dietary fish oil and docosahexaenoic acid. J Lipid Res. 2007;48: 395–404.
37. Bosner MS, Lange LG, Stenson WF, Ostlund Jr RE. Percent cholesterol absorption in normal women and men quantified with dual stable isotopic tracers and

negative ion mass spectrometry. J Lipid Res. 1999;40:302–8.
38. Nguyen TM, Sawyer JK, Kelley KL, Davis MA, Rudel LL. Cholesterol esterification by ACAT2 is essential for efficient intestinal cholesterol absorption: evidence from thoracic lymph duct cannulation. J Lipid Res. 2012;53:95–104.
39. Stieger B. Recent insights into the function and regulation of the bile salt export pump (ABCB11). Cur Opin Lipidol. 2009;20:176–81.
40. Blade AM, Fabritius MA, Hou L, Weinberg RB, Shelness GS. Biogenesis of apolipoprotein A-V and its impact on VLDL triglyceride secretion. J Lipid Res. 2011;52:237–44.
41. Simon T, Cook VR, Rao A, Weinberg RB. Impact of murine intestinal apolipoprotein A-IV expression on regional lipid absorption, gene expression, and growth. J Lipid Res. 2011;52:1984–94.
42. The third report of the national cholesterol education program (NCEP) expert panel on detection, evaluation, and treatment of high blood cholesterol in adults (Adult Treatment Panel III). Circulation. 2002;106:3145–21.
43. Miller M, Stone NJ, Ballantyne C, Bittner V, Criqui MH, Ginsberg HN, et al. Triglycerides and cardiovascular disease: a scientific statement from the American Heart Association. Circulation. 2011;123: 2292–333.
44. Otvos JD, Jeyarajah EJ, Cromwell WC. Measurement issues related to lipoprotein heterogeneity. Am J Cardiol. 2002;90(8A):22i–9.
45. Masson D, Jiang XC, Lagrost L, Tall AR. The role of plasma lipid transfer proteins in lipoprotein metabolism and atherogenesis. J Lip Res. 2009;S201–6.
46. Alaupovic P. The concept of apolipoprotein-defined lipoprotein families and its clinical significance. Curr Atheroscler Rep. 2003;5:459–67.
47. Rezaee F, Casetta B, Levels JH, Speijer D, Meijers JC. Proteomic analysis of high-density lipoprotein. Proteomics. 2006;6:721–30.
48. Blade AM, Fabritius MA, Hou L, Weinberg RB, GrShelness GS. Biogenesis of apolipoprotein A-V and its impact on VLDL triglyceride secretion. J Lipid Res. 2011;52:237–44.
49. Olivecrona G, Beisiegel U. Lipid binding of apolipoprotein CII is required for stimulation of lipoprotein lipase activity against apolipoprotein CII-deficient chylomicrons. Arterioscler Thromb Vasc Biol. 1997;17:1545–9.
50. Sundaram M, Zhong S, Bou Khalil M, Links PH, Zhao Y, Iqbal J, et al. Expression of apolipoprotein C-III in McA-RH7777 cells enhances VLDL assembly and secretion under lipid-rich conditions. J Lipid Res. 2010;51:150–61.
51. Jong MC, Hofker MH, Havekes LM. Role of ApoCs in lipoprotein metabolism functional differences between ApoC1, ApoC2, and ApoC3. Arterioscler Thromb Vasc Biol. 1999;19:472–84.
52. Green PH, Lefkowitch JH, Glickman RM, Riley JW, Quinet E, Blum CB. Apolipoprotein localization and quantitation in the human intestine. Gastroenterology. 1982;83(6):1223–30.
53. Eckel RH. Lipoprotein lipase. A multifunctional enzyme relevant to common metabolic disease. N Engl J Med. 1989;320:1060–8.
54. Wong K, Ryan RO. Characterization of apolipoprotein A-V structure and mode of plasma triacylglycerol regulation. Curr Opin Lipidol. 2007;18:319–24.
55. Dallinga-Thie GM, Franssen R, Mooij HL, Visser ME, Hassing C, Peelman F, et al. The metabolism of triglyceride-rich lipoproteins revisited: new players, new insight. Atherosclerosis. 2010;211:1–8.
56. Ory DS. Chylomicrons and lipoprotein lipase at the endothelial surface: bound and GAG-ged? Cell Metab. 2007;5:229–31.
57. Nilssona SK, Heerenb J, Olivecronaa G, Merkel M. Apolipoprotein A-V; a potent triglyceride reducer. Atherosclerosis. 2011;219:15–21.
58. Goldberg IJ, Scheraldi CA, Yacoub LK, Saxena U, Bisgaiere CL. Lipoprotein ApoC-II activation of lipoprotein lipase. Modulation by apolipoprotein A-IV. J Biol Chem. 1990;265:4266–72.
59. Niemeier A, Gafvels M, Heeren J, Meyer N, Angelin B, Beisiegell U. VLDL receptor mediates the uptake of human chylomicron remnants in vitro. J Lipid Res. 1996;37:1733–42.
60. Cohn JS, Tremblay M, Batal R, Jacques H, Veilleux L, Rodriguez C, et al. Plasma kinetics of VLDL and HDL apoC-I in normolipidemic and hypertriglyceridemic subjects. J Lipid Res. 2002;43:1680–7.
61. Bouchard C, Dubuc G, Davignon J, Bernier L, Cohn JS. Post-transcriptional regulation of apoC-I synthesis and secretion in human HepG2 cells. Atherosclerosis. 2005;178:257–64.
62. Gautier T, Masson D, de Barros JP, Athias A, Gambert P, Aunis D, et al. Human apolipoprotein C-I accounts for the ability of plasma high density lipoproteins to inhibit the cholesteryl ester transfer protein activity. J Biol Chem. 2000;75:37504–9.
63. Lenich C, Brecher B, Makrides S, Chobanian A, Zannis VI. Apolipoprotein gene expression in the rabbit: abundance, size, and distribution of apolipoprotein mRNA species in different tissues. J Lipid Res. 1988;29:755–64.
64. Mauger JF, Couture P, Bergeron N, Lamarche B. Apolipoprotein C-III isoforms: kinetics and relative implication in lipid metabolism. J Lipid Res. 2006;47:1212–8.
65. Chan DC, Chen MM, Ooi EM, Watts GF. An ABC of apolipoprotein C-III: a clinically useful new cardiovascular risk factor? Int J Clin Pract. 2008; 62:799–809.
66. Brewer Jr HB, Increasing HDL. Cholesterol levels. N Engl J Med. 2004;350:1491–4.
67. Otvos JD, Jeyarajah EJ, Cromwell WC. Measurement issues related to lipoprotein heterogeneity. Am J Cardiol. 2002;90(Suppl):23i–9.
68. Sniderman AD, De Graaf J, Couture P, Williams K, Kiss RS, Watts GF. Regulation of plasma LDL: the apoB paradigm. Clin Sci (Lond). 2009;118:333–9.

69. Morton RE, Gnizak HM, Greene DJ, Cho KH, Paromov VM. Lipid transfer inhibitor protein (apolipoprotein F) concentration in normolipemic and hyperlipidemic subjects. J Lip Res. 2008;49:127–35.
70. Schonfeld G. Familial hypobetalipoproteinemia: a review. J Lip Res. 2003;44:878–83.
71. Yokoyama S. HDL biogenesis and cellular cholesterol homeostasis. Ann Med. 2008;40:29–38.
72. Brewer Jr HB, Remaley AT, Neufeld EB, Basso F, Joyce C. Regulation of plasma high-density lipoprotein levels by the ABCA1 transporter and the emerging role of high-density lipoprotein in the treatment of cardiovascular disease. Arterioscler Thromb Vasc Biol. 2004;24:1755–60.
73. McGillicuddy FC, Reilly MP, Rader DJ. Adipose modulation of high-density lipoprotein cholesterol: implications for obesity, high-density lipoprotein metabolism, and cardiovascular disease. Circulation. 2011;124:1602–5.
74. Imachi H, Murao K, Sayo Y, Hosokawa H, Sato M, Niimi M, et al. Evidence for a potential role for HDL as an important source of cholesterol in human adrenocortical tumors via the CLA-1 pathway. Endocr J. 1999;46:27–34.
75. Nielson MJ, Nielson LB, Moestrup S. High density lipoprotein and innate immunity. Future Lipidol. 2006;1:729–34.
76. Lewis GF, Rader DJ. New insights into the regulation of HDL metabolism and reverse cholesterol transport. Circ Res. 2005;96:1221–32.
77. Martinez LO, Jacquet S, Esteve JP, Rolland C, Cabezon E, Champagne E, et al. Ectopic beta-chain of ATP synthase is an apolipoprotein A-I receptor in hepatic HDL endocytosis. Nature. 2003;421:75–9.
78. Duffy D, Rader DJ. Emerging therapies targeting high-density lipoprotein metabolism and reverse cholesterol transport. Circulation. 2006;113:1140–50.
79. Dayspring T. High-density lipoproteins: emerging knowledge. J Cardiometab Syndr. 2007;2:59–62.
80. Moestrup SK, Kozyraki R. Cubilin, a high-density lipoprotein receptor. Curr Opin Lipidol. 2000;11: 133–40.
81. DeFronzo RA. Insulin resistance, lipotoxicity, type 2 diabetes and atherosclerosis: the missing links. The Claude Bernard Lecture 2009. Diabetologia. 2010;53:1270–87.
82. Matthan NR, Pencina M, LaRocque JM, Jacques PF, D'Agostino RB, Schaefer EJ, et al. Alterations in cholesterol absorption/synthesis markers characterize Framingham offspring study participants with CHD. J Lipid Res. 2009;50:1927–35.
83. Assmann G, Cullen P, Erbey J, Ramey DR, Kannenberg F, Schulte H. Plasma sitosterol elevations are associated with an increased incidence of coronary events in men: results of a nested case–control analysis of the Prospective Cardiovascular Münster (PROCAM) study. Nutr Metab Cardiovasc Dis. 2006;16:13–21.
84. Miettinen TA, Gylling H, Hallikainen M, Juonala M, Räsänen L, Viikari J, et al. Relation of non-cholesterol sterols to coronary risk factors and carotid intima-media thickness: the Cardiovascular Risk in Young Finns Study. Atherosclerosis. 2010;209(2):592–7.
85. Miettinen TA, Gylling H, Strandberg T, Sarna S. Baseline serum cholestanol as predictor of recurrent coronary events in subgroup of Scandinavian simvastatin survival study. Finnish 4S investigators. BMJ. 1998;316(7138):1127–30.
86. Strandberg TE, Tilvis RS, Pitkala KH, Miettinen TA. Cholesterol and glucose metabolism and recurrent cardiovascular events among the elderly: a prospective study. J Am Coll Cardiol. 2006;48:708–14.
87. Gylling H, Miettinen TA. Cholesterol absorption, synthesis, and LDL metabolism in NIDDM. Diabetes Care. 1997;20:90–5.
88. Gylling H, Miettinen TA. Cholesterol absorption and lipoprotein metabolism in type II diabetes mellitus with and without coronary artery disease. Atheroscerosis. 1996;126:325–32.
89. Paramsothy P, Knopp RH, Kahn SE, Retzlaff BM, Fish B, Ma L, et al. Plasma sterol evidence for decreased absorption and increased synthesis of cholesterol in insulin resistance and obesity. Am J Clin Nutr. 2011;94:1182–8.
90. O'Meara NM, Devery RA, Owens D, et al. Cholesterol metabolism in alloxan-induced diabetic rabbits. Diabetes. 1990;39:626–33.
91. Lally S, Owens D, Tomkin GH. Genes that affect cholesterol synthesis, cholesterol absorption, and chylomicron assembly: the relationship between the liver and intestine in control and streptozotosin diabetic rats. Metabolism Clin Exp. 2007;56:430–8.
92. Lally S, Tan CY, Owens D, Tomkin GH. Messenger RNA levels of genes involved in dysregulation of postprandial lipoproteins in type 2 diabetes: the role of Niemann-Pick C1-like 1, ATP-binding cassette, transporters G5 and G8, and of microsomal triglyceride transfer protein. Diabetologia. 2006;49:1008–16.
93. Tomkin GH. The intestine as a regulator of cholesterol homeostasis in diabetes. Atherosclerosis. 2011;Suppl 9:27–32.
94. Gaudiani LM, Lewin A, Meneghini L, Perevozskaya I, Plotkin D, Mitchel Y, et al. Efficacy and safety of ezetimibe co-administered with simvastatin in thiazolidinedione-treated type 2 diabetic patients. Diabetes Obes Metab. 2005;7:88–97.
95. van Himbergen TM, Matthan NR, Resteghini NA, Otokozawa S, Ai M, Stein EA, et al. Comparison of the effects of maximal dose atorvastatin and rosuvastatin therapy on cholesterol synthesis and absorption markers. J Lipid Res. 2009;50:730–9.
96. Szapary PO, Rader DJ. The triglyceride-high-density lipoprotein axis: an important target of therapy? Am Heart J. 2004;148:211–21.
97. Angulo P. Nonalcoholic fatty liver disease. N Engl J Med. 2002;346:1221–31.
98. Browning JD, Horton JD. Molecular mediators of hepatic steatosis and liver injury. J Clin Invest. 2004;114:147–52.

99. Allister EM, Borradaile NM, Edwards JY, Huff MW. Inhibition of microsomal triglyceride transfer protein expression and apolipoprotein B100 secretion by the citrus flavonoid naringenin and by insulin involves activation of the mitogen-activated protein kinase pathway in hepatocytes. Diabetes. 2005;54:1676–83.
100. Shelness GS, Sellers JA. Very-low-density lipoprotein assembly and secretion. Curr Opin Lipidol. 2001;12:151–7.
101. Gill JM, Brown JC, Bedford D, Wright DM, Cooney J, Hughes DA, et al. Hepatic production of VLDL1 but not VLDL2 is related to insulin resistance in normoglycaemic middle-aged subjects. Atherosclerosis. 2004;176:49–56.
102. Chan DC, Watts GF, Gan SK, Wong ATY, Ooi EMM, Barrett PHR. Nonalcoholic fatty liver disease as the transducer of hepatic oversecretion of very-low-density lipoprotein–apolipoprotein B-100 in obesity. Arterioscler Thromb Vasc Biol. 2010;30: 1043–50.
103. Stanhope KL, Bremer AA, Medici V, Nakajima K, Ito Y, Nakano T, et al. Consumption of fructose and high fructose corn syrup increase postprandial triglycerides, LDL-cholesterol, and apolipoprotein-B in young men and women. J Clin Endocrinol Metab. 2011;96(10):E1596–605.
104. Adiels M, Boren J, Caslake MJ, Stewart P, Soro A, Westerbacka J, et al. Overproduction of VLDL1 driven by hyperglycemia is a dominant feature of diabetic dyslipidemia. Arterioscler Thromb Vasc Biol. 2005;25:1697–703.
105. Adiels M, Olofsson SO, Taskinen MR, Boren J. Diabetic dyslipidaemia. Curr Opin Lipidol. 2006; 17:238–46.
106. Asp L, Claesson C, Boren J, Olofsson S-O. ADP-ribosylation factor 1 and its activation of phospholipase D are important for the assembly of very low density lipoproteins. J Biol Chem. 2000;275: 26285–92.
107. Brown AM, Gibbons GF. Insulin inhibits the maturation phase of VLDL assembly via a phosphoinositide 3-kinase-mediated event. Arterioscler Thromb Vasc Biol. 2001;21:1656–61.
108. Packard CJ, Demant T, Stewart JP, Bedford D, Caslake MJ, Schwertfeger G, et al. Apolipoprotein B metabolism and the distribution of VLDL and LDL subfractions. J Lipid Res. 2000;41:305–18.
109. Adiels M, Olofsson SO, Taskinen MR, Boren J. Overproduction of very low-density lipoproteins is the hallmark of diabetic dyslipidemia. Arterioscler Thromb Vasc Biol. 2008;28:1225–36.
110. Garvey WT, Kwon S, Zheng D, Shaughnessy S, Wallace P, Hutto A, et al. Effects of insulin resistance and type 2 diabetes on lipoprotein subclass particle size and concentration determined by nuclear magnetic resonance. Diabetes. 2003;52:453–62.
111. Goldberg IJ, Scheraldi CA, Yacoub LK, Saxena U, Bisgaiere CL. Lipoprotein ApoC-II activation of lipoprotein lipase: modulation by apolipoprotein A-IV. J Biol Chem. 1990;265:4266–72.
112. Pruneta-Deloche V, Ponsin G, Groisne L, Fruchart-Najib J, Lagarde M, Moulin P. Postprandial increase of plasma apoAV concentrations in type 2 diabetic patients. Atherosclerosis. 2005;181:403–5.
113. Kahri J, Fruchart-Najib J, Matikainen N, Fruchart JC, Vakkilainen J, Taskinen MR. The increase of apolipoprotein A-V during postprandial lipemia parallels the response of triglyceride-rich lipoproteins in type 2 diabetes: no relationship between apoA-V and postheparin plasma lipolytic activity. Diabetes Care. 2007;8:2083–5.
114. Talmud PJ, Cooper JA, Hattori H, Miller IP, Miller GJ, Humphries SE. The apolipoprotein A-V genotype and plasma apolipoprotein A-V and triglyceride levels: prospective risk of type 2 diabetes. Results from the Northwick Park Heart Study II. Diabetologia. 2006;49:2337–40.
115. Moen CJ, Tholens AP, Voshol PJ, de Haan W, Havekes LM, Gargalovic P, et al. The Hyplip2 locus causes hypertriglyceridemia by decreased clearance of triglycerides. J Lipid Res. 2007;48:2182–92.
116. van der Ham RL, Alizadeh Dehnavi R, Berbée JF, Putter H, de Roos A, Romijn JA, et al. Plasma apolipoprotein CI and CIII levels are associated with increased plasma triglyceride levels and decreased fat mass in men with the metabolic syndrome. Diabetes Care. 2009;32:184–6.
117. Twickler T, Dallinga-Thie GM, Chapman MJ, Cohn JS. Remnant lipoproteins and atherosclerosis. Curr Atheroscler Rep. 2005;7:140–7.
118. Björkegren J. Dual roles of apolipoprotein CI in the formation of atherogenic remnants. Curr Atheroscler Rep. 2006;8:1–2.
119. Hamsten A, Silveira A, Boquist S, Tang R, Bond G, de Faire U, et al. The apolipoprotein CI content of triglyceride-rich lipoproteins independently predicts early atherosclerosis in healthy middle-aged men. J Am Coll Cardiol. 2005;45:1013–7.
120. Huang S, Qiao J, Li R, Wang L, Li M, Wang L, et al. Can serum apolipoprotein C-I demonstrate metabolic abnormality early in women with polycystic ovary syndrome? Fertil Steril. 2010;94:205–10.
121. Cohn JS, Patterson BW, Uffelman KD, Davignon J, Steiner G. Rate of production of plasma and very-low-density lipoprotein (VLDL) apolipoprotein C-III is strongly related to the concentration and level of production of VLDL triglyceride in male subjects with different body weights and levels of insulin sensitivity. J Clin Endocrinol Metab. 2004;89: 3949–55.
122. Sacks FM, Alaupovic P, Moye LA, Cole TG, Sussex B, Stampfer MJ, et al. VLDL, apolipoproteins B, CIII, and E, and risk of recurrent coronary events in the cholesterol and recurrent events (CARE) trial. Circulation. 2000;102:1886–92.
123. Lee SJ, Moye LA, Campos H, Williams GH, Sacks FM. Hypertriglyceridemia but not diabetes status is associated with VLDL containing apolipoprotein CIII in patients with coronary heart disease. Atherosclerosis. 2003;167:293–302.

124. Chen M, Breslow JL, Li W, Leff T. Transcriptional regulation of the apoC-III gene by insulin in diabetic mice: correlation with changes in plasma triglyceride levels. J Lipid Res. 1994;35:1918–24.
125. Altomonte J, Cong L, Harbaran S, Richter A, Xu J, Meseck M, et al. Foxo1 mediates insulin action on apoC-III and triglyceride metabolism. J Clin Invest. 2004;114:1493–503.
126. Ladias JAA, Hadzopoulou-Cladaras M, Kardassis D, Cardot P, Cheng J, Zannis V, et al. Transcriptional regulation of human apolipoprotein genes ApoB, ApoCIII, and ApoAII by members of the steroid hormone receptor superfamily HNF-4, ARP-1, EAR-2, and EAR-3. J Biol Chem. 1992;267:15849–60.
127. Caron S, Verrijken A, Mertens I, Samanez CH, Mautino G, Haas JT, et al. Transcriptional activation of apolipoprotein CIII expression by glucose may contribute to diabetic dyslipidemia. Arterioscler Thromb Vasc Biol. 2011;31(3):513–9.
128. Ginsberg HN, Brown WV. Apolipoprotein CIII 42 years old and even more interesting. Arterioscler Thromb Vasc Biol. 2011;31:471–3.
129. Ruby MA, Goldenson B, Orasanu G, Johnston TP, Plutzky J, Krauss RM. VLDL hydrolysis by LPL activates PPAR-α through generation of unbound fatty acids. J Lipid Res. 2010;51:2275–81.
130. Mendivil CO, Zheng C, Furtado J, Lel J, Sack FM. Metabolism of very-low-density lipoprotein and low-density lipoprotein containing apolipoprotein C-III and not other small apolipoproteins. Arterioscler Thromb Vasc Biol. 2010;30:239–45.
131. Tian L, Wu J, Fu M, Xu Y, Jia L. Relationship between apolipoprotein C-III concentrations and high-density lipoprotein subclass distribution. Metabolism Clin Exp. 2009;58:668–74.
132. Sacks FM, Zheng C, Cohn JS. Complexities of plasma apolipoprotein C-III metabolism. J Lipid Res. 2011;52:1066–70.
133. Tomiyasu K, Walsh BW, Ikewaki K, Judge H, Sacks FM. Differential metabolism of human VLDL according to content of ApoE and ApoC-III. Arterioscler Thromb Vasc Biol. 2001;21:1494–500.
134. Khoo C, Campos H, Judge H, Sacks FM. Effects of estrogenic oral contraceptives on the lipoprotein B particle system defined by apolipoproteins E and C-III content. J Lipid Res. 1999;40:202–12.
135. Asztalos BF, Schaefer EJ, Horvath KV, Yamashita S, Miller M, Franceschini G, et al. Role of LCAT in HDL remodeling: investigation of LCAT deficiency states. J Lipid Res. 2007;48:592–9.
136. Shin MJ, Krauss RM. Apolipoprotein CIII bound to apoB-containing lipoproteins is associated with small, dense LDL independent of plasma triglyceride levels in healthy men. Atherosclerosis. 2010;211:337–41.
137. Bobik A. Apolipoprotein CIII and atherosclerosis: beyond effects on lipid metabolism. Circulation. 2008;118:702–4.
138. Kawakami A, Osaka M, Tani M, Azuma H, Sacks FM, Shimokado K, et al. Apolipoprotein C-III links hyperlipidemia with vascular endothelial cell dysfunction. Circulation. 2008;118:731–42.
139. Abe Y, Kawakami A, Osaka M, Uematsu S, Akira S, Shimokado K, et al. Apolipoprotein CIII induces monocyte chemoattractant protein-1 and interleukin 6 expression via Toll-like receptor 2 pathway in mouse adipocytes. Arterioscler Thromb Vasc Biol. 2010;30:2242–8.
140. Libby P. Fat fuels the flame: triglyceride-rich lipoproteins and arterial inflammation. Circ Res. 2007;100:299–301.
141. Dugue-Pujol S, Rousset X, Pastier D, Quang NT, Pautre V, Chamba J, et al. Human apolipoprotein A-II associates with triglyceride-rich lipoproteins in plasma and impairs their catabolism. J Lipid Res. 2006;47:2631–9.
142. Brewer Jr HB. Hypertriglyceridemia: changes in the plasma lipoproteins associated with an increased risk of cardiovascular disease. Am J Cardiol. 1999;83:3F–12.
143. Castellani LW, Nguyen CN, Charugundla Weinstein MM, Doan CX, Blaner WS, Wongsiriroj N, et al. Apolipoprotein AII is a regulator of very low density lipoprotein metabolism and insulin resistance. J Bio Chem. 2008;283:11633–44.
144. Johnson LA, Arbones-Mainar JM, Fox RG, Pendse AA, Altenburg MK, Kim HS, et al. Apolipoprotein E4 exaggerates diabetic dyslipidemia and atherosclerosis in mice lacking the LDL receptor. Diabetes. 2011;60:2285–94.
145. Davis WA, Chin E, Jee A, Martins J, Bruce DG, Beilby J, et al. Apolipoprotein E genotype and mortality in Southern European and Anglo-Celt patients with type 2 diabetes: the Fremantle Diabetes Study. Eur J Endocrinol. 2010;163:559–64.
146. Anthopoulos PG, Hamodrakas SJ, Bagos PG. Apolipoprotein E polymorphisms and type 2 diabetes: a meta-analysis of 30 studies including 5423 cases and 8197 controls. Mol Genet Metab. 2010;100:283–91.
147. Ward H, Mitrou PN, Bowman R, Luben R, Wareham NJ, Khaw KT, et al. APOE genotype, lipids, and coronary heart disease risk: a prospective population study. Arch Intern Med. 2009;169:1424–9.
148. Camsari A, Tamer L, Aras Ateş N, Pekdemir H, Çiçek D, Ercan B, et al. Apolipoprotein E polymorphism in diabetic and non-diabetic patients: does it really contribute to atherosclerosis? Acta Cardiol. 2005;60:409–14.
149. Duchateau PN, Pullinger CR, Orellana RE, Kunitake ST, Naya-Vigne J, O'Connor PM, et al. Apolipoprotein L, a new human high density lipoprotein apolipoprotein expressed by the pancreas. Identification, cloning, characterization, and plasma distribution of apolipoprotein L. J Biol Chem. 1997;272:25576–82.
150. Albert TS, Duchateau PN, Deeb SS, Pullinger CR, Cho MH, Heilbron DC, et al. Apolipoprotein L-I is positively associated with hyperglycemia and plasma triglycerides in CAD patients with low HDL. J Lipid Res. 2005;46:469–74.

151. Roubtsova A, Munkonda MN, Awan Z, Marcinkiewicz J, Chamberland A, Lazure C, et al. Circulating proprotein convertase subtilisin/kexin 9 (PCSK9) regulates VLDLR protein and triglyceride accumulation in visceral adipose tissue. Arterioscler Thromb Vasc Biol. 2011;31:785–91.
152. Longato L, Tong M, Wands JR, de la Monte SM. High fat diet induced hepatic steatosis and insulin resistance: role of dysregulated ceramide metabolism. Hepatol Res. 2011. doi: 10.1111/j.1872-034X.2011.00934.x [Epub ahead of print].
153. Chan DC, Barrett PH, Ooi EM, Ji J, Chan DT, Watts GF. Very low density lipoprotein metabolism and plasma adiponectin as predictors of high-density lipoprotein apolipoprotein A-I kinetics in obese and nonobese men. J Clin Endocrinol Metab. 2009;94:989–97.
154. Ooi EM, Watts GF, Farvid MS, Chan DC, Allen MC, Zilko SR, et al. High-density lipoprotein apolipoprotein A-I kinetics in obesity. Obes Res. 2005;13:1008–16.
155. Julia Z, Duchene E, Fournier N, Bellanger N, Chapman MJ, Le Goff W, et al. Postprandial lipemia enhances the capacity of large HDL2 particles to mediate free cholesterol efflux via SR-BI and ABCG1 pathways in type IIB hyperlipidemia. J Lipid Res. 2010;51:3350–8.
156. Yancey PG, Kawashiri MA, Moore R, Glick JM, Williams DL, Connelly MA, et al. In vivo modulation of HDL phospholipid has opposing effects on SR-BI- and ABCA1-mediated cholesterol efflux. J Lipid Res. 2004;45:337–46.
157. Sarwar N, Danesh J, Eiriksdottir G, Sigurdsson G, Wareham N, Bingham S, et al. Triglycerides and the risk of coronary heart disease: 10,158 incident cases among 262,525 participants in 29 Western prospective studies. Circulation. 2007;115:450–8.
158. Tirosh A, Rudich A, Shochat T, Tekes-Manova D, Israeli E, Henkin Y, et al. Changes in triglyceride levels and risk for coronary heart disease in young men. Ann Intern Med. 2007;147:377–85.
159. Tirosh A, Shai I, Bitzur R, Kochba I, Tekes-Manova D, Israeli E, et al. Changes in triglyceride levels over time and risk of type 2 diabetes in young men. Diabetes Care. 2008;31:2032–7.
160. Mohanlal N, Holman RR. A standardized triglyceride and carbohydrate challenge: the oral triglyceride tolerance test. Diabetes Care. 2004;27:89–94.
161. Rosenson RS, Davidson MH, Pourfarzib R. Underappreciated opportunities for low-density lipoprotein management in patients with cardiometabolic residual risk. Atherosclerosis. 2010;213:1–7.
162. Nakajima K, Nakajima Y, Takeichi S, Fujita MQ. ApoB-100 carrying lipoprotein, but not apoB-48, is the major subset of proatherogenic remnant-like lipoprotein particles detected in plasma of sudden cardiac death cases. Atherosclerosis. 2007;194:473–82.
163. Nakajima K, Nakano T, Tokita Y, Nagamine T, Inazu A, Kobayashi J, et al. Postprandial lipoprotein metabolism: VLDL vs chylomicrons. Clin Chim Acta. 2011;412:1306–18.
164. Nakajima K, Nakano T, Moon HD, Nagamine T, Stanhope KL, Havel PJ, et al. The correlation between TG vs remnant lipoproteins in the fasting and postprandial plasma of 23 volunteers. Clin Chim Acta. 2009;404:124–7.
165. Langsted A, Nordestgaard BG. Nonfasting lipids, lipoproteins, and apolipoproteins in individuals with and without diabetes: 58 434 individuals from the Copenhagen General Population Study. Clin Chem. 2011;57:482–9.
166. Nakajima K, Nakano T, Tanaka A. The oxidative modification hypothesis of atherosclerosis: the comparison of atherogenic effects on oxidized LDL and remnant lipoproteins in plasma. Clin Chim Acta. 2006;367:36–47.
167. März W, Scharnagl H, Winkler K, Tiran A, Nauck M, Boehm BO, et al. Low-density lipoprotein triglycerides associated with low-grade systemic inflammation, adhesion molecules, and angiographic coronary artery disease: the Ludwigshafen Risk and Cardiovascular Health study. Circulation. 2004;110:3068–74.
168. Nigon F, Lesnik P, Rouis M, Chapman MJ. Discrete subspecies of human low density lipoproteins are heterogeneous in their interaction with the cellular LDL receptor. J Lipid Res. 1991;32:1741–53.
169. Prassl R, Laggner P. Molecular structure of low density lipoprotein: current status and future challenges. Eur Biophys J. 2009;38(2):145–58.
170. van Antwerpen R, Chen GC, Pullinger CR, Kane JP, Labelle M, Krauss RM, et al. Cryo-electron microscopy of low density lipoprotein and reconstituted discoidal high density lipoprotein: imaging of the apolipoprotein moiety. J Lipid Res. 1997;38:659–69.
171. Skalen K, Gustafsson M, Rydberg EK, Hulten LM, Wiklund O, Innerarity TL, et al. Subendothelial retention of atherogenic lipoproteins in early atherosclerosis. Nature. 2002;417:750–4.
172. Gazi I, Lourida ES, Filippatos T, Tsimihodimos V, Elisaf M, Tselepis AD. Lipoprotein-associated phospholipase A2 activity is a marker of small, dense LDL particles in human plasma. Clin Chem. 2005;51:2264–73.
173. Gaubatz JW, Gillard BK, Massey JB, Hoogeveen RC, Huang M, Lloyd EE, et al. Dynamics of dense electronegative low density lipoproteins and their preferential association with lipoprotein phospholipase A(2). J Lipid Res. 2007;48:348–57.
174. Mora S, Szklo M, Otvos JD, Greenland P, Psaty BM, Goff Jr DC, et al. LDL particle subclasses, LDL particle size, and carotid atherosclerosis in the Multi-Ethnic Study of Atherosclerosis (MESA). Atherosclerosis. 2007;192:211–7.
175. Cromwell WC, Otvos JD, Keyes MJ, Pencina MJ, Sullivan L, Vasan RS, et al. LDL particle number and risk of future cardiovascular disease in the Framingham offspring study—implications for LDL management. J Clin Lipidol. 2007;1:583–92.

176. Otvos JD, Mora S, Shalaurova I, Greenland P, Mackey RH, Goff Jr DC. Clinical implications of discordance between low-density lipoprotein cholesterol and particle number. J Clin Lipidol. 2011;5: 105–13.
177. Cromwell WC, Otvos JD. Heterogeneity of low-density lipoprotein particle number in patients with type 2 diabetes mellitus and low-density lipoprotein cholesterol <100 mg/dl. Am J Cardiol. 2006;98: 1599–602.
178. Sniderman AD, Williams K, McQueen MJ, Furberg CD. When is equal not equal? J Clin Lipidol. 2010;4:83–8.
179. Kathiresan S, Otvos JD, Sullivan LM, Keyes MJ, Schaefer EJ, Wilson PW, et al. Increased small low-density lipoprotein particle number: a prominent feature of the metabolic syndrome in the Framingham Heart Study. Circulation. 2006;113(1):20–9.
180. Brown RJ, Rader DJ. When HDL gets fat. Circ Res. 2008;103:131–2.
181. McGillicuddy FC, Muredach MP, Rader DF. Adipose tissue modulation of high-density lipoprotein cholesterol. Implications for obesity, high-density lipoprotein metabolism, and cardiovascular disease. Circulation. 2011;124:1602–5.
182. Jaye M, Krawiec J. Endothelial lipase and HDL metabolism. Curr Opin Lipidol. 2004;15:183–9.
183. Moestrup SK, Nielsen LB. The role of the kidney in lipid metabolism. Curr Opin Lipidol. 2005;16:301–6.
184. Moestrup SK, Kozyraki R. Cubilin, a high-density lipoprotein receptor. Curr Opin Lipidol. 2000;11:133–40.
185. Barrans A, Collet X, Barbaras R, Jaspard B, Manent J, Vieu C, et al. Hepatic lipase induces the formation of pre-beta 1 high density lipoprotein (HDL) from triacylglycerol-rich HDL2. A study comparing liver perfusion to in vitro incubation with lipases. J Biol Chem. 1994;269:11572–7.
186. Asztalos BF, Collins D, Cupples LA, Demissie S, Horvath KV, Bloomfield HE, et al. Value of high-density lipoprotein (HDL) subpopulations in predicting recurrent cardiovascular events in the Veterans Affairs HDL Intervention Trial. Arterioscler Thromb Vasc Biol. 2005;25:2185–91.
187. Lamon-Fava S, Herrington DM, Reboussin DM, Sherman M, Horvath KV, Cupples LA, et al. Plasma levels of HDL subpopulations and remnant lipoproteins predict the extent of angiographically-defined coronary artery disease in postmenopausal women. Arterioscler Thromb Vasc Biol. 2008;28:575–9.
188. Söderlund S, Soro-Paavonen A, Ehnholm C, Jauhiainen M, Taskinen MR. Hypertriglyceridemia is associated with prebeta-HDL concentrations in subjects with familial low HDL. J Lipid Res. 2005;46:1643–51.
189. Jonkers IJ, Smelt AH, Hattori H, Scheek LM, van Gent T, de Man FH, et al. Decreased PLTP mass but elevated PLTP activity linked to insulin resistance in HTG: effects of bezafibrate therapy. J Lipid Res. 2003;44:1462–9.
190. Lee M, Kim JQ, Kim J, Oh H, Park M. Studies on the plasma lipid profiles, and LCAT and CETP activities according to hyperlipoproteinemia phenotypes (HLP). Atherosclerosis. 2001;159:381–9.
191. Sorrentino SA, Besler C, Rohrer L, Meyer M, Heinrich K, Bahlmann FH, et al. Endothelial-vasoprotective effects of high-density lipoprotein are impaired in patients with type 2 diabetes mellitus but are improved after extended-release niacin therapy. Circulation. 2010;121:110–22.
192. McQueen MJ, Hawken S, Wang X, Ounpuu S, Sniderman A, Probstfield J, et al. INTERHEART study investigators. Lipids, lipoproteins, and apolipoproteins as risk markers of myocardial infarction in 52 countries (the INTERHEART study): a case–control study. Lancet. 2008;372:224–33.
193. Otvos JD, Collins D, Freedman DS, Shalaurova I, Schaefer EJ, McNamara JR, et al. Low-density lipoprotein and high-density lipoprotein particle subclasses predict coronary events and are favorably changed by gemfibrozil therapy in the Veterans Affairs High-Density Lipoprotein Intervention Trial. Circulation. 2006;113:1556–63.
194. Blake GJ, Otvos JD, Rifai N, Ridker PM. Low-density lipoprotein particle concentration and size as determined by nuclear magnetic resonance spectroscopy as predictors of cardiovascular disease in women. Circulation. 2002;106:1930–7.
195. Gasevic D, Frohlich J, Mancini GB, Lear SA. The association between triglyceride to high-density-lipoprotein cholesterol ratio and insulin resistance in a multiethnic primary prevention cohort. Metabolism. 2011.
196. Hanak V, Munoz J, Teague J, Stanley Jr A, Bittner V. Accuracy of the triglyceride to high-density lipoprotein cholesterol ratio for prediction of the low-density lipoprotein phenotype B. Am J Cardiol. 2004;94:219–22.
197. Bittner V, Johnson BD, Zineh I, Rogers WJ, Vido D, Marroquin OC, et al. The triglyceride/high-density lipoprotein cholesterol ratio predicts all-cause mortality in women with suspected myocardial ischemia: a report from the Women's Ischemia Syndrome Evaluation (WISE). Am Heart J. 2009;157:548–55.
198. Carey VJ, Bishop L, Laranjo N, Harshfield BJ, Kwiat C, Sacks FM. Contribution of high plasma triglycerides and low high-density lipoprotein cholesterol to residual risk of coronary heart disease after establishment of low-density lipoprotein cholesterol control. Am J Cardiol. 2010;106:757–63.
199. Cordero A, Andrés E, Ordoñez B, León M, Laclaustra M, Grima A, et al. Usefulness of triglycerides-to-high-density lipoprotein cholesterol ratio for predicting the first coronary event in men. Am J Cardiol. 2009;104:1393–7.
200. Zoppini G, Negri C, Stoico V, Casati S, Pichiri I, Bonora E. Triglyceride-high-density lipoprotein cholesterol is associated with microvascular complications in type 2 diabetes mellitus. Metabolism. 2012;61:22–9.

201. Di Bonito P, Moio N, Scilla C, Cavuto L, Sibilio G, Sanguigno E, et al. Usefulness of the high triglyceride-to-HDL cholesterol ratio to identify cardiometabolic risk factors and preclinical signs of organ damage in outpatient children. Diabetes Care. 2012;35:158–62.
202. Patel DC, Albrecht C, Pavitt D, Paul V, Pourreyron C, Newman SP, et al. Type 2 diabetes is associated with reduced ATP-binding cassette transporter A1 gene expression, protein and function. PLoS One. 2011;6:e22142.
203. Passarelli M, Tang C, McDonald TO, O'Brien KD, Gerrity RG, Heinecke JW, et al. Advanced glycation end product precursors impair ABCA1-dependent cholesterol removal from cells. Diabetes. 2005;54:2198–205.
204. Mora S, Otvos JD, Rosenson RS, Pradhan A, Buring JE, Ridker PM. Lipoprotein particle size and concentration by nuclear magnetic resonance and incident type 2 diabetes in women. Diabetes. 2010;59:1153–60.
205. Koo SH, Dutcher AK, Towle HC. Glucose and insulin function through two distinct transcription factors to stimulate expression of lipogenic enzyme genes in liver. J Biol Chem. 2001;276:9437–45.

# Lipoprotein Metabolism and Alterations Induced by Insulin Resistance and Diabetes

5

Gerald H. Tomkin and Daphne Owens

Global warming continues to excite the imagination even though in Ireland we have had the coldest summer on record, and it is now fashionable to talk not about global warming but climate change. Similarly there is tremendous enthusiasm and interest in the explosion of obesity and diabetes that has occurred in the past 30 years, yet at the same time people are living longer and we worry how to fund pension plans that will cover this increase in longevity. Obesity without diabetes, hypertension or dyslipidemia may be less of a risk factor for cardiovascular disease than was originally thought, but with accompanying risk factors, it is certainly a dangerous condition with an increase in risk for diabetes mellitus, cardiovascular disease, cancer, stroke and osteoarthritis [1]. The link between obesity, insulin resistance and diabetes is complex and poorly understood, and the coining of the term "metabolic syndrome" has not helped to foster understanding of this complex disease process. Diabetes is primarily a disease of beta cells leading to partial or complete loss of insulin production. It is an ongoing process with little evidence of reversibility, and we have yet to find a robust method of reversing the destruction of the beta cell whether it is due to apoptosis or necrosis. Obesity plays a major part in insulin resistance and it is rare to find insulin resistance without obesity. Insulin resistance without a defect in pancreatic function (recognised by hyperinsulinemia in the absence of hyperglycemia) is also associated with increased risk for atherosclerotic disease. The purpose of this chapter is to explore the relationship between insulin and lack of insulin in the presence or absence of insulin resistance on lipid metabolism and secondly to explore the effect of insulin resistance in the absence of a defect in the beta cell on lipid metabolism.

The lipoprotein level in the blood depends on the balance of synthesis and degradation or turnover. Synthesis of the lipoprotein particle depends on cholesterol and fat absorption, de novo cholesterol synthesis and de novo fatty acid synthesis. Cholesterol absorption depends on the availability of cholesterol in the diet and the availability of recirculated cholesterol via the enterohepatic circulation. De novo cholesterol synthesized in the intestine is also included in the cholesterol pool since it also enters the lipoprotein pool through the intestinal villi [2]. De novo synthesis of cholesterol occurs mainly in the liver, but virtually every cell in the body has the ability to synthesize cholesterol and the intestine is an important site of cholesterol synthesis. The larger lipoprotein particles consist of a triglyceride-rich core and fatty acids which have been esterified to form phospholipid and cholesterol esters [2]. Phospholipids play

G.H. Tomkin, M.D., F.R.C.P., F.R.C.P.I., F.A.C.P. (✉)
D. Owens
Diabetes Institute of Ireland, Beacon Hospital, Sandyford, Dublin 18, Ireland

Trinity College Dublin, Dublin 2, Ireland
e-mail: gerald.tomkin@tcd.ie

A.J. Jenkins et al. (eds.), *Lipoproteins in Diabetes Mellitus*, Contemporary Diabetes,
DOI 10.1007/978-1-4614-7554-5_5, © Springer Science+Business Media New York 2014

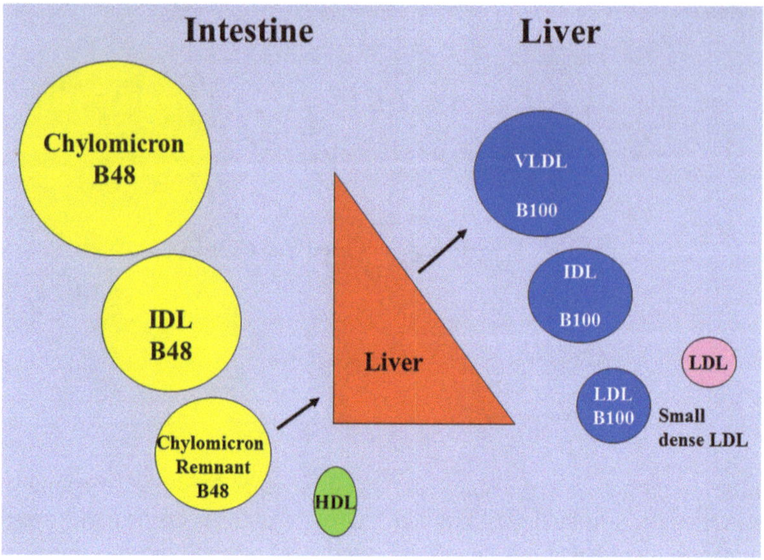


**Fig. 5.1** The lipoprotein cascade

an important part in the outer coat of the chylomicron particle, and the particle is solubilised by the addition of intestinally derived apolipoprotein (apo) B48 which is a better carrier protein for large amounts of triglyceride than apo B100 [3]. Apo B100 is the structural protein for very-low-density lipoprotein (VLDL), the major hepatically derived triglyceride-containing lipoprotein. VLDL is converted to low-density lipoprotein (LDL) by delipidation in the circulation. The VLDL particle acquires its cholesterol from the cholesterol which is taken up into the liver through the receptors such as the LDL B/E receptor, VLDL receptor, LDL receptor-related protein (LRP) and perhaps other receptors such as the apo E receptor 2 (apo ER2) [4]. Cholesterol that has been newly synthesised in the liver is the other source of cholesterol for the VLDL particle. Some cholesterol is also derived from high-density lipoprotein (HDL) which is a cellular scavenger of cholesterol and transports it back to the liver from the peripheral tissue. The HDL cholesterol may be directly taken up by the liver through the scavenger receptor class B type1 (SR-B1) [5] (Fig. 5.1).

## Apolipoproteins and Triglyceride-Rich Lipoprotein Metabolism

So far we have given a very simplified version of lipoprotein metabolism. Apolipoproteins other than apo B48 and apo B100 are important for the chylomicron and VLDL story. Apo E, for example, which is synthesised in the liver and other extrahepatic tissues including macrophages, is transferred to the chylomicron and VLDL particles in the circulation. Apo E is necessary for clearance of the triglyceride-rich particles by the B/E receptor in the liver. Chylomicrons from diabetic patients have less apo E per particle than those from control subjects [6]. Once released from the chylomicron particle, or indeed from the VLDL particle since apo E is also attached to VLDL and is involved in its uptake by the liver, apo E is transferred to HDL. Apo E is a very interesting protein in that it appears also to mediate cellular cholesterol efflux when attached to apo B [7]. (Many extrahepatic cells including the macrophage secrete apo E) [8].

Apo E recycling in the hepatocyte is associated with an increase in ABCA1, a mechanism by which apo E increases cholesterol uptake by the liver [7]. Apo CI is another apolipoprotein attached to the chylomicron and VLDL; 70 % of apo CI is associated with HDL. During the postprandial rise of triglyceride-rich lipoproteins in serum, apo CI is transferred from HDL to VLDL [9]. Apo CI, at least experimentally, modulates lipoprotein production by increasing the production rate of hepatic VLDL, inhibiting lipoprotein lipase activity, interfering with apo E-mediated uptake of VLDL and inhibiting cholesteryl ester transfer protein (CETP). CETP transfers cholesterol from HDL to VLDL in exchange for triglyceride (for review see Tall [10]). Apo CII on the other hand is a cofactor for lipoprotein lipase which hydrolyses the triglyceride in chylomicrons and VLDL and promotes their uptake by the liver receptors and thus is associated with a decrease in triglyceride-rich lipoproteins. ApoC-III is yet another constituent of triglyceride-rich lipoproteins which impairs lipoprotein uptake and is involved in hypertriglyceridemia and fatty liver disease [11]. It has also been shown to enhance hepatic triglyceride-rich VLDL assembly and secretion under lipid-rich conditions [12].

## Low-Density Lipoprotein

The LDL particle is a cholesterol-rich, triglyceride-poor particle (Fig. 5.2). LDL is composed of a hydrophilic surface layer of phospholipid, free cholesterol and hepatically derived apo B100 which packages the particle and adds stability. The core of the LDL particle includes esterified cholesterol and triglyceride together with the fatty acid tails of the phospholipid. LDL may act as a carrier for other insoluble particles such as free fatty acids and proteins which may be loosely attached [13]. Perhaps more importantly, lipoprotein lipase attaches to the particle and facilitates attachment of the particle onto the endothelial cell surface.

LDL can be subdivided into sizes by gradient gel electrophoresis and separated into a pattern A and a pattern B, pattern B being termed small dense LDL [14]. This pattern has been associated with an increase in atherosclerosis, but it has been difficult to define changes in composition of the LDL that create the increased atherogenicity. The usual way to separate the different sizes of apo B-containing lipoproteins is by ultracentrifugation, but the correlation between the denser particles on ultracentrifugation and electrophoresis is uncertain. The most recent addition to the methods to investigate lipoproteins is magnetic resonance (MR) spectroscopy which can sort particle size in large numbers of samples over very short time, but this technique still does not define small dense LDL [15]. Some years ago a subfraction of LDL with oxidised characteristics was described and was named electronegative LDL ($LDL^-$) based on its properties of electrical mobility [16]. It was later renamed minimally oxidised LDL. More heavily oxidised LDL is more electronegative than $LDL^-$ and is identified as $LDL^{--}$. It now appears that electronegative LDL may also be produced by phospholipase

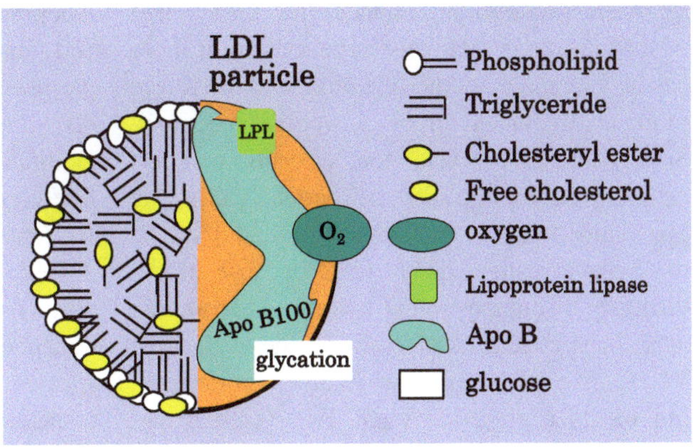


**Fig. 5.2** The LDL particle

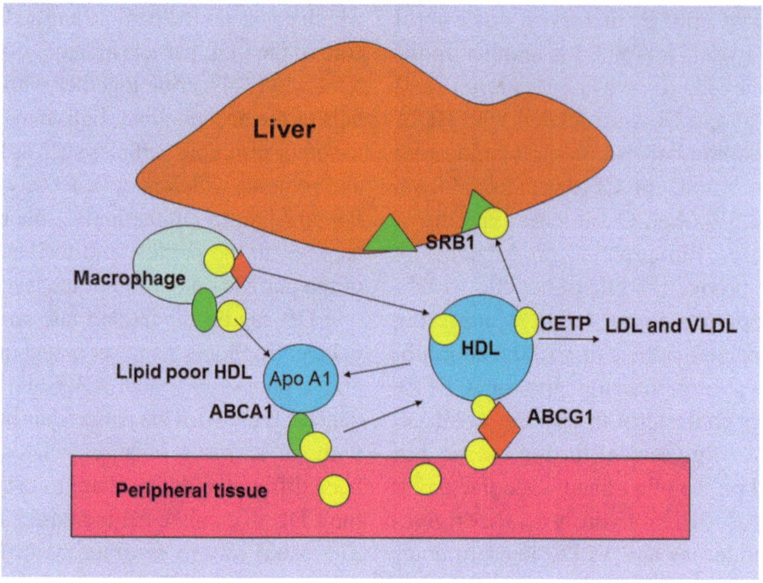


**Fig. 5.3** HDL cholesterol uptake by the liver. Cholesterol uptake by HDL from macrophages and peripheral tissue is facilitated by ABCA1 and ABCG1 receptors. The HDL particle then docks with the liver giving up free cholesterol and lipid through the scavenger receptor (SR) B1 pathway and becomes free to circulate as nascent HDL

(PL) A2. Rosenson et al. in the PLASMA11 Trial [17] showed that an inhibitor of PLA2 reduced LDL by 7 % and small dense LDL by 11 %. Enrichment of LDL with apoC-III contributes to the electronegativity [18]. Anti-LDL-monoclonal antibody had a protective effect against atherosclerosis in LDL receptor knockout mice [19]. It has been suggested that $LDL^-$ is a potential stress biomarker present in health and disease [20]. Small dense LDL isolation by various methods has been compared by Cheung [21]. The suggestion is that LDL's atherogenicity resides in the large amount of cholesterol being packaged in a relatively small volume; hence, the surface area of the particle is relatively large making it more easily amenable to modification and therefore more avidly taken up by scavenger receptors. Small dense LDL is also more susceptible to glycation even in non-diabetic people [22]. The association between small dense LDL and VLDL has been investigated, not least because of the difficulty of demonstrating hypertriglyceridemia as an independent risk factor for atherosclerosis. VLDL, like LDL, comes in many sizes depending on its triglyceride load. The Scottish and Finnish groups [23, 24] many years ago demonstrated the relationship between large triglyceride-rich VLDL and small dense LDL: the larger the VLDL, the smaller and denser the LDL. Oxidation of the LDL particle depends on oxidation of its constituent protein and/or fatty acids. Polyunsaturated but not monounsaturated fatty acids are amenable to oxidation; hence, a particle rich in linoleic acid is more susceptible to oxidation than one rich in oleic acid [25] (Fig. 5.3).

## High-Density Lipoprotein

Apoprotein AI is the major apoprotein in HDL and functions as a cholesterol acceptor in the periphery through a complex set of interactions. ATP-binding cassette transporter A1 (ABCA1) facilitates the efflux of cellular phospholipid and free cholesterol to assemble with apolipoprotein AI (apo A-I), forming nascent HDL particles. ABCG1 is another protein involved in cholesterol efflux from peripheral tissue to apo A-I for reverse transport and binds larger, more spherical HDL species. Lipid-poor apo A-I accepts cholesterol released from macrophages forming nascent HDL [26]. The esterification of cholesterol to cholesteryl esters by lecithin/cholesterol acyltransferase (LCAT) is important for the process of mobilizing cholesterol from the periphery. And once HDL becomes mature, it may transfer cholesterol and phospholipid, through the action of cholesteryl ester transfer protein (CETP) and phospholipid transfer protein (PLTP) to apo B-containing lipoproteins, in exchange for triglyceride which is then hydrolyzed by the action of hepatic lipase [27]. The HDL particle docks with the liver and gives up its remaining cholesterol and lipid through the scavenger receptor (SR) B1 pathway and becomes free to circulate as nascent HDL. There is an inverse relationship between HDL cholesterol and hepatic expression of SR-B1 [28]. In passing it should be noted that the kidney plays an important part in apo A-I metabolism by both synthesis and clearance [29]. Apo AII is another apoprotein constituent of HDL and facilitates cholesterol efflux, HDL remodelling and cholesteryl ester uptake. Apo AII has been found to be a strong risk factor for cardiovascular disease, and it has been suggested that variation in Apo AII production may exert an influence on apo B production [30]. The composition of HDL reflects on its various functions. For example, its ability to act as an antioxidant to apo B-containing lipoproteins through PON-I [31] and reconstituted HDL has been shown to have an anti-thrombotic effect [32]. HDL may play a role in inflammation, and recently it has been shown that serum amyloid A, which is elevated in inflammation and may be deposited in atheroma plaque, may promote endothelial dysfunction. HDL may reverse this process at least to some extent [33]. More recent studies have suggested that HDL may modulate glucose metabolism in the muscle and affect insulin secretion [34].

## Diabetes, Insulin Resistance and the Metabolic Syndrome

### The Chylomicron

To explore the effect of diabetes and insulin resistance on lipoproteins, we will start at the beginning. In this chapter the beginning must be the chylomicron and its synthesis, since without food there would be little interest in diabetes or insulin resistance and in the rural areas of the world where starvation occurs, there is little talk of type 2 diabetes or insulin resistance. The apo B48-containing chylomicron transports both cholesterol and triglyceride from the intestine to the circulation and has a dominant role in distributing fatty acids/triglyceride to the tissues prior to being taken up by the liver [35]. The second function of the chylomicron is to transport cholesterol to the liver, although on the way the cholesterol may be taken up by tissues including the atheromatous plaque where the macrophage sits in waiting with a specific apo B48 receptor [36] as well as VLDL and scavenger receptors [35]. Apo B48 has been demonstrated in plaque by a number of workers [37–40]. Apo B48 is the solubilising protein necessary for the transport of cholesterol and lipid in aqueous solution in humans. The amount of triglyceride available for the chylomicron particle is limitless, the normal gut managing to limit the amount of triglyceride/fatty acids in the stool to under 5 g/day. On the other hand serum cholesterol is very tightly regulated and varies very little throughout one's lifetime due to a hugely efficient regulatory process. Absorbed cholesterol varies considerably from person to person, and high absorbers of cholesterol have been shown to have low synthesis rates and to be less sensitive to cholesterol lowering with statin therapy [41]. The mechanism that regulates cholesterol absorption in the intestine is complex and both diabetes and insulin resistance have been shown to affect the regulation [42, 43], causing the initiation of the dyslipidemia of insulin resistance and diabetes (Fig. 5.4).

### Intestinal Niemann-Pick C1-Like 1 Protein

The first step in cholesterol absorption in the intestine appears to be through the multi-transmembrane protein Niemann-pick C1-like 1 (NCP1-L1) which is highly expressed in the jejunum. In humans it is localised to the brush borders of the enterocytes and acts as a

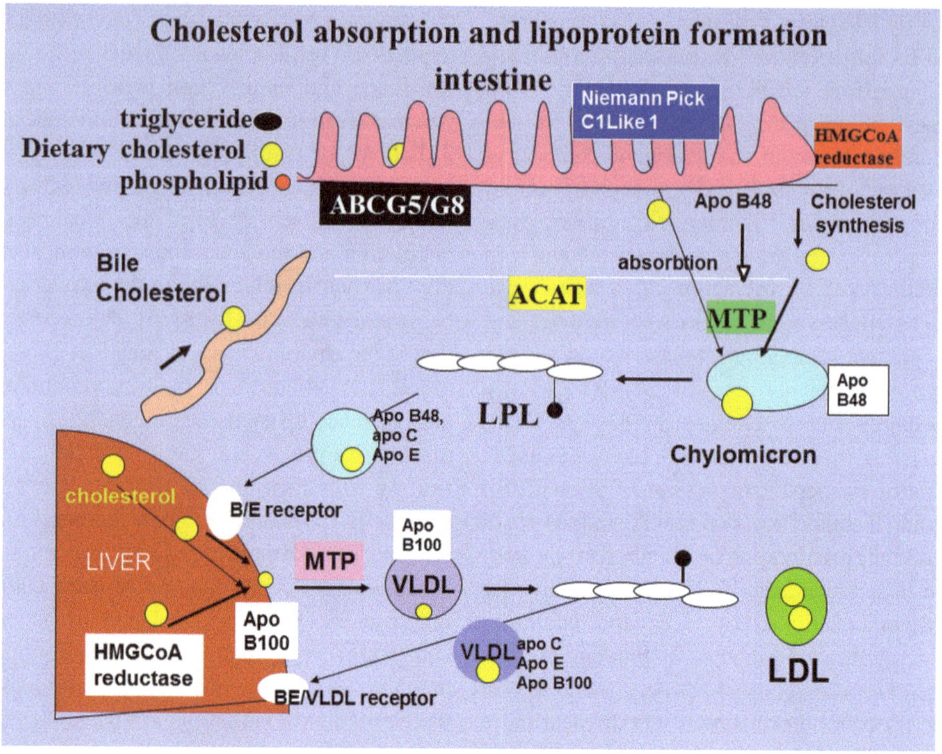


**Fig. 5.4** Cholesterol absorption and lipoprotein formation. Dietary cholesterol, biliary cholesterol and cholesterol synthesized in the intestine for which HMGCoA is the rate-limiting enzyme, is transported across the cell membrane by NCP1-L1 and, together with triglyceride, phospholipid and the intestinally derived apoB48 protein, is assembled, under the influence of MTP into the triglyceride-rich chylomicron. Some of the absorbed cholesterol is excreted back into the lumen of the intestine under the influence of ABC G5/G8. The chylomicron is partially hydrolyzed in the circulation by lipoprotein lipase and acquires apoC-III and apo E. The resulting chylomicron remnant is taken up by the B/E receptor in the liver. The cholesterol and triglyceride released are reassembled with hepatically synthesized cholesterol and apo B100 to form VLDL. Lipoprotein lipase in the artery wall releases the triglyceride from VLDL and it acquires apoC-III and apo E. Some of the VLDL is taken up again by the liver, and the rest is further hydrolysed and looses apoC-III and E to become IDL and then LDL

unidirectional transporter of cholesterol and non-cholesterol sterols [44, 45]. The mechanism of action of NCP1-L1 has been elucidated. It has been shown that cholesterol promotes the formation and endocytosis of NCP1-L1-flotillin-cholesterol membrane microdomains which is an early step in cholesterol uptake. Zang et al. [46] discovered that it is the N-terminal domain of NCP1-L1 that binds cholesterol. It is interesting that this domain does not bind to plant sterols; thus, it now seems that plasma membrane-bound NCP1-L1 binds exogenous cholesterol, and this binding facilitates the formation of the NCP1-L1-flotillin-cholesterol microdomains that are then internalised into cells through the clathrin adaptor protein 2 pathway. Twenty rare NCP1L1 alleles have been found in the low cholesterol absorbers and appear to impair NCP1-L1 cholesterol uptake through various mechanism ([47, 48]; for review see Calandera [49]). It has been shown that the effectiveness of ezetimibe, which blocks NCP1-L1 and inhibits cholesterol absorption, depends on the NCP1-L1 genotype [50].

There are other transporters of cholesterol; for example, SR-B1 is located both in the apical and basolateral membranes of the enterocyte [51]. Scavenger receptors (SR) are cell surface proteins that can bind and internalise modified lipoproteins. SR-B1, which is involved in cholesterol uptake in the intestine and may play an important part in intestinal chylomicron production, and the fatty acid transporter CD36, which is also involved in the uptake of oxidised LDL, are members of the class B scavenger receptor family [52]. Hiashi et al. [53] investigated gene expression of key proteins involved in the active absorption of dietary fat and cholesterol in response to the development of insulin resistance. They used two models of diet-induced insulin resistance, the fructose-fed hamster and the high-fat-fed mouse. Expression of SR-B1 was increased in both the fructose-fed hamster and the high-fat-fed mouse models of insulin resistance. In CaCo2 adenocarcinoma cell line, SR-B1 over-expression increased apo B100 and apo B48 secretion. The authors conclude that apical or basolateral SR-B1 may have an important role in cholesterol absorption and may play a part in cholesterol over-absorption in insulin-resistant states. SR-B1 in the intestine may play an important role in chylomicron production. Cdc42, a member of the Rho family of small guanidine triphosphatases with numerous functions, has been shown by Xia et al. [54] to interact with NCP1-L1 and to control its movement from the endocytic recycling compartment to plasma membranes in a cholesterol-dependent manner. Glucose-stimulated Cdc42 signalling appears to be essential for second stage insulin secretion [55]. It is probable that in insulin resistance the signalling of NCP1-L1 is disturbed through this pathway, but we have been unable to find any studies in the intestine that have explored the pathway in diabetes/insulin resistance. In animal studies we have demonstrated an increase in cholesterol absorption in diabetes [56]. We then asked the question as to whether diabetes might be associated with an increase in cholesterol absorption through stimulation of NCP1-L1. We demonstrated in animal models of diabetes that NCP1-L1 was upregulated [57], and in diabetic patients we demonstrated an increase in NCP1-L1 mRNA [58], suggesting a mechanism for an increase in cholesterol absorption. In the Psammomys obesus, a model of type 2 diabetes, the animals exhibiting weight gain, hyperinsulinaemia and hypercholesterolaemia, NCP1-L1 protein and gene expression were both significantly reduced in the intestine, and the authors found a lower capacity to absorb cholesterol compared to controls [59]. This may suggest interspecies variation, but it is a surprising finding considering that this animal model of diabetes has been shown to have increased production of intestinal apo B48-containing lipoproteins [60]. Ezetimibe has been shown to bind to the brush border and to NCP1-L1 expressing cells [61]. There is a sterol regulatory element in the promoter and a sterol-sensing domain of NCP1-L1 which appears to regulate cholesterol absorption in response to cholesterol intake. Huff et al. [62] have shown that NCP1-L1 is suppressed in mice given a cholesterol-rich diet and increased in the cholesterol-depleted porcine intestine. The nuclear receptor, peroxisome proliferator-activated receptor (PPAR) δ/β, appears to control the expression of NCP1-L1. Activation by a synthetic agonist of PPARδ has been shown to reduce cholesterol absorption and reduce expression of NCP1-L1 without altering expression of the adenosine triphosphate (ATP)-binding membrane cassette transport proteins ABC G5/G8 [63]. ABC G5/G8 is a transmembrane heterodimer that transports plant sterols and excess cholesterol out of jejunal enterocytes (discussed in greater detail below). Fenofibrate, a PPARα agonist, has been shown to inhibit cholesterol absorption; the mechanism has been shown to be through reduced NCP1L1 transcription by binding to a PPARα response element upstream of the human NCP1-L1 gene. In a human construct, Iwayanagi et al. [64] showed that PPARα positively regulated human NCP1-L1 transcription, and Valasek et al. [65] showed that fenofibrate reduced intestinal cholesterol absorption by PPARα modulation of NCP1-L1. Tremblay et al. [66] have shown that atorvastatin increases NCP1-L1 in the intestine and decreased ABC G5/G8 which leads to an increase in cholesterol absorption. These findings were accompanied by an increase in the transcription factors, sterol regulatory element-binding protein (SREBP) 2 and hepatic nuclear factor (HNF)-4.

## Intestinal ATP-Binding Cassette Proteins G5/G8

Once cholesterol has been transported across the brush border membrane, it faces another regulatory process and may be excreted back into the intestinal lumen rather than being further processed for absorption into the perimesenteric lymphatic circulation. ABC G5/G8 expression is mostly confined to the human small intestine and liver [67]. These two proteins act in tandem to re-excrete both cholesterol and, in particular, non-cholesterol sterols such as plant sterols from the body. Much of the understanding of ABC G5/G8 comes from the rare mutations that cause a defect in ABC G5/G8 and result in high levels of sitosterol in the blood. Beta-sitosterolemia is a condition which manifests itself in children as tendon xanthomas or in young adults as severe CHD with massive accumulation of sterols and stanols in monocyte-derived macrophages [68]. Ma et al. [69] found in an animal model that dietary calcium had a beneficial effect on lipoprotein profile by upregulating the mRNA levels of intestinal ABC G5/G8 and cholesterol-7α-hydroxylase (CYP7A1), whereas it downregulated the intestinal NCP1-L1 and microsomal triacylglyceride transport protein (MTP) due to enhanced biliary cholesterol excretion. Mendes Gonzales et al. [70] investigated the effect of ABC G5/G8 deficiency on lipoproteins in mice. They found that postprandial triglycerides were fivefold higher in the ABC G5/G8$^{--}$ mice due to a lower fractional catabolic rate with lower post-heparin lipoprotein lipase activities. They also showed that liver triglyceride secretion and intestinal triglyceride secretion were higher and there was a relationship between this and the HOMA index as a measure of insulin resistance. Since diabetes is so frequently associated with dyslipidaemia and atherosclerosis, the ABC translocases became a target for research. Blocks et al. [71] examined mRNA and protein expression of ABC G5/G8 in the intestine of streptozotocin diabetic rats and found significant reduction in expression of both ABC G5/G8. They found that levels were partially normalised on insulin supplementation. We have shown that ABC G5/G8 were reduced by more than 50 % in the intestine of Zucker diabetic fa/fa rats compared with lean rats although these changes did not reach statistical significance [58]. Insulin treatment caused a nonsignificant increase in ABC G5/G8 mRNA. In another study of streptozotocin diabetic rats, ABC G5/G8 were both very significantly reduced in the intestine [57]. There was a negative correlation between ABC G5/G8 and chylomicron cholesterol [57]. In the Psammomys obesus, another model of diabetes, Levy et al. [59, 60] showed a reduction in ABC G5/G8 in the intestine. In the intestine of human subjects with type 2 diabetes, ABC G5/G8 mRNA were both significantly lower compared to controls [58]. There was a negative correlation between ABC G5/G8 and NCP1L1 in the combined diabetic and control subjects, and there was a significant negative correlation between chylomicron cholesterol and both ABC G5/G8 [57]. These two genes appear to play an important role in the dysregulation of cholesterol metabolism in diabetes.

## Microsomal Triglyceride Transport Protein

The cholesterol that has evaded ABC G5/G8 in the intestine is now ready to be solubilised for transport through the lymphatic system. The assembly of the chylomicron occurs under the direction of microsomal triglyceride transfer protein (MTP). MTP has the ability to combine cholesterol, triglyceride and phospholipid into the triglyceride-rich chylomicron particle. The cholesterol that becomes available however not only is cholesterol that has been absorbed from the diet but is also cholesterol that has been excreted through the bile duct under the influence of hepatic ABC G5/G8. Finally, there is the cholesterol that has been synthesised in the intestine through the 3-hydroxy-3-methylglutaryl coenzyme A (HMGCoA) reductase pathway. This pathway in the intestine accounts for up to 25 % of body-synthesised cholesterol, the amount varying depending on whether the patients are high or low cholesterol absorbers. Intestinal MTP plays a major role in the assembly of the chylomicron particle and therefore of cholesterol and triglyceride metabolism. MTP has become a hot topic since inhibitors of intestinal MTP have been shown to lower triglyceride without causing hepatic steatosis at least in animal studies [72, 73]. In short-term human studies, a specific intestinal MTP inhibitor did not appear to effect liver function tests [74]. Although many polymorphisms of MTP have been described, some of which have considerable impact on LDL cholesterol in both nondiabetic and diabetic subjects, it is difficult to know whether the results mainly stemmed from the effect in the liver rather than the intestine [75, 76]. The intestinal inhibitors of MTP which have no effect on the liver should answer this question in the future. In animal studies, diabetes is associated with an increase in MTP mRNA with close correlation between MTP mRNA and chylomicron cholesterol [77–80]. In the diabetic rabbit, increased intestinal MTP mRNA is associated with an increase in chylomicron particle numbers [77], but in the rat it is associated with larger particles [78]. The fructose-fed insulin-resistant hamster model had an increase in MTP protein mass, and this was associated with an increase in the triglyceride-rich intestinally derived lipoproteins [79]. Zolotowska et al. [80] in 2003 [80] examined the B48-containing lipoprotein assembly in the small intestine of *Psammomys obesus*, a model of nutritionally induced diabetes and insulin resistance. De novo triglyceride synthesis, apo B48 biogenesis and triglyceride-rich lipoprotein assembly were all increased. MTP activity and protein expression, however, were not altered. In the enterocyte of fructose-fed golden hamster, MTP mRNA and protein mass were increased by TNFα, but apo B levels in the enterocyte were not effected suggesting that there is considerable interspecies variation [80]. In humans with type 2 diabetes, we demonstrated an increase in MTP mRNA in intestinal biopsies [58, 81]. Diabetic patients who were on statin therapy had lower MTP mRNA compared to those not on statins [81]. We found positive correlations between MTP mRNA and chylomicron fraction cholesterol and apo B48 [81]. A novel intestinal-specific inhibitor of MTP has been shown to ameliorate impaired glucose and lipid metabolism in Zucker diabetic fatty rats, but whether this effect was due to impairment of food intake or to inhibition of fat absorption is not clear [82].

The signals that upregulate chylomicron formation to cope with excess fat in the diet are slowly being elucidated. Another non-specific inhibitor of MTP, which reduced serum levels of triglycerides by more than 70 %, was also associated with significant improvements in glucose tolerance and insulin sensitivity in Zucker fatty rats [83]. Hepatic MTP mRNA expression is negatively regulated by insulin, and it is suggested that insulin might also directly inhibit apo B48 secretion independently of MTP even though it is probable that upregulation of MTP stimulates apo B secretion [84]. The membrane glycoprotein CD36 binds long-chain fatty acids. CD36 deficiency reduces chylomicron production [84]. It has recently been shown that binding of lipid by CD36 upregulates apo B48 and MTP through CD36 signalling via the ERK-1/ERK-2 pathway [85]. Interestingly polymorphisms of MTP which have been associated with differences in serum lipids appear to alter cholesterol absorption but not synthesis in women [86].

## Apolipoprotein B48 and B100

Apo B48, the structural protein for the chylomicron, is produced in the intestine by editing of the hepatic version, apo B100 [87]. The enzyme apobec cuts the apo B100 form into the shorter version, apo B48. It has been suggested that apo B is in excess of body needs. In the liver recent work has demonstrated that insulin silences apo B translation by introducing intracellular traffic into mRNA granules [88]. The authors showed that the availability of apo B mRNA for translation was regulated by the rate of release from translationally silenced mRNPs processing bodies (p bodies). Insulin specifically silences apo B mRNA translation by reprogramming its mRNA into p bodies and reducing the size of translationally competent mRNA pools. Translational control via traffic into cytoplasmic RNA granules may be an important mechanism for controlling the rate of apo B synthesis and hepatic lipoprotein production, the authors suggest. It is however not clear that this silencing plays a part in reducing chylomicron production or influences nascent chylomicron size. In diabetes it may be that there is an increase in apo B48 production, but then if meaningful, one would expect smaller chylomicron particles containing less triglyceride per particle to be produced. Our studies in an animal model demonstrated that the particles in the cannulated lymphatic duct of the rabbit were associated with an increase in chylomicron particle numbers [89], but in the rat it was associated with larger particles [56]. In patients with type 2 diabetes, apo B48 is increased, but it is difficult to ascertain whether the increase is due to delayed delipidation, increased synthesis or both [90]. We injected labelled chylomicrons, collected by cannulation of the lymph duct into diabetic and nondiabetic rabbits, into another group of diabetic and nondiabetic rabbits and found evidence of both increased synthesis and delayed clearance [89]. Our animal research therefore suggests that the increase in apo B48 particles in diabetes may be due to both an increase in synthesis and a decrease in turnover.

## Cholesterol Synthesis and HMGCoA Reductase

Cholesterol synthesis is regulated by HMGCoA reductase, the rate-limiting enzyme in the synthetic pathway. Sterol regulatory element-binding protein-2 (SREBP-2) is a regulatory protein of cholesterol homeostasis and regulates HMGCoA gene expression. In isolated rat hepatocytes, we demonstrated significant reduction in HMGCoA reductase activity in the presence of insulin [91]. In animal studies we have recently reported the different effects of pioglitazone, an insulin sensitizer which acts through peroxisome proliferator-activated receptor (PPAR) gamma, as compared to insulin on expression of hepatic HMGCoA reductase mRNA [42]. We found a highly significant increase in expression of HMGCoA reductase in the liver of diabetic animals (Zucker diabetic fatty fa/fa rats). There was a small but insignificant reduction in HMGCoA reductase mRNA in the intestine when the animals were treated with insulin [42]. There was a larger reduction in HMGCoA reductase in the liver of the insulin-treated animals, but this reduction did not reach statistical significance [42]. In type 1 diabetes Sittiwet et al. [92] presented some evidence to suggest that improved glycaemic control increases cholesterol synthesis. However, the study was perhaps a little unsatisfactory in that, although there was a significant increase in cholesterol synthesis, there was no change in serum or lipoprotein cholesterol nor was there any change in markers of cholesterol absorption. Inhibition of HMGCoA reductase with a statin has been shown to decrease ABC G5/G8 as well as increasing NCP1L1, thus increasing cholesterol absorption [81].

Hepatic steatosis is common in diabetes, insulin resistance and obesity. Inflammatory stress is present in these conditions and is also associated with obesity, insulin resistance and diabetes. It is therefore of interest that Zhao et al. [93] demonstrated that interleukin 1b and interleukin 6 stimulation of Hep G2 cells increased SREBP2 and HMGCoA mRNA. Further high-fat loading in mice or LDL loading in Hep G2 cells suppressed the above genes, but this suppression could be overridden by the above inflammatory proteins [93]. Severe calorie restriction in patients with steatosis results in rapid reduction of liver fat, insulin resistance and improvement in diabetes control. In contrast, insulin resistance and the accompanying hyperinsulinaemia are associated with an upregulation of SREPB2 through extracellular signal-regulated pathways involving the kinases ERK-1 and ERK-2, another example of the interaction between fat and carbohydrate metabolism [94] (for review, see Van Rooyen and Farrell [95]).

## Very-Low-Density Lipoprotein

Before discussing clearance of the chylomicron particle with reference to insulin resistance and diabetes, it is necessary to discuss VLDL, the other major triglyceride transport particle which is produced by the liver and has as its structural protein apo B100. The synthesis of the VLDL particle in the liver is somewhat similar to that of the chylomicron in the intestine. Through a series of steps, the lipid and cholesterol are assembled under the influence of MTP with apo B100 yielding VLDL. The VLDL particle will contain some de novo synthesized cholesterol.

As with the chylomicron, apo E attaches itself to the particle and is necessary for clearance by the liver through the LDL B/E receptor. The VLDL particle is distinguished from the LDL particle, not only by its triglyceride content which is much higher than LDL, but also by the attachment of apo E onto the particle. There are three common polymorphisms of apo E. Apo E2/2, although rare, is associated with hypercholesterolemia but E4/4 with hypertriglyceridemia [96]. Compared with individuals with the E3/3 genotype, E2 carriers have a 20 % lower risk of coronary heart disease, and E4 carriers have a slightly higher risk [97]. It has been suggested that the apo E4 allele is a risk factor for the metabolic syndrome [98]. ApoC-III can be present on apo B-containing lipoproteins but is not integral to the basic lipoprotein particle structure; thus, lipoproteins exist both with and without apoC-III. Apo B-containing lipoproteins with apoC-III are enriched in triglyceride and cholesterol and have slow clearance from plasma. The concentration of apoC-III in VLDL and LDL is highly and independently predictive of coronary heart disease, more so than triglyceride alone [99]. LDL particles with apoC-III, a remnant particle produced by partial lipolysis in plasma of VLDL [100], is the lipoprotein particle type most predictive of CVD in type 2 diabetes [101]. ApoC-III inhibits lipoprotein lipase and triglyceride hydrolysis as well as direct clearance of VLDL particles from plasma, resulting in the formation of less LDL.

In passing one might mention apo A5, a key gene regulating triglyceride levels and was thought to be exclusively in the liver. Recently Guardiola et al. [102] have described the expression of the gene in the mouse and human small intestine. The function here has yet to be explained. Dallinger Thie et al. [103] examined apo A5 in diabetes in relation to triglycerides and found the same positive relationship between apo A5 as in non-diabetic subjects. They found in a group of 215 subjects with type 2 diabetes taken from the Diabetes Atorvastatin Intervention Study that 6 % of the variation in plasma triglycerides was due to apo A5 whereas 52 % was explained by apoC-III. Diabetes sometimes results from pancreatitis which may be caused by severe hypertriglyceridemia. Apo A5 has not been shown to play a part in diabetes secondary to pancreatitis [104].

## Cholesterol Synthesis and Transport in the Liver

Cholesterol either may be synthesized in the liver through the HMGCoA reductase pathway and packaged for transport by association with apo B100 or may have been delivered to the liver by the chylomicron particle. Insulin plays a major part in regulating many of the steps in the production of cholesterol [105]. HMGCoA reductase is increased in animal models of diabetes in the liver [91]. In isolated rat hepatocytes, we have demonstrated significant reduction in HMGCoA reductase activity in the presence of insulin [106]. In animal studies we have more recently reported the different effects of pioglitazone, an insulin sensitiser through peroxisome proliferator-activated receptor (PPAR) gamma, as compared to insulin on expression of intestinal and hepatic HMGCoA reductase mRNA [42]. In that study we also found a highly significant increase in expression of HMGCoA reductase in the liver of diabetic animals (Zucker diabetic fatty fa/fa rats). There was a large reduction in HMGCoA reductase in the liver of insulin-treated animals, but this reduction did not reach statistical significance (116+122 vs. 143+48 arbitrary units $n+10$) [42]. The liver, like the intestine, can regulate, at least to some extent, the amount of cholesterol in the VLDL particle by regulating the excretion of cholesterol in bile.

## Hepatic NCP1-L1

NCP1-L1 is localised to the canalicular membrane in hepatocytes where it plays a part in the regulation of cholesterol transport. Hepatic nuclear factor-1 (HNF-1) alpha and sterol regulatory element-binding protein-2 (SREBP-2) appear to be important regulators of NCP1-L1 in the liver [107]. It has also been shown that they have important binding sites within the human NCP1-L1 promoter. The role of NCP1-L1 in the liver is probably to divert cholesterol away from excretion in the bile [108]. A recent study in female Chinese women with gallstones has shown reduced NCP1-L1 mRNA and protein in the liver and supersaturation of cholesterol in the bile [109]. Ezetimibe has not been shown to increase the risk of gallstones perhaps because the drug has its primary effect in reducing cholesterol absorption. Indeed in the golden Syrian hamster, ezetimibe reduced the diet-induced increase in biliary cholesterol [110], and in gallstone-susceptible mice fed lithogenic diets, ezetimibe prevented gallstone formation [111]. Inhibition of NCP1-L1 by ezetimibe is associated with an improvement in hepatic steatosis. Jia et al. [112] investigated the mechanism by deleting NCP1-L1 in mice and inducing hepatic steatosis with a high-fat diet. The knockout mice did not develop steatosis. Hepatic fatty acid synthesis and mRNA for genes regulating lipogenesis were reduced and the knockout animals did not develop hyperinsulinaemia. Nomura et al. [113] demonstrated in Zucker rats that ezetimibe improved hepatic insulin signalling as well as hepatic steatosis both in the liver and in cultured steatotic hepatocytes. The drug recovered insulin-induced Akt activation and reduced gluconeogenic genes. The relevance of this study to humans is not clear as patients with diabetes who are treated with ezetimibe do not improve blood sugar control [114]. Over-expression of NCP1-L1 in the liver inhibits biliary cholesterol secretion and raises serum cholesterol suggesting that inhibitors of NCP1-L1 may have a role in the liver [115]. NCP1-L1 mRNA has been shown to be increased in the liver of diabetic rats with a positive correlation between NCP1-L1 mRNA and VLDL cholesterol [57]. Interestingly, we found that although pioglitazone significantly reduced NCP1-L1 in the liver of diabetic fa/fa rats, insulin had no effect [42]. ABC G5/G8 play a role in the regulation of cholesterol excretion by promoting excretion of neutral steroids into the bile. Diet-induced lipid loading into the liver causes a significant increase in the expression of ABC G5/G8 in the bile canaliculi [116].

## Hepatic ABC G5/G8

The liver X receptor (LXR) helps to regulate expression of ABC G5/G8 [117], and ABC G5/G8 expression is also stimulated by LXR agonists but not to the same extent as by feeding. It has recently been demonstrated that NCP2, a cholesterol-binding protein secreted by the biliary system, positively regulates biliary secretion of cholesterol through stimulation of ABC G5/G8. It is well documented that there is a relationship between gallstones, diabetes and the metabolic syndrome. Under conditions of obesity and insulin resistance, the serine/threonine protein kinase Akt/PKB is required for lipid accumulation in liver. Two forkhead transcription factors, FOXA2 and O1, have been suggested to function downstream of, and to be negatively regulated by, Akt and are proposed as key determinants of hepatic triglyceride content [118]. In mice with isolated insulin resistance, there was an increased expression of biliary transporter ABC G5/G8 through the disinhibition of the forkhead transcription factor FOX 01 [119]. However, these findings do not fit well with the increased VLDL synthesis that has been described in insulin resistance and diabetes [120–122] even if they explain the increased gallstones found in diabetes [123, 124]. In diabetic fa/fa rats insulin but not pioglitazone significantly increased hepatic expression of ABC G5/G8 [42].

## MTP in the Liver

The final stage for the production of the VLDL particle is the assembly of the cholesterol, triglyceride and phospholipid with apo B100 under the regulation of MTP. In animal studies MTP mRNA is increased in streptozotocin diabetic rats in the liver [57]. We have shown modest suppression with insulin treatment in the liver of Zucker diabetic rats [42]. In the alloxan diabetic rabbit model, we found no difference in MTP mRNA or activity in the liver, whereas there was a significant increase in the intestine [77]. The disturbances in chylomicron and VLDL production reflect the increase in chylomicron and VLDL particles found in diabetes. Although chylomicron production has only been measured in animal models of diabetes and insulin resistance, VLDL overproduction has been shown in diabetes in humans as well [120–122, 125], the driving force being the non-supressability of FFA postprandially due to the malfunction of adipose tissue by adipose triglyceride lipase (ATGL) leading to an increase in postprandial triglycerides which are taken up by the liver and re-secreted in the VLDL [126]. VLDL overproduction is also found in insulin resistance [127].

## Triglyceride-Rich Lipoproteins in Diabetes

One of the causes of the disturbance in the metabolism of the triglyceride-rich lipoproteins in diabetes is the inhibition of lipoprotein lipase (LL) activity. Lipoprotein lipase is an insulin-sensitive enzyme. In type 2 diabetes insulin treatment significantly increases LPL activity in adipose tissue [128, 129]. Among the causes of lipoprotein lipase dysfunction is the effect of glucose on enzyme dimerization and has been related to the severity of diabetes [130]. Clearance of both VLDL and chylomicrons is severely impeded due to the inability of lipoprotein lipase to function in a relative or absolute insulin-deficient environment. The VLDL remnant is cleared by the LDL B/E receptor or the VLDL lipoprotein receptor (VLDLr) which is found mainly in the adipocyte and muscle cells [131]. The LDL receptor-related protein which clears postprandial lipoproteins is also insulin dependent [132]. Perhaps one of the most important results of this delay in clearance is the influence that the triglyceride-rich lipoproteins have on LDL size and atherogenicity [133]. Large triglyceride-rich VLDL is associated with both increased small dense LDL and reductions in HDL.

## LDL in Diabetes

The concentration of LDL is often normal in diabetic when compared to non-diabetic patients of similar BMI. However, since turnover of the LDL particle is increased in diabetes [134] and production is increased through the increase in hepatic VLDL secretion, a similar serum level of LDL in diabetes should not be taken as meaning that the atherogenic risk of LDL should be presumed to be similar to that in the non-diabetic and is one of the reasons why emphasis is placed on maximum reduction of LDL in diabetes. HMGCoA reductase and the LDL receptor are insulin sensitive and the receptor is down-regulated and HMGCoA reductase is up-regulated in the setting of insulin resistance [135]. As stated previously, small dense LDL is more common in diabetes [133], and small dense LDL has been shown to promote macrophage foam cell formation [136]. LDL composition is abnormal in other ways, i.e. it contains more esterified cholesterol [137], an increase in linoleic acid and more FFA [13]. However, a more recent study suggests that patients with diabetes and the metabolic syndrome have lower cholesterol ester and lower linoleic acid in the cholesteryl esters [138]. This may of course be due to differences in diets between the 2 studies. Both studies agree that markers of lipid peroxidation are increased in diabetes. Colas et al. [138] have also shown that LDL from metabolic syndrome and type 2 diabetic patients was potent in activating the platelet arachadonic acid-signalling cascade, potentiating platelet aggregation as compared to control LDL. An increase of free radical production occurs in hyperglycemia of diabetes [139] causing LDL glycation, and glycated LDL is more susceptible to oxidation, one reason for the increased LDL oxidation that occurs in poorly controlled diabetes [140]. The foam cell is perhaps the hallmark of the atherosclerotic lesion. The development of the foam cell depends on macrophage uptake of cholesterol. A novel mechanism has recently been described which

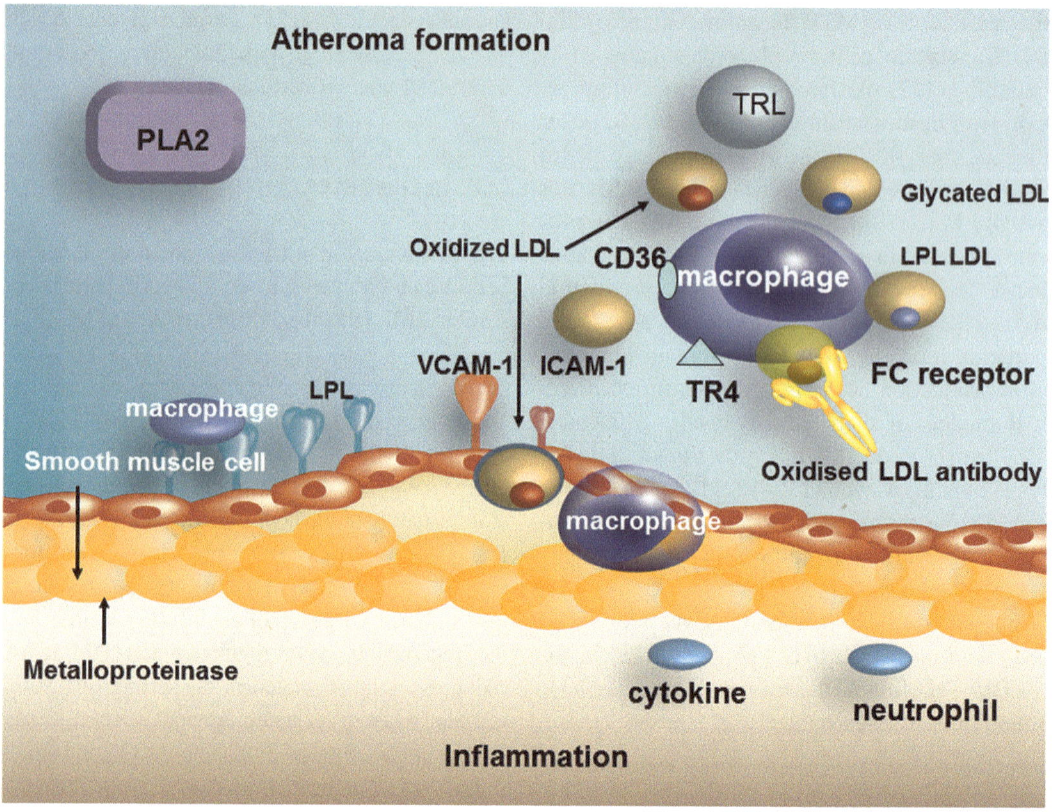


**Fig. 5.5** Atherosis formation. The atherosclerotic plaque is composed of a lipid-rich core containing cholesterol, fatty acids and necrotic tissue and is covered by a fibrous smooth muscle cell cap. Low-density lipoprotein (LDL) is the major contributor to plaque cholesterol. LDL may attach to the endothelium through lipoprotein lipase and heparin sulphate proteoglycans (HPSG) which facilitate their uptake into the subendothelial space. Macrophages, which have accumulated large amounts of cholesterol, attach to chemotactic factors such as VCAM and ICAM on the artery wall and slip between the endothelial cells into the intima where they are trapped, mature into foam cells and eventually disintegrate providing the cholesterol for the lipid-rich atherosclerotic core

facilitated uptake of oxidised LDL through uptake by the toll-like receptor 4 (TR4) which is found on the macrophage surface [141, 142]. It has been demonstrated that cholesterol ester hydroperoxides are an indigenous ligand for TR4. The increase in free fatty acids in poorly controlled diabetes is associated with an increase in fatty acids attached to the LDL particle, a further potential cause for increased oxidation of the particle [13]. Oxidized LDL can be taken up by the macrophage through scavenger receptors in an unregulated manner. We have shown that lipoprotein lipase mass is increased on diabetic LDL [13], a factor which also increases LDL uptake into plaque (Fig. 5.5).

Normally LDL is cleared through the LDL receptor which is downregulated by receptor-mediated cholesterol uptake into the cell. The LDL receptor is upregulated by insulin. Insulin signalling via Akt2 and mTORC1 has emerged as having a key role in the regulation of hepatic lipogenesis in obese mice. The underlying mechanism involves induction of proprotein convertase subtilisin kexin type 9 (PCSK9) via mTORC1 leading to post-transcriptional downregulation of hepatic LDL receptors. The glucose-insulin pathway is perhaps another story but very exciting since it involves both an understanding of how glucose stimulates insulin secretion in the beta cell and how insulin stimulates

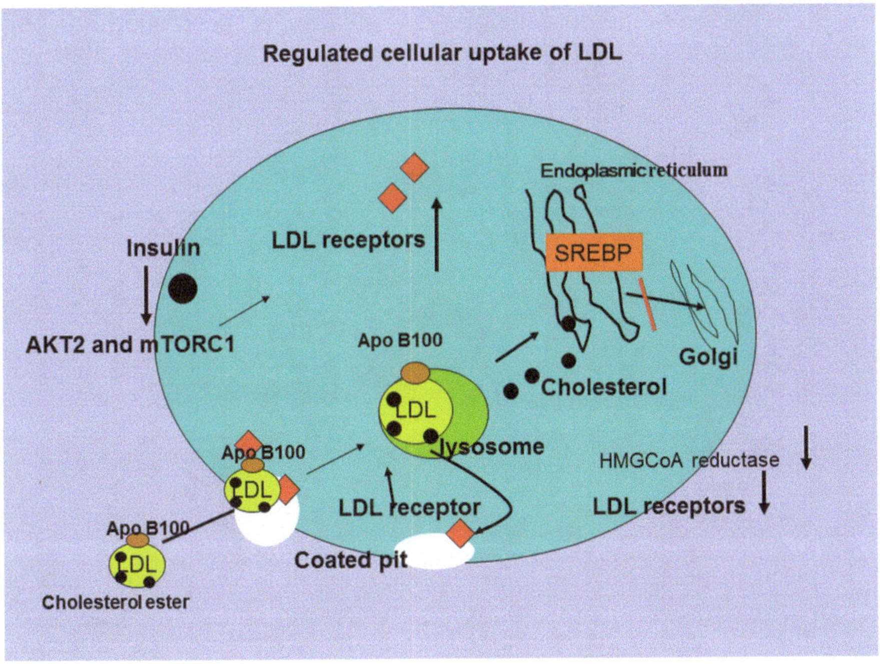


**Fig. 5.6** Receptor-mediated LDL clearance. LDL is normally taken into the cell through the LDL receptor pathway. In the lysosome the apo B is degraded and the cholesterol released is transferred to the endoplasmic reticulum. This blocks the transport of SREBP to the Golgi complex preventing transcription of HMGCoA reductase thus reducing de novo cholesterol synthesis and also blocking LDL receptor synthesis, preventing further LDL uptake

glucose disposal in all other cells. Protein kinase C (PKC) is involved in insulin signalling and glucose transportation. PKC1 is also involved in stimulation of SREBP, and in another pathway stimulates AKT2 under the influence of insulin. In this way insulin both regulates glucose and lipid metabolism explaining the link between hyperglycemia and insulin in diabetes. A few years ago PKCs were all the rage and an editorial in Diabetologia on The Rising Star of PKC started with the sentence "In the pubs of Ireland there is talk of little else". PKCs are involved in insulin signalling and glucose transport but in another pathway, and in particular a pathway involved in glucose disposal in exercise is signalled by Akt2. Thus, the understanding that Akt2 is also involved in cholesterol lowering through its effect on the LDL receptor is another link in the chain tightening the link between dyslipidemia and hyperglycemia in diabetes (and of course supports the idea diabetes mellitus being renamed diabetes lipidus) (Fig. 5.6).

The excitement of this new information, apart from a better understanding of the control mechanism for the receptor, is that it opens up new avenues for pharmacological intervention. An example of translational science at its best might become the discovery of antibodies that inhibit PCSK9. PCSK9 is the gene which regulates recycling of the LDL receptor, diverting it to the lysosomal compartment for degradation. PCSK9 binds tightly to the LDL receptor and channels it towards the lysosomal compartment for degradation which results in decreased LDL receptor numbers and increased plasma LDL levels. An interesting loss of function polymorphism of PCSK9 increases the number of LDL receptors and increases LDL removal from the plasma, reducing LDL levels. There is strong evidence that PCSK9 and LDLR transcription are both activated by cellular cholesterol depletion via sterol regulatory element-binding protein-2 (SREBP-2). This notion is supported by human studies that plasma PCSK9 concentration is increased with

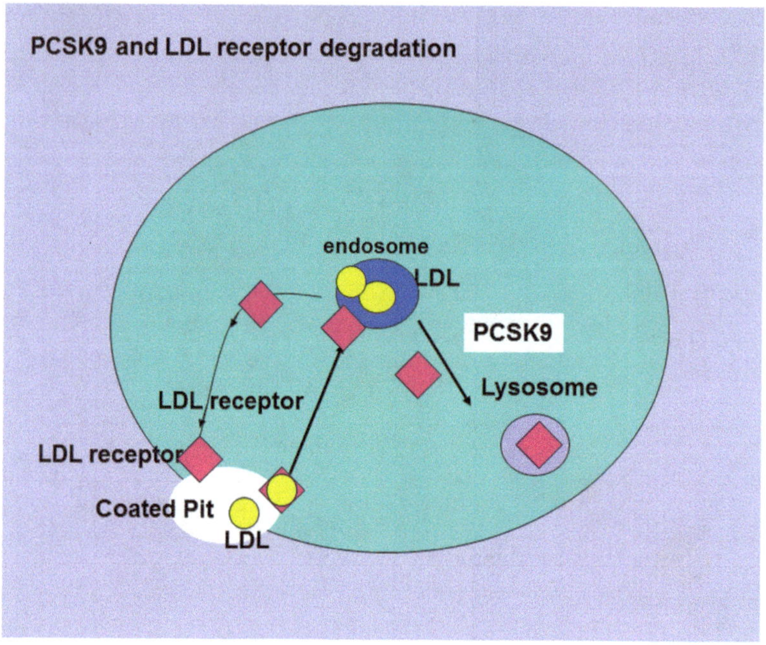


**Fig. 5.7** PCSK9. PCSK9 is a regulator of liver LDL receptor expression. Normally the LDL receptor, once it has delivered LDL to the lysosome, recirculates to the coated pit on the cell surface. Insulin signalling via Akt2 and mTORC1 induces PCSK9 which binds tightly to the LDL receptor and instead channels it towards the lysosomal compartment for degradation resulting in decreased LDL receptor numbers and increased plasma LDL cholesterol

statin therapy. It has been shown that fibrates also significantly increase circulating PCSK9 levels. Thus, an inhibitor of PCSK9 would be a useful addition to statin and fibrate therapy. Dramatic lowering of LDL cholesterol has been described in non-human primates using monoclonal antibodies (mAB) against PCSK9, and the New England Journal of Medicine has recently reported on a clinical trial of mAB against PCSK9. They showed in healthy volunteers, up to 65 % reduction in LDL cholesterol. These experiments were repeated in patients with familial hypercholesterolemia (FH) who were already on atorvastatin, and the results were similar to healthy volunteers. The authors found a good correlation between reduction in free PCSK9 and reduction in LDL cholesterol, and they demonstrated that the drug had an additive rather than synergistic effect since the mean reductions were similar between normal and FH patients when administered alone or in subjects receiving atorvastatin. This is to be expected since atorvastatin increases hepatic LDL receptor activity by enhancing production of LDL receptors, whereas the antibody decreases the degradation of receptors. There was a significant increase in HDL cholesterol. There was no clear evidence of drug-related events which perhaps was the most important finding in the study. New blockbusters appear to be very hard to come by these days, but perhaps PCSK9 inhibitors may help at least one pharmaceutical company to be optimistic at least in the short term! For patients and practising physicians, it may help to take the burden of guilt away since so often LDL targets are not being met and in particular not being met in patients who already have had a myocardial infarction (Fig. 5.7).

## High-Density Lipoprotein in Diabetes

The lipoprotein cascade which starts with the chylomicron ends with HDL, the smallest of the particles and the only non-apo B-containing particle. The solubilising proteins for HDL are apo A-I and AII, although no HDL species contain only apo AII. Diabetes is associated with low HDL, and in many studies low HDL has been associated with premature/accelerated atherosclerosis. The reasons for the low HDL in diabetes include an increase in apo A-I catabolism. Chan et al. [30] examined the relationship between the fractional catabolic rate between apo A-I and VLDL kinetics in a group of obese men compared to non-obese men. They found that variations in VLDL apo B production and therefore triglyceride concentrations exerted a major effect on the catabolism of apo A-I. They further found that insulin resistance and adiponectin, a hormone associated with insulin sensitivity and reduced in obesity, were contributing factors. They found that in a study of 87 non-diabetic men, plasma adiponectin was one of the best predictors of HDL apo AI fractional catabolic rate (FCR). The significant relationship between plasma adiponectin and HDL apo A-I FCR was independent of HOMA IR score, an index of insulin sensitivity. The authors suggest that adiponectin may have a direct role in HDL catabolism. It has been shown that low plasma adiponectin levels are associated with enhanced hepatic lipase activity in vivo, so lower adiponectin levels may enhance the catabolism of HDL apo A-I by an increase in the lipolysis of HDL triglyceride and the dissociation of apo A-I from the HDL particles [143].

The causes and consequences of low levels of HDL in patients with diabetes have recently been reviewed by Barter [144]. The low HDL is associated with smaller and denser particles, again thought to be secondary to the elevated level of plasma triglycerides. Patel et al. [145] studied the influence of plasma glucose on expression and function of a key mediator in reverse cholesterol transport, the ATP-binding cassette transporter-A1 (ABCA1) and expression of its regulators liver X receptor-α (LXRα) and peroxisome proliferator-activated receptor-γ (PPARγ). They found that ABCA1 expression and protein concentrations in leukocytes, as well as function in cultured skin fibroblasts, were reduced in type 2 diabetes. ABCA1 protein concentration and function were associated with HDL-C levels. These findings indicate a glycemia-related, persistent disruption of a key component of reverse cholesterol transport. Cholesteryl ester transfer protein (CETP) is increased in diabetes and may account, at least in part, for the lower cholesteryl ester and higher level of triglyceride in diabetic HDL [146].

Hepatic lipase is increased in diabetes and insulin resistance [147] and accounts for the increased catabolism of triglyceride giving a smaller, less active HDL particle. There are about 100 HDL-associated proteins which make the function, or rather functions, of HDL extremely complex. In diabetes glycation and oxidation of HDL are increased and may affect HDL function [148]. The formation of advanced glycation end products impairs HDL function and its ability to activate LCAT [148]. Hyperglycemia increased LCAT activity and lowered PON-I activity which was suggested to contribute to the impaired antioxidant capacity of HDL [148]. Interestingly, Loued et al. [149] have recently shown that the anti-inflammatory effect of PON-I appears to depend on its association with HDL. A recent study in type 2 diabetic subjects showed that the antioxidative function of HDL was impaired because of lower HDL cholesterol [150]. Phospholipid transfer protein (PLTP) is elevated in type 2 diabetes. Dullart et al. [151] found that it was raised in diabetic patients, particularly in those with enlarged waist compared to control subjects. HDL with low clusterin (apo J) may be associated with insulin resistance. Apo J is low in patients with reduced insulin sensitivity, perhaps related to alteration in the anti-inflammatory function of HDL [152]. There has recently been interest in the relationship between HDL and retinopathy [153]. Sasongko [154] have demonstrated that apo A-I and B are stronger biomarkers of diabetic retinopathy than traditional lipids. This has recently been confirmed by Deguchy [155] who also showed a relationship between apo B/A1 and retinopathy. The beta cell in the pancreas contains LDL receptors, and it has been suggested that increased oxidation of LDL as occurs in diabetes due to increased free radical production may lead to further destruction of the already damaged beta cell. HDL in diabetes is functionally abnormal and often low and thus can be considered to be an accomplice in the death of the beta cell due to its inability to prevent LDL oxidation. Recently Fryirs et al. [156] have demonstrated that lipid-free and lipid-associated apo AI and apo AII increase beta cell insulin secretion, and it has also been shown that HDL can decrease beta cell apoptosis [157]. It is interesting that insulin sensitivity is affected by the hormone adiponectin secreted by the adipocyte. HDL has been shown to mediate release of adiponectin [158]; hence, dysfunctional HDL may play a part in insulin resistance and type 2 diabetes.

## Conclusion

The complexity of the lipoproteins has meant that it has been possible to study many aspects of the pathways in diabetes and insulin resistance [159]. A recent review of lipoproteins entitled "Mechanisms of disease: the human lipodome" compounds the complexity in an exciting and intimidating way [160]. It is clear that diabetes and insulin resistance play a major part in disturbing lipoprotein metabolism, and many of the disturbances have been shown to be atherogenic either directly or indirectly through the influence on the lipoprotein cascade. Evidence continues to accumulate that improvement in glycemic and lipid control influences atherosclerosis disease progression.

## References


1. Wang YC, McPherson K, Marsh T, Gortmaker SL, Brown M. Health and economic burden of the projected obesity trends in the USA and the UK. Lancet. 2011;378:815–25.
2. Pan X, Hussain MM. Gut triglyceride production. Biochim Biophys Acta. 2012;1821(5):727–35. doi:10.1016/j.bbalip.2011.09.013.
3. Lo CM, Nordskog BK, Nauli AM, Zheng S, Vonlehmden SB, Yang Q, Lee D, Swift LL, Davidson NO, Tso P. Why does the gut choose apolipoprotein B48 but not B100 for chylomicron formation? Am J Physiol Gastrointest Liver Physiol. 2008;294: G344–52.
4. Guttman M, Prieto JH, Croy JE, Komives EA. Decoding of lipoprotein-receptor interactions: properties of ligand binding modules governing interactions with apolipoprotein E. Biochemistry. 2010;49: 1207–16.
5. Sacks FM, Rudel LL, Conner A, Akeefe H, Kostner G, Baki T, Rothblat G, de la Llera-Moya M, Asztalos B, Perlman T, Zheng C, Alaupovic P, Maltais JA, Brewer HB. Selective delipidation of plasma HDL enhances reverse cholesterol transport in vivo. J Lipid Res. 2009;50:894–907.
6. Madigan C, Ryan M, Owens D, Collins P, Tomkin GH. Postprandial lipoprotein particles are deficient in apo E in type 2 diabetes: a cause of postprandial hyperlipidaemia? Ir J Med Sci. 2005;174: 8–21.
7. Zhao Y, Chen X, Yang H, Zhou L, Okoro EU, Guo Z. A novel function of apolipoprotein E: upregulation of ATP-binding cassette transporter A1 expression. PLoS One. 2011;6:e21453.
8. Mahley RW. Apolipoprotein E: cholesterol transport protein with expanding role in cell biology. Science. 1988;240(4852):622–30.
9. Hansen JB, Fernández JA, Notø AT, Deguchi H, Björkegren J, Mathiesen EB. The apolipoprotein C-I content of very-low-density lipoproteins is associated with fasting triglycerides, postprandial lipemia, and carotid atherosclerosis. J Lipids. 2011;2011: 271062.
10. Tall AR. Functions of cholesterol ester transfer protein and relationship to coronary artery disease risk. J Clin Lipidol. 2010;4:389–93.
11. Petersen KF, Dufour S, Hariri A, Nelson-Williams C, Foo JN, Zhang XM, Dziura J, Lifton RP. Shulman GI Apolipoprotein C3 gene variants in nonalcoholic fatty liver disease. N Engl J Med. 2010;362:1082–9.
12. Sundaram M, Zhong S, Bou Khalil M, Links PH, Zhao Y, Iqbal J, Hussain MM, Parks RJ, Wang Y, Yao Z. Expression of apolipoprotein C-III in McA-RH7777 cells enhances VLDL assembly and secretion under lipid-rich conditions. J Lipid Res. 2010;51:150–61.
13. Phillips C, Owens D, Mullan K, Tomkin GH. Low density lipoprotein non-esterified fatty acids and lipoprotein lipase in diabetes. Atherosclerosis. 2005; 181:100–14.
14. Krauss RM, Burke DJ. Identification of multiple subclasses of plasma low density lipoprotein in normal humans. J Lipid Res. 1982;23:97–104.
15. Blake GJ, Otvos JD, Rifai N, Ridker PM. Low-density lipoprotein particle concentration and size as determined by nuclear magnetic resonance spectroscopy as predictors of cardiovascular disease in women. Circulation. 2002;8(106):1930–7.
16. Avogaro P, Bon GB, Cazzolato G. Presence of a modified low density lipoprotein in humans. Arteriosclerosis. 1988;8:79–87.
17. Rosenson RS, Elliott M, Stasiv Y, Hislop C, PLASMA II Investigators. Randomized trial of

inhibitor of secretory phospholipase A2 on atherogenic lipoprotein subclasses in statin-treated patients with coronary heart disease. Eur Heart J. 2011;32: 999–1005.

18. Hiukka A, Ståhlman M, Pettersson C, Levin M, Adiels M, Teneberg S, Leinonen ES, Hultén LM, Wiklund O, Oresic M, Olofsson SO, Taskinen MR, Ekroos K, Borén J. ApoCIII enriched LDL in type 2 diabetes displays altered lipid composition, increased susceptibility for sphingomyelinase, and increased binding to biglycan. Diabetes. 2009;58: 2018–26.
19. Grosso DM, Ferderbar S, Wanschel AC, Krieger MH, Higushi ML, Abdalla DS. Antibodies against electronegative LDL inhibit atherosclerosis in LDLr-/- mice. Braz J Med Biol Res. 2008;41:1086–92.
20. Mello AP, da Silva IT, Abdalla DS, Damasceno NR. Electronegative low-density lipoprotein: origin and impact on health and disease. Atherosclerosis. 2011;215:257–65.
21. Chung M, Lichtenstein AH, Ip S, Lau J, Balk EM. Comparability of methods for LDL subfraction determination: a systematic review. Atherosclerosis. 2009;20:342–8.
22. Younis N, Charlton-Menys V, Sharma R, Soran H, Durrington PN. Glycation of LDL in non-diabetic people: small dense LDL is preferentially glycated both in vivo and in vitro. Atherosclerosis. 2009;202: 162–8.
23. Gaw A, Packard CJ, Lindsay GM, Griffin BA, Caslake MJ, Lorimer AR, Shepherd J. Overproduction of small very low density lipoproteins (Sf 20-60) in moderate hypercholesterolemia: relationships between apolipoprotein B kinetics and plasma lipoproteins. J Lipid Res. 1995;36:158–71.
24. Adiels M, Borén J, Caslake MJ, Stewart P, Soro A, Westerbacka J, Wennberg B, Olofsson SO, Packard C, Taskinen C. Overproduction of VLDL1 driven by hyperglycemia is a dominant feature of diabetic dyslipidemia. Arterioscler Thromb Vasc Biol. 2005;25: 1697–703.
25. Dimitriadis E, Griffin M, Owens D, Johnson A, Collins P, Tomkin GH. Lipoprotein composition in NIDDM. The effect of dietary oleic acid on composition and oxidisability and function of low and high density lipoproteins. Diabetologia. 1996;39:667–76.
26. Zhao Y, Pennings M, Vrins CL, Calpe-Berdiel L, Hoekstra M, Kruijt JK, Ottenhoff R, Hildebrand RB, van der Sluis R, Jessup W, Le Goff W, Chapman MJ, Huby T, Groen AK, Van Berkel TJ, Van Eck M. Hypocholesterolemia, foam cell accumulation, but no atherosclerosis in mice lacking ABC-transporter A1 and scavenger receptor BI. Atherosclerosis. 2011;218:314–22.
27. Soyal SM, Sandhofer A, Hahne P, Oberkofler H, Felder T, Iglseder B, Miller K, Krempler F, Patsch JR, Paulweber B, Patsch W. Cholesteryl ester transfer protein and hepatic lipase gene polymorphisms: effects on hepatic mRNA levels, plasma lipids and carotid atherosclerosis. Atherosclerosis. 2011;216:374–80.
28. West M, Greason E, Kolmakova A, Jahangiri A, Asztalos B, Pollin TI, Rodriguez A. Scavenger receptor class B type I protein as an independent predictor of high-density lipoprotein cholesterol levels in subjects with hyperalphalipoproteinemia. J Clin Endocrinol Metab. 2009;94:1451–7.
29. Krikken JA, Gansevoort RT, Dullaart RP, PREVEND Study Group. Lower HDL-C and apolipoprotein A-I are related to higher glomerular filtration rate in subjects without kidney disease. J Lipid Res. 2010;51: 1982–90.
30. Chan DC, Barrett PH, Ooi EM, Ji J, Chan DT, Watts GF. Very low density lipoprotein metabolism and plasma adiponectin as predictors of high-density lipoprotein apolipoprotein A-I kinetics in obese and nonobese men. J Clin Endocrinol Metab. 2009;94: 989–97.
31. Liu Y, Mackness B, Mackness M. Comparison of the ability of paraoxonases 1 and 3 to attenuate the in vitro oxidation of low-density lipoprotein and reduce macrophage oxidative stress. Free Radic Biol Med. 2008;45:743–8.
32. Calkin AC, Drew BG, Ono A, Duffy SJ, Gordon MV, Schoenwaelder SM, Sviridov D, Cooper ME, Kingwell BA, Jackson SP. Reconstituted high-density lipoprotein attenuates platelet function in individuals with type 2 diabetes mellitus by promoting cholesterol efflux. Circulation. 2009;120: 2095–104.
33. Witting PK, Song C, Hsu K, Hua S, Parry SN, Aran R, Geczy C, Freedman SB. The acute-phase protein serum amyloid A induces endothelial dysfunction that is inhibited by high-density lipoprotein. Free Radic Biol Med. 2011;51:1390–8.
34. Drew BG, Duffy SJ, Formosa MF, Natoli AK, Henstridge DC, Penfold SA, Thomas WG, Mukhamedova N, de Courten B, Forbes JM, Yap FY, Kaye DM, van Hall G, Febbraio MA, Kemp BE, Sviridov D, Steinberg GR, Kingwell BA. High-density lipoprotein modulates glucose metabolism in patients with type 2 diabetes mellitus. Circulation. 2009;119:2103–11.
35. Botham KM, Moore EH, de Pascale C, Bejta F. The induction of macrophage foam cell formation by chylomicron remnants. Biochem Soc Trans. 2007; 35(Pt 3):454–8.
36. Gianturco SH, Ramprasad MP, Lin AH, Song R, Bradley WA. Cellular binding site and membrane binding proteins for triglyceride-rich lipoproteins in human monocyte-macrophages and THP-1 monocytic cells'. J Lipid Res. 1994;35:1674–87.
37. Elsegood CL, Mamo JC. An investigation by electron microscopy of chylomicron remnant uptake by human monocyte-derived macrophages. Atherosclerosis. 2006;188:251–9.
38. Proctor SD, Mamo JC. Intimal retention of cholesterol derived from apolipoprotein B100- and apolipoprotein B48-containing lipoproteins in carotid arteries of Watanabe heritable hyperlipidemic rabbits. Arterioscler Thromb Vasc Biol. 2003;23:1595–600.

39. Pal S, Semorine K, Watts GF, Mamo J. Identification of lipoproteins of intestinal origin in human atherosclerotic plaque. Clin Chem Lab Med. 2003;41:792–5.
40. Nakano T, Nakajima K, Niimi M, Fujita MQ, Nakajima Y, Takeichi S, Kinoshita M, Matsushima T, Teramoto T, Tanaka A. Detection of apolipoproteins B-48 and B-100 carrying particles in lipoprotein fractions extracted from human aortic atherosclerotic plaques in sudden cardiac death cases. Clin Chim Acta. 2008;390:38–43.
41. Miettinen TA, Gylling H, Tuominen J, Simonen P, Koivisto V. Low synthesis and high absorption of cholesterol characterize type 1 diabetes. Diabetes Care. 2004;27:53–8.
42. Lally S, Owens D, Tomkin GH. The different effect of pioglitazone as compared to insulin on expression of hepatic and intestinal genes regulating postprandial lipoproteins in diabetes. Atherosclerosis. 2007;193:343–51.
43. Federico LM, Naples M, Taylor D, Adeli K. Intestinal insulin resistance and aberrant production of apolipoprotein B48 lipoproteins in an animal model of insulin resistance and metabolic dyslipidemia: evidence for activation of protein tyrosine phosphatase-1B, extracellular signal-related kinase, and sterol regulatory element- binding protein-1c in the fructose-fed hamster intestine. Diabetes. 2006; 55:1316–26.
44. Altmann SW, Davis Jr HR, Zhu LJ, Yao X, Hoos LM, Tetzloff G, Iyer SP, Maguire M, Golovko A, Zeng M, Wang L, Murgolo N, Graziano MP. Niemann-Pick C1 like 1 protein is critical for intestinal cholesterol absorption. Science. 2004;303: 1201–4.
45. Sané AT, Sinnett D, Delvin E, Bendayan M, Marcil V, Ménard D, Beaulieu JF, Levy E. Localization and role of NPC1L1 in cholesterol absorption in human intestine. J Lipid Res. 2006;47:2112–20.
46. Zhang JH, Ge L, Qi W, Zhang L, Miao HH, Li BL, Yang M, Song BL. The N-terminal domain of NPC1L1 binds cholesterol and plays essential roles in cholesterol uptake. J Biol Chem. 2011;286(28): 25088–97.
47. Fahmi S, Yang C, Esmail S, Hobbs HH, Cohen JC. Functional characterization of genetic variants in NPC1L1 supports the sequencing extremes strategy to identify complex trait genes. Hum Mol Genet. 2008;17:2101–7.
48. Wang LJ, Wang J, Li N, Ge L, Li BL, Song BL. Molecular characterization of the NPC1L1 variants identified from cholesterol low absorbers. J Biol Chem. 2011;286:7397–408.
49. Calandra S, Tarugi P, Speedy HE, Dean AF, Bertolini S, Shoulders CC. Mechanisms and genetic determinants regulating sterol absorption, circulating LDL levels and sterol elimination: implications for classification and disease risk. J Lipid Res. 2011;52: 1885–926.
50. Wang LJ, Song BL. Niemann-Pick C1-Like 1 and cholesterol uptake. Biochim Biophys Acta. 2012;1821:964–72.
51. Wiersma H, Nijstad N, Gautier T, Iqbal J, Kuipers F, Hussain MM, Tietge UJ. Scavenger receptor BI facilitates hepatic very low density lipoprotein production in mice. J Lipid Res. 2010;51:544–53.
52. Iqbal J, Hussain MM. Intestinal lipid absorption. Am J Physiol Endocrinol Metab. 2009;296:E1183–94.
53. Hayashi AA, Webb J, Choi J, Baker C, Lino M, Trigatti B, Trajcevski KE, Hawke TJ, Adeli K. Intestinal SR-BI is upregulated in insulin-resistant states and is associated with overproduction of intestinal apoB48-containing lipoproteins. Am J Physiol Gastrointest Liver Physiol. 2011;301:G326–37.
54. Xie C, Li N, Chen ZJ, Li BL, Song BL. The small GTPase Cdc42 interacts with Niemann-Pick C1-like 1 (NPC1L1) and controls its movement from endocytic recycling compartment to plasma membrane in a cholesterol-dependent manner. J Biol Chem. 2011;286:35933–42.
55. Wang Z, Thurmond DC. Differential phosphorylation of RhoGDI mediates the distinct cycling of Cdc42 and Rac1 to regulate second-phase insulin secretion. J Biol Chem. 2010;285:6186–97.
56. Gleeson A, Owens D, Collins P, Johnson A, Tomkin GH. The relationship between cholesterol absorption and intestinal cholesterol synthesis in the diabetic rat model. Int J Exp Diabetes Res. 2000;1:203–10.
57. Lally S, Owens D, Tomkin GH. Genes that affect cholesterol synthesis, cholesterol absorption and chylomicron assembly. The relationship between the liver and intestine in control and streptozotosin diabetic rats. Metabolism. 2007;56:430–8.
58. Lally S, Tan CY, Owens D, Tomkin GH. Messenger RNA levels of genes involved in dysregulation of postprandial lipoproteins in type 2 diabetes: the role of Niemann-Pick C1-like 1, ATP-binding cassette, transporters G5 and G8, and of microsomal triglyceride transfer protein. Diabetologia. 2006;49: 1008–16.
59. Levy E, Lalonde G, Delvin E, Elchebly M, Précourt LP, Seidah NG, Spahis S, Rabasa-Lhoret R, Ziv E. Intestinal and hepatic cholesterol carriers in diabetic *Psammomys obesus*. Endocrinology. 2010;151: 958–70.
60. Levy E, Spahis S, Ziv E, Marette A, Elchebly M, Lambert M, Delvin E. Overproduction of intestinal lipoprotein containing apolipoprotein B-48 in *Psammomys obesus*: impact of dietary n-3 fatty acids. Diabetologia. 2006;49:1937–45.
61. Garcia-Calvo M, Lisnock J, Bull HG, Hawes BE, Burnett DA, Braun MP, Crona JH, Davis Jr HR, Dean DC, Detmers PA, Graziano MP, Hughes M, Macintyre DE, Ogawa A, O'Neill KA, Iyer SP, Shevell DE, Smith MM, Tang YS, Makarewicz AM, Ujjainwalla F, Altmann SW, Chapman KT, Thornberry NA. The target of ezetimibe is Niemann-

Pick C1-like 1 (NPC1L1). Proc Natl Acad Sci USA. 2005;102:8132–7.
62. Huff MW, Pollex RL, Hegele RA. NPC1L1: evolution from pharmacological target to physiological sterol transporter. Arterioscler Thromb Vasc Biol. 2006;26:2433–8.
63. van der Veen JN, Kruit JK, Havinga R, Baller JF, Chimini G, Lestavel S, Staels B, Groot PH, Groen AK, Kuipers F. Reduced cholesterol absorption upon PPAR delta activation coincides with decreased intestinal expression of NPC1L1. J Lipid Res. 2005;46:526–34.
64. Iwayanagi Y, Takada T, Tomura F, Yamanashi Y, Terada T, Inui K, Suzuki H. Human NPC1L1 expression is positively regulated by PPARα. Pharm Res. 2011;28:405–12.
65. Valasek MA, Clarke SL, Repa JJ. Fenofibrate reduces intestinal cholesterol absorption via PPAR alpha-dependent modulation of NPC1L1 expression in mouse. J Lipid Res. 2007;48:2725–35.
66. Tremblay AJ, Lamarche B, Lemelin V, Hoos L, Benjannet S, Seidah NG, Davis Jr HR, Couture P. Atorvastatin increases intestinal expression of NPC1L1 in hyperlipidemic men. J Lipid Res. 2011;52:558–65.
67. Berge KE, Tian H, Graf GA, et al. Accumulation of dietary cholesterol in sitosterolemia caused by mutations in adjacent ABC transporters. Science. 2000;290:1771–5.
68. Silbernagel G, Fauler G, Renner W, Landl EM, Hoffmann MM, Winkelmann BR, Boehm BO, März W. The relationships of cholesterol metabolism and plasma plant sterols with the severity of coronary artery disease. J Lipid Res. 2009;50:334–41.
69. Ma KY, Yang N, Jiao R, Peng C, Guan L, Huang Y, Chen ZY. Dietary calcium decreases plasma cholesterol by down-regulation of intestinal Niemann-Pick C1 like 1 and microsomal triacylglycerol transport protein and up-regulation of CYP7A1 and ABCG 5/8 in hamsters. Mol Nutr Food Res. 2011;55: 247–58.
70. Méndez-González J, Julve J, Rotllan N, Llaverias G, Blanco-Vaca F, Escolà-Gil JC. ATP-binding cassette G5/G8 deficiency causes hypertriglyceridemia by affecting multiple metabolic pathways. Biochim Biophys Acta. 1811;2011:1186–93.
71. Blocks VW, Bakker-Van Waarde WM, Verkade HJ, Kema IP, Wolters H, Vink E, Groen AK, Kuipers F. Down-regulation of hepatic and intestinal ABCG5 and ABCG8 expression associated with altered sterol fluxes in rats with streptozotocin-induced diabetes. Diabetologia. 2004;47:104–12.
72. Aggarwal D, West KL, Zern TL, Shrestha S, Vergara-Jimenez M, Fernandez ML. JTT-130, a microsomal triglyceride transfer protein (MTP) inhibitor lowers plasma triglycerides and LDL cholesterol concentrations without increasing hepatic triglycerides in guinea pigs. BMC Cardiovasc Disord. 2005;5:30.
73. Hata T, Mera Y, Ishii Y, Tadaki H, Tomimoto D, Kuroki Y, Kawai T, Ohta T, Kakutani M. JTT-130, a novel intestine-specific inhibitor of microsomal triglyceride transfer protein, suppresses food intake and gastric emptying with the elevation of plasma peptide YY and glucagon-like peptide-1 in a dietary fat-dependent manner. J Pharmacol Exp Ther. 2011;336:850–6.
74. Kim E, Campbell S, Schueller O, Wong E, Cole B, Kuo J, Ferkany J, Ellis J, Sweetnam P. A small molecule inhibitor of enterocytic microsomal triglyceride transfer protein; SLx-4090, biochemical, pharmacodynamic, pharmacokinetic and safety profile. J Pharmacol Exp Ther. 2011;337:775–85.
75. Phillips C, Mullan K, Owens D, Tomkin GH. A common microsomal triglyceride transfer protein polymorphism significantly reduces low density lipoprotein cholesterol in type 2 diabetic patients through its effect on the triglyceride-rich lipoproteins. QJM. 2004;97:211–8.
76. Karpe F, Lundahl B, Ehrenborg E, Eriksson P, Hamsten A. A common functional polymorphism in the promoter region of the microsomal triglyceride transfer protein gene influences plasma LDL levels. Atheroscler Thromb Vasc Biol. 1998;18:756–61.
77. Phillips C, Anderton K, Bennett A, et al. Intestinal rather than hepatic microsomal triglyceride transfer protein as a cause of postprandial dyslipidaemia in diabetes. Metabolism. 2002;51:847–52.
78. Gleeson A, Anderton K, Owens D, et al. The role of microsomal triglyceride transfer protein and dietary cholesterol in chylomicron production in diabetes. Diabetologia. 1999;42:944–9.
79. Qin B, Qiu W, Avramoglu RK, Adeli K. Tumor necrosis factor-alpha induces intestinal insulin resistance and stimulates the overproduction of intestinal apolipoprotein B48-containing lipoproteins. Diabetes. 2007;56:450–61.
80. Zoltowska M, Ziv E, Delvin E, Sinnett D, Kalman R, Garofalo C, Seidman E, Levy E. Cellular aspects of intestinal lipoprotein assembly in *Psammomys obesus*: a model of insulin resistance and type 2 diabetes. Diabetes. 2003;52:2539–45.
81. Phillips C, Mullan K, Owens D, Tomkin GH. Intestinal microsomal triglyceride transfer protein in type 2 diabetic and non-diabetic subjects: the relationship to triglyceride-rich postprandial lipoprotein composition. Atherosclerosis. 2006;187:57–64.
82. Hata T, Mera Y, Kawai T, Ishii Y, Kuroki Y, Kakimoto K, Ohta T, Kakutani M. JTT-130, a novel intestine-specific inhibitor of microsomal triglyceride transfer protein, ameliorates impaired glucose and lipid metabolism in Zucker diabetic fatty rats. Diabetes Obes Metab. 2011;13:629–38.
83. Dhote V, Joharapurkar A, Kshirsagar S, Dhanesha N, Patel V, Patel A, Raval S, Jain M. Inhibition of microsomal triglyceride transfer protein improves insulin sensitivity and reduces atherogenic risk in

Zucker fatty rats. Clin Exp Pharmacol Physiol. 2011;38:338–44.

84. Sparks JD, Chamberlain JM, O'Dell C, Khatun I, Hussain MM, Sparks CE. Acute suppression of apo B secretion by insulin occurs independently of MTP. Biochem Biophys Res Commun. 2011;406:252–6.
85. Tran TT, Poirier H, Clément L, Nassir F, Pelsers MM, Petit V, Degrace P, Monnot MC, Glatz JF, Abumrad NA, Besnard P, Niot I. Luminal lipid regulates CD36 levels and downstream signaling to stimulate chylomicron synthesis. J Biol Chem. 2011;286:25201–10.
86. Wolff E, Vergnes MF, Defoort C, Planells R, Portugal H, Nicolay A, Lairon D. Cholesterol absorption status and fasting plasma cholesterol are modulated by the microsomal triacylglycerol transfer protein -493 G/T polymorphism and the usual diet in women. Genes Nutr. 2011;6:71–9.
87. Ashur-Fabian O, Har-Zahav A, Shaish A, Wiener Amram H, Margalit O, Weizer- Stern O, Dominissini D, Harats D, Amariglio N, Rechavi G. apoB and apobec1, two genes key to lipid metabolism, are transcriptionally regulated by p53. Cell Cycle. 2010(18):3761–70.
88. Karimian Pour N, Adeli K. Insulin silences apolipoprotein B mRNA translation by inducing intracellular traffic into cytoplasmic RNA granules. Biochemistry. 2011;50(32):6942–50.
89. Phillips C, Madigan C, Owens D, Collins P, Tomkin GH. Defective chylomicron synthesis as a cause of delayed particle clearance in diabetes? Int J Exp Diabetes Res. 2002;2:171–8.
90. Curtin A, Deegan P, Owens D, Collins P, Johnson A, Tomkin GH. Alterations in apolipoprotein B-48 in the post-prandial state in non-insulin-dependent diabetes. Diabetologia. 1994;37:1259–64.
91. Devery R, O'Meara N, Collins P, Johnson A, Scott L, Tomkin GH. A comparative study of the rate-limiting enzymes of cholesterol synthesis, esterification and catabolism in the alloxan-induced diabetic rat and rabbit. Comp Biochem Physiol. 1987;87:697–702.
92. Sittiwet C, Gylling H, Hallikainen M, Pihlajamäki J, Moilanen L, Laaksonen DE, Niskanen L, Agren JJ, Laakso M, Miettinen TA. Cholesterol metabolism and non-cholesterol sterol distribution in lipoproteins of type 1 diabetes: the effect of improved glycemic control. Atherosclerosis. 2007;194:465–72.
93. Zhao L, Chen Y, Tang R, Chen Y, Li Q, Gong J, Huang A, Varghese Z, Moorhead JF, Ruan XZ. Inflammatory stress exacerbates hepatic cholesterol accumulation via increasing cholesterol uptake and de novo synthesis. J Gastroenterol Hepatol. 2011; 26:875–83.
94. Xie X, Liao H, Dang H, Pang W, Guan Y, Wang X, Shyy JY, Zhu Y, Sladek FM. Down-regulation of hepatic HNF4alpha gene expression during hyperinsulinemia via SREBPs. Mol Endocrinol. 2009;23: 434–43.
95. Van Rooyen DM, Farrell GC. SREBP-2: a link between insulin resistance, hepatic cholesterol, and inflammation in NASH. J Gastroenterol Hepatol. 2011;26:789–92.
96. Song Y, Stampfer MJ, Liu S. Meta-analysis: apolipoprotein E genotypes and risk for coronary heart disease. Ann Intern Med. 2004;141:137–47.
97. Bennet AM, Di Angelantonio E, Ye Z, Wensley F, Dahlin A, Ahlbom A, et al. Association of apolipoprotein E genotypes with lipid levels and coronary risk. JAMA. 2007;298:1300–11.
98. Tao MH, Liu JW, LaMonte MJ, Liu J, Wang L, He Y, Li XY, Wang LN, Ye L. Different associations of apolipoprotein E polymorphism with metabolic syndrome by sex in an elderly Chinese population. Metabolism. 2011;60:1488–96.
99. Sacks FM, Alaupovic P, Moye LA, et al. VLDL, apolipoproteins B, CIII, and E, and risk of recurrent coronary events in the Cholesterol and Recurrent Events (CARE) trial. Circulation. 2000;102:1886–92.
100. Zheng C, Khoo C, Ikewaki K, Sacks FM. Rapid turnover of apolipoprotein C-III- containing triglyceride rich lipoproteins contributing to the formation of LDL subfractions. J Lipid Res. 2007;48:1190–203.
101. Lee SJ, Campos H, Moye LA, Sacks FM. LDL containing apolipoprotein CIII is an independent risk factor for coronary events in diabetic patients. Arterioscler Thromb Vasc Biol. 2003;23:853–8.
102. Guardiola M, Alvaro A, Vallvé JC, Rosales R, Solà R, Girona J, Serra N, Duran P, Esteve E, Masana L, Ribalta J. APOA5 gene expression in the human intestinal tissue and its response to in vitro exposure to fatty acid and fibrate. Nutr Metab Cardiovasc Dis. 2011;22(9):756–62 [PMID:21489765].
103. Dallinga-Thie GM, van Tol A, Hattori H, van Vark-van der Zee LC, Jansen H, Sijbrands EJ, DALI study group. Plasma apolipoprotein A5 and triglycerides in type 2 diabetes. Diabetologia. 2006;49:1505–11.
104. Coca-Prieto I, Valdivielso P, Olivecrona G, Ariza MJ, Rioja J, Font-Ugalde P, García- Arias C, González-Santos P. Lipoprotein lipase activity and mass, apolipoprotein C-II mass and polymorphisms of apolipoproteins E and A5 in subjects with prior acute hypertriglyceridaemic pancreatitis. BMC Gastroenterol. 2009;9:46.
105. Kamagate A, Dong HH. FoxO1 integrates insulin signaling to VLDL production. Cell Cycle. 2008;7: 3162–70.
106. Scott L, Tomkin GH. Regulatory effects of insulin on cholesterol metabolism. Diabetologia. 1984;27: 330.
107. Pramfalk C, Jiang ZY, Cai Q, Hu H, Zhang SD, Han TQ, Eriksson M, Parini P. HNF1 alpha and SREBP2 are important regulators of NPC1L1 in human liver. J Lipid Res. 2010;51:1354–62.
108. Jia L, Betters JL, Yu L. Niemann-pick C1-like 1 (NPC1L1) protein in intestinal and hepatic cholesterol transport. Annu Rev Physiol. 2011;73:239–59.

109. Cui W, Jiang ZY, Cai Q, Zhang RY, Wu WZ, Wang JC, Fei J, Zhang SD, Han TQ. Decreased NPC1L1 expression in the liver from Chinese female gallstone patients. Lipids Health Dis. 2010;9:17.
110. Valasek MA, Repa JJ, Quan G, Dietschy JM, Turley SD. Inhibiting intestinal NPC1L1 activity prevents diet-induced increase in biliary cholesterol in Golden Syrian hamsters. Am J Physiol Gastrointest Liver Physiol. 2008;295:G813–22.
111. Zúñiga S, Molina H, Azocar L, Amigo L, Nervi F, Pimentel F, Jarufe N, Arrese M, Lammert F, Miquel JF. Ezetimibe prevents cholesterol gallstone formation in mice. Liver Int. 2008;28:935–47.
112. Jia L, Ma Y, Rong S, Betters JL, Xie P, Chung S, Wang N, Tang W, Yu L. Niemann- Pick C1-Like 1 deletion in mice prevents high-fat diet-induced fatty liver by reducing lipogenesis. J Lipid Res. 2010; 51:3135–44.
113. Nomura M, Ishii H, Kawakami A, Yoshida M. Inhibition of hepatic Neimann-Pick C1-like 1 improves hepatic insulin resistance. Am J Physiol Endocrinol Metab. 2009;297:E1030–8.
114. Kishimoto M, Sugiyama T, Osame K, Takarabe D, Okamoto M, Noda M. Efficacy of ezetimibe as monotherapy or combination therapy in hypercholesterolemic patients with and without diabetes. J Med Invest. 2011;58:86–94.
115. Tang W, Jia L, Ma Y, Xie P, Haywood J, Dawson PA, Li J, Yu L. Ezetimibe restores biliary cholesterol excretion in mice expressing Niemann-Pick C1-like 1 only in liver. Biochim Biophys Acta. 1811;2011:549–55.
116. Yamanashi Y, Takada T, Yoshikado T, Shoda J, Suzuki H. NPC2 regulates biliary cholesterol secretion via stimulation of ABCG5/G8-mediated cholesterol transport. Gastroenterology. 2011;140: 1664–74.
117. Repa JJ, Berge KE, Pomajzl C, Richardson JA, Hobbs H, Mangelsdorf DJ. Regulation of ATP-binding cassette sterol transporters ABCG5 and ABCG8 by the liver X receptors alpha and beta. J Biol Chem. 2002;277:18793–800.
118. Wan M, Leavens KF, Saleh D, Easton RM, Guertin DA, Peterson TR, Kaestner KH, Sabatini DM, Birnbaum MJ. Postprandial hepatic lipid metabolism requires signaling through Akt2 independent of the transcription factors FoxA2, FoxO1, and SREBP1c. Cell Metab. 2011;14:516–27.
119. Biddinger SB, Haas JT, Yu BB, Bezy O, Jing E, Zhang W, Unterman TG, Carey MC, Kahn CR. Hepatic insulin resistance directly promotes formation of cholesterol gallstones. Nat Med. 2008;14: 778–82.
120. Cummings MH, Watts GF, Umpleby AM, Hennessy TR, Naoumova R, Slavin BM, Thompson GR, Sonksen PH. Increased hepatic secretion of very-low-density lipoprotein apolipoprotein B-100 in NIDDM. Diabetologia. 1995;38:959–67.
121. Watts GF, Ooi EM, Chan DC. Therapeutic regulation of apoB100 metabolism in insulin resistance in vivo. Pharmacol Ther. 2009;123:281–91.
122. Subramanian S, Chait A. Hypertriglyceridemia secondary to obesity and diabetes. Biochim Biophys Acta. 2012;1821(5):819–25 [PMID:22005032].
123. Ata N, Kucukazman M, Yavuz B, Bulus H, Dal K, Ertugrul DT, Yalcin AA, Polat M, Varol N, Akin KO, Karabag A, Nazligul Y. The metabolic syndrome is associated with complicated gallstone disease. Can J Gastroenterol. 2011;25:274–6.
124. Weikert C, Weikert S, Schulze MB, Pischon T, Fritsche A, Bergmann MM, Willich SN, Boeing H. Presence of gallstones or kidney stones and risk of type 2 diabetes. Am J Epidemiol. 2010;15(171): 447–54.
125. Sørensen LP, Andersen IR, Søndergaard E, Gormsen LC, Schmitz O, Christiansen JS, Nielsen S. Basal and insulin mediated VLDL-triglyceride kinetics in type 2 diabetic men. Diabetes. 2011;60:88–96.
126. Pavlic M, Xiao C, Szeto L, Patterson BW, Lewis GF. Insulin acutely inhibits intestinal lipoprotein secretion in humans in part by suppressing plasma free fatty acids. Diabetes. 2010;59:580–7.
127. Taskinen MR. Diabetic dyslipidaemia: from basic research to clinical practice. Diabetologia. 2003;46: 733–49.
128. Taskinen MR. Lipoprotein lipase in diabetes. Diabetes Metab Rev. 1987;3:551–70.
129. Costabile G, Annuzzi G, Di Marino L, De Natale C, Giacco R, Bozzetto L, Cipriano P, Santangelo C, Masella R, Rivellese AA. Fasting and post-prandial adipose tissue lipoprotein lipase and hormone-sensitive lipase in obesity and type 2 diabetes. J Endocrinol Invest. 2011;34:e110–4.
130. Wang Y, Puthanveetil P, Wang F, Kim MS, Abrahani A, Rodrigues B. Severity of diabetes governs vascular lipoprotein lipase by affecting enzyme dimerization and disassembly. Biochim Biophys Acta. 2011;60:2041–50.
131. Tao H, Hajri T. Very low density lipoprotein receptor promotes adipocyte differentiation and mediates the proadipogenic effect of peroxisome proliferator-activated receptor gamma agonists. Biochem Pharmacol. 2011;15(82):1950–62.
132. Laatsch A, Merkel M, Talmud PJ, Grewal T, Beisiegel U, Heeren J. Insulin stimulates hepatic low density lipoprotein receptor-related protein 1 (LRP1) to increase postprandial lipoprotein clearance. Atherosclerosis. 2009;204:105–11.
133. Mikhailidis DP, Elisaf M, Rizzo M, Berneis K, Griffin B, Zambon A, Athyros V, de Graaf J, März W, Parhofer KG, Rini GB, Spinas GA, Tomkin GH, Tselepis AD, Wierzbicki AS, Winkler K, Florentin M, Liberopoulos E. "European panel on low density lipoprotein (LDL) subclasses": a statement on the pathophysiology, atherogenicity and clinical significance of LDL subclasses: executive summary. Curr Vasc Pharmacol. 2011;9:531–2.
134. Deegan P, Owens D, Collins P, Johnson A, Tomkin GH. The relationship between diabetic control, low density lipoprotein glycosylation and turnover. Diabetologia. 1994;37:A67.

135. Devery R, Tomkin GH. The effect of insulin and catecholamines on the activities of 3- hydroxy-3-methyl glutaryl coenzyme A reductase and acyl-coenzyme A: cholesterol-o- acyltransferase in isolated rat hepatocytes. Diabetologia. 1986;29:122–4.
136. Tani M, Kawakami A, Mizuno Y, Imase R, Ito Y, Kondo K, Ishii H, Yoshida M. Small dense LDL enhances THP-1 macrophage foam cell formation. J Atheroscler Thromb. 2011;18:698–704.
137. Tomkin GH, Owens D. Abnormalities of cholesterol metabolism in diabetes. Proc Nutr Soc. 1991;50: 583–9.
138. Colas R, Sassolas A, Guichardant M, Cugnet-Anceau C, Moret M, Moulin P, Lagarde M, Calzada C. LDL from obese patients with the metabolic syndrome show increased lipid peroxidation and activate platelets. Diabetologia. 2011;54:2931–40.
139. Pitocco D, Zaccardi F, Di Stasio E, Romitelli F, Santini SA, Zuppi C, Ghirlanda G. Oxidative stress, nitric oxide, and diabetes. Rev Diabet Stud. 2010;7: 15–25. Review.
140. Bowie A, Owens D, Collins P, Johnson A, Tomkin GH. Glycosylated low density lipoprotein is more sensitive to oxidation: implications for the diabetic patient? Atherosclerosis. 1993;102:63–7.
141. Miller YI, Choi SH, Fang L, Harkewicz R. Toll-like receptor-4 and lipoprotein accumulation in macrophages. Trends Cardiovasc Med. 2009;19(7): 227–32. Review.
142. Geng H, Wang A, Rong G, Zhu B, Deng Y, Chen J, Zhong R. The effects of ox-LDL in human atherosclerosis may be mediated in part via the toll-like receptor 4 pathway. Mol Cell Biochem. 2010;342(1-2):201–6.
143. Schneider JG, von Eynatten M, Schiekofer S, Nawroth PP, Dugi KA. Low plasma adiponectin levels are associated with increased hepatic lipase activity in vivo. Diabetes Care. 2005;28:2181–6.
144. Barter PJ. The causes and consequences of low levels of high density lipoproteins in patients with diabetes. Diabetes Metab J. 2011;35:101–6.
145. Patel DC, Albrecht C, Pavitt D, Paul V, Pourreyron C, Newman SP, Godsland IF, Valabhji J, Johnston DG. 2 diabetes is associated with reduced ATP-binding cassette transporter A1 gene expression, protein and function. PLoS One. 2011;6:e22142.
146. Jones R, Brennan K, Owens D, Collins P, Johnson A, Tomkin GH. Increase esterification of cholesterol and transfer of cholesteryl esters to apo B containing lipoproteins in type 2 diabetes—relationship to serum free cholesterol, HDL cholesterol and LDL composition. Atherosclerosis. 1996;119:151–7.
147. López-Ríos L, Nóvoa FJ, Chirino R, Varillas F, Boronat-Cortés M, Wägner AM. Interaction between cholesteryl ester transfer protein and hepatic lipase encoding genes and the risk of type 2 diabetes: results from the Telde study. PLoS One. 2011;6:e27208.
148. Kappelle PJ, de Boer JF, Perton FG, Annema W, de Vries R, Dullaart RP, Tietge UJ. Increased LCAT activity and hyperglycaemia decrease the antioxidative functionality of HDL. Eur J Clin Invest. 2012; 42(5):487–95.doi:10.1111/j.1365-2362.2011.02604.x.
149. Loued S, Isabelle M, Berrougui H, Khalil A. The anti-inflammatory effect of paraoxonase 1 against oxidized lipids depends on its association with high density lipoproteins. Life Sci. 2012;90(1–2):82–8. PMID:22067439.
150. Morgantini C, Natali A, Boldrini B, Imaizumi S, Navab M, Fogelman AM, Ferrannini E, Reddy ST. Anti-inflammatory and antioxidant properties of HDLs are impaired in type 2 diabetes. Diabetes. 2011;60(10):2617–23. PMID:21852676.
151. Dullaart RP, Vergeer M, de Vries R, Kappelle PJ, Dallinga-Thie GM. Type 2 diabetes mellitus interacts with obesity and common variations in PLTP to affect plasma phospholipid transfer protein activity. J Intern Med. 2012;271(5):490–8. doi:10.1111/j.1365-2796.2011.02465.x.
152. Hoofnagle AN, Wu M, Gosmanova AK, Becker JO, Wijsman EM, Brunzell JD, Kahn SE, Knopp RH, Lyons TJ, Heinecke JW. Low clusterin levels in high-density lipoprotein associate with insulin resistance, obesity, and dyslipoproteinemia. Arterioscler Thromb Vasc Biol. 2010;30:2528–34.
153. Chait A, Montes VN. Apolipoproteins and diabetic retinopathy. Diabetes Care. 2011;34:529–31.
154. Sasongko MB, Wong TY, Nguyen TT, Kawasaki R, Jenkins A, Shaw J, Wang JJ. Serum apolipoprotein AI and B are stronger biomarkers of diabetic retinopathy than traditional lipids. Diabetes Care. 2011;34:474–9.
155. Deguchi Y, Maeno T, Saishin Y, Hori Y, Shiba T, Takahashi M. Relevance of the serum apolipoprotein ratio to diabetic retinopathy. Jpn J Ophthalmol. 2011;55:128–31.
156. Fryirs MA, Barter PJ, Appavoo M, Tuch BE, Tabet F, Heather AK, Rye KA. Effects of high-density lipoproteins on pancreatic beta-cell insulin secretion. Arterioscler Thromb Vasc Biol. 2010;30: 1642–8.
157. Rütti S, Ehses JA, Sibler RA, Prazak R, Rohrer L, Georgopoulos S, Meier DT, Niclauss N, Berney T, Donath MY, von Eckardstein A. Low- and high-density lipoproteins modulate function, apoptosis, and proliferation of primary human and murine pancreatic beta-cells. Endocrinology. 2009;150: 4521–30.
158. Van Linthout S, Foryst-Ludwig A, Spillmann F, Peng J, Feng Y, Meloni M, Van Craeyveld E, Kintscher U, Schultheiss HP, De Geest B, Tschöpe C. Impact of HDL on adipose tissue metabolism and adiponectin expression. Atherosclerosis. 2010;210: 438–44.
159. Getz GS, Reardon CA. High-density lipoprotein function in regulating insulin secretion: possible relevance to metabolic syndrome. Arterioscler Thromb Vasc Biol. 2010;30:1497–9.
160. Quehenberger O, Dennis EA. The human plasma lipidome. N Engl J Med. 2011;365:1812–23.

# 6 Production and Metabolism of Triglyceride-Rich Lipoproteins in Both the Normal and Diabetic States

Angela Pirillo, Giuseppe D. Norata, and Alberico L. Catapano

Apolipoprotein B (apoB)-containing lipoproteins are believed to be atherogenic and include chylomicrons, very low-density lipoproteins (VLDL), and low-density lipoproteins (LDL). Chylomicrons, which transport lipids derived from diet, are produced by the intestine, while VLDL, which transport endogenous lipids, are produced by the liver. Both are produced at the surface of the endoplasmic reticulum (ER). After secretion of these lipoproteins, triglycerides are hydrolyzed by lipoprotein lipase, and fatty acids are taken up by the cells to provide energy (in the muscle) or to be stored (in adipose tissue). Remnant lipoproteins are enriched in cholesterol and can be taken up by cells, and VLDL can be converted to LDL. Plasma triglycerides are mainly produced in the liver and the intestine.

A. Pirillo
Center for the Study of Atherosclerosis, E. Bassini Hospital, Cinisello Balsamo, and IRCCS Multimedica, Milan, Italy

G.D. Norata
Department of Pharmacological and Biomolecular Sciences, University of Milan and Center for the Study of Atherosclerosis, E. Bassini Hospital, Cinisello Balsamo, Italy

A.L. Catapano (✉)
Department of Pharmacological and Biomolecular Sciences, University of Milan, Milan, Italy

Center for the Study of Atherosclerosis, E. Bassini Hospital, Cinisello Balsamo, and IRCCS Multimedica, Milan, Italy
e-mail: alberico.catapano@unimi.it

## TG-Rich Lipoproteins Secretion by Liver and Intestine

TG-rich lipoproteins (TGRLs) comprise both hepatically derived apoB100-containing very low-density lipoprotein (VLDL) and intestinally derived apoB48-containing chylomicrons [1, 2]. TGRLs are assembled in the liver by hepatocytes and in the intestine by jejunal enterocytes. These lipoproteins are spherical particles, consisting of a neutral lipid core (mainly cholesteryl esters and TG) surrounded by a monolayer of lipids (phospholipids and free cholesterol) and apolipoproteins. Apolipoprotein B (apoB) is the main protein in both VLDL and chylomicrons; each particle contains a single apoB molecule. Human apoB100 is secreted exclusively by the liver in VLDL, while apoB48 is secreted exclusively by the intestine in chylomicrons. ApoB is synthesized in two isoforms: apoB100 in the liver and apoB48 (deriving from the same gene of apoB100) in the intestine [3, 4]. ApoB is synthesized in coordination with MTP (microsomal triglyceride transfer protein) expression and activity [5]. In the presence of lipids, nascent apoB is quickly lipidated by MTP; in the absence of lipids, nascent apoB is ubiquitinylated and degraded. ApoB levels are in fact highly regulated by multiple distinct degradative pathways [6]. When lipid availability is low or MTP activity is reduced, apoB is cotranslationally targeted for ubiquitinylation and degradation by the proteasome [7–9]. Alternatively, fully assembled apoB

A.J. Jenkins et al. (eds.), *Lipoproteins in Diabetes Mellitus*, Contemporary Diabetes,
DOI 10.1007/978-1-4614-7554-5_6, © Springer Science+Business Media New York 2014

particles can undergo reuptake by cells through interaction with the LDL receptor or with specific proteoglycans [10]. In addition, dietary polyunsaturated fatty acids (PUFAs) induce the degradation of newly synthesized apoB through a non-proteasome, post-ER pathway [6]; this process occurs in the presence of normal triglyceride levels, resulting in reduced VLDL secretion.

Lipoprotein assembly starts with apoB transcription and translocation into the lumen of the endoplasmic reticulum (ER). Here, lipid droplets are added to apoB, facilitated by the activity of MTP, thus resulting in a premature form of apoB-containing particle. Next, the addition of neutral lipids increases the size of the nascent particle that is then transported through the Golgi and secreted into the hepatic vein for the hepatic lipoproteins and in the lymphatic system for intestinal lipoproteins.

## VLDL Assembly and Secretion

ApoB100 is the major structural protein of VLDL, exhibits a highly lipophilic nature, and contains two domains able to interact irreversibly with the neutral lipids present in the lipoprotein core [11]. The intrahepatic assembly of apoB into VLDL can be divided into two steps (Fig. 6.1). Due to its lipophilic nature, apoB folding and stability depends upon the simultaneous addition of lipids; this process is related to the activity of MTP [12, 13]. MTP is an ER-resident protein that, following heterodimerization with the small subunit protein disulfide isomerase (PDI), catalyzes the transfer of polar (phospholipids) and neutral (triglycerides) lipids to nascent apoB during its translocation through a protein channel in the membrane of the rough ER [14, 15]. MTP is also expressed in the intestine and plays a key role in the lipidation of apoB48 during chylomicron assembly [16, 17]. This lipidation step results in the formation of a relatively small (max 25 nm), dense particle. Maturation of these precursors to VLDL particles with 30–80 nm diameter involves the post-translational acquisition of the bulk of triglycerides by fusion of the apoB-containing precursor with large triglyceride droplets produced in the smooth endoplasmic reticulum [18], giving rise to TG-rich VLDL. The size of the VLDL particles secreted by the liver is determined by the size of the TG pool [19], which mainly derives from lipolytic mobilization of the hepatic storage pool [20] rather than from newly formed TG [21].

VLDL assembly and secretion is a process highly regulated by the availability of triglycerides in the liver [22]; TG may derive from different sources, including uptake of albumin-bound fatty acids, uptake of circulating remnants of VLDL and chylomicrons, and de novo hepatic synthesis. Beside apoB and MTP, TG availability

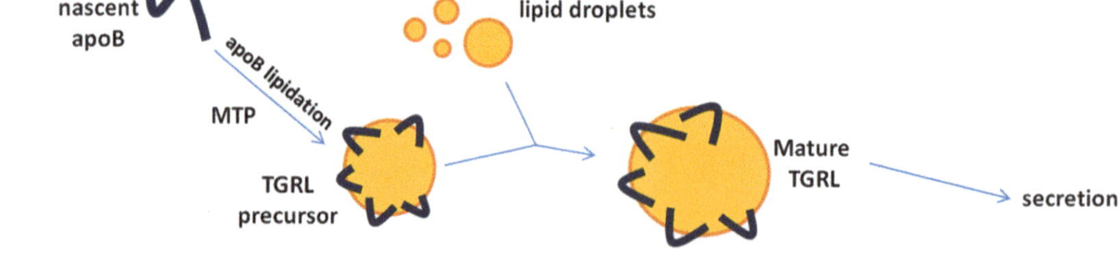


**Fig. 6.1** Intrahepatic assembly of apoB into VLDL

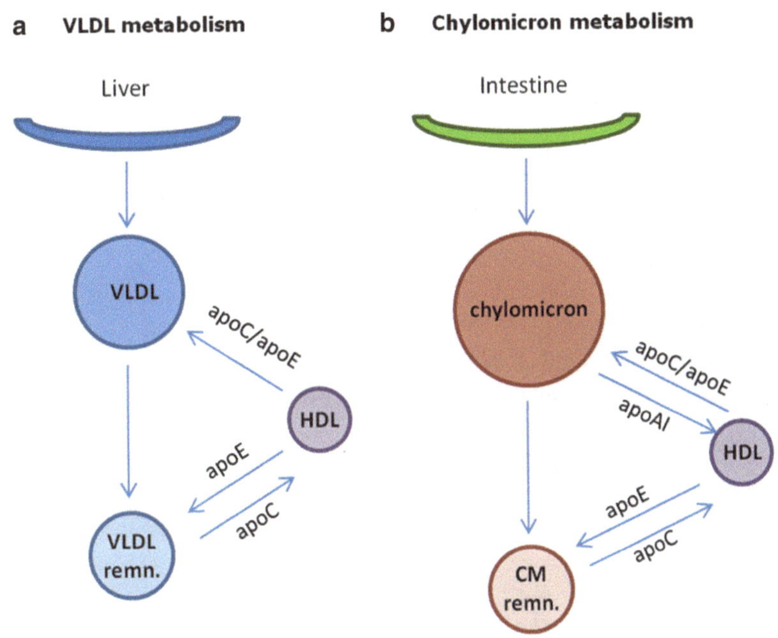


**Fig. 6.2** Metabolism of VLDL (**a**) and chylomicrons (**b**)

determines the efficiency of apoB-lipoprotein formation. In fact, reduced lipid availability results in targeting of apoB for degradation and decreased VLDL secretion [23]. Fatty acids derived from diet or released from adipose tissue enter the liver where they are re-esterified, forming triglyceride droplets [24]. Not all mobilized TGs enter into the secretory pool to contribute to VLDL formation; a relatively large proportion (determined by MTP and insulin activity) is returned back to the cytosolic pool. Newly synthesized VLDL contain little apoC; after secretion in the circulation, they acquire apoE and additional apoC from HDL (Fig. 6.2).

Two major subfractions of VLDL exist, large VLDL1 and smaller VLDL2. VLDL1 secretion is dependent on fatty acid availability, and insulin inhibits VLDL1 secretion [25]; this does not seem to be true for VLDL2. After secretion, VLDL1 are delipidated, following hydrolysis of TG through lipoprotein lipase; the delipidation process of VLDL1 is not complete, and only a minor fraction is converted to LDL, most remnants being directly removed from plasma [26]. On the contrary, most VLDL2 particles are delipidated and converted to LDL [27].

## Chylomicron Assembly and Secretion

Three proteins play a key role in the process of chylomicron assembly: apoB48, MTP, and apoA-IV. ApoB48 is produced from the same gene of apoB100 in the small intestine and is formed by post-transcriptional mRNA editing in intestinal enterocytes; it lacks the LDLR-binding domain and is essential for the assembly of chylomicrons. MTP is a lipid-transfer protein that transports ER membrane-bound lipid (mainly TG) to newly synthesized apoB48, a step that prevents apoprotein degradation; moreover, MTP facilitates the successive lipidation of chylomicron precursors. ApoA-IV is a lipid-binding protein expressed mainly in the small intestine and incorporated early into nascent chylomicrons; after chylomicron secretion, apoA-IV dissociates from the particles to circulate as lipid-free protein.

Chylomicrons are responsible for the transport of dietary cholesterol and medium- and long-chain fatty acids from the intestinal lumen to the liver. The main lipids in chylomicrons are triacylglycerols. They are assembled mainly in the ER and then transported to the Golgi via specialized vesicles (PCTVs, prechylomicron transport vesicles). During the first assembly step, apoB48, synthesized by the small intestine, is translated into the ER lumen and immediately lipidated through the action of intestinal MTP (Fig. 6.1), resulting in the formation of a precursor particle. The lipidation can occur both by transfer of lipid from the ER membrane to apoB48 or by binding of MTP to apoB48 to facilitate the protein folding and lipid acquisition. During the second step, MTP mediates further addition of lipids to the precursor. In this phase apoA-IV is added at the particle surface; apoA-IV increases MTP activity and increases chylomicron lipidation [28].

## Lipoprotein Lipase-Mediated Lipolysis

VLDL and chylomicrons leave the liver and intestine and enter the circulation where they acquire apoC-II and apoE from plasma HDL. In the capillaries of adipose tissue and muscle, triacylglycerols are hydrolyzed by endothelial lipoprotein lipase (LPL, activated by apoC-II) to produce free fatty acids which are then absorbed by the tissues. During the removal of fatty acids, a large percentage of the phospholipids and apoproteins are transferred to HDL, converting the lipoproteins to VLDL and chylomicron remnants (Fig. 6.2).

## Hepatic Clearance of Remnants

The main organ involved in the clearance of remnant lipoprotein is the liver, where hepatocytes express LDL receptor (LDLR), LDL receptor-related protein 1 (LRP1), and heparan sulfate proteoglycans (HSPGs) in high amounts. In concert with LPL and hepatic lipase (HL), these surface molecules facilitate the rapid hepatic clearance of remnant lipoproteins [29–32] that are extremely atherogenic [33] (Fig. 6.3). The most critical molecule in the remnant clearance is apoE, involved in the binding of lipoprotein to the LDLR family and HSPGs [31]. Multiple steps are involved in the uptake of remnants by hepatocytes. HSPGs interact with apoE present on the remnant surface and sequester them in the space of Disse [32]; moreover, HSPGs can bind LPL and HL that eventually may continue their lipolytic activity and prepare the particles for the successive internalization process [32, 34], which is mediated by LDLR, HSPGs, and the HSPGs/LRP complex.

Chylomicron remnants contain mainly cholesteryl esters, apoE, and apoB48 and return to the liver where they are taken up by hepatocytes via interaction with the LDL receptor which requires apoE [35]. Moreover, chylomicron remnants can acquire additional apoE, allowing the remnants to be taken up via the chylomicron remnant receptor, a member of the LDL receptor-related protein (LRP) family [35]. Alternatively, chylomicron remnants can remain sequestered in the space of Disse by binding of apoE to heparan sulfate proteoglycans and/or binding of apoB48 to hepatic lipase [35]. During this phase, chylomicron remnants may be further metabolized which increases apoE and lysophospholipid content, allowing for transfer to LDL receptors or LRP for hepatic uptake. VLDL remnant particles are immediately cleared by the liver or, alternatively, further modified by HL and cholesteryl ester transfer protein (CETP) to generate LDL.

## The Role of Insulin in TGRLs Metabolism

The VLDL assembly process in the liver is tightly regulated by insulin [36, 37]: under fasting conditions, VLDL production in the liver is induced; on the contrary, in response to post-prandial insulin release, hepatic VLDL production is repressed [25, 38, 39]. This tight regulation allows the liver to rapidly adapt to metabolic shifts between fasting and feeding and to maintain plasma lipids within the physiological range [25, 39, 40] (Fig. 6.4).

Several observations suggest that insulin inhibits apoB secretion by inducing its degradation [41–44]; alternatively, insulin reduced free fatty acid (FFA) availability by reducing FFA mobilization from adipose tissue, resulting in apoB secretion inhibition [45]. The apoB gene is believed to be constitutively expressed as hepatic mRNA

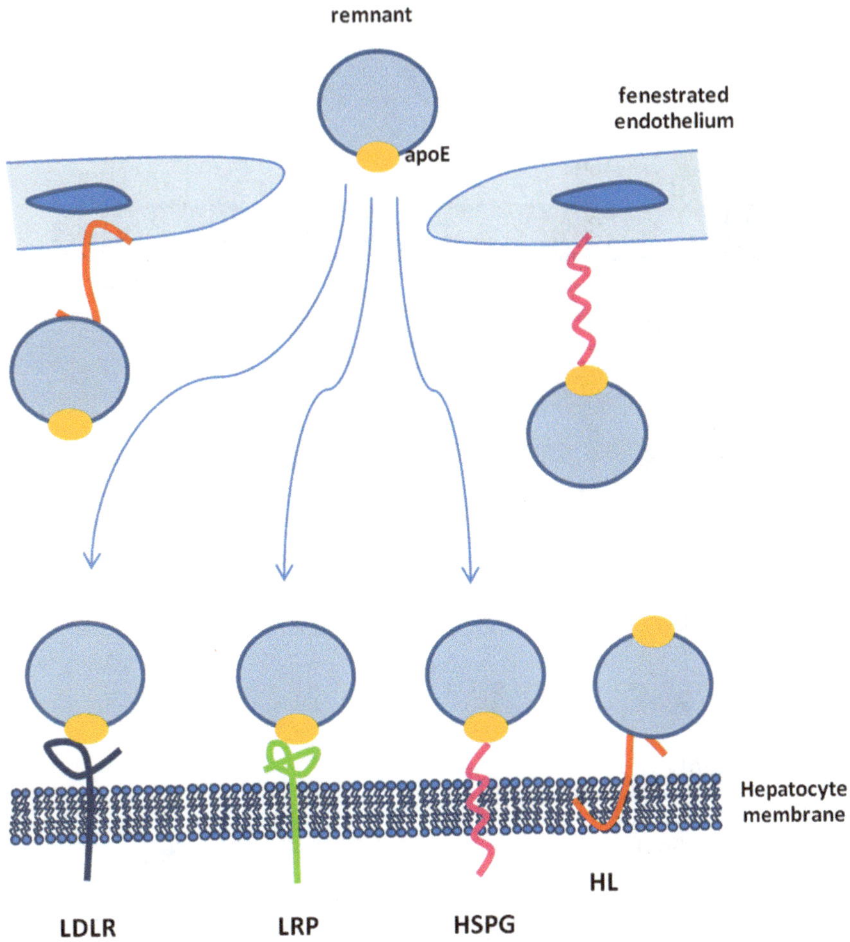


**Fig. 6.3** Pathways of hepatic clearance of remnants

levels in vivo tend to be stable in most animal systems. However, several studies suggest that apoB mRNA abundance can be influenced by insulin in vivo [46, 47]. Hepatic apoB production is mainly regulated at the post-translational level by lipid availability, a process that is inhibited by insulin, resulting in an acute inhibitory effect of insulin on hepatic VLDL-triglyceride secretion to limit postprandial plasma lipid excursion. Hepatic apoB mRNA is stimulated by forkhead box O1 (FoxO1) and inhibited by insulin in a cell system [48]; moreover, hepatic activity of FoxO1 is increased during fasting and inhibited in response to feeding [49]. These observations suggest an additional mechanism by which the liver controls hepatic apoB production at the transcriptional level.

In the liver, insulin acts on fatty acids similarly to glucose: it promotes the storage of glucose as glycogen, and fatty acids as triglycerides during feeding. This will result in decreased hepatic VLDL secretion and decreased hepatic glucose release. Moreover, a decreased VLDL secretion during feeding limits the increase of plasma triglycerides during the prandial phase, when intestinal fats are absorbed to produce chylomicrons, which in turn deliver fatty acids to adipose tissue.

FoxO1 (forkhead box O1) is a transcription factor that plays a role in regulating hepatic glucose metabolism during fasting by inducing the expression of genes involved in gluconeogenesis [50]. In addition, FoxO1 may regulate lipid metabolism by inducing hepatic MTP expression, resulting in increased secretion of VLDL [48]. Under physiological conditions, this effect is reversed by insulin [48]. In the absence of

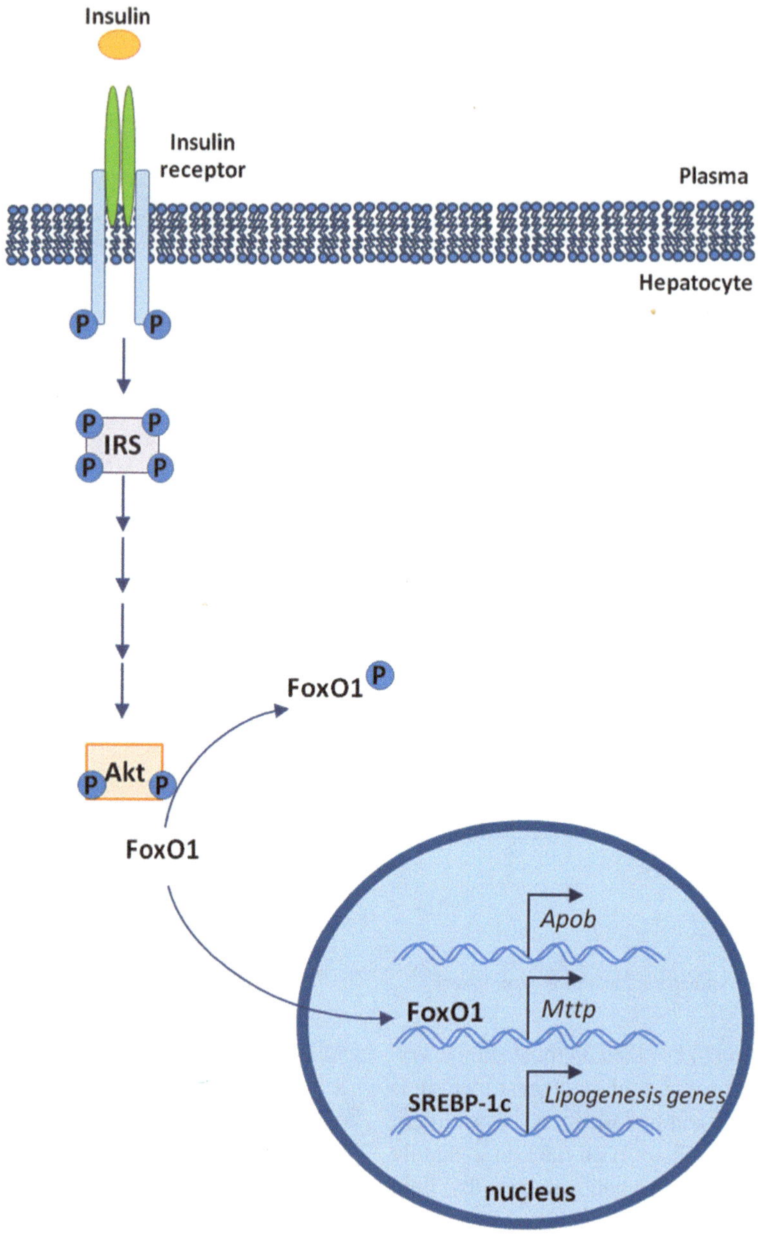


**Fig. 6.4** Insulin regulation of FoxO1 activity

insulin, FoxO1 is localized in the nucleus in a transcriptionally active form and induces the expression of MTP; after insulin release, FoxO1 is phosphorylated and translocated out of the nucleus, resulting in inhibition of FoxO1 transcriptional activity [51] (Fig. 6.4).

## Insulin Resistance

Diabetes is characterized by hyperglycemia due to either defects in insulin secretion and/or insulin properties. Patients with insulin resistance are at high risk of developing diabetes and cardiovascular (CV) disease [52]. Insulin resistance is a condition of reduced responsiveness of tissues (liver, muscle, and adipose tissue) to normal circulating levels of insulin [53, 54], a condition present in different diseases, including type 2 diabetes [55], obesity, hypertension, and dyslipidemia [56]. As a result, insulin production increases to maintain normal levels of blood glucose. Insulin is a hormone essential for the maintenance of glucose homeostasis, secreted by the pancreatic β-cells mainly in response to increased circulating glucose levels after a meal [57].

When the concentration of blood glucose increases, the pancreas releases insulin into the circulation. In muscle and adipose tissues, insulin binds to cell surface receptors [58]. Following this binding, several biochemical signals are activated within the cells to take up glucose and convert it to energy [59]. If the pancreas fails to produce enough insulin or the insulin receptors do not function properly, the cells cannot uptake glucose and the level of glucose in the blood remains high.

Several defects can determine insulin resistance, including insulin receptor defects, insulin signaling defects [59, 60], mutations in insulin signaling molecules [61], and mitochondrial dysfunction [60]. In the early stages of insulin resistance, the pancreas compensates by producing more insulin to control the increased levels of glucose in the blood. This results in high blood glucose levels and high blood insulin levels (a condition known as hyperinsulinemia) at the same time. If this condition is not treated, the islets of Langerhans (the insulin-secreting groups of cells) in the pancreas may eventually shut down and decrease in number. When an insulin-resistant subject cannot maintain the degree of hyperinsulinemia required to bypass the defective action of insulin, type 2 diabetes develops.

## The Role of Insulin Resistance in TGRLs Metabolism

In animal models of insulin resistance, hepatic MTP mRNA levels are significantly higher with simultaneous increase in VLDL levels [62–64]; finally, treatments that ameliorate insulin resistance and dyslipidemia determined reduced MTP expression and VLDL levels [49, 65, 66]. These observations suggest that in insulin-resistant subjects, MTP expression is no longer regulated by insulin, resulting in VLDL overproduction.

Insulin resistance is considered mainly a carbohydrate metabolism disorder; however, lipid and lipoprotein abnormalities are observed in individuals with insulin resistance [67]. These abnormalities include (1) increased plasma levels of VLDL triglyceride and apoB100, (2) reduced plasma levels of HDL and apoA-I, and (3) relatively normal LDL levels with increase of small dense LDL particles.

Acute insulin infusion reduces production of TG-rich VLDL in healthy non-obese humans [25, 40, 68, 69]; this effect can result from several mechanisms, including inhibition of hepatic MTP expression [70], increased apoB degradation [43], and inhibition of VLDL particle maturation [71]. This suppressive effect of insulin is, however, attenuated or even reversed [41, 72] when exposure to insulin is prolonged (such as in conditions of insulin resistance [68, 69]), where an increase in VLDL (mainly in the VLDL1 fraction) production is observed [73–75]. These observations suggest that chronic hyperinsulinemia plays a role in mediating the increased production of hepatic VLDL. In addition, insulin resistance of adipose tissue increases the levels of circulating free fatty acids that can enter into the liver, thus stimulating VLDL production [76]. Finally, loss of insulin inhibition of FoxO1 activity in insulin resistance increases the production of both glucose and VLDL-TG, contributing to the dual pathogenesis of hyperglycemia and hypertriglyceridemia in diabetes.

## Hepatic TG in Insulin Resistance

Fatty acid flux to the liver is increased in insulin resistance [77, 78], due to a failure of insulin to inhibit TG lipolysis in adipose tissue [79]. Increased levels of fasting and post-prandial TG are features of insulin resistance [80]. The increase in post-prandial TG is due both to defective lipolysis of VLDL and chylomicrons, combined with increased VLDL secretion [80], and to increased production of chylomicrons [81]. In addition, insulin resistance also reduces lipoprotein lipase activity secondary to increased apoC-III (an inhibitor of LPL) secretion [82], resulting in reduced lipolysis of VLDL and chylomicron TG.

Another source of hepatic TG is de novo lipogenesis that contributes significantly to VLDL lipidation and production in insulin-resistant subjects. The main transcription factor of de novo lipogenesis is SREBP-1c (sterol response element-binding protein-1c) [83] that in turn is regulated by LXR (liver X receptor) [84]. Insulin plays a key role in the expression of hepatic SREBP-1c, in part by stimulating LXR expression [85, 86]; furthermore, insulin promotes the maturation of SREBP-1c independently of LXR [87].

Intestinal lipoprotein production is increased in insulin resistance; chylomicron overproduction is in fact a consequence of impaired insulin regulation. Under physiological conditions, chylomicron production is inhibited by insulin; this inhibitory process is lost or reduced in the presence of impaired insulin responsiveness. Increased postprandial TG was thought to be due to reduced chylomicron and VLDL lipolysis, combined with increased VLDL secretion [80, 88]. However, increased assembly and secretion of apoB48-containing chylomicrons has been observed in hyperinsulinemic conditions [81]. The elevation of free fatty acids in plasma increases not only hepatic, but also intestinal, lipoprotein production [81, 89], suggesting that the intestine responds to insulin resistance similarly to the liver [90].

## Diabetes and Hepatic Uptake of Remnant Lipoproteins

Diabetes impairs hepatic uptake of remnant lipoproteins [29, 91, 92]. Under these pathological conditions, LDLR does not seem to significantly contribute to the reduced uptake of remnant lipoprotein [93, 94]. The major contribution to this effect appears to be related to HSPGs; as they are not proteins, a high number of genes involved in their assembly and disassembly must be regulated, both at translational and at posttranslational levels [95, 96]. In type 1 diabetes, hepatic HSPGs exhibit sulfation defects [97, 98], due to the suppression of a crucial enzyme in HSPG assembly [96]; moreover, the farnesoid X receptor, a known inducer of HSPG expression [99], is suppressed [100]. In type 2 diabetes and other diseases characterized by insulin resistance, proteoglycans exhibit several defects, including decreased sulfation [101, 102]. Insulin resistance also induces the hepatic overexpression of the heparan sulfate glucosamine 6-O-endosulfatase-2 (SULF2), an enzyme that degrades cell surface and matrix HSPGs, thus reducing the catabolism of remnant lipoprotein and contributing to postprandial dyslipoproteinemia in type 2 diabetes [103].

## Triglyceride-Rich Lipoproteins and Vascular Dysfunction

The elevation in circulating free fatty acids impairs endothelium-dependent vasodilatation [104], and the decreased endothelial function may be dependent on enhanced oxidative stress [105]. The changes induced by TGRLs in the post-prandial phase are even more deleterious in terms of endothelial dysfunction and inflammation; indeed, several in vivo studies have demonstrated that post-prandial hypertriglyceridemia impairs endothelial function [106, 107]. Postprandial hypertriglyceridemia is also associated with an inflammatory state and enhanced levels of tumor necrosis factor (TNF)-α, interleukin (IL)-6, soluble intercellular adhesion molecule (sICAM)-1, and soluble vascular cell adhesion molecule (sVCAM)-1 [108–110].

The molecular mechanisms underlying these effects of TGRLs have only recently been studied in detail. There are a few key issues that should be taken into account when analyzing the vascular effects of TGRLs. TGRLs derive either from an exogenous pathway (chylomicrons and chylomicron remnants containing apolipoprotein apoB48) or from a liver-derived pathway (VLDL and VLDL remnants containing apoB100). Under fasting conditions, however, chylomicrons are rapidly metabolized, thus the TGRL fraction is mainly composed of apoB100-rich particles, and the remnants derive mainly from the catabolism of VLDL (small VLDL and intermediate-density lipoprotein). In several dyslipidemic conditions, chylomicrons are metabolized at a lower rate, resulting in the accumulation of chylomicron remnants in the fasting state. In the post-prandial state, an enormous production of TGRLs containing both apoB48 and apoB100 occurs, leading to an impaired endothelial function. This dysfunction rapidly fades away in normotriglyceridemic subjects where the TGRLs are efficiently metabolized, whereas the condition persists in hypertriglyceridemic patients where TGRLs accumulate in the circulation. TGRLs undergo lipolysis mediated by lipoprotein lipase (LPL), generating different biologically active products that may affect endothelial cell function [111].

Early studies using HepG2 cells investigated the intracellular signaling pathway induced by VLDL exposure [112]. VLDL-induced protein kinase C activity results in the activation of mitogen-activated protein kinase (MAPK). Studies conducted in endothelial cells (ECs) indicate that VLDL can also activate nuclear factor (NF)-κB [113], a transcription factor that plays an important role in the phenotypic modulation of ECs in a pro-inflammatory condition. To date, plasminogen activator inhibitor-1 is the only gene that has been shown to be consistently induced in ECs to a larger extent when comparing VLDL from patients with hypertriglyceridemic type IV and type II versus VLDL from normolipidemic subjects [114]. Both in human umbilical vein ECs and human aortic ECs, TGRLs from hypertriglyceridemic subjects induce an increased mRNA expression of adhesion molecules, such as VCAM-1, platelet/endothelial cell adhesion molecule (PECAM)-1, and endothelial/leukocyte adhesion molecule (ELAM)-1, while TGRLs from normolipidemics induced VCAM-1 expression in both the cell lines and ELAM-1 selectively in the aortic ECs, but to a lesser extent [115]. Specific inhibition of p38 mitogen-activated protein kinase and NF-κB suggests a major involvement of these factors in adhesion molecule expression induced by TGRLs in both NTG and HTG patients. Furthermore, TGRLs induced monocyte chemoattractant protein (MCP)-1 expression in ECs, suggesting that activation of the endothelium by TGRLs could support both adhesion and transmigration of leukocytes. In addition, TGRLs from hypertriglyceridemic patients induced IL-6 expression. Again, these effects are mainly dependent on NF-κB activation.

The composition of the TGRL particles plays a key role in determining the pro-inflammatory response to TGRLs [116]. A different composition of VLDL (fatty acid, lipids, and apoproteins) may be responsible for the differences observed between normolipidemic and hypertriglyceridemic TGRLs. TGRLs isolated following a meal enriched in saturated fatty acids induced E-selectin and VCAM-1 expression to a higher extent than TGRLs isolated after a meal enriched in monounsaturated and polyunsaturated fatty acids [116]. Furthermore, lipolysis products from TGRLs increase endothelial permeability, perturb zonula occludens-1 and F-actin, and induce apoptosis [111]. One could speculate that, in the presence of hypertriglyceridemia, the reduced activity of LPL may promote the presence of pro-inflammatory TGRLs.

Although hypertriglyceridemia is an independent risk factor for coronary artery disease [117], accumulating evidence suggests that post-prandial (hyper)lipidemia contributes to the development of atherosclerosis and coronary artery disease [118]. Several studies have demonstrated that post-prandial hypertriglyceridemia impairs endothelial function, suggesting a role for triglycerides in the initiation and further progression of atherosclerosis [106, 107]. Post-prandial hypertriglyceridemia is associated with an inflammatory state and enhanced levels of TNF-α, IL-6, sICAM-1, and sVCAM-1 [108–110]. Although TGRLs isolated from fasting plasma samples of hypertriglyceridemic subjects induce an inflammatory response in ECs [115], ECs incubated with post-prandial TGRL demonstrated an increased mRNA expression of VCAM-1, ELAM-1, P-selectin, PECAM-1, and ICAM-1. Similarly, post-prandial TGRLs increased ICAM-1 and VCAM-1 protein

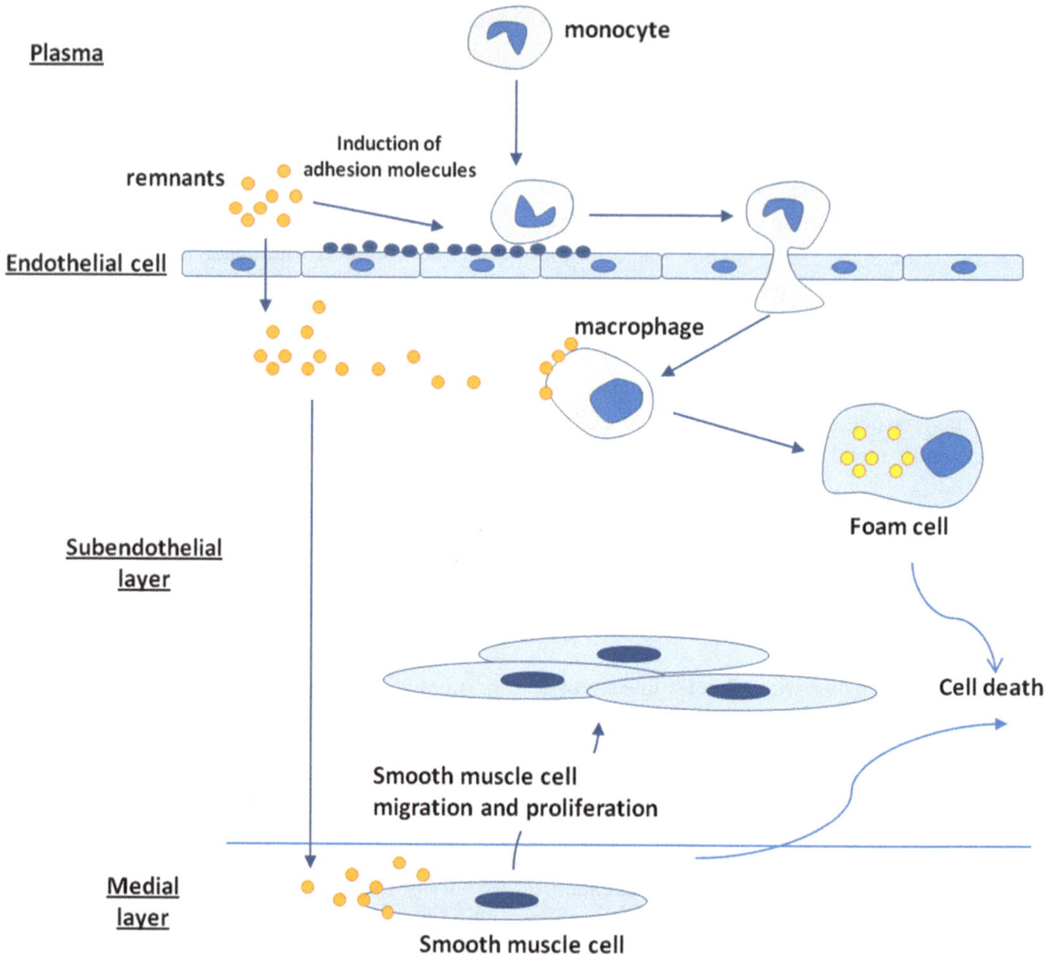


**Fig. 6.5** Remnant contribution to the atherosclerotic lesion development

expression [119]. Also fasting TGRLs increase adhesion molecule expression, however, the effect observed with post-prandial TGRL is much more pronounced. Furthermore, ICAM-1 expression was induced solely upon incubation with post-prandial TGRLs. Likewise, MCP-1 and IL-6 expression was induced upon incubation with post-prandial TGRLs; again, this effect is more pronounced than that observed with fasting TGRLs. As the induction of adhesion molecules and the increased release of cytokines and chemokines have been associated with endothelial dysfunction [120], our data suggest that endothelial activation by TGRL occurs during the post-prandial phase and may promote the endothelial dysfunction observed after a meal. Notably, a single high-fat meal led to a significant elevation of endothelial microparticles, known to be a sensitive indicator of endothelial disturbance, in healthy normolipidemic subjects [107]. This observation suggests that endothelial microparticles may be an indirect marker of endothelial dysfunction or injury induced by postprandial TGRL.

TGRLs and their remnants are present within human and experimental atherosclerotic lesions [121–123]: chylomicron remnants directly penetrate the endothelial cell layer and are entrapped within the subendothelial space, leading to focal accumulation [122] (Fig. 6.5). TGRLs may directly contribute to the atherosclerotic process by inducing endothelial dysfunction [124], by enhancing monocyte adhesion [125], and by triggering lipid accumulation within the artery wall [126]. Exposure to TGRLs, especially those isolated from patients with type 2 diabetes [127], leads to the intracellular accumulation of triglyceride and/or cholesteryl ester in human monocyte- [127] and murine-derived macrophages [126, 128]. Abnormal reverse cholesterol transport and low levels of high-density lipoprotein associated with hypertriglyceridemia [129, 130] can accelerate the lipid deposition process within arterial macrophages. The interaction of TGRLs with cholesterol-loaded human macrophages increases the cell lipid content while compromising the subsequent efflux of cholesterol to lipid-poor apoA-I [131]. These aspects may contribute significantly to the generation of macrophage foam cells in vivo and might account for the accelerated atherogenesis observed in patients with type 2 diabetes. Finally, remnant lipoproteins induce smooth muscle cell activation and proliferation [132, 133].

Most of the available evidence suggests that in normolipidemic subjects either in the fasting state or in the post-prandial phase, TGRL may affect endothelial function only when a pro-inflammatory environment is already present and may perhaps contribute to accelerating the damage induced by other lipid and non-lipid factors. However, in hypertrygliceridemic patients, TGRLs from the fasting state and postprandial phase can both induce endothelial dysfunction by promoting a pro-inflammatory activation of the endothelium. These findings are in line with the idea that these lipoproteins may play a significant role in the early stages of atherogenesis.

## References


1. Karpe F, Bell M, Bjorkegren J, Hamsten A. Quantification of postprandial triglyceride-rich lipoproteins in healthy men by retinyl ester labeling and simultaneous measurement of apolipoproteins B-48 and B-100. Arterioscler Thromb Vasc Biol. 1995;15: 199–207.
2. Taskinen MR. Diabetic dyslipidaemia: from basic research to clinical practice. Diabetologia. 2003;46: 733–49.
3. Chen SH, Habib G, Yang CY, et al. Apolipoprotein B-48 is the product of a messenger RNA with an organ-specific in-frame stop codon. Science. 1987;238:363–6.
4. Powell LM, Wallis SC, Pease RJ, Edwards YH, Knott TJ, Scott J. A novel form of tissue-specific RNA processing produces apolipoprotein-B48 in intestine. Cell. 1987;50:831–40.
5. Pan X, Hussain MM. Diurnal regulation of microsomal triglyceride transfer protein and plasma lipid levels. J Biol Chem. 2007;282:24707–19.
6. Fisher EA, Pan M, Chen X, et al. The triple threat to nascent apolipoprotein B. Evidence for multiple, distinct degradative pathways. J Biol Chem. 2001; 276:27855–63.
7. Benoist F, Grand-Perret T. Co-translational degradation of apolipoprotein B100 by the proteasome is prevented by microsomal triglyceride transfer protein. Synchronized translation studies on HepG2 cells treated with an inhibitor of microsomal triglyceride transfer protein. J Biol Chem. 1997;272:20435–42.
8. Dixon JL, Furukawa S, Ginsberg HN. Oleate stimulates secretion of apolipoprotein B-containing lipoproteins from Hep G2 cells by inhibiting early intracellular degradation of apolipoprotein B. J Biol Chem. 1991;266:5080–6.
9. Zhou M, Fisher EA, Ginsberg HN. Regulated Co-translational ubiquitination of apolipoprotein B100. A new paradigm for proteasomal degradation of a secretory protein. J Biol Chem. 1998;273: 24649–53.
10. Williams KJ, Brocia RW, Fisher EA. The unstirred water layer as a site of control of apolipoprotein B secretion. J Biol Chem. 1990;265:16741–4.
11. Schumaker VN, Phillips ML, Chatterton JE. Apolipoprotein B and low-density lipoprotein structure: implications for biosynthesis of triglyceride-rich lipoproteins. Adv Protein Chem. 1994;45:205–48.
12. Gordon DA, Wetterau JR, Gregg RE. Microsomal triglyceride transfer protein: a protein complex required for the assembly of lipoprotein particles. Trends Cell Biol. 1995;5:317–21.
13. Rustaeus S, Stillemark P, Lindberg K, Gordon D, Olofsson SO. The microsomal triglyceride transfer protein catalyzes the post-translational assembly of apolipoprotein B-100 very low density lipoprotein in McA-RH7777 cells. J Biol Chem. 1998;273: 5196–203.
14. Hussain MM, Shi J, Dreizen P. Microsomal triglyceride transfer protein and its role in apoB-lipoprotein assembly. J Lipid Res. 2003;44:22–32.
15. Jamil H, Chu CH, Dickson Jr JK, et al. Evidence that microsomal triglyceride transfer protein is limiting in the production of apolipoprotein B-containing lipoproteins in hepatic cells. J Lipid Res. 1998;39: 1448–54.
16. Hui TY, Olivier LM, Kang S, Davis RA. Microsomal triglyceride transfer protein is essential for hepatic secretion of apoB-100 and apoB-48 but not triglyceride. J Lipid Res. 2002;43:785–93.
17. Manchekar M, Richardson PE, Forte TM, Datta G, Segrest JP, Dashti N. Apolipoprotein B-containing lipoprotein particle assembly: lipid capacity of the nascent lipoprotein particle. J Biol Chem. 2004;279: 39757–66.

18. Alexander CA, Hamilton RL, Havel RJ. Subcellular localization of B apoprotein of plasma lipoproteins in rat liver. J Cell Biol. 1976;69:241–63.
19. Wu X, Shang A, Jiang H, Ginsberg HN. Low rates of apoB secretion from HepG2 cells result from reduced delivery of newly synthesized triglyceride to a "secretion-coupled" pool. J Lipid Res. 1996;37:1198–206.
20. Gibbons GF, Islam K, Pease RJ. Mobilisation of triacylglycerol stores. Biochim Biophys Acta. 2000;1483:37–57.
21. Gibbons GF, Bartlett SM, Sparks CE, Sparks JD. Extracellular fatty acids are not utilized directly for the synthesis of very-low-density lipoprotein in primary cultures of rat hepatocytes. Biochem J. 1992;287(Pt 3):749–53.
22. Fisher EA, Ginsberg HN. Complexity in the secretory pathway: the assembly and secretion of apolipoprotein B-containing lipoproteins. J Biol Chem. 2002;277:17377–80.
23. Pan M, Liang Js JS, Fisher EA, Ginsberg HN. The late addition of core lipids to nascent apolipoprotein B100, resulting in the assembly and secretion of triglyceride-rich lipoproteins, is independent of both microsomal triglyceride transfer protein activity and new triglyceride synthesis. J Biol Chem. 2002;277:4413–21.
24. Wiggins D, Gibbons GF. The lipolysis/esterification cycle of hepatic triacylglycerol. Its role in the secretion of very-low-density lipoprotein and its response to hormones and sulphonylureas. Biochem J. 1992;284(Pt 2):457–62.
25. Malmstrom R, Packard CJ, Watson TD, et al. Metabolic basis of hypotriglyceridemic effects of insulin in normal men. Arterioscler Thromb Vasc Biol. 1997;17:1454–64.
26. Packard CJ, Munro A, Lorimer AR, Gotto AM, Shepherd J. Metabolism of apolipoprotein B in large triglyceride-rich very low density lipoproteins of normal and hypertriglyceridemic subjects. J Clin Invest. 1984;74:2178–92.
27. Gaw A, Packard CJ, Lindsay GM, et al. Overproduction of small very low density lipoproteins (Sf 20-60) in moderate hypercholesterolemia: relationships between apolipoprotein B kinetics and plasma lipoproteins. J Lipid Res. 1995;36:158–71.
28. Black DD. Development and physiological regulation of intestinal lipid absorption. I. Development of intestinal lipid absorption: cellular events in chylomicron assembly and secretion. Am J Physiol Gastrointest Liver Physiol. 2007;293:G519–24.
29. Williams KJ, Chen K. Recent insights into factors affecting remnant lipoprotein uptake. Curr Opin Lipidol. 2010;21:218–28.
30. Fuki IV, Kuhn KM, Lomazov IR, et al. The syndecan family of proteoglycans. Novel receptors mediating internalization of atherogenic lipoproteins in vitro. J Clin Invest. 1997;100:1611–22.
31. Mahley RW, Huang Y. Atherogenic remnant lipoproteins: role for proteoglycans in trapping, transferring, and internalizing. J Clin Invest. 2007;117: 94–8.
32. Mahley RW, Ji ZS. Remnant lipoprotein metabolism: key pathways involving cell-surface heparan sulfate proteoglycans and apolipoprotein E. J Lipid Res. 1999;40:1–16.
33. Mahley RW, Weisgraber KH, Innerarity TL, Rall Jr SC. Genetic defects in lipoprotein metabolism. Elevation of atherogenic lipoproteins caused by impaired catabolism. JAMA. 1991;265:78–83.
34. Williams KJ, Fuki IV. Cell-surface heparan sulfate proteoglycans: dynamic molecules mediating ligand catabolism. Curr Opin Lipidol. 1997;8:253–62.
35. Cooper AD. Hepatic uptake of chylomicron remnants. J Lipid Res. 1997;38:2173–92.
36. Lewis GF, Uffelman KD, Szeto LW, Weller B, Steiner G. Interaction between free fatty acids and insulin in the acute control of very low density lipoprotein production in humans. J Clin Invest. 1995;95: 158–66.
37. den Boer MA, Voshol PJ, Kuipers F, Romijn JA, Havekes LM. Hepatic glucose production is more sensitive to insulin-mediated inhibition than hepatic VLDL-triglyceride production. Am J Physiol Endocrinol Metab. 2006;291:E1360–4.
38. Lewis GF, Steiner G. Acute effects of insulin in the control of VLDL production in humans. Implications for the insulin-resistant state. Diabetes Care. 1996;19:390–3.
39. Sparks JD, Sparks CE. Insulin regulation of triacylglycerol-rich lipoprotein synthesis and secretion. Biochim Biophys Acta. 1994;1215:9–32.
40. Malmstrom R, Packard CJ, Caslake M, et al. Effects of insulin and acipimox on VLDL1 and VLDL2 apolipoprotein B production in normal subjects. Diabetes. 1998;47:779–87.
41. Dashti N, Williams DL, Alaupovic P. Effects of oleate and insulin on the production rates and cellular mRNA concentrations of apolipoproteins in HepG2 cells. J Lipid Res. 1989;30:1365–73.
42. Sparks CE, Sparks JD, Bolognino M, Salhanick A, Strumph PS, Amatruda JM. Insulin effects on apolipoprotein B lipoprotein synthesis and secretion by primary cultures of rat hepatocytes. Metabolism. 1986;35:1128–36.
43. Sparks JD, Sparks CE. Insulin modulation of hepatic synthesis and secretion of apolipoprotein B by rat hepatocytes. J Biol Chem. 1990;265:8854–62.
44. Sparks JD, Sparks CE, Miller LL. Insulin effects on apolipoprotein B production by normal, diabetic and treated-diabetic rat liver and cultured rat hepatocytes. Biochem J. 1989;261:83–8.
45. Stein DT, Esser V, Stevenson BE, et al. Essentiality of circulating fatty acids for glucose-stimulated insulin secretion in the fasted rat. J Clin Invest. 1996;97:2728–35.
46. Sparks JD, Collins HL, Chirieac DV, et al. Hepatic very-low-density lipoprotein and apolipoprotein B production are increased following in vivo induction of betaine-homocysteine S-methyltransferase. Biochem J. 2006;395:363–71.
47. Sparks JD, Sparks CE, Bolognino M, Roncone AM, Jackson TK, Amatruda JM. Effects of nonketotic streptozotocin diabetes on apolipoprotein B synthesis and secretion by primary cultures of rat hepatocytes. J Clin Invest. 1988;82:37–43.

48. Kamagate A, Qu S, Perdomo G, et al. FoxO1 mediates insulin-dependent regulation of hepatic VLDL production in mice. J Clin Invest. 2008;118:2347–64.
49. Qu S, Su D, Altomonte J, et al. PPAR{alpha} mediates the hypolipidemic action of fibrates by antagonizing FoxO1. Am J Physiol Endocrinol Metab. 2007;292:E421–34.
50. Matsumoto M, Pocai A, Rossetti L, Depinho RA, Accili D. Impaired regulation of hepatic glucose production in mice lacking the forkhead transcription factor Foxo1 in liver. Cell Metab. 2007;6:208–16.
51. Manning BD, Cantley LC. AKT/PKB signaling: navigating downstream. Cell. 2007;129:1261–74.
52. Catapano AL, Reiner Z, De Backer G, et al. ESC/EAS Guidelines for the management of dyslipidaemias The Task Force for the management of dyslipidaemias of the European Society of Cardiology (ESC) and the European Atherosclerosis Society (EAS). Atherosclerosis. 2011;217:3–46.
53. Petersen KF, Shulman GI. Etiology of insulin resistance. Am J Med. 2006;119:S10–6.
54. Reaven GM. Why Syndrome X? From Harold Himsworth to the insulin resistance syndrome. Cell Metab. 2005;1:9–14.
55. American Diabetes Association (2007) Diagnosis and classification of diabetes mellitus. Diabetes Care 30(Suppl 1):S42–47
56. Eckel RH, Grundy SM, Zimmet PZ. The metabolic syndrome. Lancet. 2005;365:1415–28.
57. Sesti G. Pathophysiology of insulin resistance. Best Pract Res Clin Endocrinol Metab. 2006;20:665–79.
58. Taniguchi CM, Emanuelli B, Kahn CR. Critical nodes in signalling pathways: insights into insulin action. Nat Rev Mol Cell Biol. 2006;7:85–96.
59. DeFronzo RA. Insulin resistance, lipotoxicity, type 2 diabetes and atherosclerosis: the missing links. The Claude Bernard Lecture 2009. Diabetologia. 2010; 53:1270–87.
60. Morino K, Petersen KF, Shulman GI. Molecular mechanisms of insulin resistance in humans and their potential links with mitochondrial dysfunction. Diabetes. 2006;55 Suppl 2:S9–15.
61. Schinner S, Scherbaum WA, Bornstein SR, Barthel A. Molecular mechanisms of insulin resistance. Diabet Med. 2005;22:674–82.
62. Bartels ED, Lauritsen M, Nielsen LB. Hepatic expression of microsomal triglyceride transfer protein and in vivo secretion of triglyceride-rich lipoproteins are increased in obese diabetic mice. Diabetes. 2002;51:1233–9.
63. Kuriyama H, Yamashita S, Shimomura I, et al. Enhanced expression of hepatic acyl-coenzyme A synthetase and microsomal triglyceride transfer protein messenger RNAs in the obese and hypertriglyceridemic rat with visceral fat accumulation. Hepatology. 1998;27:557–62.
64. Taghibiglou C, Carpentier A, Van Iderstine SC, et al. Mechanisms of hepatic very low density lipoprotein overproduction in insulin resistance. Evidence for enhanced lipoprotein assembly, reduced intracellular ApoB degradation, and increased microsomal triglyceride transfer protein in a fructose-fed hamster model. J Biol Chem. 2000;275:8416–25.
65. Carpentier A, Taghibiglou C, Leung N, et al. Ameliorated hepatic insulin resistance is associated with normalization of microsomal triglyceride transfer protein expression and reduction in very low density lipoprotein assembly and secretion in the fructose-fed hamster. J Biol Chem. 2002;277:28795–802.
66. Chong T, Naples M, Federico L, et al. Effect of rosuvastatin on hepatic production of apolipoprotein B-containing lipoproteins in an animal model of insulin resistance and metabolic dyslipidemia. Atherosclerosis. 2006;185:21–31.
67. Chahil TJ, Ginsberg HN. Diabetic dyslipidemia. Endocrinol Metab Clin North Am. 2006;35:491–510. vii–viii.
68. Malmstrom R, Packard CJ, Caslake M, et al. Defective regulation of triglyceride metabolism by insulin in the liver in NIDDM. Diabetologia. 1997;40:454–62.
69. Lewis GF, Uffelman KD, Szeto LW, Steiner G. Effects of acute hyperinsulinemia on VLDL triglyceride and VLDL apoB production in normal weight and obese individuals. Diabetes. 1993;42:833–42.
70. Au WS, Kung HF, Lin MC. Regulation of microsomal triglyceride transfer protein gene by insulin in HepG2 cells: roles of MAPKerk and MAPKp38. Diabetes. 2003;52:1073–80.
71. Brown AM, Gibbons GF. Insulin inhibits the maturation phase of VLDL assembly via a phosphoinositide 3-kinase-mediated event. Arterioscler Thromb Vasc Biol. 2001;21:1656–61.
72. Bartlett SM, Gibbons GF. Short- and longer-term regulation of very-low-density lipoprotein secretion by insulin, dexamethasone and lipogenic substrates in cultured hepatocytes. A biphasic effect of insulin. Biochem J. 1988;249:37–43.
73. Cummings MH, Watts GF, Pal C, et al. Increased hepatic secretion of very-low-density lipoprotein apolipoprotein B-100 in obesity: a stable isotope study. Clin Sci (Lond). 1995;88:225–33.
74. Gill JM, Brown JC, Bedford D, et al. Hepatic production of VLDL1 but not VLDL2 is related to insulin resistance in normoglycaemic middle-aged subjects. Atherosclerosis. 2004;176:49–56.
75. Riches FM, Watts GF, Naoumova RP, Kelly JM, Croft KD, Thompson GR. Hepatic secretion of very-low-density lipoprotein apolipoprotein B-100 studied with a stable isotope technique in men with visceral obesity. Int J Obes Relat Metab Disord. 1998;22:414–23.
76. Sniderman AD, Cianflone K. Substrate delivery as a determinant of hepatic apoB secretion. Arterioscler Thromb. 1993;13:629–36.
77. Basu A, Basu R, Shah P, Vella A, Rizza RA, Jensen MD. Systemic and regional free fatty acid metabolism in type 2 diabetes. Am J Physiol Endocrinol Metab. 2001;280:E1000–6.
78. Fabbrini E, Mohammed BS, Magkos F, Korenblat KM, Patterson BW, Klein S. Alterations in adipose tissue and hepatic lipid kinetics in obese men and

women with nonalcoholic fatty liver disease. Gastroenterology. 2008;134:424–31.
79. Jafri H, Alsheikh-Ali AA, Karas RH. Baseline and on-treatment high-density lipoprotein cholesterol and the risk of cancer in randomized controlled trials of lipid-altering therapy. J Am Coll Cardiol. 2010;55:2846–54.
80. Ginsberg HN, Zhang YL, Hernandez-Ono A. Regulation of plasma triglycerides in insulin resistance and diabetes. Arch Med Res. 2005;36:232–40.
81. Duez H, Lamarche B, Uffelman KD, Valero R, Cohn JS, Lewis GF. Hyperinsulinemia is associated with increased production rate of intestinal apolipoprotein B-48-containing lipoproteins in humans. Arterioscler Thromb Vasc Biol. 2006;26:1357–63.
82. Cohn JS, Patterson BW, Uffelman KD, Davignon J, Steiner G. Rate of production of plasma and very-low-density lipoprotein (VLDL) apolipoprotein C-III is strongly related to the concentration and level of production of VLDL triglyceride in male subjects with different body weights and levels of insulin sensitivity. J Clin Endocrinol Metab. 2004;89:3949–55.
83. Horton JD, Goldstein JL, Brown MS. SREBPs: activators of the complete program of cholesterol and fatty acid synthesis in the liver. J Clin Invest. 2002;109:1125–31.
84. Schultz JR, Tu H, Luk A, et al. Role of LXRs in control of lipogenesis. Genes Dev. 2000;14:2831–8.
85. Cha JY, Repa JJ. The liver X receptor (LXR) and hepatic lipogenesis. The carbohydrate-response element-binding protein is a target gene of LXR. J Biol Chem. 2007;282:743–51.
86. Chen G, Liang G, Ou J, Goldstein JL, Brown MS. Central role for liver X receptor in insulin-mediated activation of Srebp-1c transcription and stimulation of fatty acid synthesis in liver. Proc Natl Acad Sci USA. 2004;101:11245–50.
87. Hegarty BD, Bobard A, Hainault I, Ferre P, Bossard P, Foufelle F. Distinct roles of insulin and liver X receptor in the induction and cleavage of sterol regulatory element-binding protein-1c. Proc Natl Acad Sci USA. 2005;102:791–6.
88. Brunzell JD, Hazzard WR, Porte Jr D, Bierman EL. Evidence for a common, saturable, triglyceride removal mechanism for chylomicrons and very low density lipoproteins in man. J Clin Invest. 1973;52:1578–85.
89. Duez H, Lamarche B, Valero R, et al. Both intestinal and hepatic lipoprotein production are stimulated by an acute elevation of plasma free fatty acids in humans. Circulation. 2008;117:2369–76.
90. Adeli K, Lewis GF. Intestinal lipoprotein overproduction in insulin-resistant states. Curr Opin Lipidol. 2008;19:221–8.
91. Dane-Stewart CA, Watts GF, Barrett PH, et al. Chylomicron remnant metabolism studied with a new breath test in postmenopausal women with and without type 2 diabetes mellitus. Clin Endocrinol (Oxf). 2003;58:415–20.
92. Georgopoulos A, Phair RD. Abnormal clearance of postprandial Sf 100-400 plasma lipoproteins in insulin-dependent diabetes mellitus. J Lipid Res. 1991;32:1133–41.
93. Han S, Liang CP, Westerterp M, et al. Hepatic insulin signaling regulates VLDL secretion and atherogenesis in mice. J Clin Invest. 2009;119:1029–41.
94. Niesen M, Bedi M, Lopez D. Diabetes alters LDL receptor and PCSK9 expression in rat liver. Arch Biochem Biophys. 2008;470:111–5.
95. Grobe K, Esko JD. Regulated translation of heparan sulfate N-acetylglucosamine N-deacetylase/n-sulfotransferase isozymes by structured 5′-untranslated regions and internal ribosome entry sites. J Biol Chem. 2002;277:30699–706.
96. Williams KJ, Liu ML, Zhu Y, et al. Loss of heparan N-sulfotransferase in diabetic liver: role of angiotensin II. Diabetes. 2005;54:1116–22.
97. Kjellen L, Bielefeld D, Hook M. Reduced sulfation of liver heparan sulfate in experimentally diabetic rats. Diabetes. 1983;32:337–42.
98. Ebara T, Conde K, Kako Y, et al. Delayed catabolism of apoB-48 lipoproteins due to decreased heparan sulfate proteoglycan production in diabetic mice. J Clin Invest. 2000;105:1807–18.
99. Anisfeld AM, Kast-Woelbern HR, Meyer ME, et al. Syndecan-1 expression is regulated in an isoform-specific manner by the farnesoid-X receptor. J Biol Chem. 2003;278:20420–8.
100. Duran-Sandoval D, Mautino G, Martin G, et al. Glucose regulates the expression of the farnesoid X receptor in liver. Diabetes. 2004;53:890–8.
101. Olsson U, Egnell AC, Lee MR, et al. Changes in matrix proteoglycans induced by insulin and fatty acids in hepatic cells may contribute to dyslipidemia of insulin resistance. Diabetes. 2001;50:2126–32.
102. Rohrbach DH, Hassell JR, Kleinman HK, Martin GR. Alterations in the basement membrane (heparan sulfate) proteoglycan in diabetic mice. Diabetes. 1982;31:185–8.
103. Chen K, Liu ML, Schaffer L, et al. Type 2 diabetes in mice induces hepatic overexpression of sulfatase 2, a novel factor that suppresses uptake of remnant lipoproteins. Hepatology. 2010;52:1957–67.
104. Steinberg HO, Tarshoby M, Monestel R, et al. Elevated circulating free fatty acid levels impair endothelium-dependent vasodilation. J Clin Invest. 1997;100:1230–9.
105. Anderson RA, Evans ML, Ellis GR, et al. The relationships between post-prandial lipaemia, endothelial function and oxidative stress in healthy individuals and patients with type 2 diabetes. Atherosclerosis. 2001;154:475–83.
106. Maggi FM, Raselli S, Grigore L, Redaelli L, Fantappie S, Catapano AL. Lipoprotein remnants and endothelial dysfunction in the postprandial phase. J Clin Endocrinol Metab. 2004;89:2946–50.
107. Ferreira AC, Peter AA, Mendez AJ, et al. Postprandial hypertriglyceridemia increases circulating levels of endothelial cell microparticles. Circulation. 2004;110:3599–603.

108. Burdge GC, Calder PC. Plasma cytokine response during the postprandial period: a potential causal process in vascular disease? Br J Nutr. 2005;93:3–9.
109. Lundman P, Eriksson MJ, Silveira A, et al. Relation of hypertriglyceridemia to plasma concentrations of biochemical markers of inflammation and endothelial activation (C-reactive protein, interleukin-6, soluble adhesion molecules, von Willebrand factor, and endothelin-1). Am J Cardiol. 2003;91:1128–31.
110. Nappo F, Esposito K, Cioffi M, et al. Postprandial endothelial activation in healthy subjects and in type 2 diabetic patients: role of fat and carbohydrate meals. J Am Coll Cardiol. 2002;39:1145–50.
111. Eiselein L, Wilson DW, Lame MW, Rutledge JC. Lipolysis products from triglyceride-rich lipoproteins increase endothelial permeability, perturb zonula occludens-1 and F-actin, and induce apoptosis. Am J Physiol Heart Circ Physiol. 2007;292:H2745–53.
112. Banfi C, Mussoni L, Rise P, et al. Very low density lipoprotein-mediated signal transduction and plasminogen activator inhibitor type 1 in cultured HepG2 cells. Circ Res. 1999;85:208–17.
113. Dichtl W, Nilsson L, Goncalves I, et al. Very low-density lipoprotein activates nuclear factor-kappaB in endothelial cells. Circ Res. 1999;84:1085–94.
114. Stiko-Rahm A, Wiman B, Hamsten A, Nilsson J. Secretion of plasminogen activator inhibitor-1 from cultured human umbilical vein endothelial cells is induced by very low density lipoprotein. Arteriosclerosis. 1990;10:1067–73.
115. Norata GD, Grigore L, Raselli S, et al. Triglyceride-rich lipoproteins from hypertriglyceridemic subjects induce a pro-inflammatory response in the endothelium: Molecular mechanisms and gene expression studies. J Mol Cell Cardiol. 2006;40:484–94.
116. Williams CM, Maitin V, Jackson KG. Triacylglycerol-rich lipoprotein-gene interactions in endothelial cells. Biochem Soc Trans. 2004;32:994–8.
117. Austin MA, Hokanson JE, Edwards KL. Hypertriglyceridemia as a cardiovascular risk factor. Am J Cardiol. 1998;81:7B–12.
118. Sniderman AD. Postprandial hypertriglyceridemia(s): time to enlarge our pathophysiologic perspective. Eur J Clin Invest. 2000;30:935–7.
119. Norata GD, Grigore L, Raselli S, et al. Post-prandial endothelial dysfunction in hypertriglyceridemic subjects: molecular mechanisms and gene expression studies. Atherosclerosis. 2007;193:321–7.
120. Constans J, Conri C. Circulating markers of endothelial function in cardiovascular disease. Clin Chim Acta. 2006;368:33–47.
121. Mamo JC, Wheeler JR. Chylomicrons or their remnants penetrate rabbit thoracic aorta as efficiently as do smaller macromolecules, including low-density lipoprotein, high-density lipoprotein, and albumin. Coron Artery Dis. 1994;5:695–705.
122. Proctor SD, Mamo JC. Retention of fluorescent-labelled chylomicron remnants within the intima of the arterial wall–evidence that plaque cholesterol may be derived from post-prandial lipoproteins. Eur J Clin Invest. 1998;28:497–503.
123. Rapp JH, Lespine A, Hamilton RL, et al. Triglyceride-rich lipoproteins isolated by selected-affinity anti-apolipoprotein B immunosorption from human atherosclerotic plaque. Arterioscler Thromb. 1994;14:1767–74.
124. Sattar N, Petrie JR, Jaap AJ. The atherogenic lipoprotein phenotype and vascular endothelial dysfunction. Atherosclerosis. 1998;138:229–35.
125. Carantoni M, Abbasi F, Chu L, et al. Adherence of mononuclear cells to endothelium in vitro is increased in patients with NIDDM. Diabetes Care. 1997;20:1462–5.
126. Bates SR, Murphy PL, Feng ZC, Kanazawa T, Getz GS. Very low density lipoproteins promote triglyceride accumulation in macrophages. Arteriosclerosis. 1984;4:103–14.
127. Saito M, Eto M, Okada M, Iwashima Y, Makino I. Remnant-like particles (RLP) from NIDDM patients with apolipoprotein E3/3 phenotype stimulate cholesteryl ester synthesis in human monocyte-derived macrophages. Artery. 1996;22:155–63.
128. Fujioka Y, Cooper AD, Fong LG. Multiple processes are involved in the uptake of chylomicron remnants by mouse peritoneal macrophages. J Lipid Res. 1998;39:2339–49.
129. Cavallero E, Brites F, Delfly B, et al. Abnormal reverse cholesterol transport in controlled type II diabetic patients. Studies on fasting and postprandial LpA-I particles. Arterioscler Thromb Vasc Biol. 1995;15:2130–5.
130. Syvanne M, Castro G, Dengremont C, et al. Cholesterol efflux from Fu5AH hepatoma cells induced by plasma of subjects with or without coronary artery disease and non-insulin-dependent diabetes: importance of LpA-I:A-II particles and phospholipid transfer protein. Atherosclerosis. 1996;127:245–53.
131. Palmer AM, Murphy N, Graham A. Triglyceride-rich lipoproteins inhibit cholesterol efflux to apolipoprotein (apo) A1 from human macrophage foam cells. Atherosclerosis. 2004;173:27–38.
132. Kawakami A, Tanaka A, Nakano T, Saniabadi A, Numano F. Stimulation of arterial smooth muscle cell proliferation by remnant lipoprotein particles isolated by immuno-affinity chromatography with anti-apo A-I and anti-apo B-100. Horm Metab Res. 2001;33:67–72.
133. Kawakami A, Tanaka A, Chiba T, Nakajima K, Shimokado K, Yoshida M. Remnant lipoprotein-induced smooth muscle cell proliferation involves epidermal growth factor receptor transactivation. Circulation. 2003;108:2679–88.

# Lipoprotein(a): Structure, Metabolism, and Pathophysiology

7

Alicia J. Jenkins, Karam M. Kostner, and Gerhard M. Kostner

## Introduction

Lipoprotein(a) [Lp(a)] was first described by K. Berg in 1963. Originally, it was believed to represent a genetic variant of β-lipoproteins [1]. Despite of intensive research, the physiological function of Lp(a) remains elusive. There is mounting evidence that elevated plasma Lp(a) levels contribute significantly to the incidence of cardiovascular diseases [2]. First reports of the 1970s were based on case control studies with only few patients and on observational reports of single families. Based on the results from several more recent prospective studies with large sample size, it became clear that the risk for developing coronary artery diseases (CAD) in the Western population is more than two times higher in individuals with increased plasma Lp(a) levels [3]. In addition, a causal relationship between plasma Lp(a) levels and CAD and myocardial infarction (MI) has been assessed. Unfortunately, there are still many gaps in understanding Lp(a) biosynthesis and catabolism, and this hampers the development of specific Lp(a)-lowering medications. Today, there is hardly any safe medication that selectively reduces plasma Lp(a) with high efficacy.

Alicia J. Jenkins (✉)
Section of Endocrinology and Diabetes, University of Oklahoma Health Sciences Center, Oklahoma City, OK, USA

NHMRC Clinical Trials Centre, University of Sydney, Sydney, NSW, Australia
e-mail: alicia-jenkins@ouhsc.edu

K.M. Kostner
University of Queensland, Mater Hospital, Brisbane, Australia

G.M. Kostner
Medical University of Graz, Graz, Austria

## The Structures of Lp(a) and Apo(a)

Lp(a) is composed of an LDL-like core lipoprotein and of the glycoprotein apo(a) complexed to each other by a disulfide bridge (Fig. 7.1). The disulfide bridge links Cys 4326 in apoB100 with the only free Cys 4057 in apo(a), that is located in kringle four Type 9. The lipid core of Lp(a) is almost indistinguishable from that of LDL. Table 7.1 shows the average composition of Lp(a) in comparison to LDL isolated from the same individuals.

Apo(a), the characteristic glycoprotein component of Lp(a), has a unique structure. It consists of repetitive protein segments, so called kringles (K) that are highly homologous to the K-four (K-IV) in plasminogen. K-IV contain approx. 110 amino acids forming a secondary structure, which resembles "Danish kringles" [4]. The N-terminal part of apo(a) consists of numerous repetitive copies of these kringle-IVs. Apo(a) in addition has one copy of a K-V-like kringle and a protease-like domain similar to plasminogen. In humans, there exist probably 30 and more genetically determined apo(a) isoforms, giving rise to a great size heterogeneity. The smallest

A.J. Jenkins et al. (eds.), *Lipoproteins in Diabetes Mellitus*, Contemporary Diabetes, DOI 10.1007/978-1-4614-7554-5_7, © Springer Science+Business Media New York 2014

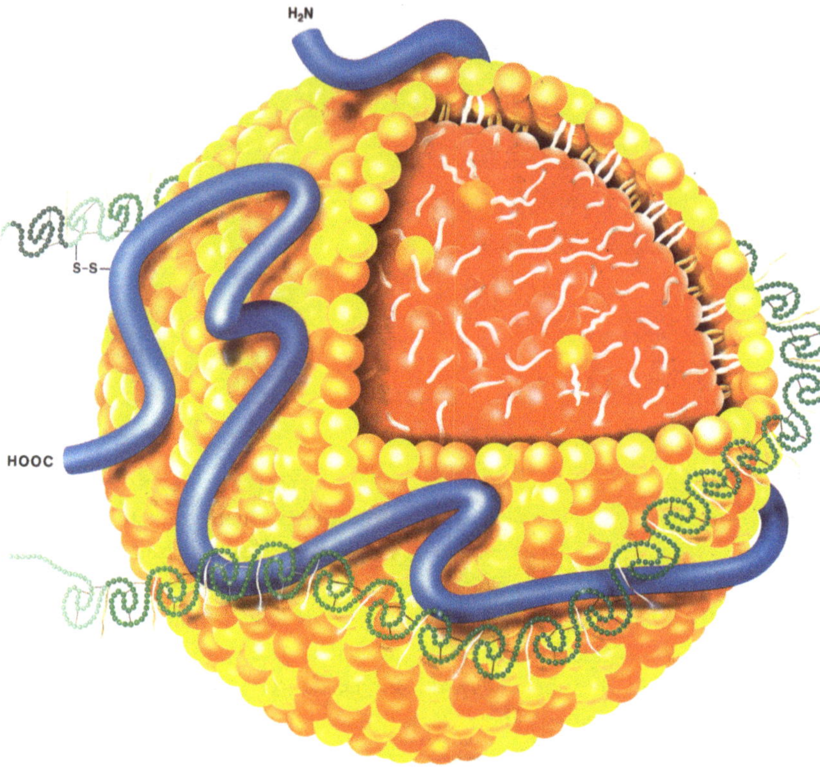


**Fig. 7.1** Schematic view of Lp(a)

**Table 7.1** Average composition of Lp(a) in comparison to LDL

| | Lp(a) (%) | LDL (%) |
|---|---|---|
| Protein | 30.0 | 21.0 |
| Carbohydrates | 10.0 | 1.3 |
| Cholesteryl esters | 31.5 | 42.0 |
| Free cholesterol | 7.0 | 9.0 |
| Phospholipids | 16.0 | 20.7 |
| Triglycerides | 5.5 | 6.0 |

It should be pointed out that the major protein in Lp(a), apo(a), exhibits a great size polymorphism that strongly impacts on the % distribution shown below

apo(a) isoform contains the protease domain, one copy of K-V and 11 K-IVs of which K-IV Type 1 (T-1) and T-(3–10) are unique in their primary structure, whereas K-IV T-2 is present in two identical copies. Larger isoforms differ by the number of K-IV T-2s; the largest apo(a) described so far had 52–54 K-IVs. Between the K-IV domains, there are linker regions, which are highly glycosylated by *N*- and *O*-linked sugars. Although the majority of apo(a) is complexed to LDL, there are small and variable amounts, which are present in plasma in the free form [5] and found in the bottom fraction after ultracentrifugation. Free apo(a) is prone to proteolytic degradation, and the generated fragments are secreted into urine (see below).

## Lp(a) Metabolism

### Assembly of Lp(a)

Lp(a) is biosynthesized only in humans and old world monkeys which poses some problems in studying its metabolism in detail. Apo(a) expression takes place primarily in the liver, yet small amounts of APOA mRNA have also been detected in testis and brain. Their role on the overall Lp(a) metabolism is unknown. Hepatocytes from primates have been found to synthesize a preform of apo(a) with a lower

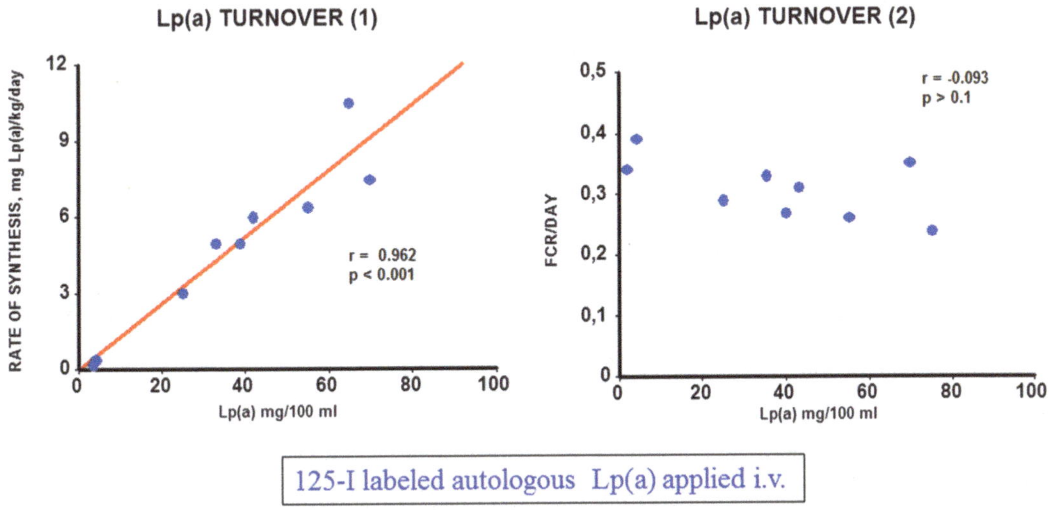


**Fig. 7.2** Turnover of Lp(a) in humans. $^{125}$I radiolabeled Lp(a) was injected into 9 volunteers with plasma concentrations ranging from 5 to 75 mg/dl and the decay of the specific radioactivity was followed over time (details are found in [9])

degree of glycosylation. Upon maturation, intracellular apo(a) reaches the Golgi apparatus and is secreted in mature form as a glycoprotein most probably without attached LDL. The genetically determined size of apo(a) reflecting the number of K-IV repeats correlates with the intracellular residence time, and thus, small isoforms are secreted much faster as compared to large isoforms. This appears to be the reason for the existence of the negative correlation between apo(a) size and plasma Lp(a) concentration. We and others have found that the assembly of Lp(a) from apo(a) and LDL is a two-step process [6]. In the first step, specific K-IVs of apo(a), mostly K-IV T3-6, bind non-covalently to Lys groups on apoB of LDL. This binding is reversible and may be dissociated by Lys analogues such as epsilon aminocaproic acid, tranexamic acid, and others [7]. It has been argued that by interfering with the first step of Lp(a) assembly, plasma Lp(a) levels may be reduced, as free apo(a) is degraded faster than LDL-bound apo(a). In the in vivo and in vitro experiments, however, this assumption has been refuted, and plasma apo(a) and Lp(a) levels went in opposite directions, i.e., were twofold and higher elevated [7]. The reason for these observations may be explained by the fact that free apo(a) binds to the surface of liver cells and upon contact with LDL forms the first Lp(a) complex. Apo(a) which does not find its way to LDL is internalized and degraded. We actually could demonstrate that cell bound apo(a) dissociates upon treatment with Lys analogues and assembles with LDL more efficiently.

When recombinant apo(a) was mixed with LDL in vitro, a fast assembly took place, characterized by stable disulfide bridging. This mechanism that most probably also occurs in vivo does not need any enzymatic activity and leads to the formation of the final mature Lp(a). Interestingly, apo(a) has a preponderance for binding apoB100 from humans and few animal species, yet apoB100 from rodents, in particular from mice, hardly form any Lp(a) upon incubation with apo(a). Thus, the metabolism of Lp(a) might be studied only in double transgenic human apo(a):apoB100 mice or in monkeys.

Although the evidence for an extracellular assembly is favored by many investigators, there are still experimental data that may be only interpreted if an intracellular assembly of Lp(a) is assumed [8]. Further experiments will be needed to reach a definite conclusion.

## In Vivo Metabolism of Lp(a)

As common laboratory animals do not express apo(a), the Lp(a) metabolism had to be studied in humans. We actually were the first to demonstrate that plasma Lp(a) concentrations highly significantly correlate with the production rate, yet the Lp(a) catabolism does not control Lp(a) levels [9].

This is demonstrated in Fig. 7.2, where we studied 9 probands with Lp(a) levels ranging from 5 to 75 mg/dl. Our results have been confirmed subsequently by other investigators using radioactive Lp(a) tracers or stable isotope precursors [10].

Concerning the catabolism of Lp(a), the liver appears to be the major organ of Lp(a) degradation. This has been proven by turnover studies in several animal species including rats, rabbits, mice, and hedgehogs. The latter animal model has been chosen since it synthesizes a lipoprotein that resembles Lp(a) [11]. In the in vivo studies, we found that approx. 50 % of Lp(a) is taken up by the liver, followed by kidney, spleen, and muscle. Unfortunately, the mechanism of in vivo cellular uptake of Lp(a) is mostly unknown. In the in vitro experiments, Lp(a) has been shown to bind to the LDL receptor—yet with a greatly reduced affinity as compared to LDL. There have been also reports suggesting an in vitro binding of Lp(a) to other receptors such as VLDL receptor, Gp-330 (megalin), asialoglycoprotein receptor, and scavenger receptors, yet their relevance for the in vivo metabolism remains to be established.

## Regulation of Apo(a) Transcription

The transcription of genes involved in lipid and lipoprotein metabolism is heavily influenced by nuclear receptors including PPARs, RXR, CAR, PXR, LXR, and FXR, in addition to others [12]. These nuclear receptors in concert with other transcription factors coordinate pathways involved in lipid absorption, de novo biosynthesis, cell excretion from different organs, and conversion of cholesterol to steroid hormones and bile acids. In the bile acid metabolism, FXR is of major importance as it controls for the overproduction of bile acids and detoxification of liver and cells from the biliary tract. FXR is also involved in glucose homeostasis, intestinal bacterial infection, and tumorigenesis of liver [13]. Although the molecular mechanism of FXR action is not elucidated in full detail, one may say the following: FXR is mainly expressed in the liver, intestine, kidney, and adrenals and binds to response elements in the promoter as heterodimer together with RXR, thereby transactivating or transrepressing cognate target genes. Of key importance is the transactivation of small heterodimer partner (SHP) and of FGF-15/19. SHP is a transcriptional repressor that has no DNA binding capability but rather interacts with the DNA binding and/or activating factor domain of numerous nuclear receptors, among them HNF4, LRH-1, estrogen receptor (ER), and RXR, thereby interfering with gene transcription [14]. Mouse FGF-15 that is expressed almost exclusively in the intestine and its human orthologue FGF-19 expressed in the small intestine but also in the liver are also transactivated by FXR-RXR heterodimers. It has been demonstrated that FGF-15/19 signals from intestine to liver to repress the transcription of key enzymes of bile acid biosynthesis. Inagaki et al. [15], for example, provided evidence that FGF-15 represses CYP7A1 in wild-type mice but did not affect CYP7A1 mRNA levels in SHP−/− mice. It was suggested that in the FGF15/19 pathway, post-transcriptional activation of SHP may take place. It was also shown that FGF binding to its receptor, FGFR4, signals via the MAP-kinase pathway, thereby interfering with CYP7A1 transcription [16]. In a recent report, Song et al. [17] published that the MAPK-ERK1/2 pathway is a major trigger of FGF19-mediated inhibition of CYP7A1. Binding of FGF19 to FGF4R led to Tyr phosphorylation of the latter and in turn to a phosphorylation cascade of RAS, c-RAF, MEK1/2, and MAPK/ERK1/2 and finally to the transcriptional inhibition of CYP7A1. This pathway was independent of SHP.

In our recent studies, we made the observations that patients suffering from obstructive cholestasis with high plasma bile acid concentrations had comparatively low plasma Lp(a) levels. When patients were treated by surgery, plasma bile acid levels normalized, and plasma Lp(a) rose significantly to levels compatible with their individual isoform [18] (Table 7.2). This led us to hypothesize that FXR might be responsible for these observed changes in plasma Lp(a). We therefore performed a serious in vivo studies with transgenic mice expressing apo(a) under the control of its native human promoter, in addition to in vitro studies using cultured primary hepatocytes

**Table 7.2** Influence of drugs and other substances on plasma Lp(a) concentrations

| Substance | % Decrease |
|---|---|
| Omega-3 fatty acids | 5–20 |
| Palm oil | 10–25 |
| Vegetarian diet | 10 |
| Nicotinic acid and derivatives | 15–35 |
| Aspirin | 15–20 |
| L-carnitine | 10–15 |
| Lp(a)/LDL apheresis | 60–80 |
| ACE inhibitors | 10–40 |

from these mice, aimed at elucidating the role of FXR ligands in apo(a) transcription. In a first report published in JCI [18], we show that the apo(a) promoter contains at nucleotide 814–826 upstream to the transcription initiation site, a direct repeat (DR-1) that binds HNF4a with high affinity, thereby transactivating apo(a) transcription. FXR upon activation by bile acids or synthetic ligands is transported from the cytosol to the nucleus and competes with the HNF4a binding to the DR-1, thereby downregulating apo(a) transcription. This pathway was further proven by reporter assays using a 2kB promoter sequence of apo(a) in front of the luciferase gene.

Feeding mice with a diet containing 0.2 % cholic acid, the mouse ligand for FXR, led to a reduction of plasma apo(a) to almost zero. The pathway described above however accounted for only approx. 60 % of the downregulation of apo(a) transcription. We therefore performed additional experiments exploring the possibility that SHP and/or FGF-15/19 might be responsible for the remaining 40 % repression of apo(a) transcription. Overexpression of SHP in primary hepatocytes from transgenic apo(a) mice did not downregulate apo(a) biosynthesis. These findings were backed up also by promoter studies using a luciferase reporter assay. On the other hand, we could show that the addition of FGF-19 to primary hepatocytes of the apo(a) transgenic mice downregulated apo(a) transcription and protein biosynthesis. Knockdown of the FGF-15/19 receptor (FGFR4) on the primary hepatocytes by a specific siRNA abolished the effect of FGF15/19. We also could prove that in this pathway, FGF15/19 binding to FGFR4 activates a phosphorylation cascade involving RAS-RAF-MEK1/2 ERK1/2 that leads to ELK-1 phosphorylation and translocation to the nucleus. Using luciferase reporter assays in combination with site directed mutagenesis, we finally identified an ETS domain at nt −1,615 to −1,630 that was responsible for P-ELK-1 binding and repression of APOA transcription [19]. These two pathways are schematically displayed in Fig. 7.3. We believe that the clarification of these pathways may serve as basis for developing new medications to treat individuals with elevated plasma Lp(a) levels that are at high risk for CAD and MI.

Although bile acids are capable in downregulating apo(a) transcription almost completely by the two pathways described above, there are numerous additional regulatory sequences in the apo(a) promoter that need to be addressed in future investigations.

## Genetics of Lp(a)

Lp(a) concentrations in human plasma range from <1 mg/dl to >250 mg/dl and are to >90 % genetically determined. The gene for apo(a) is located on chromosome 6q26–q27. Utermann et al. were first to recognize that apo(a) shows a tremendous size heterogeneity that is based on the number of K-IV repeats [20]. This size heterogeneity correlates with plasma Lp(a) levels. Large isoforms were found to correlate with low plasma Lp(a) levels and vice versa. The molecular mechanism of these findings is based on one hand on the fact that large apo(a) isoforms are trapped and degraded during biosynthesis in the rough endoplasmatic reticulum and in the Golgi compartment to a much greater extent than small isoforms [21].

The promoter region of apo(a) contains a variable number of tandem repeats (VNTR) with the pentanucleotide TTTTA in addition to the +93 C/T polymorphism of the untranslated region in the apo(a) gene. Further mutations and polymorphisms are abundant in the apo(a) gene that explain many but not all variations in plasma Lp(a) levels. Ichinose [22], for example, identified two additional functional SNPs in the distal

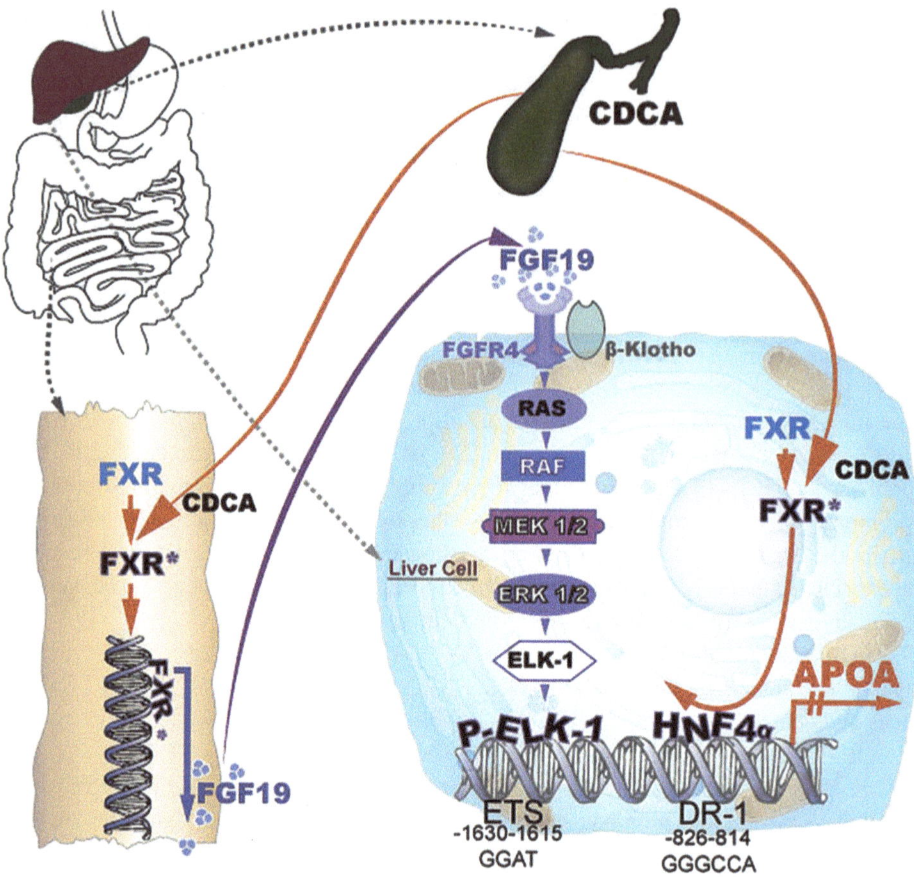


**Fig. 7.3** Cartoon of the transcriptional regulation of apo(a)

enhancer region 20 kB upstream of the apo(a) gene. In addition, numerous polymorphisms were identified in the K-IV domains of the apo(a) gene that showed significant impacts on apo(a) plasma concentrations. As mentioned above, in the proximal apo(a) promoter region contains numerous regulatory sequences including binding sites for HNF1 and HNF4, IL-6, SREBPs, CREB, and many more. It will be interesting to study the influence of genetic variations in these transcription factors in addition to their DNA binding sites in apo(a) in view of their impact on genetically determined variations of plasma Lp(a) levels.

Another point that needs attention is the fact that there exist great ethnic differences in the distribution of plasma Lp(a) levels. Africans and African Americans, for example, have much higher Lp(a) levels than the white population, considering the individual size polymorphism. The opposite is the case with Chinese individuals and other Asian populations. The reason for these differences has never been explored at a molecular basis and will need much more attention in future.

## Factors Affecting Plasma Lp(a)

There are numerous factors that have been described to permanently or transiently modulate plasma Lp(a) concentrations [23]. A comprehensive list of most of these factors is shown in Table 7.3.

In addition to the apo(a) gene, other genes involved in lipid metabolism such as apoE, LDL-R, and HNF1 and HNF4 have variable effects. Among the secondary factors, renal and liver diseases appear to be the most striking ones. In kidney diseases, Lp(a) is elevated two- to three-fold, and it appears that nephrotic syndrome

**Table 7.3** Factors affecting plasma Lp(a) concentrations

| | | |
|---|---|---|
| Genes and diseases | | |
| Genes | Effect | |
| APOA | Size polymorphism (50 %); other 40 % | |
| APOE | Variable | |
| LDL-R | Increase | |
| MODY (HNF1/4a) | Variable | |
| Diseases | | |
| Acute phase | Increase | |
| Renal disease | Increase | |
| Diabetes mellitus | Increase | |
| Cancer: different forms | Increase | |
| Gout | Increase | |
| Antiphospholipid antibodies | Increase | |
| Liver disease | Decrease | |
| Hyperthyroidism | Decrease | |
| Hypothyroidism | Increase | |
| Others | | |
| Alcohol | Decrease | |
| Menopause | Increase | |
| Hormones | | |
| Compound | Effect | Comment |
| Estrogens | Up to 35 % reduction | Rebound effects have been observed |
| Progesterone | 30–40 % reduction | Only few studies reported |
| Tamoxifen | 35 % reduction | Antiestrogen |
| Tibolone | 35 % reduction | Synthetic steroid hormone |
| Raloxifene | 18 % reduction | Estrogen-R modulator |
| Testosterone | 30–40 % reduction | Only short observations |
| Pregnancy | Two-fold increase | Normalized postpartum |
| Anabolic steroids | 60–70 % reduction | Not for clinical use |
| ACTH | 30–40 % reduction | Few observations |
| Conventional drugs | | |
| Compound | Effect | Comment |
| Niacin | 20–30 % reduction | Currently most recommended |
| Fibrates | <20 % reduction | Large study with gemfibrozil |
| Statins | Inconsistent | Significant increases in Lp(a) were reported |
| Neomycin (2 g/d) | 24 % decrease | Interferes with release of apo(a) from liver cell surface |
| *N*-act-cys | Controversial | Antioxidant, reduces –S–S– bonds |
| L-carnitine | 10–20 % decrease | Mitochondrial FA transport |
| ASA | 10–20 % reduction | Even at low dose efficient |
| Apheresis | 50–80 % reduction | Independent of the system except for AB column |
| New medications under investigation | | |
| Compound | Effect on Lp(a) | Mechanism |
| Mipomersen | >30 % reduction | siRNA against apoB |
| Eprotirome | Up to 40 % reduction | Thyroid mimetic |
| PSK-9 inhibitor | ? | PSK-9 antibody |
| Lomitapide | ? | MTP inhibitor |
| Anacetrapib | 30–50 % reduction | CETP inhibitor |
| Different factors | | |
| HGH treatment | 2× increase | |
| Smoking | 10–20 % reduction | |
| Obesity | 10–20 % reduction | |
| Omega-3 FA | 10–20 % reduction | |
| Stearic acid | Up to 25 % increase | |
| Trans-FA | Up to 25 % increase | |
| Conjugated linoleic acid | Up to 25 % increase | |
| Cyclosporine | 2× increase | |

and end-stage renal disease have a different etiology for elevating Lp(a). While in nephrotic syndrome the rate of Lp(a) biosynthesis was found to be increased, end-stage renal disease is characterized by a reduced Lp(a) catabolism.

Since liver is the almost only organ for Lp(a) biosynthesis, it is not astonishing that liver diseases are characterized by a gross reduction of plasma Lp(a). This was observed at first instance in patients with cholestasis, yet their Lp(a) reduction is transient if the patients are successfully treated. Other substances that are liver toxic including alcohol and several drugs have been also shown to significantly reduce Lp(a).

Steroid hormones including estrogens, progesterone, and testosterone, in addition to synthetic sex hormone-like compounds, reduce plasma Lp(a) up to 40 %, yet these effects are partly transient. Anabolic steroids in particular reportedly have a great reducing effect on plasma Lp(a), whose mechanism has not been elucidated so far.

There are numerous reports in the literature suggesting that conventional lipid-lowering drugs including niacin, statins, fibrates, and drugs interfering with cholesterol absorption (Neomycin, Ezetimibe) significantly reduce plasma Lp(a). Unfortunately, these effects are by for not consistent and great individual differences have been observed. In numerous cases, these compounds even led to an increase of plasma Lp(a). The only compound of this list that consistently reduces Lp(a) is nicotinic acid or its derivatives. Unfortunately, the recent reports of large intervention studies using nicotinic acid, AIM-HIGH [24] did not show the expected results on the reduction of primary endpoints. There are numerous new drugs in the pipeline of many companies, among them CETP inhibitors, thyroid mimetics, PSK-9, and MTP inhibitors as well as siRNA analogues that look promising from results of phase I and phase II clinical trials. Today, the only measure used in some countries to drastically reduce elevated plasma Lp(a) is LDL—or Lp(a) apheresis. This treatment has been shown to be effective not only to lower plasma Lp(a) from 50 to 80 % but also to reduce the risk for cardiovascular diseases and MI.

Finally, there are several anecdotal reports with very low numbers of cases that suggest other treatment regimes to lower Lp(a). These include different forms of dietary fatty acids, aspirin (ASA), L-carnitine, ascorbic acid, and others. There is no doubt that the ideal drug for reducing Lp(a) has not been found so far, and additional work will be necessary to achieve this goal.

## The Role of the Kidney in Lp(a) Metabolism

As mentioned above, detailed knowledge on the site and mechanism of Lp(a) catabolism is still missing. When we infused radiolabeled Lp(a) into animals that per se do not express a human orthologue of apo(a), approx. 50 % of the radioactivity was found in liver and bile and 20 % in the kidney. The question of the role of kidney in Lp(a) metabolism was studied by Kronenberg et al. [25] who reported on a 10 % renovascular arteriovenous difference in Lp(a) plasma concentrations in healthy individuals. If these findings can be backed up by additional work, the kidney may turn out as an important organ in humans for Lp(a) catabolism.

Another interesting point is that apo(a) immune reactivity is found in urine [26]. As Lp(a) is by far too large to pass the kidney, only apo(a) fragments of various size are found in urine. Irrespective of the apo(a) isoform present in patient's plasma, consistently more than 10 distinct apo(a) bands in urine with molecular masses between 50 and 160 kD have been reported. These secreted apo(a) fragments are glycosylated and not complexed to apoB. Most importantly there is a highly significant correlation between urinary apo(a) concentrations and plasma Lp(a) levels. We also observed that diurnal urinary apo(a) levels normalized to creatinine remained constant over months within single individuals. It is not fully clear where and how these fragments are formed, but it appears that a large portion might be formed extrarenally, followed by excretion by the kidney in a possible selective pathway. Urinary apo(a) excretion is rapid and depends on plasma Lp(a) levels: Reduction of plasma Lp(a) by LDL apheresis leads to an immediate reduction of urinary apo(a) fragment concentration [27]. Studies from our laboratory showed that under normal physiological conditions, a constant amount of apo(a) is excreted into urine, depending on the plasma Lp(a) level. The excretion rate of apo(a) into urine was not altered by changes in glomerular filtration rate and renal plasma flow in healthy males [28]. Urinary apo(a) was significantly decreased in a large study of kidney patients and this was even more pronounced in patients with a creatinine clearance of <70 ml/min [29]. Because urinary apo(a) excretion is highly dependent on plasma Lp(a) levels, patient and control group were matched for plasma Lp(a) levels, and it was found that with increasing plasma Lp(a) levels, kidney patients excreted significantly less apo(a) into urine as compared to controls [30]. Whether or not this mechanism might be responsible for the grossly increased Lp(a) values in kidney patients remains to be established. Above a plasma Lp(a) concentration of 30 mg/dl, urinary apo(a) excretion was highly diminished: There was a reduction of apo(a) excretion in patients to one fifth in comparison to controls. Interestingly, 30 mg/dl is the cutoff level for Lp(a) that best discriminates coronary heart disease patients from controls.

Subjects with small apo(a) isoforms in addition to higher plasma Lp(a) levels also exhibit significantly higher urinary apo(a) excretion as compared to patients with large apo(a) isoforms [26]. This observation and the fact that a good correlation of plasma Lp(a) and urinary apo(a) in both proteinuric patients and healthy controls exists led us to believe that urinary apo(a) excretion highly depends on plasma Lp(a) levels but not on apo(a) isoforms. Our earlier observation that after rapid reduction of plasma Lp(a) with LDL apheresis, urinary apo(a) is also rapidly reduced supports this hypothesis.

Because of the significant correlation between plasma and urinary apo(a) concentration, it should be possible to discriminate coronary artery disease patients (CAD) from normals by measuring urinary apo(a). In one study, 225 patients and controls were analyzed for plasma and urinary apo(a), and urinary apo(a) turned out to be a better discriminator for CAD than plasma Lp(a) [31]. Since the analysis of these kringle-IV fragments found in urine is not biased by the apo(a) phenotype, it might be appropriate to include the measurement of apo(a) fragments into future studies. In this regard, it is noteworthy that free apo(a) in serum, which consists of these fragments, as measured by a recently described new ELISA [32], has a better diagnostic test performance than total Lp(a).

## Lp(a) and the Risk for Atherosclerotic Diseases

In the original work from the laboratory of K. Berg, Lp(a) was described as "sinking pre-β-lipoprotein" [33], and a semiquantitative relation of this fraction with CAD was suggested. Our laboratory in fact was the first to quantify Lp(a) immunochemically by rocket electrophoresis, and we suggested a cutoff level 30 mg/dl for patients at an increased risk for MI [34]. We also could show in this report that individuals with elevated LDL and in particular those with a phenotype IIA hyperlipoproteinemia were at a 10-fold or higher MI risk. Later studies also demonstrated that the combination of high Lp(a) plasma levels with low HDL-C strongly increases the risk for CAD. In a prospective population study involving almost 800 male participants of the PROCAM cohort, von Eckhardstein et al. [35] reported that Lp(a) increases the coronary risk particularly in men with high LDL-C and low HDL-C in addition to high blood pressure and high global CAD risk. Even more importantly, it has been found that polymorphisms in the apo(a) promoter were associated with an increased risk for MI [3]. In the following, several hundred reports appeared in the literature dealing with one or the other aspect of atherosclerosis such as myocardial infarction, stroke, and peripheral vascular diseases in relation to elevated plasma levels or various isoforms of apo(a). The majority of them strongly suggest that Lp(a) in fact is a severe risk factor—in several studies even the best discriminator for the atherogenic risk. As Lp(a) metabolism is quite distinct from that of other plasma lipoprotein, it is not surprising that the atherogenicity of Lp(a) is independent of other factors.

It should be mentioned at this point that several prospective studies in the past, such as the Physicians Health Study, have shown contrasting results [36]. In some of these reports, Lp(a) was measured in long-term frozen samples with insufficiently evaluated test kits. Moreover, due to the extremely wide range of plasma Lp(a) levels from less than 0.1 mg/dl to more than 300 mg/dl and the highly skewed distribution, studies that include a small number of cases/controls are prone to random deviations. Another reason why studies on Lp(a) are sometimes controversial is the fact that due to its heterogeneity, it is difficult to standardize the measurement of Lp(a). Starting in 2009, a series of papers have been published that demonstrate beyond any doubt that Lp(a) not only is a risk indicator for atherosclerotic diseases but even more so that a causal relationship exists between elevated Lp(a) and CAD risk. The first report of this series was published by Tregouet et al. who studied 2700 CAD patients and > 4500 control individuals by an SNP analysis using the 500 K Affymetrix chip [37]. In this haplotype association study, the authors identified the LPA gene cluster as a strong susceptibility locus for CAD. Kamstrup et al. [38] published in the same year their data of the Copenhagen Heart study comprising > 40,000 individuals. There was a significant correlation between plasma Lp(a) levels, KIV-2 genotype, and the risk for myocardial infarction which they interpreted as proof for causality. Erqou et al. [39] finally performed a meta-analysis including 40 studies with >58,000 participants and found that individuals with smaller isoforms are at a >two-fold risk for coronary heart diseases.

Another important finding is that Lp(a) may play a role in acute coronary syndromes. Shindo et al. [40] found significantly higher apo(a) and PAI-1 stainable areas in atherectomy specimens of patients with unstable than in those with stable angina. Cerebral vascular disease, peripheral vascular disease, and more recently carotid atherosclerosis have also been associated with elevated Lp(a) levels. Finally, it appears that Lp(a) may also be involved as a cofactor in essential hypertension [41].

## Impact of Lp(a) on Hemostasis

Apo(a) has a striking homology with plasminogen, and thus it was suggested that Lp(a) interferes with fibrinolysis in several ways [42]. Lp(a) competitively inhibited plasminogen binding to fibrinogen and fibrin. Lp(a) interferes with plasminogen conversion to plasmin. It was also found that plasminogen activator inhibitor (PAI-1) biosynthesis in endothelial cells is stimulated by Lp(a). Lp(a) upregulated PAI-2 expression in blood monocytes [43]. Another link between Lp(a) and thrombosis is the binding and inactivation of tissue factor pathway inhibitor (TFPI) [44]. On the other hand, there is evidence that Lp(a) binds platelet-activating factor acetyl hydrolase (PAF-AH) with high affinity and specificity. Thus, Lp(a) not only inactivates one of the strongest factors known for platelet aggregation, PAF, but also hydrolyzes short-chain phospholipids which are generated during lipid peroxidation [45]. Lp(a) also attenuated collagen-mediated platelet aggregation and in turn reduced thromboxane secretion. Taken together, it appears that many of the proposed prothrombotic properties of Lp(a) are weighed off by some quite significant antithrombotic effects, and it remains to be determined which effect prevails under different in vivo situations.

## Lp(a) and Diabetes Mellitus

There are more than 100 papers and abstracts published in the literature on this topic. In 1993, Haffner [46] reviewed the literature available until then and summarized the available data on insulin dependent diabetes mellitus (IDDM) by stating that IDDM (Type 1) patients have "probably" elevated Lp(a) concentrations, and these concentrations might be related to metabolic control. Lp(a) levels in addition are increased in patients with microalbuminuria. Literature data even today on the role of IDDM as a causal modulator of plasma Lp(a) levels are not consistent. A relationship has not been found in young children with type 1 diabetes mellitus, and it appears that the positive correlation with IDDM in adulthood is mostly indirect. The latter group of patients in many cases suffers from impaired kidney function which causes increased Lp(a) levels in a similar manner as kidney diseases of other etiology. In a more recent work, Kollerits et al. [47] asked the question as to what extent Lp(a) might be an independent predictor of CVD in IDDM patients. More than 400 IDDM patients were followed over an observation period of 10.7 years. Since renal disease is a severe risk factor for CAD, patients with kidney impairments were excluded from the study. Although this study did not answer the question per se whether or not IDDM patients have increased Lp(a) levels, it was concluded that Lp(a) values > 30 mg/dl contribute significantly to the CAD risk in type 1 DM.

The relationship of non-insulin-dependent diabetes mellitus (NIDDM) with elevated plasma Lp(a) levels is more complicated since this disease has many facets and multiple etiologies, many of them related to mutations or polymorphisms of genes involved in lipid and lipoprotein metabolism. A good example for this complex situation is found in the article of Shih et al. [48] who studied the Q268X mutation in the MODY gene in relation to plasma apoAII, apoCIII, and Lp(a) levels. MODY stands for maturity onset diabetes of the young, and MODY genes are nuclear receptors (HNF1a and HNF4a), known as master regulators of genes expressed in the liver that are involved in lipid metabolism. As mentioned in the paragraph "transcriptional regulation of apo(a)," the expression of apo(a) is highly dependent on the binding of HNF4a to a DR-1 in the promoter. Thus, any mutation in HNF4a that affects the transactivation of genes must have an influence on plasma lipid and lipoprotein levels. In fact, it was found that carrier of the Q268X mutation not only suffer from MODY but also have reduced plasma concentrations of Lp(a), apoAII, and apoCIII. There are other mutations and polymorphisms known in the MODY genes that may have similar effects on plasma Lp(a).

On the other hand, the etiology of NIDDM is multifactorial, and thus it is unlikely that Lp(a) levels are affected in all NIDDM patients to the same extent. This explains that in the past, unaltered, higher or lower Lp(a) plasma concentrations have been reported in this group of patients. In 2010, Kamstrup et al. published a study on > 35,000 US and Danish participants adjusted for numerous well-established CAD risk factors including HbA1c, CRP, and lipids [49]. Lp(a) levels were inversely associated with the incidence of type 2 diabetes mellitus with hazard ratios for quintiles 2–5 vs. quintile 1 of 0.87. The authors concluded that Lp(a) is inversely related with the risk of type 2 DM independently of risk factors. This is in discordance to previous reports that suggest positive associations of Lp(a) with CVD.

From our own studies, it appears that Lp(a) is mainly elevated in patients with impaired renal function [23].

### Treatment of Elevated Lp(a) Levels

Even though Lp(a) has been established as an independent risk factor for coronary artery disease and cerebrovascular disease, it is still not clear whether lowering of Lp(a) is beneficial. This is mainly due to the fact that to date no practical treatment is available to reduce elevated Lp(a) levels. Furthermore, most effective treatments like LDL apheresis also affect LDL levels. Most lipidologists and clinicians recommend to lower LDL cholesterol more aggressively to levels below 100 mg/dl in case of elevated Lp(a) levels above 30 mg/dl, even though the hard evidence for this is also lacking.

### Diet

Dietary influences on plasma Lp(a) levels are variable and moderate, yet measurable. Polyunsaturated fatty acids and saturated fatty acids found in palm oil have a mild, although significant, reducing effect. Dietary intake of omega 3 fatty acids has shown to decrease plasma Lp(a) levels in some studies. A diet rich in coconut oil has also been shown to reduce plasma Lp(a) levels [50]. In a similar way, trans-fatty acids were suggested to have a lowering effect on Lp(a). Taking all published studies on dietary treatment of hyper-Lp(a) patients together, it is fair to say that the effects are moderate and transient in many cases and appear to vary among individuals, depending on their type of hyperlipoproteinemia. Long-term studies on this topic in fact are lacking.

### Statins

Statin treatment may have a variable effect on plasma Lp(a) concentrations. In most studies, Lp(a) remains unchanged after treatment with HMG-CoA reductase inhibitors. Treatment of hypercholesterolemic patients for 6 weeks revealed that approx. one third responded with a reduction of plasma Lp(a); in one third, there was no change; and in the remaining third, Lp(a) was significantly increased [51]. Some studies have shown lowering of Lp(a) by long-term treatment of FH patients with statins [52]. Importantly aggressive LDL reduction with statins removes some of the risk associated with elevated Lp(a) levels.

### Nicotinic Acid

Nicotinic acid and its derivatives can reduce Lp(a) levels by up to 35 % [53]. Niceritrol, a nicotinic acid derivative, has also been shown to reduce plasma Lp(a) levels in patients with chronic renal disease and hyperlipidemia. From all lipid-lowering drugs described so far, nicotinic acid and its derivatives appear to be the most efficient Lp(a)-lowering agent. Studies however are missing addressing the question of dose response and long-term efficacy. The Heart Protection Study 2: Treatment of HDL to Reduce the Incidence of Vascular Events (HPS2-THRIVE) is testing simvastatin plus extended-release niacin plus a D prostanoid 1 receptor antagonist, MK 0524, to inhibit the flushing side effect in comparison with simvastatin monotherapy in 20,000 patients with coronary disease.

### Fibrates

There are numerous reports in the literature concerning the influence of fibrates, which include clofibrate, fenofibrate, and gemfibrozil on plasma Lp(a) levels. In essence, it appears that there is no uniform response as part of the treated patients respond with approx. 25 % decreases in plasma Lp(a); in some, there are no changes, and there are also numerous individuals whose plasma Lp(a) increase upon fibrate therapy. The latter group of patients is characterized by rather high plasma triglycerides and VLDL, and respond upon fibrate therapy with elevations of LDL in addition to elevations of Lp(a). The pathomechanism of this phenomenon remains to be elucidated.

### Other Agents

All ACE inhibitors in monotherapy lower elevated Lp(a) plasma concentrations in proteinuric patients by reversing proteinuria and in turn enhanced Lp(a) production by the liver [54]. Fosinopril seems to be the only ACE inhibitor to reduce Lp(a) concentrations also in non-proteinuric patients, probably by increasing apo(a) fragmentation and excretion into the urine (Kostner K et al. unpublished results).

Lp(a)-lowering steroid hormones are not indicated for treatment due to side effects. Likewise, tranexamic acid is able to lower Lp(a) plasma concentrations in vivo, but cannot be used in the majority of patients due to possible side effects. The anti-estrogen tamoxifen has also an interesting Lp(a)-lowering effect [55]. The synthetic steroid tibolone reportedly reducted in Lp(a) by about 35 %; however, this was accompanied by a concomitant reduction of the anti-atherogenic HDLs by about 20 %. Raloxifene is a selective estrogen receptor modulator and an alternative to estrogen replacement as it obviates the need for a progestin and does not increase C-reactive protein levels. In a recent study, it was reported that raloxifene significantly reduced Lp(a) by 18 % [56].

As mentioned previously, ACTH has been found to decrease Lp(a) by more than 50 % and also resulted in lower total cholesterol, LDL, and apoB levels in hemodialysis patients and steroid-treated, healthy, and hyperlipemic individuals.

Recently, L-carnitine was shown to reduce elevated Lp(a) levels by about 10 % in patients with and without diabetes mellitus [57]. There are also reports indicating that aspirin and vitamin C lower elevated Lp(a) levels.

### Apheresis

The most effective therapy for lowering Lp(a) known today is extracorporeal elimination with apheresis. LDL apheresis and selective Lp(a) apheresis using antibody-coupled columns, precipitation and complex formation at low pH, double filtration, and direct absorption have been demonstrated to lower plasma Lp(a) to the same extent as LDL cholesterol (up to 80 %). However, these treatments are expensive and accessible only to a small number of high-risk patients [58, 59].

## Novel Lipid-Lowering Compounds

*ApoB Antisense and MTP Inhibitors*: ApoB antisense inhibits only production of ApoB100-containing lipoproteins such as Lp(a) which are found in the liver, whereas MTP inhibitors generally reduce both hepatic ApoB100-containing lipoproteins and ApoB48 lipoproteins which are produced in the intestine and transport dietary fat via chylomicrons. Even though MTP inhibitors have shown to reduce apoB-containing lipoproteins in humans, the future of systemic MTP appears uncertain because of their poor tolerability, transaminase elevations and probable hepatic steatosis, and significant negative impact on ApoA1 lipoprotein and HDL-C.

The most advanced ApoB antisense drug in clinical development is mipomersen. Phase 2 studies in patients on statins and other lipid-lowering agents showed mipomersen dose-dependently reduced LDL, Lp(a), and triglycerides [60].

*Proprotein Convertase Subtilisin/Kexin Type 9 (PCSK9) Inhibitors*: In 2003, Abifadel and colleagues described a new form of autosomal dominant hypercholesterolemia (ADH), which was not associated with mutations in the genes coding for the receptor or its ligand, apoB. They reported two mutations in the gene encoding proprotein convertase subtilisin/kexin type 9 (PCSK9) that were responsible for hypercholesterolemia [61]. PCSK9 inhibitors have shown to reduce LDL and Lp(a) in phase II clinical trials and are currently being investigated in several phase III trials.

## References


1. Berg K. A new serum type system in man: the Lp system. Acta Pathol Microbiol Scand. 1963;59:362–82.
2. Catapano AL, Reiner Z, De Backer G, Graham I, Taskinen MR, Wiklund O, Agewall S, Alegria E, Chapman M, Durrington P, Erdine S, Halcox J, Hobbs R, Kjekshus J, Filardi PP, Riccardi G, Storey RF, Wood D. ESC/EAS Guidelines for the management of dyslipidaemias. The Task Force for the management of dyslipidaemias of the European Society of Cardiology (ESC) and the European Atherosclerosis Society (EAS). Atherosclerosis. 2011;217:3–46.
3. Holmer SR, Hengstenberg C, Kraft HG, Mayer B, Poll M, Kurzinger S, Fischer M, Lowel H, Klein G, Riegger GA, Schunkert H. Associations of polymorphisms of the apo(a) gene with Lp(a) and myocardial infarction. Circulation. 2003;107:696–701.
4. McLean JW, Tomlinson JE, Kuang WJ, Eaton DL, Chen EY, Fless GM, Scanu AM, Lawn RM. cDNA sequence of human apolipoprotein(a) is homologous to plasminogen. Nature. 1987;330:132–7.
5. Gries A, Nimpf J, Nimpf M, Wurm H, Kostner GM. Free and apoB-associated Lp(a) specific protein in human serum. Clin Chim Acta. 1987;164:93–100.
6. Frank S, Krasznai K, Durovic S, Lobentanz EM, Dieplinger H, Wagner E, Zatloukal K, Cotten M, Utermann G, Kostner GM. High-level expression of various apolipoprotein(a) isoforms by "transferrinfection": the role of kringle IV sequences in the extracellular association with low-density lipoprotein. Biochemistry. 1994;33:12329–39.
7. Frank S, Durovic S, Kostner K, Kostner GM. Inhibitors for the in vitro assembly of Lp(a). Arterioscler Thromb Vasc Biol. 1995;15:1774–80.
8. Dieplinger H, Utermann G. The seventh myth of lipoprotein (a): where and how is it assembled. Curr Opinion Lipidol. 1999;10:275–83.
9. Krempler F, Kostner GM, Bolzano K, Sandhofer F. Turnover of lipoprotein (a) in man. J Clin Invest. 1980;65:1483–90.
10. Kronenberg F, Ikewaki K, Schaefer JR, Konig P, Dieplinger H. Kinetic studies of atherogenic lipoproteins in hemodialysis patients: do they tell us more about their pathology? Semin Dial. 2007;20:554–60.
11. Rouy D, Laplaud PM, Saboureau M, Angles-Cano E. Hedgehog lipoprotein(a) is a modulator of activation of plasminogen at the fibrin surface. An in vitro study. Arterioscler Thromb. 1992;12:146–54.
12. Chawla A, Repa JJ, Evans RM, Mangelsdorf DJ. Nuclear receptors and lipid physiology: opening the X-files. Science. 2001;294:1866–70.
13. Yanqiao Zhang Y, Edwards PA. FXR signaling in metabolic disease. FEBS Lett. 2008;582:10–8.
14. Lee YK, Dell H, Dowhan DH, Hadzopoulou-Cladaras M, Moore DD. The orphan nuclear receptor SHP inhibits hepatocyte nuclear factor 4 and retinoid X receptor transactivation: two mechanisms for repression. Mol Cell Biol. 2000;20:187–95.
15. Inagaki T, Choi M, Moschetta A, Peng L, Cummins CL, McDonald JG, Luo G, Jones SA, Goodwin B, Richardson JA, Gerard RD, Repa JJ, Mangelsdorf DJ, Kliewer SA. Fibroblast growth factor 15 functions as an enterohepatic signal to regulate bile acid homeostasis. Cell Metab. 2005;2:217–25.
16. Holt JA, Luo G, Billin AN, Bisi J, McNeill YY, Kozarsky KF, Donahee M, Yuan WD, Mansfield TA, Kliewer SA, Goodwin B, Jones SA. Definition of a novel growth factor dependent signal cascade for the suppression of bile acid biosynthesis. Genes Dev. 2003;17:1581–91.
17. Kwang-Hoon Song KH, Li T, Owsley E, Strom S, Chiang JYL. Bile acids activate fibroblast growth factor 19 signaling in human hepatocytes to inhibit cholesterol 7a-hydroxylase gene expression. Hepatology. 2009;49:297–305.
18. Chennamsetty I, Claudel T, Kostner KK, Baghdasaryan A, Kratky D, Levak-Frank S, Gnzalez FJ, Trauner M, Kostner GM. Farnesoid X receptor

represses hepatic human *APOA* gene expression. J Clin Invest. 2011;121:3724–34.
19. Chennamsetty I, Claudel T, Kostner KM, Trauner M, Kostner GM. FGF19 Signaling cascade suppresses *APOA* gene expression. Arterioscler Thromb Vasc Biol. 2012;32:1220–7.
20. Utermann G, Menzel HJ, Kraft HG, Duba HC, Kemmler HG, Seitz C. Lp(a) glycoprotein phenotypes: inheritance and relation to Lp(a)- lipoprotein concentrations in plasma. J Clin Invest. 1987;80: 458–65.
21. White AL, Hixon JE, Rainwater DL, Lanford RE. Molecular basis for "null" lipoprotein(a) phenotypes and the influence of apolipoprotein(a) size on plasma lipoprotein(a) level in the baboon. J Biol Chem. 1994;269:9060–6.
22. Ichinose A. Hyperlipoprotein (a)-emia determined by genetic polymorphisms in apolipoprotein (a) gene. Brain Nerve. 2008;60:1307–17.
23. Kostner KM, Kostner GM. Factors affecting plasma Lp(a) levels. Semin Vasc Med. 2004;4:211–4.
24. Investigators AIM-HIGH. The role of niacin in raising high-density lipoprotein cholesterol to reduce cardiovascular events in patients with atherosclerotic cardiovascular disease and optimally treated low-density lipoprotein cholesterol: baseline characteristics of study participants. The Atherothrombosis Intervention in Metabolic syndrome with low HDL/high triglycerides: impact on Global Health outcomes (AIM-HIGH) trial. Am Heart J. 2011;161:538–43.
25. Kronenberg F, Trenkwalder E, Lingenhel A. Renovascular arteriovenous differences in Lp(a) plasma concentrations suggest removal of Lp(a) from the renal circulation. J Lipid Res. 1997;38:1755–6.
26. Kostner KM, Maurer G, Huber K, Stefenelli T, Dieplinger H, Steyrer E, Kostner GM. Urinary excretion of apo(a) fragments: role in apo(a) catabolism. Arterioscler Thromb Vasc Biol. 1996;16:905–11.
27. Kostner K, Jansen M, Maurer G, Derfler K. LDL-apheresis significantly reduces urinary apo(a) excretion. Eur J Clin Invest. 1997;27:93–5.
28. Kostner K, Clodi M, Maurer G, Hörl W. Urinary apo(a) excretion is not altered by changes in glomerular filtration rate in healthy males. Wien Klin Wochenschr. 2000;112:121–5.
29. Kostner K, Clodi M, Bodlaj G, Watschinger B, Hörl W, Derfler K, Huber K. Decreased urinary apo(a) excretion in patients with impaired renal function. Eur J Clin Invest. 1998;28:447–52.
30. Kostner KM, Banyai S, Banyai M, Maurer G, Hörl W, Oberbauer R. Urinary apo(a) excretion in patients with proteinuria. Ann Med. 1998;30:497–502.
31. Kostner KM, Huber K, Stefenelli T, Rinner H, Maurer G. Urinary apo(a) discriminates coronary artery disease patients from controls. Atherosclerosis. 1997; 129:103–10.
32. Herrmann W, Quast S, Wolter K, Eger S, Kiessig S, Hahmann H, Kreuter J, Molinari E. Determination of free Apo(a) in serum by immunoassay and its significance for risk assessment in patients with coronary artery disease. Clin Chem Lab Med. 1999;37:21–6.
33. Berg K, Dahlen G, Frick MH. Lp(a) lipoprotein and pre-beta1-lipoprotein in patients with coronary heart disease. Clin Genet. 1974;6:230–5.
34. Kostner GM, Avogaro P, Cazzolato G, Marth E, Bittolo-Bon G, Qunici GB. Lipoprotein Lp(a) and the risk for myocardial infarction. Atherosclerosis. 1981;38:51–61.
35. Von Eckardstein A, Schulte H, Cullen P, Assmann G. Lipoprotein(a) further increases the risk of coronary events in men with high global cardiovascular risk. J Am Coll Cardiol. 2001;37:434–9.
36. Ridker PM, Hennekens CA, Stampfer MJ. A prospective study of Lp(a) and the risk of myocardial infarction. JAMA. 1993;270:2195–9.
37. Tregouet DA, König IR, Jeanette Erdmann J. Genome-wide haplotype association study identifies the SLC22A3-LPAL2-LPA gene cluster as a risk locus for coronary artery disease. Nat Genet. 2009;41:283–5.
38. Kamstrup PR, Tybjaerg-Hansen A, Nordestgaard BG. Lipoprotein(a) and risk of myocardial infarction-genetic epidemiologic evidence of causality. Scand J Clin Lab Invest. 2011;71:87–93.
39. Erqou S, Thompson A, Di Angelantonio E, Saleheen D, Kaptoge S, Marcovina S, Danesh J. Apolipoprotein(a) isoforms and the risk of vascular disease: systematic review of 40 studies involving 58,000 participants. J Am Coll Cardiol. 2010;55: 2160–7.
40. Shindo J, Ishibashi T, Kijima M, Nakazato K, Nagata K, Yokoyama K, Hirosaka A, Sato E, Kunii H, Yamaguchi N, Watanabe N, Saito T, Maehara K, Maruyama Y. Increased plasminogen activator inhibitor-1 and apolipoprotein (a) in coronary atherectomy specimens in acute coronary syndromes. Coron Artery Dis. 2001;12:573–9.
41. Antonicelli R, Testa R, Bonfigli AR, Sirolla C, Pieri C, Marra M, Marcovina SM. Relationship between lipoprotein (a) levels, oxidative stress and blood pressure levels in patients with essential hypertension. Clin Exp Med. 2001;1:145–50.
42. Harpe P, Hermann A, Zhang X, Ostfeld I, Borth W. Lipoprotein (a), plasmin modulation and atherogenesis. Thromb Haemost. 1995;74:382–6.
43. Buechler C, Ullrich H, Ritter M, Porsch-Oezcueruemez M, Lackner KJ, Barlage S, Friedrich SO, Kostner GM, Schmitz G. Lipoprotein(a) upregulates the expression of the plasminogen activator inhibitor 2 in human blood monocytes. Blood. 2001;97:981–6.
44. Caplice NM, Panetta C, Peterson TE, Kleppe LS, Mueske CS, Kostner GM, Broze GJ, Simari RD. Lipoprotein(a) binds and inactivates tissue factor pathway inhibitor. A novel link between lipoproteins and thrombosis. Blood. 2001;98:2980–7.
45. Blencowe C, Hermetter A, Kostner GM, Deigner HP. Enhanced association of platelet activating factor acetylhydrolase with Lipoprotein(a) in comparison to Low Density Lipoprotein. J Biol Chem. 1995; 270:31151–7.
46. Haffner SM. Lipoprotein(a) and diabetes. Diabetes Care. 1993;16:835–40.

47. Kollerits B, Auinger M, Reisig V, Kästenbauer T, Lingenhel A, Irsigler K, Prager R, Kronenberg F. Lipoprotein(a) as a predictor of cardiovascular disease in a prospectively followed cohort of patients with type 1 diabetes. Diabetes Care. 2006;29:1661–3.
48. Shih DQ, Dansky HM, Fleisher M, Assmann G, Fajans SS. Genotype/phenotype relationships in HNF-4alpha/MODY1: haploinsufficiency is associated with reduced apolipoprotein (AII), apolipoprotein (CIII), lipoprotein(a), and triglyceride levels. Diabetes. 2000;49:832–7.
49. Mora S, Kamstrup PR, Rifai N, Nordestgaard BG, Buring JE, Ridker PM. Lipoprotein(a) and risk of type 2 diabetes. Clin Chem. 2010;56:1252–60.
50. Muller H, Lindman AS, Blomfeldt A, Seljeflot I, Pedersen JI. A diet rich in coconut oil reduces diurnal postprandial variations in circulating tissue plasminogen activator antigen and fasting lipoprotein (a) levels compared to a diet rich in unsaturated fat in women. J Nutr. 2003;133(11):3422–7.
51. Kostner GM, Gavish D, Leopold B, Bolzano K, Weintraub MS, Breslow JL. HMG CoA reductase inhibitors lower LDL cholesterol without reducing Lp(a) levels. Circulation. 1989;80(5):1313–9.
52. Van Wissen S, Smilde TJ, Trip MD, De Boo T, Kastelein JJ, Stalenhoef AF. Long term statin treatment reduces lipoprotein(a) concentrations in heterozygous FH. Heart. 2003;89:893–6.
53. Carlson LA, Hamsten A, Asplund A. Pronounced lowering of serum levels of Lp(a) in hyperlipidemic subjects with nicotinic acid. J Intern Med. 1989;226: 271–6.
54. Schlueter W, Keilani T, Batlle DC. Metabolic effects of ACE inhibitors: focus on the reduction of cholesterol and lipoprotein (a) by fosinopril. Am J Cardiol. 1993;72(20):37H–44.
55. Shewmon DA, Stock JL, Rosen CJ, Heiniluoma KM, Hogue MM, Morrison A, Doyle EM, Ukena T, Weale V, Baker S. Tamoxifen and estrogen lower circulating Lp(a) concentrations in healthy postmenopausal women. Arterioscler Thromb. 1994;14:1586–93.
56. Sbarouni E, Flevari P, Kroupis C, Kyriakides ZS, Koniavitou K, Kremastinos DT. The effects of raloxifene and simvastatin on plasma lipids and endothelium. Cardiovasc Drugs Ther. 2003;17(4): 319–23.
57. Derosa G, Cicero AF, Gaddi A, Muggelini A, Ciccarelli L, Fogari R. The effect of L-carnitine on plasma Lp(a) levels in hypercholesterolemic patients with type 2 diabetes mellitus. Clin Ther. 2003;25(5): 1429–39.
58. Kostner K. Aggressive therapie und kombinationstherapie von hypercholesterinämien. Wien Med Wochenschr. 1999;149(5–6):146–8.
59. Hoffmann U, Derfler K, Haas M, Stadler A, Brady TJ, Kostner K. Effects of combined Low-density lipoprotein apheresis and aggressive statin therapy on coronary calcified plaque as measured by computed tomography. Am J Cardiol. 2003;91:461–4.
60. Kastelein JJ, Wedel MK, Baker BF, et al. Potent reduction of apolipoprotein B and low-density lipoprotein cholesterol by short-term administration of an antisense inhibitor of apolipoprotein B. Circulation. 2006;114:1729–35.
61. Abifadel M, Varret M, Rabès JP, Allard D, Ouguerram K, Devillers M, Cruaud C, Benjannet S, Wickham L, Erlich D, Derré A, Villéger L, Farnier M, Beucler I, Bruckert E, Chambaz J, Chanu B, Lecerf JM, Luc G, Moulin P, Weissenbach J, Prat A, Krempf M, Junien C, Seidah NG, Boileau C. Mutations in PCSK9 cause autosomal dominant hypercholesterolemia. Nat Gene. 2003;34:154–6.

# Lipoprotein Glycation in Diabetes Mellitus

**8**

Alicia J. Jenkins, Richard L. Klein, and Andrzej S. Januszewski

## Introduction

The prevalence of both Type 1 and Type 2 diabetes mellitus is increasing in both developed and developing nations, and in spite of modern measures to control blood glucose, blood pressure, lipid levels, and thrombosis the vascular complications of diabetes affect large numbers of people and society as a whole [1]. Diabetes is conservatively associated with a two- to four-fold increased risk of coronary artery, cerebrovascular, and peripheral vascular disease [2]. Diabetes usually accounts for over a third of all patients with end stage renal disease (ESRD), and in the Western world is the most common cause of blindness in working age adults [2]. Over 60 % of people with diabetes will likely die of macrovascular disease [2, 3], which is particularly common in those subjects with microvascular damage, in particular diabetic nephropathy. Multiple genetic, biochemical and lifestyle risk factors are recognized, with hyperglycemia and dyslipidemia being major risk factors. These two factors independently have deleterious effects, but together they result in lipoprotein glycation, which can aggravate lipoprotein dysfunction. There is generally more circulating glycated LDL than oxidatively modified LDL, yet the literature has mainly focused on lipoprotein oxidation. There is relatively little research related to glycated lipoproteins. Either directly or indirectly via effects on metabolism, oxidation and inflammation, lipoprotein glycation has deleterious effects on lipoprotein function, thrombosis and cellular function in many tissues prone to the chronic sequelae of diabetes.

A.J. Jenkins, M.D., F.R.A.C.P. (✉)
Section of Endocrinology and Diabetes, University of Oklahoma Health Sciences Center, 941 Stanton L. Young Blvd., BSEB 302F, Oklahoma City, OK 73104, USA

NHMRC Clinical Trials Centre, University of Sydney, Sydney, NSW, Australia
e-mail: alicia-jenkins@ouhsc.edu

R.L. Klein
Division of Endocrinology, Diabetes, and Medical Genetics, Medical University of South Carolina, Charleston, SC, USA

A.S. Januszewski
Department of Medicine, The University of Melbourne, St. Vincent's Hospital, Melbourne, VIC, Australia

NHMRC Clinical Trials Centre, University of Sydney, Sydney, NSW, Australia

## Lipids and Lipoproteins in Diabetes

Dyslipidemia is a well-accepted risk factor for atherosclerosis in the diabetic and nondiabetic population and in both Type 1 and Type 2 diabetes is also a risk factor for diabetic retinopathy and nephropathy. As both *quantitative* and *qualitative* changes occur in lipoproteins and can affect lipoprotein related apolipoproteins and enzymes we prefer the more encompassing term of dyslipoproteinemia rather than dyslipidemia. Hyperglycemia and therefore dyslipoproteinemia, including lipoprotein glycation, also occurs in gestational diabetes and secondary forms of diabetes

A.J. Jenkins et al. (eds.), *Lipoproteins in Diabetes Mellitus*, Contemporary Diabetes,
DOI 10.1007/978-1-4614-7554-5_8, © Springer Science+Business Media New York 2014

(such as iatrogenic (corticosteroid-induced) diabetes or that secondary to pancreatitis or pancreatectomy), but research studies of lipoprotein glycation in these clinical settings are lacking [4].

In Type 2 diabetes there is a characteristic lipid profile with increased triglycerides, normal to high Low Density Lipoprotein (LDL)-cholesterol, and reduced High Density Lipoprotein (HDL)-cholesterol levels. In people with Type 1 diabetes with moderate to good glycemic control, normal renal function and the absence of other risk factors such as obesity, smoking or coexistent familial dyslipidemia, the lipid profile is relatively normal, but vascular disease is still accelerated [5, 6]. Even with good glycemic control, which in clinical practice can be difficult to achieve, and with good lipid control, which often requires pharmacologic intervention, discussed elsewhere in this book, residual vascular risk often remains in diabetic patients. Residual risk is the remaining risk of vascular damage after optimal control of the known risk factors, such as related to glycemia, blood pressure, and the traditional lipid profile. Many factors may be contributory to residual risk, including qualitative changes in lipoproteins such as post-translational lipoprotein glycation. Other subtle lipoprotein abnormalities, such as oxidation, which can occur concurrently with glycation, alterations in lipoprotein composition, size and immunogenicity, which are also discussed in other chapters in this book, may also contribute [4, 7].

Adverse biological effects of lipoprotein glycation may be direct, and/or indirect via modulating coagulation, fibrinolysis, vascular tone, matrix binding, inflammation, altered susceptibility to oxidation and cellular and tissue responses, including angiogenesis.

## The Chemistry of Lipoprotein Glycation

The glycation process can be divided into early and late glycation, summarized in Fig. 8.1.

In 1912 French food chemist Loius C. Maillard first described the formation of brown-colored substances from non-enzymatic reactions between reducing sugars and proteins [8], and such reactions are also relevant to the human body. A simplified view of the chemistry is that carbonyl groups and amino groups react to form Schiff bases and then Amadori compounds, (early glycation products), which are potentially reversible. Early glycation product formation may be followed by irreversible dehydration, condensation, and cross-linking reactions, resulting in a large, and likely incompletely known heterogeneous family of derivatives termed Advanced Glycation End-Products (AGEs). AGEs are also known as late glycation products, Maillard products, or glycoxidation products (as formation of many AGEs involves oxidative chemistry, see Fig. 8.2) [9]. Similar reactions can occur, by both enzymatic and non-enzymatic pathways, without glucose, providing the non-glucose materials contain an aldehyde group. Reactive metabolites such as the dicarbonyls (methylglyoxal (MG), glyoxal, and 3-deoxyglucosone (3DG)) from the glycolysis pathway, and from the metabolism of lipids and ketones can also interact with protein residues to form AGEs, including in lipoproteins [10]. Increased production of reactive dicarbonyls or their reduced detoxification by the glyoxalase system or by endogenous scavengers leads to increased carbonyl stress, which is a major driving force for AGE formation and accumulation [11]. AGE formation occurs in many extracellular and intracellular proteins, including lipoproteins, and AGEs are present in all people. AGE levels in long-lived tissues, such as skin, usually increase with chronologic age [12]. AGE formation is accelerated by hyperglycemia as in diabetes [13] and also by renal impairment, even in the non-diabetic milieu [14].

AGEs are chemically heterogeneous groups of both fluorescent and nonfluorescent compounds with over 25 fully characterized AGE structures [15]. The (type and concentration) of glycation products formed depends on both the range and concentration of substrates available and the duration of their interaction. Nε-carboxymethyl-lysine (CML) is the simplest and best characterized AGE and the main epitope for many commercially available antibodies used for AGE detection and quantification. Many of these products such as CML (thought to be the most abundant AGE in vivo), pentosidine, and erythronic acid

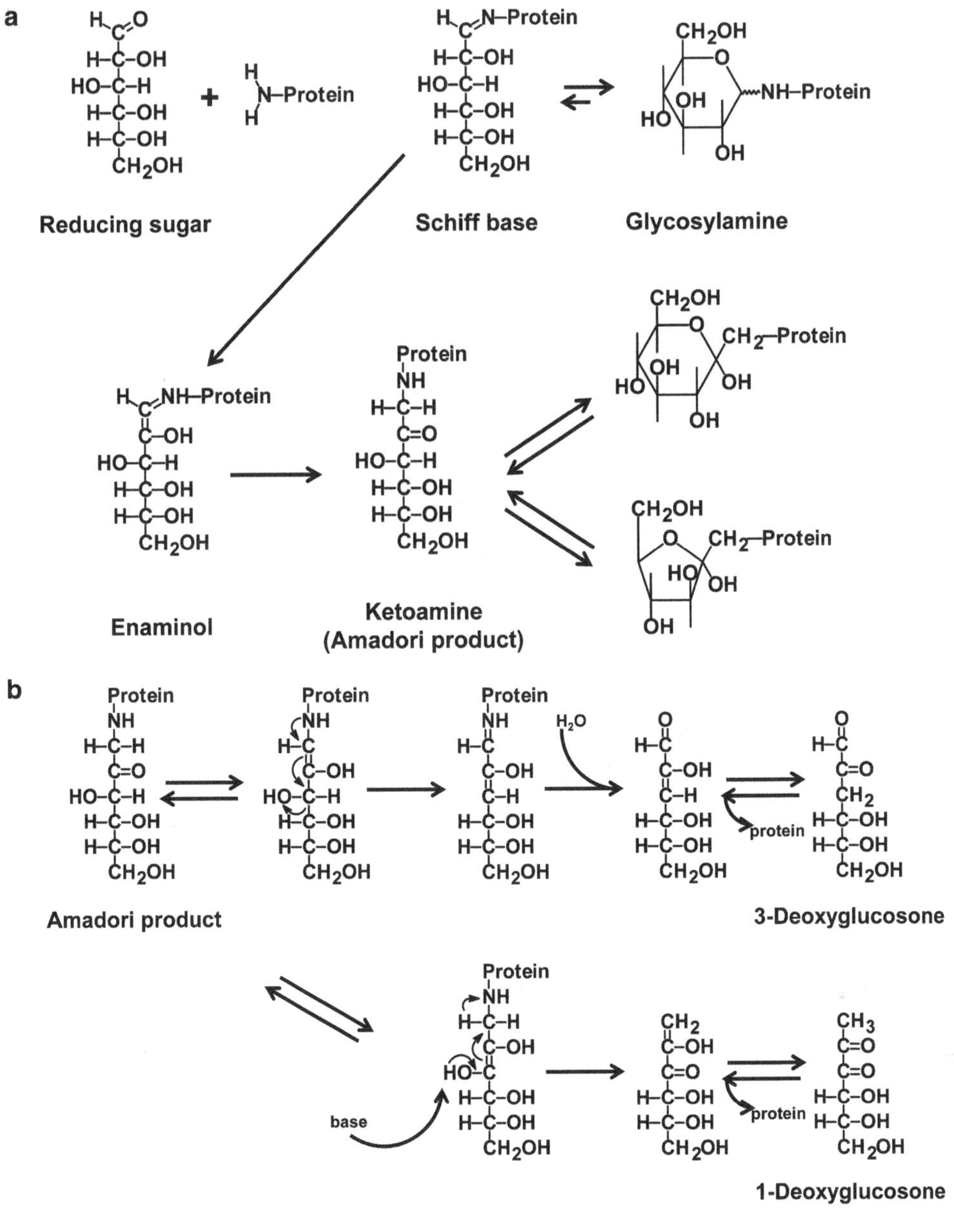


**Fig. 8.1** Biochemistry of early and late glycation. (**a**) Early steps of the Maillard reaction. The reducing sugars in open chain form reacting an amino groups on proteins to form a reversible Schiff base. The Schiff base then form a cyclic glycosylamine or can rearrange to an enaminol and then to a ketoamine (Amadori compound). The Amadori compound is also stabilized by its cyclization to a furanose or pyranose ring. (**b**) The Amadori compound fructoselysine can undergo decomposition to form both 1- and 3-deoxyglucosone (1-DG and 3-DG). 3-DG is more reactive than glucose in the formation of AGEs. (**c**) Various pathways leading to the formation of AGEs. The Maillard pathway involves the reaction of a reducing sugar with an amine on a protein to form a ketoamine, which can break down to form AGEs. Alternatively, the autoxidation of glucose forms reactive compounds like arabinose and glyoxal that can further react with amino groups and form AGEs (Wolff pathway). The Schiff base intermediate can also form reactive carbonyl compounds under oxidizing conditions and can also react with an amine leading to AGE formation (Namiki pathway). Lastly, the ketoamine, under both oxidative and non-oxidative conditions, can fragment to form reactive deoxyosones that can form AGEs (Hodge pathway). Reproduced with modifications from: J.W. Baynes, "The role of AGEs in aging: causation or correlation", Exp. Gerontol. (2001) 36(9), 1527–1537

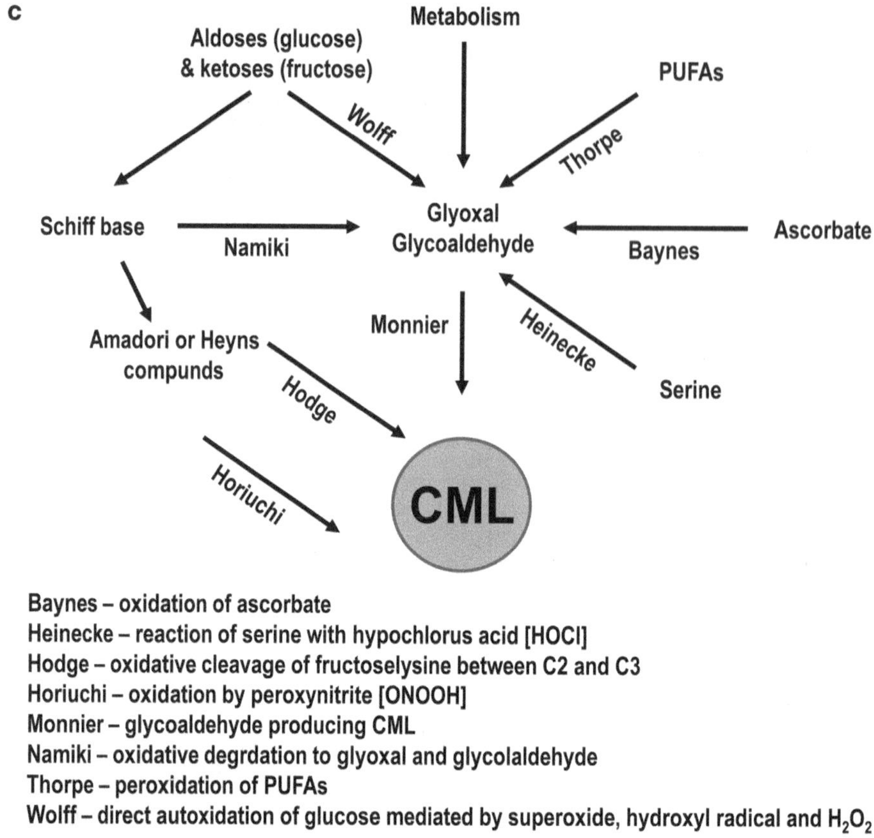


**Fig. 8.1** (continued)

are formed oxidatively [16]. Non-oxidatively derived AGEs such as the imidazolones and pyrraline have also been identified and characterized [17, 18]. Pyrraline is formed by the reaction of 3-deoxyglucasone with lysine, and imidazolone-type AGEs are formed by the reaction of 3-deoxyglucasone with arginine. The value of each specific AGE, or group of AGEs, as a marker or mediator of diabetic microvascular and macrovascular damage is not fully elucidated.

AGEs can also be derived exogenously, such as from the diet and smoking [19–21]. Dietary AGEs, which are abundant in foods such as (all as per 100 g of product) fried pork bacon, roast chicken skin, sesame oil, parmesan cheese, sweet butter cream, pan fried beef or pizza [22]. AGEs in food are partially absorbed from the gastrointestinal tract, and approximately two-thirds are thought to remain in contact with tissues for several days, whereas the rest is rapidly excreted by the kidneys [23]. AGE restriction in mice, without energy or nutrient change, alleviates inflammation, prevents vascular complications, and extends their normal life span [24]. Human studies have showed that a low-AGE diet reduces inflammatory markers (C-reactive protein (CRP), Tumor Necrosis Factor alpha (TNFα)) and vascular cell adhesion molecule (VCAM-1) levels [25]. In Type 2 diabetes high-AGE meals have been shown to acutely impair vascular reactivity as measured by flow mediated dilation (FMD) [26]. HDL does suppress TNF-α induced VCAM-1 suppression in vitro, but it is not known how much of the low AGE diet benefit, in animals or in humans, relates to effects on AGE modified lipoproteins.

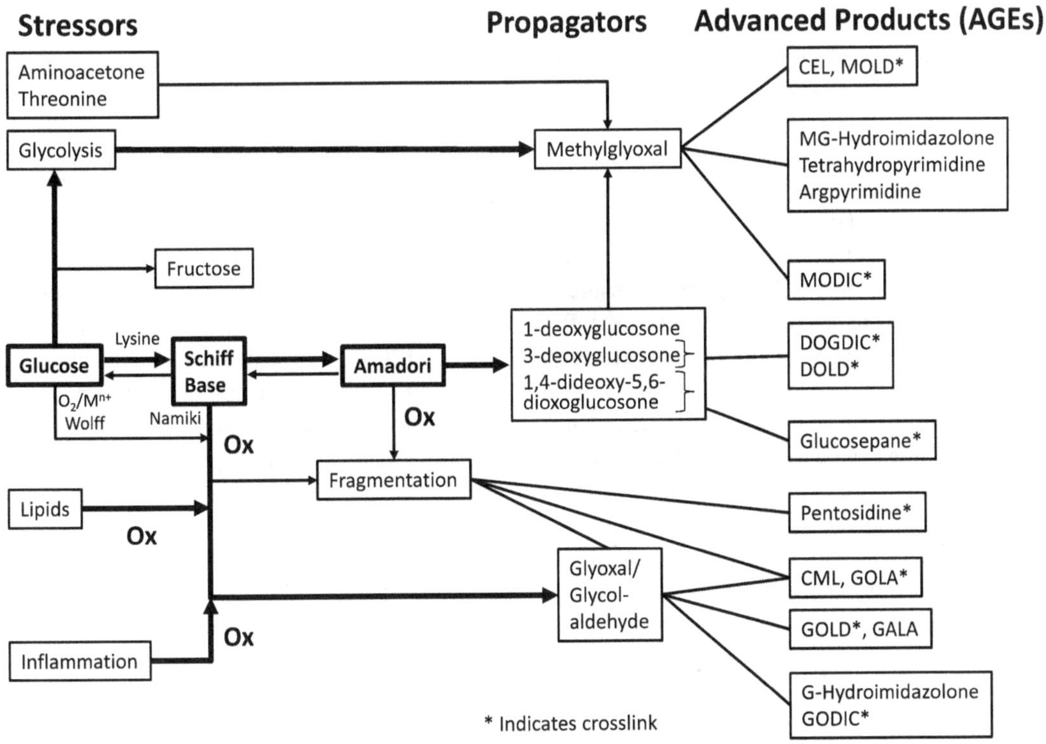


**Fig. 8.2** Factors affecting AGEs formation and accumulation. Reproduced from: V.M. Monnier and X. Wu, "Enzymatic deglycation with amadoriase enzymes from Aspergillus sp. as a potential strategy against the complications of diabetes and aging" Biochem. Soc. Trans. (2003) 31, 1349–1353

## Differences Between Glycation and Glycosylation

The term "glycation" refers to non-enzymatic reactions between amino acid residues of proteins and reducing sugars. Glycosylation is a different set of usually enzymatic chemical reactions. Glycosylation is a major post-translational modification of both intracellular and extracellular proteins. Most intracellular proteins in humans contain sugars and are also known as glycoconjugates. Depending on the nature of the covalent attachment glycosylated proteins can be divided into glycoproteins (in which the major component is a protein) and proteoglycans (in which typically >95 % mass is a carbohydrate). Glycoproteins are an integral part of plasma membranes, and serve important functions such as hormones, receptors and mediators in intercellular interactions. Proteoglycans are major components of the extra cellular matrix (ECM) [27]. These ECM proteins can also become modified by (early and late) glycation, which is discussed elsewhere in this book.

## Glycation of Apolipoproteins in Lipoproteins

Within lipoproteins apolipoproteins are major sites of glycation. Theoretically any amino compound with at least one hydrogen atom on its nitrogen can participate in the Maillard reaction. Chemically, within a protein moiety only amino acids with one or more nucleophilic residues (lysine (Lys), arginine (Arg), cysteine (Cys), methionine (Met), and histidine (His)) are likely to become glycated. Although the amino acid cysteine is the strongest nucleophile, Lys residues are particularly abundant in apolipoproteins [28] and thus are the preferred site of glycation. For example, ApoA-I, found in HDL, contains 243 amino acids residues, including three Met, 21 Lys, five His, and 16 Arg residues, but no Cys residues. ApoB-100, found in VLDL, LDL, and Lp(a), contains 4,563 amino acids residues: 79 Met, 356 Lys, 114 His, 150 Arg, and only 25 Cys (0.5 %). The extent of lipoprotein glycation will depend on (1) the time of lipoprotein exposure to the glycating agent, which may in turn be influenced by the location of the lipoprotein being glycated (e.g., intra- or extravascular); (2) the concentration of glycating agent; (3) the potency of the glycating agent; and (4) the efficacy of any deglycating or anti-glycating factors. The nature of the glycating agent determines the type of glycation products formed. For example protein glycation with glucose leads to the formation of the late glycation produce CML, whereas protein glycation with methylglyoxal results in formation of CEL [29]. In humans the major circulating glycating agent is glucose in an open chain form [27]. Circulating levels of glucose in non-diabetic subjects averaging at 5 mmol/l whilst that of methylglyoxal is 147 nmol/l [30], in addition several glycating agents may act on amino acids (in both the extracellular and intracellular milieu).

## Extent of Lipoprotein Glycation

The extent of lipoprotein glycation usually correlates with other measures of glycemia such as HbA1c and fructosamine [4, 31, 32]. Any inconsistencies may relate to differences in half-lives of the glycated protein moieties, methodologies for the quantification of lipoprotein glycation (discussed below) and the range of glycemia related values in the study group. The half-life of lipoproteins is days, whilst HbA1c from within red blood cells, reflects glycemia over the previous 2–3 months, hence it is probable that the extent of lipoprotein glycation is more strongly correlated with shorter term measures of glycemia over days, such as mean glucose levels (perhaps measured by Continuous (Interstitial Fluid) Glucose Monitoring or blood glucose monitoring), or 1,5 anhydroglucitol levels [33], but such a comparative studies are not yet available.

## The Measurement of Lipoprotein Glycation

The quantification of glycated lipoproteins is currently a research laboratory tool. Various techniques have been used, and have been predominantly applied to LDL and HDL. The most specific measure is the direct quantification of *fructoselysine* (an early glycation product) in lipoproteins by High Pressure Liquid Chromatography (HPLC) [34], which requires the physical separation of lipoproteins by ultracentrifugation. We have utilized this technique to study lipoproteins from diabetes patients [35, 36].

Glycated proteins, such as albumin, and glycated lipoproteins bind to boronate, so *boronate affinity chromatography* has been used in both a preparative manner [37] and in a rapid relatively simple HPLC and gel permeation column based assay, developed by Tanaka et al. [38] which has been used to quantify glycated LDL and HDL from low volumes (5 $\mu$l) of serum.

*Antibodies to glycated apoB* have also been developed and used in in-house ELISA assays [39] and in a commercially available indirect competitive ELISA (Glyacor, Exocell, Philadel-phia, PA). A monoclonal antibody (ES12) is directed against a specific epitope in apoB in glycated LDL and does not cross-react with other human plasma proteins including non-glycated LDL. The assay range is 3–40 $\mu$g/ml (corresponding to 0.3–4 mg/dl) in serum. Other antibodies have also been used to quantify glycated HDL and glycated Lp(a) [40].

Unlike purely glycated unoxidized lipoproteins AGE modified lipoproteins have increased electrophoretic mobility [41], a technique usually used for the characterization of physically separated isolated lipoproteins. AGEs can also be quantified by Gas Chromatography/Mass Spectroscopy (GC/MS) [42] in separated lipoproteins. An AGE-LDL antibody based capture assay has also been developed [43] and used to quantify AGE-LDL in Type 1 diabetes.

A less specific biochemical tool to measure the extent of lipoprotein glycation is the TNBS (trinitrobenzene sulfonic acid) assay [44]. The TNBS assay measures the amount of free Lys in a protein. As mentioned earlier Lys is the most abundant amino group in human lipoproteins and is a strong nucleophile (Lys is the only one amino acid with two amino groups: alpha and epsilon). Unfortunately, due to the secondary and tertiary structure of proteins not all Lys residues (regardless of whether free or modified) are always available for reaction and therefore detection by the TNBS assay.

The development and validation of low cost high throughput assays of lipoprotein glycation would expedite this area of clinical research.

## General Consequences of Lipoprotein Glycation

The potential consequences of increased lipoprotein glycation are summarized in Table 8.1. These include effects on lipoprotein metabolism (such as on their half-life in the circulation) and on cell interactions and responses, including effects related to important processes (e.g., inflammation, thrombosis, vasoreactivity) relevant to the vascular complications of diabetes. Lipoproteins modified by glycation and by oxidation and extravasated are more likely to bind to vascular matrix, such as proteoglycans, than unmodified lipoproteins [45]. Tsmikas et al. demonstrated that the concentration of oxidized LDL in the arterial wall is 70-fold that in the circulation [46], but we are not aware of similar studies related to glycated lipoproteins. Matrix binding of lipoproteins is discussed in more detail in another chapter.

**Table 8.1** Adverse effects of lipoprotein glycation

| |
|---|
| Effects on circulating half-life of lipoproteins |
| Foam cell formation |
| Increased matrix binding |
| Pro-oxidant and reduction of antioxidant effects |
| Pro-inflammatory or reduced anti-inflammatory effects |
| Pro-thrombotic effects |
| Pro-apoptotic effects |
| Effects on lipoprotein related enzyme activities |
| Altered lipoprotein receptor interactions |
| Cell signaling effects |
| Effects on gene expression |
| Promotion of antibody and immune complex formation |
| Altered reactivity in assays |

It is important to recognize that even normoglycemic people have some lipoproteins that undergo glycation, and that more extensively modified (late glycation or AGE modified) lipoproteins, may not remain in the circulation very long. Indeed AGE-modified lipoproteins are likely to exist predominantly outside the potent antioxidant milieu of blood in the extravascular spaces (of arteries, the retina, and renal beds), being rapidly removed from the circulation by pathways such as scavenger receptors in liver and in white blood cells. Antioxidants in blood include albumin, urate, bilirubin, and vitamin C [47], all of which are water soluble. Some fat soluble vitamins, which can be carried within the lipoproteins (e.g., Vitamin E) are also antioxidants [48]. The low concentrations of modified lipoproteins in the circulation (relative to unmodified lipoproteins) may reflect both that formed within blood and that has effluxed from the extravascular bed.

Another challenge in this area of research is that in vitro modified lipoproteins studied in the laboratory setting may be differentially or more extensively modified than that occurring in vivo. Often the glucose or reactive intermediate (e.g., methylglyoxal) concentrations and incubation times used in the laboratory are well beyond that present in people. Later in this chapter we will point out some studies in which both in vivo and in vitro glycated lipoproteins were studied, with divergent responses.

In the literature related to in vitro modified lipoproteins the term glycation is often used loosely, not specifying if it is early or late glycation. The effects of early glycation and late glycation often differ. For example, in in vitro studies of modified LDL on cultured retinal or renal cells by Lyons et al. both LDL modified by early glycation (glycated LDL) and LDL modified by late glycation (Heavily oxidized glycated LDL (HOG-LDL)) have been studied. HOG-LDL effects were generally significantly greater than that of less extensively modified glycated LDL [49–52]. Ideally researchers should present data related to the preparation and characterization of the modified lipoproteins they have studied. The in vitro modification of lipoproteins by early glycation alone requires the presence of metal chelating antioxidants, such as EDTA and DTPA in adequate concentrations and reduced exposure to oxygen such as may be achieved by incubation under nitrogen or argon and dialysis against nitrogen purged buffers [7]. In general, if there is increased electrophoretic mobility of lipoproteins on agarose gels, or increased AGEs or lack of recognition of modified LDL by the classical LDL receptor, then the glycation is more advanced (late glycation).

Whilst in vivo studies, including longitudinal human or animal studies, can also be informative as to the effects of lipoprotein glycation, we must evaluate their findings whilst also recognizing that improved glycemic control may use lifestyle changes and drugs which may have direct effects on lipoprotein related gene or protein expression or other pleiotropic effects, and that more than just glycemia (and lipoprotein glycation) may change. Some of the particularly relevant sites of change, such as within the vascular wall, in the retina or within glomeruli or renal tubules, may not be accessible for sampling, particularly in living humans.

## Human Studies of Glycated Lipoproteins

Glycated lipoproteins, particularly those modified by early glycation, are present in the circulation of both non-diabetic and diabetic people at relatively high concentrations [53, 54] Durrington et al. have demonstrated that circulating levels of glycated apoB (which may reflect glycated apolipoprotein B within LDL, VLDL, Lp(a), and chylomicrons) are increased in primary conditions in which LDL is raised, such as heterozygous familial hypercholesterolemia. As with hyperglycemia itself, the hallmark of diabetes mellitus, enhanced lipoprotein glycation occurs from diabetes onset, and likely reflects both an increase in the number of glycated amino acids per lipoprotein particle and also a greater proportion of lipoprotein particles with glycated residues. Based on our studies of in vivo glycated LDL as assessed by boronate affinity chromatography, in non-diabetic subjects approximately 5 % of LDL particles are sufficiently glycated to bind to these columns (and have increased fructoselysine levels) whereas in people with diabetes (depending on their level of glycemic control) up to 25 % of LDL may bind [35, 37]. Even within an individual the extent of glycation of lipoproteins will likely vary, in the same way that not all LDL, HDL or VLDL particles are the same size [55, 56]. At any given time the circulating lipoproteins will include some that are newly secreted, hence are likely to be less glycated, and lipoproteins that are several days older, hence more likely to be more glycated. Ambient glucose levels and lipoprotein size, apolipoprotein content and chemical composition are also likely to affect the extent of lipoprotein glycation. For example, Durrington et al. demonstrated that small LDL is more likely to undergo in vitro glycation than larger LDL [54].

## Glycation of Specific Major Lipoprotein Classes

### VLDL Glycation

Whilst hypertriglyceridemia is common in people with Type 2 diabetes and in those with Type 1 diabetes and poor glycemic control, obesity or renal damage there are few studies of VLDL glycation.

#### Levels of Glycated VLDL

Using a simple and non-specific agarose gel electrophoresis assay for glycated lipoproteins in sera from diabetic and non-diabetic subjects levels of glycated VLDL were estimated to be fourfold higher in diabetes subjects and higher in diabetic patients with vs. without clinically evident atherosclerosis [57].

#### Effects on Lipoprotein Metabolism

Hypertriglyceridemia may relate to both increased hepatic VLDL production and delayed VLDL clearance. In keeping, in in vivo VLDL kinetic studies in rodents the clearance of triglyceride and apoB of in vitro glycated VLDL was slower than that from normal VLDL. and in in vitro studies the glycated VLDL was a poorer substrate for lipoprotein lipase [58].

There are several studies comparing VLDL from diabetic subjects and non-diabetic subjects which demonstrate that VLDL from people with Type 1 and Type 2 diabetes has a different lipid and apolipoprotein content from that of non-diabetic subjects, and within the same Type 1 or Type 2 diabetic patient can differ when their glycemic control is poor vs. improved, and is associated with increased rates of cholesteryl ester synthesis by human monocyte derived macrophages [59–61] and endothelial cells [59–62]. Levels of or the extent of VLDL glycation were not quantified in these studies of modified VLDL.

## LDL Glycation

Studies of LDL glycation are more numerous than those of other lipoprotein fractions, likely because LDL is highly atherogenic, especially when modified, and is usually the most abundant lipoprotein in blood and in atherosclerotic plaque.

### Levels of Glycation

Relative to non-diabetic people the levels of glycated LDL are increased (by approximately 50 % to several fold) in Type 1 and Type 2 diabetes subjects, and usually correlate with other measures of glycemia or with LDL-C levels, two required substrates for LDL glycation [39, 55, 63–65]. In Type 2 diabetes patients levels of AGE-LDL were also elevated (about three-fold) relative to non-diabetic subjects, and were lower in diabetic patients taking metformin than in those not on metformin [65]. Levels of circulating glycated LDL have been found to be higher in Type 2 diabetic patients fed a high AGE diet than in low AGE diet fed diabetic patients and non-diabetic subjects [66].

### LDL Size and Glycation

Small dense LDL is more atherogenic than larger more buoyant LDL particles [4]. There are divergent results from studies relating LDL size and LDL glycation. Glycated LDL (in the absence of LDL antibodies) has a longer residence time in the circulation [67], thus may be smaller due to further lipolysis and lipid exchange. By evaluating in vivo modified and in vitro glycated LDL particles some studies have suggested that small dense LDL is more susceptible to glycation [54, 68]. Isolated LDL modified in vitro with methylgloxal to form AGE-LDL was also significantly smaller than the native LDL [69]. However, in Type 1 diabetic patients, using NMR spectroscopy we found no significant difference in the size of in vivo glycated and relatively non-glycated LDL separated by boronate affinity chromatography [35].

### Susceptibility to Oxidation

Oxidized LDL is more pathogenic than unmodified (native) LDL. Results of studies of the effects of LDL glycation on LDL's susceptibility to oxidation are divergent, perhaps related to differences between in vivo and in vitro modification, the type, concentration and exposure time to the pro-oxidant, and the assays used to quantify oxidation. Tsai et al. demonstrated increased susceptibility of LDL from Type 1 diabetic patients with poor glycemic control to in vitro (copper-induced) oxidation [70]. This was not so in our study of complication-free Type 1 diabetic subjects with relatively good glycemic control [71]. We also determined the in vitro susceptibility to copper induced oxidation of relatively glycated LDL (G-LDL) and relatively non-glycated LDL (G-LDL) prepared by boronate affinity chromatography from 13 subjects with Type 1 diabetes. Lipid soluble antioxidant levels did not differ between the two subfractions, in keeping with a lack of increased oxidative stress to G-LDL in plasma. The lag time to oxidation of the G-LDL was significantly less than that of the non-glycated LDL subfraction. There were no significant differences in the rate of or extent of lipid oxidation during the reaction, nor did the lag time, rate or extent of protein oxidation of the two LDL subfractions differ [35]. In cross-sectional analyses of the Diabetes Control and Complications Trial/Epidemiology of Diabetes Interventions and Complications (DCCT/EDIC) cohort we did not observe any statistically significant relationship between LDL susceptibility to lipid or protein oxidation and HbA1c and severity of nephropathy or retinopathy [72].

### Glycated LDL and Immune Complex Formation

Antibodies to, and immune complexes with, modified lipoproteins such as glycated and

AGE-modified LDL are implicated in human vascular damage. Modified lipoproteins themselves are pro-inflammatory, but when in immune complexes they are even more pathogenic. Such immune complexes can increase foam cell formation and have pro-inflammatory effects, features of microvascular complications as well as atherosclerosis [73]. In Type 1 diabetes subjects of the DCCT/EDIC cohort levels of AGE-LDL in circulating immune complexes are associated with and predict progression of carotid intima-media thickness [74], and also predict progression of diabetic retinopathy [75].

## Matrix Binding

Lipoprotein matrix interactions, also discussed in another book chapter, may promote atherosclerosis and may also accelerate diabetic nephropathy by binding to glomerular matrix and affecting renal cell signaling [76]. Matrix binding and retention of LDL and of glycated and/or oxidized LDL is thought to increase LDL's likelihood of further modification by glycation, oxidation and AGE formation.

In vitro generated AGE-LDL has been found to be smaller and to bind more avidly to proteoglycans [69]. Using an in vitro model system of binding to arterial wall proteoglycans Edwards et al. demonstrated that improved glycemic control in Type 2 diabetes patients reduced LDL proteoglycan binding, even in the absence of significant improvements in lipid levels. LDL glycation (fructosamine) was the only LDL compositional variable that correlated ($r=0.95$) with the proteoglycan binding [77].

## Effects on Receptor Interactions and Cell Signaling

Lipoprotein glycation can change LDL's cell-based receptors and responsive cell signaling pathways in cells relevant to the vascular complications of diabetes. In general LDL modified by early glycation can still interact with the classical LDL receptor on cells, as does unmodified (native) LDL, but with increasing degrees of glycation major pathways of cellular uptake are via scavenger receptors, the Receptor for AGEs (RAGE), and by endocytosis [49, 78–80].

Glycated-LDL was isolated from diabetic patients and from non-diabetic subjects. In cultured human fibroblasts, which express only the classical LDL receptor the rates of receptor-mediated accumulation of relatively non-glycated LDL from both subject groups were greater than those of glycated-LDL. In contrast, when incubated with human monocyte-derived macrophages, the rates of receptor-mediated accumulation of glycated-LDL from both groups were significantly greater than those of non-glycated-LDL [37].

We exposed cultured rat mesangial cells to native LDL or to LDL modified (in vitro) by early glycation or by extensive oxidation and glycation (AGE-LDL). Glycated LDL was taken up via the classical LDL receptor, induced a transient intracellular calcium spike and marked extracellular signal–regulated protein kinase (ERK) activation. AGE-LDL, recognized by the scavenger receptor, induced a sustained rise in intracellular calcium and less marked ERK activation [49]. In cultured human vascular smooth muscle cells relative to native LDL AGE-LDL significantly increased protein and/or gene expression of receptors for modified LDL and AGE proteins (LRP1, CD36 and RAGE), which was associated with adverse cellular responses related to oxidative stress and cell proliferation [79].

## Adverse Cellular Effects

Early and late glycation of LDL has been demonstrated to have many adverse cellular effects which may promote macro- and microvascular damage in diabetes. Most studies involve cultured monocytes, or arterial, retinal and glomerular cells exposed to in vivo or in vitro glycated LDL. Adverse cellular responses include foam cell formation, cell proliferation or death (commonly by apoptosis), matrix overproduction (of particular relevance to glomerulosclerosis), pro-inflammatory effects and (discussed in subsequent sections in this chapter) impaired vasorelaxation and pro-thrombotic effects.

Macrophages are implicated in atherosclerosis and also in diabetic microvascular damage. Lopes-Virella et al. demonstrated than human monocyte derived macrophage had increased cholesteryl ester accumulation when exposed to in vivo modified LDL from diabetic subjects, or to in vitro glycated LDL [31, 36]. Several groups demonstrated increased cholesterol uptake and cholesteryl ester accumulation by macrophages in response to glycated LDL, with greater effects of more extensively modified LDL, such as AGE-LDL generated by glycoaldehyde [80–82].

In cultured human vascular endothelial cells (HUVEC) in vivo and in vitro glycated LDL can induce apoptosis [83] and in vitro generated AGE-LDL can increase expression of monocyte chemoattractant protein (MCP) [84], which may also promote atheroma. AGE-LDL induced MCP-1 expression in cultured human endothelial cells has been demonstrated to be ameliorated by the PPARα agonist lipid drug fenofibrate, and by the anti-platelet agent dilazep, both of which suppressed the AGE-LDL induction of NFκB [85].

With regard to cultured microvascular cells, Lyons et al. demonstrated reduced cell viability of retinal capillary cells after exposure to in vitro glycated vs. native LDL [86] and reduction in this cytotoxicity by LDL glycation in the presence of the AGE inhibitor aminoguanidine [87].

Whilst we found that glycated LDL did not reduce mesangial cell viability, it increased mesangial cell TGFβ mRNA expression and induced hemeoxygenase-1 (HO-1) expression, an intracellular marker of oxidative stress (personal communication A Jenkins). Others have demonstrated altered mesangial cell modified LDL binding and increased matrix (e.g., fibronectin and laminin) production by cultured mesangial cells exposed to glycated LDL than to native LDL [76, 88–91]. These changes may promote glomerulosclerosis, a major feature of diabetic nephropathy.

### Effects on Modulators of Fibrinolysis

Exposure of cultured human vascular endothelial cells to in vitro glycated LDL increases PAI-1 production [92, 93]. This process is via activation of the PAI promotor [94] and involves the Golgi apparatus [95] and RAGE [96], and decreases generation of tissue plasminogen activator (tPA) [93]. In contrast, using in vivo modified LDL from Type 1 diabetic subjects separated by boronate affinity chromatography into glycated and relatively non-glycated LDL subfractions PAI-1 and tPA production by human aortic endothelial cells exposed did not differ significantly [35]. The different responses may relate to different extents of LDL glycation and cell types.

### Effects on Platelet Reactivity

Platelet hyperactivation is a common feature of diabetes and may promote thromboses in both large and small vessels. LDL that was AGE modified in vitro and LDL from Type 2 diabetic patients with poor glycemic control stimulated platelet p38MAPK phosphorylation and thromboxane B2 production [97].

Another group demonstrated that relative to native LDL in vitro glycated LDL increased platelet TBARS levels (a measure of oxidative damage), NO production, intracellular calcium levels, and ADP-induced aggregation [98].

### Effects on Vasoreactivity

Glycated LDL can also impair vascular reactivity. Whilst early glycation of LDL (without oxidation) had no effect on aortic ring acetylcholine-induced endothelium dependent relaxation AGE-modified LDL attenuated their vasorelaxation to an even greater extent than Ox-LDL [99]. In keeping with these results, AGE-LDL impaired acetylcholine-induced endothelium-dependent vasorelaxation of isolated mouse aortas, which was prevented by pharmacological inhibition of calpain. Exposure of bovine aortic endothelial cells to this same type of AGE-LDL reduced eNOS protein levels in a dose and time-dependent manner, without altering eNOS mRNA levels, increased intracellular calcium and reactive oxygen species production [100].

In cultured porcine aortic endothelial cells exposed to in vivo glycated LDL and relatively non-glycated LDL from diabetic and non-diabetic subjects (separated by boronate affinity chromatography) the glycated LDL increased superoxide release by five-fold relative to the non-glycated LDL [101].

Both in vivo modified LDL from diabetic patients and in vitro glycated LDL caused vasoconstriction of arterioles in skeletal muscle of living mice [102], in keeping with similar adverse effects on vascular tone in the microvasculature.

## HDL Glycation

Glycation of HDL in diabetes may ameliorate the efficacy of some of HDL's vasoprotective functions, which include reverse cholesterol transport, antioxidant, anti-inflammatory, anti-thrombotic, and vasodilatory effects. As with other lipoprotein subclasses, there is an admixture of studies using in vivo and in vitro modified HDL, and some studies of in vitro modified HDL use glycating agent concentrations or incubation times which may not occur in vivo.

### Levels of Glycated HDL

Relative to that in non-diabetic subjects the level of glycation of HDL is increased about four-fold in people with Type 1 or Type 2 diabetes and correlates with other measures of glycemic control. Whilst all HDL associated apolipoproteins are glycated, about 80 % of HDL glycation is located on ApoA1. In in vitro studies for any given glucose concentration the extent of apoA1 glycation was significantly greater in the presence of phospholipids [103].

*Antioxidant effects* of HDL can be assessed by measuring the susceptibility to oxidation and also the efficacy of HDL in breaking down preformed lipid peroxides. Oxidation is implicated in the formation of late glycation (AGE) products, which also occur in HDL. The literature is divergent as to the effects of HDL glycation of its susceptibility to oxidation, which may relate to different oxidation techniques and measures of oxidation.

Using 50 mM D-glucose, aluminum, and iron, one group demonstrated increased oxidative damage in HDL [104], whilst another group found that glycated HDL was less, not more susceptible to in vitro oxidation by copper based on a xylenol orange assay, with no difference in levels of induced conjugated dienes or thiobarbituric acid reactive substances (TBARS) [105].

In Type 2 diabetic patients with diabetic nephropathy serum AGE levels were increased and isolated (in vivo modified) HDL was less effective than that from nondiabetic subjects in protecting against ex vivo LDL oxidation (induced by DCFH), however the extent of HDL glycation was not reported [106].

Using in vivo and in vitro modified HDL and oxidized red blood cell (RBC) membranes we found that the efficacy of HDL to remove preformed lipid peroxides (LPO) from RBC membranes was significantly impaired with HDL from complication-free Type 1 diabetes patients relative to healthy subjects. We did not quantify HDL glycation, but relative to unmodified HDL in vitro glycated HDL from non-diabetic subjects did not have impaired LPO removal efficacy, whilst AGE-modified HDL did, suggesting that late but not early glycation may be deleterious [107]. In a similar model system HDL from Type 2 diabetes patients with in vivo glycated paraxonase-1 (PON-1) was less able to break down preformed LPO, with in vitro AGE modification having greater function effects on this HDL function than in vitro HDL glycation [108].

### Effects on Modulators of Fibrinolysis

In people with diabetes circulating levels of PAI-1 are often increased, and in cultured vascular endothelial cells Shen et al. demonstrated that glycated HDL increased HUVEC PAI-1 production, whilst unmodified HDL had no effect. Neither native nor glycated HDL altered endothelial cell tPA production [93, 94]; however, in HUVEC cell culture the effects of HDL from non-diabetic and diabetic patients on tPA or PAI-1 production were similar. If HDL glycation has such an effect in vivo this could promote thrombosis.

### Effects on Vasoreactivity

HDL can have vasodilatory effects. In a rabbit aortic ring model HDL from Type 1 diabetic patients could not attenuate the inhibitory effects of Oxidized LDL on endothelial dependent vasodilatation as well as HDL from non-diabetic subjects. However, this effect was not correlated with HDL-fructosamine levels (reflecting HDL glycation) or other systemic measures of glycemia [109].

### Reverse Cholesterol Transport

The transport of cholesterol from cells to HDL is one of the more well-known functions of HDL. Results of studies related to the effects of HDL glycation are divergent, which again may reflect the extent of HDL glycation and the model systems used.

In general reverse cholesterol transport is thought to be impaired in people with Type 2 diabetes and in mouse models, but some investigators have reported greater cholesterol efflux with Type 2 diabetic HDL than non-diabtetic HDL, but no measures of HDL glycation were reported [110]. In a model of cholesterol efflux from mouse peritoneal macrophages HDL from Type 1 diabetes had impaired cholesterol efflux, but this did not correlate with measures of HDL glycation, nor was the function of in vitro glycated HDL impaired [111]. In another study of in vitro glycated HDL its ability to promote cholesterol efflux was not significantly altered [105].

In an in vivo model of macrophage-to-feces RCT HDL mediated cholesterol efflux was reduced (about 20 %) in Type 1 diabetic rodents vs. non-diabtetic rodents, with unchanged cholesterol efflux to diabetic HDL but lower SR-BI mediated uptake from Type 1 diabetic HDL. Both in vitro and in vivo experiments supported effects due to HDL glycation [112].

### Anti-inflammatory Effects

Another role of HDL is inhibition of vascular endothelial cell adhesion molecule expression (CAMs), such as VCAM-1 and ICAM [113, 114]. CAMs promote the attachment, rolling, and ingress of monocytes into the vascular wall, and levels of circulating forms, such as soluble (s) VCAM-1, sICAM, and sE-selectin, are increased in Type 1 and Type 2 diabetes [115], and circulating CAM levels have been correlated with circulating HDL-C levels, but correlations with glycated HDL levels have not been reported. CAM expression is also implicated in diabetic nephropathy [116] and diabetic retinopathy [117] and serum levels can be acutely lowered by intensive insulin treatment [118], but levels of glycated HDL were not reported. In our rabbit studies of collared carotid arteries the suppression of vascular CAMs was attenuated by methylglyoxal glycated ApoA1 and by ApoA1 from diabetic patients relative to unmodified ApoA1. The collars caused intima/media neutrophil infiltration and increased endothelial expression of VCAM-1) and ICAM-1. Unmodified ApoA1 infusions decreased neutrophil infiltration and CAM expression substantially, whilst in vitro glycated ApoA1 was less effective at suppressing neutrophil infiltration and did not significantly lower CAM expression. The in vivo glycated ApoA-I from diabetic patients did not inhibit neutrophil infiltration or CAM expression. These reduced anti-inflammatory properties of glycated ApoA1 were related to reduced inhibition of NFκB and reactive oxygen species (ROS) formation [119].

In keeping, another group demonstrated that in vitro glycated and AGE modified HDL, with increased levels of both fructoselysine and carboxymethylysine, had reduced PON activity and did not suppress oxidized LDL induced monocyte adhesion to human aortic endothelial cells, as did unmodified ApoA1 [120]. In contrast in vitro glycation of HDL did not impair its ability to inhibit monocyte adhesion to cultured aortic endothelial cells [120].

Perhaps also related to CAM expression glycated HDL increased breast cell adhesion to HUVEC and to extracellular matrix, implicating HDL glycation in cancer metastasis [121].

In another model of inflammation, of high glucose induced redox signaling in human monocyte-derived macrophages, apoA1 inhibited glucose-induced oxidative stress (ROS generation, NADPH expression, Nox2, SOD 1 and superoxide production) whilst in vitro glycated apoA1 and that from Type 2 diabetic subjects was less effective [122]. In THP1 cells, human monocyte derived macrophages and mouse RAW2647 cells native HDL suppresses lipopolysaccharide (LPS) induced cytokine (TNFα and interleukin-1β(IL-1β) release, whilst in vitro (28-fold) and in vivo (4-fold) glycated HDL were significantly less effective [123].

## Lipoprotein (a) Glycation

The pro-atherogenic and pro-thrombotic lipoprotein lipoprotein (a) (Lp(a)), which is discussed in another book chapter, also undergoes non-enzymatic glycation in diabetes, and this may enhance its adverse vascular effects.

### Levels of Glycated Lp(a)

In a small cross-sectional study using boronate affinity chromatography and immunonephelometry serum levels of glycated Lp(a) were found to be increased (more than double) in Type 2 diabetes patients relative to non-diabetic subjects, and higher in those with vs. without diabetes complications, but the extent of apoB glycation within Lp(a) was relatively higher [124]. In keeping, Doucet et al. demonstrated (using boronate affinity chromatography and ELISA) that levels of glycated Lp(a) were about 50 % higher in diabetic than non-diabetic patients, with apo(a) being less glycated than the apoB within Lp(a). Glycated Lp(a) levels correlated positively with HbA1c levels. Their in vitro glycation studies demonstrated that Lp(a) was less susceptible to non-enzymatic glycation by glucose than LDL [40].

### Susceptibility to Oxidation

As usually found with LDL, glycation of Lp(a) increases its susceptibility to in vitro copper induced oxidation [125].

### Effects on Modulators of Fibrinolysis

Relative to native Lp(a), glycation (including late glycation) of Lp(a) increases the production of PAI-1 and PAI-1 mRNA expression in cultured HUVEC and human coronary artery endothelial cells and suppresses tPA synthesis and secretion (but not mRNA expression). These changes are attenuated by the AGE inhibitor aminoguanidine and by the lipid soluble antioxidant butylated hydroxytoluene (BHT) [126], implicating the importance of combined glycation and oxidation (AGE modification). These changes may impair fibrinolysis and promote vascular thrombosis and clinically evident vascular events.

### Effects on Vascular Reactivity

In people with diabetes vascular reactivity is usually impaired, contributed to by reduced nitric oxide (NO) bioavailability (which is also discussed elsewhere in this book). In a model system of isolated rat aortic rings glycated Lp(a) without concomitant oxidation did not impair acetylcholine (Ach)-induced endothelium dependent vasodilation, whilst oxidized Lp(a) and AGE modified Lp(a) did, with AGE-Lp(a) having the most deleterious effects. The likely mechanism is by increased superoxide formation, which may inactivate NO [125].

## Glycation of Lipoprotein Related Enzymes

Lipoprotein related enzymes, found on the lipoproteins themselves and on cells with which they interact, mediate exchange of constituents between lipoproteins, alter lipoprotein composition (e.g., by cholesterol esterification), and have antioxidant effects. Glycation may affect these enzymes directly by modification of their amino acid components, by altering their reactivity with their glycation modified lipoprotein substrates or receptors, or by a combination thereof. The role of altered activity of these enzymes due to glycation and their potential as a therapeutic target for amelioration of diabetes vascular complications has not been fully delineated.

We now review studies of the effects of glycation on some important lipoprotein related enzymes, including Platelet Activating Factor Acetylhydrolase (PAFAH), located mainly on LDL, and of paraoxonase, Lecithin-Cholesterol Acyl Transferase (LCAT), and Cholesteryl Ester Transfer Protein (CETP), which are predominantly located on HDL.

### Platelet Activating Factor Acetylhydrolase (PAFAH)

The enzyme PAFAH, which is also known as lipoprotein-associated phospholipase A(2) hydrolyzes and inactivates the lipid mediator

Platelet-Activating Factor (PAF) and/or oxidized phospholipids. PAF is a phospholipid that activates neutrophils, macrophages, platelets, and smooth muscle cells, and increases vascular cell adhesion molecule (CAM) expression and vascular permeability. Increased PAF and/or decreased PAFAH levels or activity have been associated with atherosclerosis and inflammation [127]. PAFAH, circulates on LDL and to a lesser extent on HDL, and can inhibit lipoprotein oxidation [127, 128], but there are few studies of the effects of lipoprotein glycation on PAFAH. Serum PAFAH activity levels have been found to be increased in people with Type 1 diabetes [129–131] and with Type 2 diabetes [132] relative to non-diabetic subjects, and to be increased in renal failure [133], perhaps as a compensatory protective response. PAFAH activity in diabetes correlated with LDL-C and HDL-C levels in both forms of diabetes [129–132, 134] and correlated inversely with HbA1c levels in Type 1 diabetes [129]. Whilst serum PAFAH activity in Type 1 diabetes correlates with LDL susceptibility to oxidation and with Oxidized LDL levels [130, 134] the relationships between lipoprotein glycation and PAFAH are not yet reported.

## Paraoxonase (PON)

There are three PON genes and related proteins [135]. PON1 and PON3 proteins are located on HDL and have protective effects against LDL oxidation. PON2 is also implicated in vascular damage in diabetes [136], but is not known to be associated with lipoproteins. The glycoprotein PON1 is predominantly synthesized in the liver, is located in tissues, in particular the kidney [137, 138] and in serum is located exclusively on HDL [139], with a preference for certain apo J containing and smaller HDL subclasses [140, 141]. PON protects against exogenous organophosphate poisons and in vivo is thought to hydrolyze phospholipid oxidation products [137], homocysteine, thiolactone [142], "statins" [143] and to protect against modifications of lipoproteins and cell membranes. Acute-phase HDL is less protective against LDL oxidation: this type of HDL has greatly reduced PON1 activity [144]. PON1 activity is usually assessed in vitro by hydrolysis of the artificial substrates of paraoxon and phenylacetate [137] and lactones [145].

A major determinant of PON activity are PON genotypes, which have also been associated with cardiovascular disease in the general [137, 146] and diabetic [147, 148] populations, and with diabetic retinopathy and nephropathy [149–151]. PON genotype may also modulate glycemia in both non-diabetic [152] and diabetic subjects [153, 154], which in turn may affect glycation of all lipoprotein classes.

PON protein levels are usually normal in diabetes [155, 156], but there is reduced serum PON activity in people with Type 1 and Type 2 diabetes [150, 155, 156]. In some cross-sectional studies serum PON activity is lower in diabetic subjects with neuropathy [157], retinopathy [158] and nephropathy [159], but not in others [153]. PON activity in humans can be increased by statins and fibrates [135, 160].

Mackness et al. postulate that the low PON1 activity observed in diabetes is due to non-enzymatic glycation [153], which is in keeping with in vitro studies [156] or a circulating inhibitor of PON [155]. HbA1c and serum PON activity were not well correlated in our cross-sectional studies [150], but this may relate to differences in half-lives. Shorter term measures of glycemia (e.g., glucose records over a few days) are preferable because they correspond more closely to the (several days) half-life of PON. Longitudinal studies of improved glycemic control and PON activity and lipoprotein glycation are desirable.

*Lecithin: Cholesterol Acyl Transferase* (LCAT), a glycoprotein produced by the liver, is preferentially bound to circulating HDL, and is also found on VLDL and LDL [113]. LCAT which catalyzes esterification of free cholesterol to cholesteryl ester, and may also hydrolyze oxidized lipids, is the rate-limiting enzyme in reverse cholesterol transport [161]. LCAT activity is inhibited by $HDL_2$, lipid peroxidation products [162–164], and activated by apoAI and ApoAIV, both of which may become glycated. LCAT activity is decreased in both Type 1 and Type 2 diabetes [165, 166] and in uremia [167]. Whilst some have found that LCAT activity and glycemia do not correlate in diabetes [168] Nakhjavani et al. found that LCAT activity and HbA1c were negatively correlated (rho=0.951) in Type 2 diabetes subjects, and on multivariate analysis HbA1c was a strong independent predictor of LCAT activity. LCAT activity and Oxidized LDL levels in serum also correlated, but relationships between LCAT and glycated lipoproteins were not reported [169]. In longitudinal studies LCAT activity decreases with glycemia improved by insulin [170, 171], but not by diet or sulfonylureas [170].

In 1995 Fournier et al. reported both in vivo and in vitro modified LCAT and its reactivity to non-diabetic and diabetic (in vivo glycated) HDL [172]. The kinetics of isolated non-diabetic LCAT activity varied according to the extent of in vitro LCAT glycation. Moderate glycation (<30 % residues on the TNBS reactivity assay) increased Km and Vmax, whilst greater glycation reduced both Km and Vmax. At all levels of LCAT glycation the LCAT reactivity was lower in the presence of in vitro glycated HDL, related to the extent of lysine glycation in (the potent LCAT activator) apoA1. With in vivo modified HDL (from diabetic patients) as LCAT substrate Km values were not altered, but Vmax and LCAT reactivity were reduced by about 30 %. These differences between in vitro and in vivo glycated HDL may relate to physiochemical changes other than glycation. More recently in in vitro studies Nobecourt et al. demonstrated that methylgloxal-induced late glycation of apoA1 impaired its ability to activate LCAT, which was ameliorated by the late glycation inhibitors aminoguanidine and pyridoxamine, the AGE breaker alagebrium, and the insulin sensitizer metformin [114].

## Cholesteryl Ester Transfer Protein (CETP)

CETP, a glycoprotein, stimulates transfer of cholesteryl ester, triglycerides and phospholipids between circulating lipoproteins, such that triglyceride-rich lipoproteins lose triglyceride and gain cholesteryl esters [113], and is a key enzyme in reverse cholesterol transport [173] Synthesized by hepatocytes, adipose tissue and arterial smooth muscle cells [174] CETP binds to VLDL, LDL and HDL. CETP gene polymorphisms influence HDL levels and vascular disease [175]. The effects of glycemia and lipoprotein glycation on CETP activity have been studied. CETP activity is increased in people with Type 1 [176] and Type 2 diabetes [177] relative to non-diabetic subjects. In diabetes patients subcutaneous insulin delivery activates, while intraperitoneal delivery reduces, CETP activity [178]. Glycemia may influence CETP activity via non-enzymatic glycation of the enzyme [179] and via conformational changes which affect enzyme binding and lipid exchange. Passarelli et al. showed that in vitro glycated and in vivo glycated lipoproteins are associated with increased cholesteryl ester transfer rates from HDL to VLDL and LDL. Whilst in vitro glycation of partially purified CETP markedly impaired its activity [179], greater lipid transfer rates were observed when in vivo glycated lipoproteins from diabetic subjects were used, which was attributed to glycation of HDL protein. Lemkadem et al. demonstrated that in vitro glycation of HDL3 (with glucose concentrations up to 200 mM) increased cholesteryl ester transfer, but kinetic studies showed a paradoxical increase in CETP activity associated with a decrease of CETP affinity. HDL lipid and protein composition was unchanged but its fluidity was decreased and its electronegativity increased, which may affect CETP reactivity [180].

CETP inhibitors substantially increase HDL-C levels in people with and without diabetes, but the first major clinical trial on the cardiovascular effects of CETP inhibitors was stopped due to off-label effects (hypertension) [181, 182]. The development of other CETP inhibitors is ongoing.

## Treatment of Lipoprotein Glycation in Diabetes

Approaches that may reduce lipoprotein glycation are listed in Table 8.2. The general approaches include reduction in "substrate stress" by lowering levels of glucose (and other glycating agents) and

**Table 8.2** Potential approaches to reduce lipoprotein glycation

| |
|---|
| *Lower glucose levels* |
| Lifestyle, e.g., diets such as low AGE diets |
| Glucose control drugs, e.g., metformin, insulin, sulfonylureas, incretins |
| *Lower lipid levels* |
| Lifestyle |
| Drugs such as statins, fibrates, ezetimibe, resins |
| LDL apharesis |
| *Combined glucose and lipid lowering drugs*, e.g., colestamide |
| *Inhibit glycation reactions* |
| Early glycation, e.g., saponins, some nutrients |
| Late glycation, e.g., amadorins |
| *Removal of preformed AGEs* |
| AGE breakers? |
| *Deglycating drugs* |
| *Increase activity of deglycating enzymes* |

of lipids, the inhibition of early and late glycation reactions, the use of deglycating agents and the removal of existent AGEs. Another strategy would be to modulate adverse cellular and extracellular matrix responses to glycated lipoproteins.

*Lipid control.* Dyslipidemia, even by the traditional narrower definition related to measures of lipid levels, is a common associate of diabetes, in particular in the setting of poor glycemic control. As discussed elsewhere in this book, improving the lipid profile is an important aspect of preventing the macro- and microvascular complications of diabetes. Improved glycemic control, weight control, a healthy diet, exercise and non-smoking status are important goals which will also improve the lipid profile, but often, particularly in developed countries, lipid drugs are required. The benefits of the major lipid drug classes (statins and fibrates) for cardiovascular, retinal and renal event reductions have been shown in prospective placebo controlled randomized clinical trials, predominantly in Type 2 diabetes [183–188]. These benefits likely relate to both direct lipid lowering effects and pleiotropic effects

*Improved glycemic control*, which also reduces diabetic vascular complications [161, 189–191] will improve the traditional lipid profile and also reduce post-translational lipoprotein glycation, reducing substrate stress. Unfortunately in clinical practice achieving normoglycemia is often challenging related to availability, affordability, and efficacy of current glucose control drugs and insulin pumps, and patient and clinician fears of hypoglycemia, which may also have adverse cardiovascular effects. Strategies that can reduce lipoprotein glycation, or the adverse cellular and enzymatic responses to lipoprotein glycation, even in the setting of hyperglycemia, are desirable. Apart from glucose lowering drugs and perhaps HMG CoA reductase inhibitors (statins) [192] there are currently no therapies in clinical practice known to reduce lipoprotein glycation.

*Glucose control agents*: As discussed above several prospective longitudinal studies have demonstrated that drugs, such as insulin and metformin which improve glucose control, are associated with reduction in levels of glycated lipoproteins [193–195]. Some, such as metformin, may also have pleiotropic effects such as antioxidant or anti-AGE effects [196]. This is most likely related to effects on lowering ambient glucose levels and related improvements in the lipid profile. There is a novel class of glucose lowering agents, Sodium Glucose Transporter 2 inhibitors, which induce glycosuria via inhibition of glucose reabsorption by the renal tubules, which are currently in human clinical trials [197, 198] and are now approved in some countries for clinical use. As yet there are no published studies related to their effects on lipoprotein glycation.

*Lipid drugs* that are commonly used in clinical practice, such as the statins and fibrates, effectively improve dyslipidemia in diabetes, reduce the risk of macro- and microvascular events [199, 200], and also have pleiotropic antioxidant effects [201, 202] but there are few publications of effects on lipoprotein glycation. Whilst recent studies suggest that statins may increase Type 2 diabetes risk [203] and in a small prospective Type 2 diabetes study atorvastatin worsened glycemia [204] there is no definitive evidence that statins, fibrates or ezetemibe substantially alter circulating glucose levels in people with diabetes, which could impact lipoprotein glycation. In a cross-sectional study Younis et al. demonstrated lower levels of plasma glycated apoB in statin-treated type 2 diabetes patients compared with those not on statins [205]. This may relate to changes in LDL levels rather than a direct effect on lipoprotein glycation. Longitudinal studies are merited. Lipid drugs such as the statins and fibrates may also affect lipoprotein related enzyme activities, as discussed earlier.

The anion exchange resin colestimide improves both glycemia and lipid levels in people with Type 2 diabetes, hence could be expected to reduce lipoprotein glycation, but as yet there are no related publications [204, 206]. Conversely, nicotinic acid, particularly the rapid release preparations, whilst improving the lipid profile (in particular lowering VLDL and increasing HDL levels), can slightly worsen glycemia [207], so may increase lipoprotein glycation, but as yet there are no relevant published data of glycated lipoprotein levels.

*LDL Apharesis*. LDL apharesis, originally used for the treatment of familial hyperlipidemia, has been used for the treatment of patients with peripheral vascular disease, the nephrotic syndrome due to steroid-resistant focal glomerulosclerosis (FGS) and diabetic nephropathy. LDL apharesis (also discussed in another chapter) effectively lowers LDL and Lp(a) levels in people with diabetes, and has been shown to lower circulating levels of malondialdehyde (MDA) modified (oxidized) LDL, but again, there are no studies of the effects of apharesis on levels of glycated LDL (and other glycated lipoproteins). Interestingly LDL apharesis has been shown to lower levels of an intracellular glycated protein (Hb) (HbA1c), so it may be expected to lower glycated lipoprotein levels. LDL apharesis also has many other favorable effects beyond lipid-lowering, including improving blood viscosity, platelet aggregation, anti-inflammatory effects, vasodilatory effects and increases in (pro-angiogenic) Vascular Endothelial Growth Factor (VEGF) levels [208–211].

*Drugs which inhibit glycation reactions* directly rather than by lowering glucose levels could also reduce lipoprotein glycation. Saponins and some other compounds identified in traditional Chinese medicines used for diabetes have demonstrated in vitro anti-glycation effects against model proteins such as albumin [212, 213], but we have not identified any studies related to lipoprotein glycation.

There are more studies of the inhibition of late glycation than of early glycation of lipoproteins. Effective glycation inhibitory compounds fall into those primarily with anti-AGE effects, such as aminoguanidine and pyridoxamine, and various drugs classes, often already in common clinical usage with pleiotropic antioxidant/anti AGE effects. Progression to AGEs from the "early glycation" Amadori product requires chemical rearrangements to create reactive intermediates before the formation of AGEs, and drugs such as aminoguanidine can inhibit this process [87, 214–216]. Aminoguanidine has demonstrated favorable effects in cultured cell systems relevant to diabetes complications, including our work with LDL and retinal cells [87] and has prevented vascular complications in diabetic animal models [87, 214]. In human studies aminoguanidine achieved some success with lowering AGE-LDL [217, 218] and AGE modified-Hemoglobin, decreasing albuminuria and slowing progression of nephropathy and retinopathy [219, 220], but was poorly tolerated [221, 222]. Aminoguanidine inhibits AGE formation in a range of short and long-lived proteins, including lipoproteins [223, 224], and also inhibits a range of other important pathways, most notably nitric oxide production via eNOS [225–227], hence it is difficult to proportion benefit to its anti-AGE effects.

Another approach to AGE inhibition is to scavenge post-Amadori dicarbonyls and so inhibit conversion of the Amadori intermediates to AGEs [228]. Such agents are classed as "Amadorins." Examples include the vitamin B12 derivative pyridoxamine [229, 230] and benfotiamine, a lipophilic vitamin B1 (thiamine) derivative [231–236]. *Pyridoxamine* (Pyridorin™) inhibits formation of both AGEs and Advanced Lipoxidation End Products (ALES), including in lipoproteins. We demonstrated in in vitro studies of LDL oxidation that pyridoxamine decreased late, but not early glycation products [229]. In animal studies pyridoxamine prevented renal dysfunction [237, 238] and retinopathy [239] in diabetic rats and also had favorable effects on lipid levels [240]. Pyridoxamine and benfotiamine are well-tolerated and human trials are in progress, with a suggestion of some renal benefit for diabetic nephropathy in Type 2 diabetes patients, though levels of glycated lipoproteins have not been reported.

*Deglycating enzymes and drugs* could also reduce lipoprotein glycation. Comparisons of human and in vitro studies suggest that for a given ambient glucose level people vary in their propensity to form glycation products [241–243]. This may be tissue specific [244] and also relate to genetic and/or activity of deglycating enzymes [245, 246]. We are not aware of any studies of glycated lipoprotein levels in relationship to enzyme activities or genotypes. Whilst two categories of deglycation enzymes have been identified, fructosyl amine oxidases and fructosyl amine kinases, there are no papers related to their effects on lipoprotein glycation.

*AGE binders and decoys*. The prevention of AGEs, including those on toxic AGE modified lipoproteins, interacting with other proteins or with AGE receptors may also prevent diabetic complications. There are several potential approaches, but relatively little existent research specific to lipoprotein glycation. Antibodies to glycated albumin have prevented basement membrane thickening in db/db mice [247], but there are no studies of the effects of therapeutic antibodies to glycated lipoproteins. Lysozyme has demonstrated in vitro ability to bind in vivo generated AGEs in uremic sera and dialysate [248–250] and highly efficient lysozyme removing dialysis membranes may potentially reduce AGE levels, which may also include AGE modified lipoproteins, and vascular disease in dialysis patients.

Soluble RAGE (sRAGE) can act as a decoy for AGE binding and has shown benefit for reducing vascular damage in animal models, including vascular hyperpermeability [251], atherosclerotic lesion area and complexity [252], periodontal disease, impaired wound healing, renal dysfunction [253], and pro-inflammatory effects [254] such as CAM expression and neutrophil infiltration [255], but effects on glycated lipoproteins have not been evaluated.

*AGE or cross-link breakers* are a novel class of anti-AGE drugs, which have shown some benefit for improving vascular and renal damage and erectile dysfunction in diabetic animal models and in patients. The most well-studied is alagebrium, which has demonstrated some benefits related to peripheral arterial function [256], cardiac contractility [257], and erectile dysfunction [258], but in other studies of heart failure [259] and glaucoma [260], both of which are more common in diabetes, was ineffective. AGE breakers may also act by inhibition of AGE formation [261], effects on NO [258, 262] and on thiamine metabolism [263]. None of the studies have reported effects on AGEs in lipoproteins.

## Summary and Future Directions

Diabetes is already a major cause of morbidity and premature mortality in the developed and developing world. The onset and progression of diabetes-related micro- and macrovascular complications is likely to involve a wide range of pathogenic mechanisms, including lipoprotein glycation (of both early and late stages). Glycated lipoproteins can directly cause damage such as related to toxic effects on vascular cells, foam cell formation and pro-thrombotic and pro-inflammatory effects. Glycated lipoproteins, whilst present in all types of diabetes from its onset, and to relatively higher levels than oxidized lipoproteins, are not as well-studied as other forms of lipoproteins. Additional assays to quantify a range of glycated lipoprotein classes in the circulation and in tissues are of interest. Further clinical and basic science studies are merited as lipoprotein glycation is likely a therapeutic target that may reduce residual vascular risk. The long-term management of the ever-growing number of diabetic patients will likely involve lifestyle measures, tight glycemic, blood pressure, and lipid control in combination with additional therapies that may reduce the (early and late) glycation of lipoproteins, even in the setting of ongoing hyperglycemia and dyslipidemia.

**Acknowledgments** Grant support for studies discussed herein was provided by the Juvenile Diabetes Research Foundation, American Diabetes Association, National Institutes of Health, Department of Veterans Affairs Merit Review (RK), the Diabetes Research and Wellness Foundation, Lions SightFirst Diabetic Retinopathy Research Program, the National Health and Medical Research Foundation, and National Heart Foundation (Australia). The authors also acknowledge their collaborators, including Professors Timothy Lyons, John Baynes, Susan Thorpe, Maria Lopes-Virella, Gabe Virella, Kristian Hanssen, Bente Kilhovd, David O'Neal, Kerry-Anne Rye, Philip Barter, Michael Davies, the DCCT/EDIC Research Group, Andrea Semler, and Connie Karschimkus.

## References

1. Amos AF, McCarty DJ, Zimmet P. The rising global burden of diabetes and its complications: estimates and projections to the year 2010. Diabet Med. 1997;14 Suppl 5:S1–85.
2. American Diabetes Association. Diabetes vital statistics. Alexandria, VA: American Diabetes Association; 1996.
3. Jay RH, Betteridge DJ. The heart and macrovascular disease in diabetes mellitus. In: Pickup JC, Williams G, editors. Chronic complication of diabetes. Melbourne: Blackwell Press; 1994.
4. Jenkins AJ, Rowley KG, Lyons TJ, Best JD, Hill MA, Klein RL. Lipoproteins and diabetic microvascular complications. Curr Pharm Des. 2004;10: 3395–418.
5. Betteridge DJ. Risk factors for arterial disease in diabetes: dyslipidaemia. In: Tooke JE, editor. Diabetic angiopathy. Sydney: Arnold; 1999. p. 65–92.
6. Reckless JPD. Diabetes. In: Dunitz M, editor. Diabetes-author Reckless JPD. In: Diabetes and Lipids: Pocketbook (Martin Dunitz Medical Pocket Books) 2nd ed. London. Publisher Taylor and Francis Sept 1, 2011. p. 26–37.
7. Howard BV. Lipoprotein metabolism in diabetes mellitus. J Lipid Res. 1987;28(6):613–28.
8. Maillard LC. Réaction générale des acides aminés sur les sucres: ses conséquences biologiques. Compte-rendu Société de Biologie. 1912;tome 72 (LXXII), p. 599–601 (559–61).
9. Thorpe SR, Lyons TJ, Baynes JW. Oxidative stress and vascular disease. Boston, MA: Kluwer Academic Pub; 2000. p. 259–85.
10. Fu MX, Requena JR, Jenkins AJ, Lyons TJ, Baynes JW, Thorpe SR. The advanced glycation end product, Nepsilon-(carboxymethyl)lysine, is a product of both lipid peroxidation and glycoxidation reactions. J Biol Chem. 1996 Apr 26;271(17):9982–6.
11. Lyons TJ, Jenkins AJ. Glycation, oxidation, and lipoxidation in the development of the complications of diabetes: a carbonyl stress hypothesis. Diabetes Rev. 1997;5:365–91.
12. Lyons TJ. Glycation, oxidation, and glycoxidation reactions in the development of diabetic complications. Contrib Nephrol. 1995;112:1–10.
13. Cao Z, Cooper ME. Pathogenesis of diabetic nephropathy. J Diabetes Invest. 2011;2(4):243–7.
14. Miyata T, Fu MX, Kurokawa K, van Ypersele de Strihou C, Thorpe SR, Baynes JW. Autoxidation products of both carbohydrates and lipids are increased in uremic plasma: is there oxidative stress in uremia? Kidney Int. 1998;54(4):1290–5.
15. http://www.imars.org/online/?page_id=655, 2012 May 21
16. Fu MX, Requena JR, Jenkins AJ, Lyons TJ, Baynes JW, Thorpe SR. The advanced glycation end product, Nepsilon-(carboxymethyl)lysine, is a product of both lipid peroxidation and glycoxidation reactions. J Biol Chem. 1996;271(17):9982–6.
17. Niwa T. 3-Deoxyglucosone: metabolism, analysis, biological activity, and clinical implication. J Chromatogr B Biomed Sci Appl. 1999;731(1): 23–36.
18. Jono T, Nagai R, Lin X, Ahmed N, Thornalley PJ, Takeya M, Horiuchi S. Nepsilon-(Carboxymethyl) lysine and 3-DG-imidazolone are major AGE structures in protein modification by 3-deoxyglucosone. J Biochem. 2004;136(3):351–8.
19. Goldberg T, Cai W, Peppa M, Dardaine V, Baliga BW, Uribarri J, Vlassara H. Advanced glycoxidation end products in commonly consumed foods. J Am Diet Assoc. 2004;104:1287–91.
20. Koschinsky T, He CJ, Mitsuhashi T, Bucala R, Liu C, Buenting C, Heitmann K, Vlassara H. Orally absorbed reactive glycation products (glycotoxins): an environmental risk factor in diabetic nephropathy. Proc Natl Acad Sci USA. 1997;94:6474–9.
21. Uribarri J, Peppa M, Cai W, Goldberg T, Lu M, Baliga S, Vassalotti JA, Vlassara H. Dietary glycotoxins correlate with circulating advanced glycation end product levels in renal failure patients. Am J Kidney Dis. 2003;42:532–8.
22. Uribarri J, Woodruff S, Goodman S, Cai W, Chen X, Pyzik R, Yong A, Striker G, Vlassara H. Advanced glycation end products in foods and a practical guide to their reduction in the diet. J Am Diet Assoc. 2010;110:911–6.
23. Vlassara H, Palace MR. Diabetes and advanced glycation endproducts. J Intern Med. 2002;251: 87–101.
24. Cai W, He JC, Zhu L, Chen X, Wallenstein S, Striker GE, Vlassara H. Reduced oxidant stress and extended lifespan in mice exposed to a low glycotoxin diet: association with increased AGER1 expression. Am J Pathol. 2007;170(6):1893–902.
25. Vlassara H, Cai W, Crandall J, Goldberg T, Oberstein R, Dardaine V, Peppa M, Rayfield EJ. Inflammatory mediators are induced by dietary glycotoxins, a major risk factor for diabetic angiopathy. Proc Natl Acad Sci USA. 2002;99:15596–601.
26. Negrean M, Stirban A, Stratmann B, Gawlowski T, Horstmann T, Götting C, Kleesiek K, Mueller-Roesel M, Koschinsky T, Uribarri J, Vlassara H,

Tschoepe D. Effects of low- and high-advanced glycation endproduct meals on macro- and microvascular endothelial function and oxidative stress in patients with type 2 diabetes mellitus. Am J Clin Nutr. 2007;85:1236–43.
27. Baynes JW, Dominiczak H. Medical biochemistry. 2nd ed. New York: Elsevier Mosby; 2005.
28. Lund-Katz S, Ibdah JA, Letizia JY, Thomas MT, Phillips MC. A 13C NMR characterization of lysine residues in apolipoprotein B and their role in binding to the low density lipoprotein receptor. J Biol Chem. 1988;263(27):13831–8.
29. Shinohara M, Thornalley PJ, Giardino I, Beisswenger P, Thorpe SR, Onorato J, Brownlee M. Overexpression of glyoxalase-1 in bovine endothelial cells inhibits intracellular advanced glycation endproduct formation and prevents hyperglycemia-induced increases in macromolecular endocytosis. J Clin Invest. 1998;101(5):1142–7.
30. Lu J, Randell E, Han Y, Adeli K, Krahn J, Menq QH. Increased plasma methylglyoxal level, inflammation, and vascular endothelial dysfunction in diabetic nephropathy. Clin Biochem. 2011;44(4):307–11.
31. Lyons TJ, Klein RL, Baynes JW, Stevenson HC, Lopes-Virella MF. Stimulation of cholesteryl ester synthesis in human monocyte-derived macrophages by lipoproteins from Type I diabetic subjects: the influence of non-enzymatic glycosylation of low-density lipoproteins. Diabetologia. 1987;30:916–23.
32. Hayashi Y, Okumura K, Matsui H, Imamura A, Miura M, Takahashi R, Murakami R, Ogawa Y, Numaguchi Y, Murohara T. Impact of low-density lipoprotein particle size on carotid intima-media thickness in patients with type 2 diabetes mellitus. Metabolism. 2007;56(5):608–13.
33. Januszewski AS, Karschimkus C, Davis KE, O'Neal D, Ward G, Jenkins AJ. Plasma 1,5 anhydroglucitol levels, a measure of short-term glycaemia: assay assessment and lower levels in diabetic vs. non-diabetic subjects. Diabetes Res Clin Pract. 2012; 95(1):e17–9.
34. Ahmed MU, Thorpe SR, Baynes JW. Identification of N epsilon-carboxymethyllysine as a degradation product of fructoselysine in glycated protein. J Biol Chem. 1986;261(11):4889–94.
35. Jenkins AJ, Thorpe SR, Alderson NL, Hermayer KL, Lyons TJ, King LP, Chassereau CN, Klein RL. In vivo glycated low-density lipoprotein is not more susceptible to oxidation than nonglycated low-density lipoprotein in type 1 diabetes. Metabolism. 2004;53(8):969–76.
36. Lopes-Virella MF, Klein RL, Lyons TJ, Stevenson HC, Witztum JL. Glycosylation of low-density lipoprotein enhances cholesteryl ester synthesis in human monocyte-derived macrophages. Diabetes. 1988;37(5):550–7.
37. Klein RL, Laimins M, Lopes-Virella MF. Isolation, characterization, and metabolism of the glycated and nonglycated subfractions of low-density lipoproteins isolated from type I diabetic patients and nondiabetic subjects. Diabetes. 1995;44(9):1093–8.
38. Tanaka A, Yui K, Tomie N, Baba T, Tamura M, Makita T, Numano F, Nakatani S, Kato Y. New assay for glycated lipoproteins by high-performance liquid chromatography. Ann N Y Acad Sci. 1997;811: 385–94.
39. Cohen MP, Lautenslager G, Shea E. Glycated LDL concentrations in non-diabetic and diabetic subjects measured with monoclonal antibodies reactive with glycated apolipoprotein B epitopes. Eur J Clin Chem Clin Biochem. 1993;31(11):707–13.
40. Doucet C, Huby T, Ruiz J, Chapman MJ, Thillet J. Non-enzymatic glycation of lipoprotein(a) in vitro and in vivo. Atherosclerosis. 1995;118:135–43.
41. Makino K, Furbee JW, Scanu AM, Fless GM. Effect of glycation on the properties of lipoprotein(a). Arterioscler Thromb Vasc Biol. 1995;15:385–91.
42. Dyer DG, Dunn JA, Thorpe SR, Bailie KE, Lyons TJ, McCance DR, Baynes JW. Accumulation of Maillard reaction products in skin collagen in diabetes and aging. J Clin Invest. 1993;91(6):2463–9.
43. Virella G, Derrick MB, Pate V, Chassereau C, Thorpe SR, Lopes-Virella MF. Development of capture assays for different modifications of human low-density lipoprotein. Clin Diagn Lab Immunol. 2005;12(1):68–75.
44. Nagai R, Matsumoto K, Ling X, Suzuki H, Araki T, Horiuchi S. Glycolaldehyde, a reactive intermediate for advanced glycation end products, plays an important role in the generation of an active ligand for the macrophage scavenger receptor. Diabetes. 2000;49:1714–23.
45. Kaplan M, Aviram M. Macrophage plasma membrane chondroitin sulfate proteoglycan binds oxidized low-density lipoprotein. Atherosclerosis. 2000;149(1):5–17.
46. Tsmikas S, Shortal BP, Witztum JL, Palinski W. In vivo uptake of radiolabeled MDA2, an oxidation specific monoclonal antibody, provides an accurate measure of atherosclerotic lesions rich in oxidized LDL and is highly sensitive to their regression. Arterioscler Thromb Vasc Biol. 2000;20:689–97.
47. Cao G, Alessio HM, Cutler RG. Oxygen-radical absorbance capacity assay for antioxidants. Free Radic Biol Med. 1993;14(3):303–11.
48. Herrera E, Barbas C. Vitamin E: action, metabolism and perspectives. J Physiol Biochem. 2001;57(2): 43–56.
49. Jenkins AJ, Velarde V, Klein RL, Joyce KC, Phillips KD, Mayfield RK, Lyons TJ, Jaffa AA. Native and modified LDL activate extracellular signal-regulated kinases in mesangial cells. Diabetes. 2000;49(12): 2160–9.
50. Song W, Barth JL, Yu Y, Lu K, Dashti A, Huang Y, Gittinger CK, Argraves WS, Lyons TJ. Effects of oxidized and glycated LDL on gene expression in human retinal capillary pericytes. Invest Ophthalmol Vis Sci. 2005;46(8):2974–82.
51. Song W, Barth JL, Lu K, Yu Y, Huang Y, Gittinger CK, Argraves WS, Lyons TJ. Effects of modified low-density lipoproteins on human retinal pericyte survival. Ann N Y Acad Sci. 2005;1043:390–5.

52. Barth JL, Yu Y, Song W, Lu K, Dashti A, Huang Y, Argraves WS, Lyons TJ. Oxidised, glycated LDL selectively influences tissue inhibitor of metalloproteinase-3 gene expression and protein production in human retinal capillary pericytes. Diabetologia. 2007 Oct;50(10):2200–8.
53. Tames FJ, Mackness MI, Arrol S, Laing I, Durrington PN. Non-enzymatic glycation of apolipoprotein B in the sera of diabetic and non-diabetic subjects. Atherosclerosis. 1992;93(3):237–44.
54. Younis N, Charlton-Menys V, Sharma R, Soran H, Durrington PN. Glycation of LDL in non-diabetic people: small dense LDL is preferentially glycated both in vivo and in vitro. Atherosclerosis. 2009; 202(1):162–8.
55. Lyons TJ, Otvos JD, Klein RL, Zheng D, Garvey WT, Jenkins AJ, with The DCCT/EDIC Research Group. Nuclear magnetic resonance (NMR)-determined lipoprotein subclass profile: effects of hyperglycemia, lipoprotein glycation, and comparison with standard lipid profile. Diabetes. 2000;49 Suppl 1:A268.
56. Lyons TJ, Jenkins AJ, Zheng D, Klein RL, Otvos JD, Yu Y, Lackland DT, McGee D, McHenry MB, Lopes-Virella M, Garvey WT, DCCT/EDIC Research Group. Nuclear magnetic resonance-determined lipoprotein subclass profile in the DCCT/EDIC cohort: associations with carotid intima-media thickness. Diabet Med. 2006;23(9):955–66.
57. Yegin A, Ozben T, Yegin H. Glycation of lipoproteins and accelerated atherosclerosis in non-insulin-dependent diabetes mellitus. Int J Clin Lab Res. 1995;25(3):157–61.
58. Mamo JC, Szeto L, Steiner G. Glycation of very low density lipoprotein from rat plasma impairs its catabolism. Diabetologia. 1990;33(6):339–45.
59. Klein RL, Wohltmann HJ, Lopes-Virella MF. Influence of glycemic control on interaction of very-low- and low-density lipoproteins isolated from type I diabetic patients with human monocyte-derived macrophages. Diabetes. 1992;41(10):1301–7.
60. Klein RL, Lyons TJ, Lopes-Virella MF. Metabolism of very low- and low-density lipoproteins isolated from normolipidaemic type 2 (non-insulin-dependent) diabetic patients by human monocyte-derived macrophages. Diabetologia. 1990;33(5): 299–305.
61. Klein RL, Lyons TJ, Lopes-Virella MF. Interaction of very-low-density lipoprotein isolated from type I (insulin-dependent) diabetic subjects with human monocyte-derived macrophages. Metabolism. 1989;38(11):1108–14.
62. Klein RL, Lopes-Virella MF. Metabolism by human endothelial cells of very low density lipoprotein subfractions isolated from type 1 (insulin-dependent) diabetic patients. Diabetologia. 1993;36(3):258–64.
63. Moro E, Alessandrini P, Zambon C, Pianetti S, Pais M, Cazzolato G, Bon GB. Is glycation of low density lipoproteins in patients with Type 2 diabetes mellitus a LDL pre-oxidative condition? Diabet Med. 1999;16(8):663–9.
64. Akanji AO, Abdella N, Mojiminiyi OA. Determinants of glycated LDL levels in nondiabetic and diabetic hyperlipidaemic patients in Kuwait. Clin Chim Acta. 2002;317(1–2):171–6.
65. Rabbani N, Chittari MV, Bodmer CW, Zehnder D, Ceriello A, Thornalley PJ. Increased glycation and oxidative damage to apolipoprotein B100 of LDL cholesterol in patients with type 2 diabetes and effect of metformin. Diabetes. 2010;59(4):1038–45.
66. Chao PC, Huang CN, Hsu CC, Yin MC, Guo YR. Association of dietary AGEs with circulating AGEs, glycated LDL, IL-1α and MCP-1 levels in type 2 diabetic patients. Eur J Nutr. 2010;49(7):429–34.
67. Steinberg D, Witztum JL. Lipoproteins and atherogenesis. Current concepts. JAMA. 1990;264(23): 3047–52.
68. Soran H, Durrington PN. Susceptibility of LDL and its subfractions to glycation. Curr Opin Lipidol. 2011;22(4):254–61.
69. Rabbani N, Godfrey L, Xue M, Shaheen F, Geoffrion M, Milne R, Thornalley PJ. Glycation of LDL by methylglyoxal increases arterial atherogenicity: a possible contributor to increased risk of cardiovascular disease in diabetes. Diabetes. 2011;60(7):1973–80.
70. Tsai EC, Hirsch IB, Brunzell JD, Chait A. Reduced plasma peroxyl radical trapping capacity and increased susceptibility of LDL to oxidation in poorly controlled IDDM. Diabetes. 1994;43(8): 1010–4.
71. Jenkins AJ, Klein RL, Chassereau CN, Hermayer KL, Lopes-Virella MF. LDL from patients with well-controlled IDDM is not more susceptible to in vitro oxidation. Diabetes. 1996;45(6):762–7.
72. Jenkins AJ, Lyons TJ, Zheng D, Otvos JD, Lackland DT, McGee D, Garvey WT, Klein RL, DCC/EDIC Research Group. Serum lipoproteins in the diabetes control and complications trial/epidemiology of diabetes intervention and complications cohort: associations with gender and glycemia. Diabetes Care. 2003;26(3):810–8.
73. Lopes-Virella MF, Virella G. Clinical significance of the humoral immune response to modified LDL. Clin Immunol. 2010;134(1):55–65.
74. Lopes-Virella MF, Hunt KJ, Baker NL, Lachin J, Nathan DM, Virella G, Diabetes Control and Complications Trial/Epidemiology of Diabetes Interventions and Complications Research Group. Levels of oxidized LDL and advanced glycation end products-modified LDL in circulating immune complexes are strongly associated with increased levels of carotid intima-media thickness and its progression in type 1 diabetes. Diabetes. 2011;60(2):582–9.
75. Lopes-Virella MF, Baker NL, Hunt KJ, Lyons TJ, Jenkins AJ, Virella G, DCCT/EDIC Study Group. High concentrations of AGE-LDL and oxidized LDL in circulating immune complexes are associated with progression of retinopathy in type 1 diabetes. Diabetes Care. 2012;35(6):1333–40.
76. Gupta S, Rifici V, Crowley S, Brownlee M, Shan Z, Schlondorff D. Interactions of LDL and modified

LDL with mesangial cells and matrix. Kidney Int. 1992;41(5):1161–9.

77. Edwards IJ, Wagner JD, Litwak KN, Rudel LL, Cefalu WT. Glycation of plasma low density lipoproteins increases interaction with arterial proteoglycans. Diabetes Res Clin Pract. 1999;46(1):9–18.
78. Wang X, Bucala R, Milne R. Epitopes close to the apolipoprotein B low density lipoprotein receptor-binding site are modified by advanced glycation end products. Proc Natl Acad Sci USA. 1998;95(13):7643–7.
79. Sima AV, Botez GM, Stancu CS, Manea A, Raicu M, Simionescu M. Effect of irreversibly glycated LDL in human vascular smooth muscle cells: lipid loading, oxidative and inflammatory stress. J Cell Mol Med. 2010;14(12):2790–802.
80. Lam MC, Tan KC, Lam KS. Glycoxidized low-density lipoprotein regulates the expression of scavenger receptors in THP-1 macrophages. Atherosclerosis. 2004;177(2):313–20.
81. Brown BE, Rashid I, van Reyk DM, Davies MJ. Glycation of low-density lipoprotein results in the time-dependent accumulation of cholesteryl esters and apolipoprotein B-100 protein in primary human monocyte-derived macrophages. FEBS J. 2007;274(6):1530–41.
82. Brown BE, Dean RT, Davies MJ. Glycation of low-density lipoproteins by methylglyoxal and glycolaldehyde gives rise to the in vitro formation of lipid-laden cells. Diabetologia. 2005;48(2):361–9.
83. Artwohl M, Graier WF, Roden M, Bischof M, Freudenthaler A, Waldhäusl W, Baumgartner-Parzer SM. Diabetic LDL triggers apoptosis in vascular endothelial cells. Diabetes. 2003;52(5):1240–7.
84. Sonoki K, Yoshinari M, Iwase M, Iino K, Ichikawa K, Ohdo S, Higuchi S, Iida M. Glycoxidized low-density lipoprotein enhances monocyte chemoattractant protein-1 mRNA expression in human umbilical vein endothelial cells: relation to lysophosphatidylcholine contents and inhibition by nitric oxide donor. Metabolism. 2002;51(9):1135–42.
85. Sonoki K, Iwase M, Iino K, Ichikawa K, Yoshinari M, Ohdo S, Higuchi S, Iida M. Dilazep and fenofibric acid inhibit MCP-1 mRNA expression in glycoxidized LDL-stimulated human endothelial cells. Eur J Pharmacol. 2003;475(1–3):139–47.
86. Lyons TJ, Li W, Wells-Knecht MC, Jokl R. Toxicity of mildly modified low-density lipoproteins to cultured retinal capillary endothelial cells and pericytes. Diabetes. 1994;43(9):1090–5.
87. Lyons TJ, Li W, Wojciechowski B, Wells-Knecht MC, Wells-Knecht KJ, Jenkins AJ. Aminoguanidine and the effects of modified LDL on cultured retinal capillary cells. Invest Ophthalmol Vis Sci. 2000;41(5):1176–80.
88. Schlondorff D. Cellular mechanisms of lipid injury in the glomerulus. Am J Kidney Dis. 1993;22(1):72–82.
89. Santini E, Lupi R, Baldi S, Madec S, Chimenti D, Ferrannini E, Solini A. Effects of different LDL particles on inflammatory molecules in human mesangial cells. Diabetologia. 2008;51(11):2117–25.
90. Ha H, Kamanna VS, Kirschenbaum MA, Kim KH. Role of glycated low density lipoprotein in mesangial extracellular matrix synthesis. Kidney Int Suppl. 1997;60:S54–9.
91. Fujii Y, Iwano M, Dohi K. Effect of lipids on glomerular fibrinolysis in vitro. Contrib Nephrol. 1997;120:140–5.
92. Zhang J, Ren S, Sun D, Shen GX. Influence of glycation on LDL-induced generation of fibrinolytic regulators in vascular endothelial cells. Arterioscler Thromb Vasc Biol. 1998;18(7):1140–8.
93. Ren S, Shen GX. Impact of antioxidants and HDL on glycated LDL-induced generation of fibrinolytic regulators from vascular endothelial cells. Arterioscler Thromb Vasc Biol. 2000;20(6):1688–93.
94. Ren S, Lee H, Hu L, Lu L, Shen GX. Impact of diabetes-associated lipoproteins on generation of fibrinolytic regulators from vascular endothelial cells. J Clin Endocrinol Metab. 2002;87(1):286–91.
95. Ma GM, Halayko AJ, Stelmack GL, Zhu F, Zhao R, Hillier CT, Shen GX. Effects of oxidized and glycated low-density lipoproteins on transcription and secretion of plasminogen activator inhibitor-1 in vascular endothelial cells. Cardiovasc Pathol. 2006;15(1):3–10.
96. Sangle GV, Zhao R, Mizuno TM, Shen GX. Involvement of RAGE, NADPH oxidase, and Ras/Raf-1 pathway in glycated LDL-induced expression of heat shock factor-1 and plasminogen activator inhibitor-1 in vascular endothelial cells. Endocrinology. 2010;151(9):4455–66.
97. Calzada C, Coulon L, Halimi D, Le Coquil E, Pruneta-Deloche V, Moulin P, Ponsin G, Véricel E, Lagarde MJ. In vitro glycoxidized low-density lipoproteins and low-density lipoproteins isolated from type 2 diabetic patients activate platelets via p38 mitogen-activated protein kinase. Clin Endocrinol Metab. 2007;92(5):1961–4.
98. Ferretti G, Rabini RA, Bacchetti T, Vignini A, Salvolini E, Ravaglia F, Curatola G, Mazzanti L. Glycated low density lipoproteins modify platelet properties: a compositional and functional study. J Clin Endocrinol Metab. 2002;87(5):2180–4.
99. Galle J, Schneider R, Winner B, Lehmann-Bodem C, Schinzel R, Münch G, Conzelmann E, Wanner C. Glyc-oxidized LDL impair endothelial function more potently than oxidized LDL: role of enhanced oxidative stress. Atherosclerosis. 1998;138(1):65–77.
100. Dong Y, Wu Y, Wu M, Wang S, Zhang J, Xie Z, Xu J, Song P, Wilson K, Zhao Z, Lyons T, Zou MH. Activation of protease calpain by oxidized and glycated LDL increases the degradation of endothelial nitric oxide synthase. J Cell Mol Med. 2009;13(9A):2899–910.
101. Posch K, Simecek S, Wascher TC, Jürgens G, Baumgartner-Parzer S, Kostner GM, Graier WF. Glycated low-density lipoprotein attenuates shear stress-induced nitric oxide synthesis by inhibition of

shear stress-activated L-arginine uptake in endothelial cells. Diabetes. 1999;48(6):1331–7.
102. Nivoit P, Wiernsperger N, Moulin P, Lagarde M, Renaudin C. Effect of glycated LDL on microvascular tone in mice: a comparative study with LDL modified in vitro or isolated from diabetic patients. Diabetologia. 2003;46(11):1550–8.
103. Calvo C, Ponsin G, Berthezene F. Characterization of the non enzymatic glycation of high density lipoprotein in diabetic patients. Diabetes Metab. 1988;14(3):264–9.
104. Ferretti G, Bacchetti T, Marchionni C, Dousset N. Effect of non-enzymatic glycation on aluminium-induced lipid peroxidation of human high density lipoproteins (HDL). Nutr Metab Cardiovasc Dis. 2004;14(6):358–65.
105. Rashduni DL, Rifici VA, Schneider SH, Khachadurian AK. Glycation of high-density lipoprotein does not increase its susceptibility to oxidation or diminish its cholesterol efflux capacity. Metabolism. 1999;48(2):139–43.
106. Zhou H, Tan KC, Shiu SW, Wong Y. Increased serum advanced glycation end products are associated with impairment in HDL antioxidative capacity in diabetic nephropathy. Nephrol Dial Transplant. 2008;23(3):927–33.
107. Kalogerakis G, Baker AM, Christov S, Rowley KG, Dwyer K, Winterbourn C, Best JD, Jenkins AJ. Oxidative stress and high-density lipoprotein function in Type I diabetes and end-stage renal disease. Clin Sci (Lond). 2005;108(6):497–506.
108. Mastorikou M, Mackness B, Liu Y, Mackness M. Glycation of paraoxonase-1 inhibits its activity and impairs the ability of high-density lipoprotein to metabolize membrane lipid hydroperoxides. Diabet Med. 2008;25(9):1049–55.
109. Perségol L, Foissac M, Lagrost L, Athias A, Gambert P, Vergès B, Duvillard L. HDL particles from type 1 diabetic patients are unable to reverse the inhibitory effect of oxidised LDL on endothelium-dependent vasorelaxation. Diabetologia. 2007;50(11):2384–7.
110. Low H, Hoang A, Forbes J, Thomas M, Lyons JG, Nestel P, Bach LA, Sviridov D. Advanced glycation end-products (AGEs) and functionality of reverse cholesterol transport in patients with type 2 diabetes and in mouse models. Diabetologia. 2012;55(9): 2513–21.
111. Passarelli M, Shimabukuro AF, Catanozi S, Nakandakare ER, Rocha JC, Carrilho AJ, Quintão EC. Diminished rate of mouse peritoneal macrophage cholesterol efflux is not related to the degree of HDL glycation in diabetes mellitus. Clin Chim Acta. 2000;301(1–2):119–34.
112. de Boer JF, Annema W, Schreurs M, van der Veen JN, van der Giet M, Nijstad N, Kuipers F, Tietge UJ. Type I diabetes mellitus decreases in vivo macrophage-to-feces reverse cholesterol transport despite increased biliary sterol secretion in mice. J Lipid Res. 2012;53(3):348–57.
113. Barter P, Rye K. Lecithin:cholesterolacyltransferase. In: Betteridge D, Illingworth D, Shepherd J, editors. Lipoproteins in health and disease. New York: Oxford University Press; 1999. p. 261–76.
114. Nobecourt E, Davies MJ, Brown BE, Curtiss LK, Bonnet DJ, Charlton F, Januszewski AS, Jenkins AJ, Barter PJ, Rye KA. The impact of glycation on apolipoprotein A-I structure and its ability to activate lecithin:cholesterol acyltransferase. Diabetologia. 2007;50(3):643–53.
115. Nelson CL, Karschimkus CS, Dragicevic G, Packham DK, Wilson AM, O'Neal D, Becker GJ, Best JD, Jenkins AJ. Systemic and vascular inflammation is elevated in early IgA and type 1 diabetic nephropathies and relates to vascular disease risk factors and renal function. Nephrol Dial Transplant. 2005;20(11):2420–6.
116. Sugimoto H, Shikata K, Hirata K, Akiyama K, Matsuda M, Kushiro M, Shikata Y, Miyatake N, Miyasaka M, Makino H. Increased expression of intercellular adhesion molecule-1 (ICAM-1) in diabetic rat glomeruli: glomerular hyperfiltration is a potential mechanism of ICAM-1 upregulation. Diabetes. 1997;46(12):2075–81.
117. Khalfaoui T, Lizard G, Beltaief O, Colin D, Ben Hamida J, Errais K, Ammous I, Zbiba W, Tounsi L, Zhioua R, Anane R, Ouertani-Meddeb A. Immunohistochemical analysis of cellular adhesion molecules (ICAM-1, VCAM-1) and VEGF in fibrovascular membranes of patients with proliferative diabetic retinopathy: preliminary study. Pathol Biol (Paris). 2009;57(7–8):513–7.
118. Albertini JP, Valensi P, Lormeau B, Aurousseau MH, Ferrière F, Attali JR, Gattegno L. Elevated concentrations of soluble E-selectin and vascular cell adhesion molecule-1 in NIDDM. Effect of intensive insulin treatment. Diabetes Care. 1998;21(6): 1008–13.
119. Nobécourt E, Tabet F, Lambert G, Puranik R, Bao S, Yan L, Davies MJ, Brown BE, Jenkins AJ, Dusting GJ, Bonnet DJ, Curtiss LK, Barter PJ, Rye KA. Nonenzymatic glycation impairs the antiinflammatory properties of apolipoprotein A-I. Arterioscler Thromb Vasc Biol. 2010;30(4):766–72.
120. Hedrick CC, Thorpe SR, Fu MX, Harper CM, Yoo J, Kim SM, Wong H, Peters AL. Glycation impairs high-density lipoprotein function. Diabetologia. 2000;43(3):312–20.
121. Pan B, Ren H, He Y, Lv X, Ma Y, Li J, Huang L, Yu B, Kong J, Niu C, Zhang Y, Sun WB, Zheng L. HDL of patients with type 2 diabetes mellitus elevates the capability of promoting breast cancer metastasis. Clin Cancer Res. 2012;18(5):1246–56.
122. Tabet F, Lambert G, Cuesta Torres LF, Hou L, Sotirchos I, Touyz RM, Jenkins AJ, Barter PJ, Rye KA. Lipid-free apolipoprotein A-I and discoidal reconstituted high-density lipoproteins differentially inhibit glucose-induced oxidative stress in human macrophages. Arterioscler Thromb Vasc Biol. 2011;31(5):1192–200.
123. Liu D, Ji L, Zhang D, Tong X, Pan B, Liu P, Zhang Y, Huang Y, Su J, Willard B, Zheng L. Nonenzymatic

glycation of high-density lipoprotein impairs its anti-inflammatory effects in innate immunity. Diabetes Metab Res Rev. 2012;28(2):186–95.
124. Klaya F, Durlach V, Bertin E, Monier F, Monboisse JC, Gillery P. Evaluation of serum glycated lipoprotein(a) levels in noninsulin-dependent diabetic patients. Clin Biochem. 1997;30(3):227–30.
125. Galle J, Winner B, Conzelmann E, Wanner C. Impairment of endothelial function induced by glycoxidized lipoprotein a [Lp(a)]. Cell Mol Biol (Noisy-le-Grand). 1998;44(7):1035–45.
126. Shen GX. Impact and mechanism for oxidized and glycated lipoproteins on generation of fibrinolytic regulators from vascular endothelial cells. Mol Cell Biochem. 2003;246(1–2):69–74.
127. Caslake MJ, Packard CJ, Suckling KE, Holmes SD, Chamberlain P, Macphee CH. Lipoprotein-associated phospholipase A(2), platelet-activating factor acetylhydrolase: a potential new risk factor for coronary artery disease. Atherosclerosis. 2000;150: 413–9.
128. Prescott S, Zimmerman G, Stafforinie D, McIntryre T. Platelet activating factor and related Lipid mediators. Annu Rev Biochem. 2000;69:419–45.
129. de Castro SH, Faria Neto HC, Gomes MB. Platelet-activating factor acetylhydrolase (PAF-AH) activity in patients with type 1 diabetes mellitus. Arq Bras Cardiol. 2007;88(2):179–84.
130. Gomes MB, Cobas RA, Nunes E, Nery M, Castro-Faria-Neto HC, Tibiriçá E. Serum platelet-activating factor acetylhydrolase activity: a novel potential inflammatory marker in type 1 diabetes. Prostaglandins Other Lipid Mediat. 2008;87(1–4):42–6.
131. Gomes MB, Cobas RA, Nunes E, Castro-Faria-Neto HC, da Matta MF, Neves R, Tibiriçá E. Plasma PAF-acetylhydrolase activity, inflammatory markers and susceptibility of LDL to in vitro oxidation in patients with type 1 diabetes mellitus. Diabetes Res Clin Pract. 2009;85(1):61–8.
132. Serban M, Tanaseanu C, Kosaka T, Vidulescu C, Stoian I, Marta DS, Tanaseanu S, Moldoveanu E. Significance of platelet-activating factor acetylhydrolase in patients with non-insulin-dependent (type 2) diabetes mellitus. J Cell Mol Med. 2002;6(4): 643–7.
133. Yamashita S, Matsuzawa Y. Cholesteryl ester transfer protein. In: Betteridge D, Illingworth D, Shepherd J, editors. Lipoproteins in health and disease. New York: Oxford University Press; 1999. p. 277–300.
134. Wegner M, Araszkiewicz A, Zozulińska-Ziółkiewicz D, Wierusz-Wysocka B, Pioruńska-Mikołajczak A, Pioruńska-Stolzmann M. The relationship between concentrations of magnesium and oxidized low density lipoprotein and the activity of platelet activating factor acetylhydrolase in the serum of patients with type 1 diabetes. Magnes Res. 2010;23(2):97–104.
135. Précourt LP, Amre D, Denis MC, Lavoie JC, Delvin E, Seidman E, Levy E. The three-gene paraoxonase family: physiologic roles, actions and regulation. Atherosclerosis. 2011;214(1):20–36.
136. Mackness B, McElduff P, Mackness MI. The paraoxonase-2-310 polymorphism is associated with the presence of microvascular complications in diabetes mellitus. J Intern Med. 2005;258(4):363–8.
137. Mackness MI, Mackness B, Durrington PN, Connelly PW, Hegele RA. Paraoxonase: biochemistry, genetics and relationship to plasma lipoproteins. Genetics Mol Biol. 1996;7(2):69–76.
138. Mackness B, Durrington PN, Mackness MI. The paraoxonase gene family and coronary heart disease. Curr Opin Lipidol. 2002;13(4):357–62.
139. Tavori H, Khatib S, Aviram M, Vaya J. Characterization of the PON1 active site using modeling simulation, in relation to PON1 lactonase activity. Bioorg Med Chem. 2008;16(15):7504–9.
140. Kelso GJ, Stuart WD, Richter RJ, et al. Apolipoprotein J is associated with paraoxonase in human plasma. Biochemistry. 1994;33:832–9.
141. Gaidukov L, Tawfik DS. High affinity, stability, and lactonase activity of serum paraoxonase PON1 anchored on HDL with ApoA-I. Biochemistry. 2005;44:11843–54.
142. Jakubowski H. Calcium-dependent human serum homocysteine thiolactone hydrolase. A protective mechanism against protein N-homocysteinylation. J Biol Chem. 2000;275:3957–62.
143. Costa LG, Cole TB, Furlong CE. Paraoxonase (PON1): from toxicology to cardiovascular medicine. Acta Biomed. 2005;76 Suppl 2:50–7.
144. Van Lenten BJ, Wagner AC, Nayak DP, Hama S, Navab M, Fogelman AM. High-density lipoprotein loses its antiinflammatory properties during acute influenza A infection. Circulation. 2001;103(18): 2283–8.
145. Draganov DI, Teiber JF, Speelman A, Osawa Y, Sunahara R, La Du BN. Human paraoxonases (PON1, PON2, and PON3) are lactonases with overlapping and distinct substrate specificities. J Lipid Res. 2005;46(6):1239–47.
146. Chen Q, Reis SE, Kammerer CM, et al. Association between the severity of angiographic coronary artery disease and paraoxonase gene polymorphisms in the National Heart, Lung, and Blood Institute-Sponsored Women's Ischemia Syndrome Evaluation (WISE) Study. Am J Hum Genet. 2003;72(1):13–22.
147. Ruiz J, Blanche H, James RW, et al. Gln-Arg192 polymorphism of paraoxonase and coronary heart disease in type 2 diabetes. Lancet. 1995;346: 869–72.
148. Pfohl M, Koch M, Enderele MD, et al. Paraoxonase 192 Gln/Arg gene polymorphism, coronary artery disease, and myocardial infarction in Type 2 diabetes. Diabetes. 1999;48:623–7.
149. Kao YL, Donaghue K, Chan A, Knight J, Silink M. A variant of paraoxonase (PON1) gene is associated with diabetic retinopathy in IDDM. J Clin Endocrinol Metab. 1998;83:2589–92.
150. Jenkins AJ, Klein RL, Zheng D, et al. Paraoxonase genotype (192 Gln-Arg) and serum paraoxonase-arylesterase activity: relationship with Type I diabetes and nephropathy. Diabetes. 2000;49 Suppl 1:643P.

151. Kao Y, Donaghue KC, Chan A, Bennetts BH, Knight J, Silink M. Paraoxonase gene cluster is a genetic marker for early microvascular complications in type 1 diabetes. Diabet Med. 2002;19(3):212–5.
152. Leviev I, Kalix B, Brulhart Meynet MC, James RW. The paraoxonase PON1 promoter polymorphism C(-107)T is associated with increased serum glucose concentrations in non-diabetic patients. Diabetologia. 2001;44(9):1177–83.
153. Mackness B, Durrington PN, Boulton AJ, Hine D, Mackness MI. Serum paraoxonase activity in patients with type 1 diabetes compared to healthy controls. Eur J Clin Invest. 2002;32(4):259–64.
154. Kordonouri O, James RW, Bennetts B, et al. Modulation by blood glucose levels of activity and concentration of paraoxonase in young patients with type 1 diabetes mellitus. Metabolism. 2001;50(6): 657–60.
155. Mackness B, Mackness MI, Arrol S, Turkie W, Durrington PN. Effect of the human serum paraoxonase 55 and 192 genetic polymorphisms on the protection by HDL against LDL oxidative modification. FEBS Lett. 1998;423:57–60.
156. Ferretti G, Bacchetti T, Marchionni C, Caldarelli L, Curatola G. Effect of glycation of high density lipoproteins on their physicochemical properties and on paraoxonase activity. Acta Diabetol. 2001;38(4): 163–9.
157. Inoue M, Suehiro T, Nakamura T, Ikeda Y, Kumon Y, Hashimoto K. Serum arylesterase/diazoxonase activity and genetic polymorphisms in patients with type 2 diabetes. Metabolism. 2000;49(11):1400–5.
158. Mackness B, Abuashia B, Boulton A, Mackness M. Low PON activity in Type 2 diabetes mellitus complicated by retinopathy. Clin Sci. 2000;98:355–63.
159. Ikeda Y, Suehiro T, Inoue M, et al. Serum paraoxonase activity and its relationship to diabetic complications in patients with non-insulin-dependent diabetes mellitus. Metabolism. 1998;47(5):598–602.
160. Rajkovic MG, Rumora L, Barisic K. The paraoxonase 1, 2 and 3 in humans. Biochem Med (Zagreb). 2011;21(2):122–30.
161. Intensive blood-glucose control with sulphonylureas or insulin compared with conventional treatment and risk of complications in patients with type 2 diabetes (UKPDS 33). UK Prospective Diabetes Study (UKPDS) Group. Lancet. 1998;352(9131):837–53.
162. Peelman F, Vandekerckhove J, Rosseneu M. Structure and function of lecithin cholesterol acyl transferase: new insights from structural predictions and animal models. Curr Opin Lipidol. 2000;11(2):155–60.
163. Bieliciki JK, Forte TM, McCall MR. Minimally oxidized LDL is a potent inhibitor of LCAT activity. J Lipid Res. 1996;37:1012–21.
164. McCall M, van den Berg J, Kuypers F. Modification of LCAT activity and HDL structure. New links between cigarette smoking and coronary artery disease risk. Arterioscler Thromb. 1994;114:248–53.
165. Nakhjavani M, Asgharani F, Khalilzadeh O, Esteghamati A, Ghaneei A, Morteza A, Anvari M. Oxidized low-density lipoprotein is negatively correlated with lecithin-cholesterol acyltransferase activity in type 2 diabetes mellitus. Am J Med Sci. 2011;341(2):92–5.
166. Chang CK, Tso TK, Snook JT, Huang YS, Lozano RA, Zipf WB. Cholesteryl ester transfer and cholesterol esterification in type 1 diabetes: relationships with plasma glucose. Acta Diabetol. 2001;38(1): 37–42.
167. Gillett MP, Obineche EN, El-Rokhaimi M, Lakhani MS, Abdulle A, Sulaiman M. Lecithin: cholesterol acyltransfer, dyslipoproteinaemia and membrane lipids in uraemia. J Nephrol. 2001;14(6):472–80.
168. Nestel P, Hoang A, Sviridov D, Straznicky N. Cholesterol efflux from macrophages is influenced differentially by plasmas from overweight insulin-sensitive and -resistant subjects. Int J Obes (Lond). 2012;36(3):407–13.
169. Nakhjavani M, Esteghamati A, Esfahanian F, Ghanei A, Rashidi A, Hashemi S. HbA1c negatively correlates with LCAT activity in type 2 diabetes. Diabetes Res Clin Pract. 2008;81(1):38–41.
170. Iizuka T. Effect of anti-diabetic treatment on high density lipoprotein-composition and lecithin:cholesterol acyltransferase activity—a comparison between insulin, sulfonylurea and diet alone treatments. Jpn J Med. 1989;28(4):457–61.
171. Akyuz F, Tekin N, Aydın O, Temel HE, Isikli B. The effect of metformin and exercise on serum lipids, nitric oxide synthase and liver nitric oxide levels in streptozotocin-nicotinamide induced diabetic rats. Afr J Pharm Pharmacol. 2012;6(5):336–42.
172. Fournier N, Myara I, Atger V, Moatti N. Reactivity of lecithin-cholesterol acyl transferase (LCAT) towards glycated high-density lipoproteins (HDL). Clin Chim Acta. 1995;234(1–2):47–61.
173. Zhang Z, Yamashita S, Hirano K, Nakagawa-Toyama Y, Matsuyama A, Nishida M, Sakai N, Fukasawa M, Arai H, Miyagawa J, Matsuzawa Y. Expression of cholesteryl ester transfer protein in human atherosclerotic lesions and its implication in reverse cholesterol transport. Atherosclerosis. 2001;159(1):67–75.
174. Ishikawa Y, Ito K, Akasaka Y, Ishii T, Masuda T, Zhang L, Akishima Y, Kiguchi H, Nakajima K, Hata Y. The distribution and production of cholesteryl ester transfer protein in the human aortic wall. Atherosclerosis. 2001;156(1):29–37.
175. Kakko S, Tamminen M, Päivänsalo M, Kauma H, Rantala AO, Lilja M, Reunanen A, Kesäniemi YA, Savolainen MJ. Variation at the cholesteryl ester transfer protein gene in relation to plasma high density lipoproteins cholesterol levels and carotid intima-media thickness. Eur J Clin Invest. 2001;31(7):593–602.
176. Bagdade JD, Subbaiah PV, Ritter MC. Accelerated cholesteryl ester transfer in patients with insulin dependent diabetes mellitus. Eur J Clin Invest. 1991;21:161–7.
177. Bhatnagar D, Durrington PN, Kumar S, Mackness MI, Dean J, Boulton AJM. Effect of treatment with a

hydroxymethylglutaryl coenzyme A reductase inhibitor on fasting and postprandial plasma lipoproteins and cholesteryl ester transfer in patients with NIDDM. Diabetes. 1995;44:460–5.
178. Bagdade JD, Kelley DE, Henry RR, Eckel RH, Ritter MC. Effects of multiple daily insulin injections and intraperitoneal insulin therapy on cholesteryl ester transfer and lipoprotein lipase activities in NIDDM. Diabetes. 1997;46:414–20.
179. Passarelli M, Cantanozi S, Nakandakare ER, et al. Plasma lipoproteins from patients with poorly controlled diabetes mellitus and "in vitro" glycation of lipoproteins enhance the transfer rate of cholesteryl ester from HDL to apo-B-containing lipoproteins. Diabetologia. 1997;40:1085–93.
180. Lemkadem B, Loiseau D, Larcher G, Malthiery Y, Foussard F. Effect of the nonenzymatic glycosylation of high density lipoprotein-3 on the cholesterol ester transfer protein activity. Lipids. 1999;34(12):1281–6.
181. Connelly MA, Parry TJ, Giardino EC, Huang Z, Cheung WM, Chen C, Cools F, Van der Linde H, Gallacher DJ, Kuo GH, Sarich TC, Demarest KT, Damiano BP. Torcetrapib produces endothelial dysfunction independent of cholesteryl ester transfer protein inhibition. J Cardiovasc Pharmacol. 2010;55(5):459–68.
182. Simic B, Hermann M, Shaw SG, Bigler L, Stalder U, Dörries C, Besler C, Lüscher TF, Ruschitzka F. Torcetrapib impairs endothelial function in hypertension. Eur Heart J. 2012;33(13):1615–24.
183. Colhoun HM, Thomason MJ, Mackness MI, Maton SM, Betteridge DJ, Durrington PN, Hitman GA, Neil HA, Fuller JH, Collaborative AtoRvastatin Diabetes Study (CARDS). Design of the Collaborative AtoRvastatin Diabetes Study (CARDS) in patients with type 2 diabetes. Diabet Med. 2002;19(3):201–11.
184. Collins R, Armitage J, Parish S, Sleight P, Peto R, Heart Protection Study Collaborative Group. Effects of cholesterol-lowering with simvastatin on stroke and other major vascular events in 20536 people with cerebrovascular disease or other high-risk conditions. Lancet. 2004;363(9411):757–67.
185. Keech A, Simes RJ, Barter P, Best J, Scott R, Taskinen MR, Forder P, Pillai A, Davis T, Glasziou P, Drury P, Kesäniemi YA, Sullivan D, Hunt D, Colman P, d'Emden M, Whiting M, Ehnholm C, Laakso M, FIELD study investigators. Effects of long-term fenofibrate therapy on cardiovascular events in 9795 people with type 2 diabetes mellitus (the FIELD study): randomised controlled trial. Lancet. 2005;366(9500):1849–61.
186. Scott R, Best J, Forder P, Taskinen MR, Simes J, Barter P, Keech A, FIELD Study Investigators. Fenofibrate Intervention and Event Lowering in Diabetes (FIELD) study: baseline characteristics and short-term effects of fenofibrate [ISRCTN64783481]. Cardiovasc Diabetol. 2005;4:13.
187. Keech AC, Mitchell P, Summanen PA, O'Day J, Davis TM, Moffitt MS, Taskinen MR, Simes RJ, Tse D, Williamson E, Merrifield A, Laatikainen LT, d'Emden MC, Crimet DC, O'Connell RL, Colman PG, FIELD study investigators. Effect of fenofibrate on the need for laser treatment for diabetic retinopathy (FIELD study): a randomised controlled trial. Lancet. 2007;370(9600):1687–97.
188. Ginsberg HN, Bonds DE, Lovato LC, Crouse JR, Elam MB, Linz PE, O'connor PJ, Leiter LA, Weiss D, Lipkin E, Fleg JL, ACCORD Study Group. Evolution of the lipid trial protocol of the action to control cardiovascular risk in diabetes (ACCORD) trial. Am J Cardiol. 2007;99(12A):56i–67.
189. The effect of intensive treatment of diabetes on the development and progression of long-term complications in insulin-dependent diabetes mellitus. The Diabetes Control and Complications Trial Research Group. N Engl J Med. 1993;329(14):977–86.
190. Nathan DM, Cleary PA, Backlund JY, Genuth SM, Lachin JM, Orchard TJ, Raskin P, Zinman B, Diabetes Control and Complications Trial/Epidemiology of Diabetes Interventions and Complications (DCCT/EDIC) Study Research Group. Intensive diabetes treatment and cardiovascular disease in patients with type 1 diabetes. N Engl J Med. 2005;353(25):2643–53.
191. Lopes-Virella MF, McHenry MB, Lipsitz S, Yim E, Wilson PF, Lackland DT, Lyons T, Jenkins AJ, Virella G, DCCT/EDIC Research Group. Immune complexes containing modified lipoproteins are related to the progression of internal carotid intima-media thickness in patients with type 1 diabetes. Atherosclerosis. 2007;190(2):359–69.
192. Rutter MK, Prais HR, Charlton-Menys V, Gittins M, Roberts C, Davies RR, Moorhouse A, Jinadev P, France M, Wiles PG, Gibson JM, Dean J, Kalra PA, Cruickshank JK, Durrington PN. Protection against nephropathy in diabetes with atorvastatin (PANDA): a randomized double-blind placebo-controlled trial of high- vs. low-dose atorvastatin. Diabet Med. 2011;28(1):100–8.
193. Kelley DE, Williams KV, Price JC, et al. Plasma fatty acids, adiposity, and variance of skeletal muscle insulin resistance in type 2 diabetes mellitus. J Clin Endocrinol Metab. 2001;86:5412–9.
194. Yudkin JS. Abnormalities of coagulation and fibrinolysis in insulin resistance. Evidence for a common antecedent? Diabetes Care. 1999;22 Suppl 3:C25–30.
195. Vestergaard H, Lund S, Pedersen O. Rosiglitazone treatment of patients with extreme insulin resistance and diabetes mellitus due to insulin receptor mutations has no effects on glucose and lipid metabolism. J Intern Med. 2001;250:406–14.
196. Beisswenger PJ, Howell SK, Touchette AD, Lal S, Szwergold BS. Metformin reduces systemic methylglyoxal levels in type 2 diabetes. Diabetes. 1999;48(1):198–202.
197. Rosenstock J, Vico M, Wei L, Salsali A, List JF. Effects of dapagliflozin, an SGLT2 inhibitor, on

HbA1c, body weight, and hypoglycemia risk in patients with type 2 diabetes inadequately controlled on pioglitazone monotherapy. Diabetes Care. 2012;35(7):1473–8.
198. Abdul-Ghani MA, Norton L, DeFronzo RA. Efficacy and safety of SGLT2 inhibitors in the treatment of type 2 diabetes mellitus. Curr Diab Rep. 2012;12(3):230–8.
199. Buse J. Statin treatment in diabetes mellitus. Clin Diabetes. 2003;21(4):168–72.
200. Ansquer JC, Foucher C, Aubonnet P, Le Malicot K. Fibrates and microvascular complications in diabetes—insight from the FIELD study. Curr Pharm Des. 2009;15(5):537–52.
201. Olukman M, Sezer ED, Ulker S, Sözmen EY, Cınar GM. Fenofibrate treatment enhances antioxidant status and attenuates endothelial dysfunction in streptozotocin-induced diabetic rats. Exp Diabetes Res. 2010;201:828531.
202. Davignon J, Jacob RF, Mason RP. The antioxidant effects of statins. Coron Artery Dis. 2004;15(5): 251–8.
203. Culver AL, Ockene IS, Balasubramanian R, Olendzki BC, Sepavich DM, Wactawski-Wende J, Manson JE, Qiao Y, Liu S, Merriam PA, Rahilly-Tierny C, Thomas F, Berger JS, Ockene JK, Curb JD, Ma Y. Statin use and risk of diabetes mellitus in postmenopausal women in the Women's Health Initiative. Arch Intern Med. 2012;172(2):144–52.
204. Yamakawa T, Kaneko T, Shigematu E, Kawaguchi J, Kadonosono K, Morita S, Terauchi Y. Glucose-lowering effect of colestimide is associated with baseline HbA1c in type 2 diabetic patients with hypercholesterolemia. Endocr J. 2011;58(3):185–91.
205. Younis NN, Soran H, Sharma R, Charlton-Menys V, Greenstein A, Elseweidy MM, Durrington PN. Small-dense LDL and LDL glycation in metabolic syndrome and in statin-treated and non-statin-treated type 2 diabetes. Diab Vasc Dis Res. 2010;7(4): 289–95.
206. Suzuki T, Oba K, Futami S, Suzuki K, Ouchi M, Igari Y, Matsumura N, Watanabe K, Kigawa Y, Nakano H. Blood glucose-lowering activity of colestimide in patients with type 2 diabetes and hypercholesterolemia: a case-control study comparing colestimide with acarbose. J Nippon Med Sch. 2006;73(5):277–84.
207. Goldberg RB, Jacobson TA. Effects of niacin on glucose control in patients with dyslipidemia. Mayo Clin Proc. 2008;83(4):470–8.
208. Kobayashi S, Moriya H, Negishi K, Maesato K, Ohtake T. LDL-apheresis up-regulates VEGF and IGF-I in patients with ischemic limb. J Clin Apher. 2003;18(3):115–9.
209. Tamai O, Matsuoka H, Itabe H, Wada Y, Kohno K, Imaizumi T. Single LDL apheresis improves endothelium-dependent vasodilatation in hypercholesterolemic humans. Circulation. 1997;95(1): 76–82.
210. Pares MN, D'Amico EA, Kutner JM, Chamone Dde A, Bydlowski SP. Platelet aggregation and lipoprotein levels in a patient with familial hypercholesterolemia after selective LDL-apheresis. Sao Paulo Med J. 1997;115(3):1448–51.
211. Kobayashi S, Oka M, Moriya H, Maesato K, Okamoto K, Ohtake T. LDL-apheresis reduces P-Selectin, CRP and fibrinogen—possible important implications for improving atherosclerosis. Ther Apher Dial. 2006;10(3):219–23.
212. Xi M, Hai C, Tang H, Chen M, Fang K, Liang X. Antioxidant and antiglycation properties of total saponins extracted from traditional Chinese medicine used to treat diabetes mellitus. Phytother Res. 2008;22(2):228–37.
213. Motomura K, Fujiwara Y, Kiyota N, Tsurushima K, Takeya M, Nohara T, Nagai R, Ikeda T. Astragalosides isolated from the root of astragalus radix inhibit the formation of advanced glycation end products. J Agric Food Chem. 2009;57(17):7666–72.
214. Panagiotopoulos S, O'Brien RC, Bucala R, Cooper ME, Jerums G. Aminoguanidine has an anti-atherogenic effect in the cholesterol-fed rabbit. Atherosclerosis. 1998;136(1):125–31.
215. Ulrich P, Zhang X. Pharmacological reversal of advanced glycation end-product-mediated protein crosslinking. Diabetologia. 1997;40 Suppl 2:S157–9.
216. Thorpe SR, Baynes JW. Role of the Maillard reaction in diabetes mellitus and diseases of aging. Drugs Aging. 1996;9(2):69–77.
217. Philis-Tsimikas A, Parthasarathy S, Picard S, Palinski W, Witztum JL. Aminoguanidine has both pro-oxidant and antioxidant activity toward LDL. Arterioscler Thromb Vasc Biol. 1995;15(3):367–76.
218. Sing R, Barden A, Mori T, Beilin L. Advanced glycation end products. Diabetologia. 2001;44:129–46.
219. Bolton WK, Cattran DC, Williams ME, Adler SG, Appel GB, Cartwright K, Foiles PG, Freedman BI, Raskin P, Ratner RE, Spinowitz BS, Whittier FC, Wuerth JP, ACTION I Investigator Group. Randomized trial of an inhibitor of formation of advanced glycation end products in diabetic nephropathy. Am J Nephrol. 2004;24(1):32–40.
220. Yamagishi S, Amano S, Inagaki Y, Okamoto T, Koga K, Sasaki N, Yamamoto H, Takeuchi M, Makita Z. Advanced glycation end products-induced apoptosis and overexpression of vascular endothelial growth factor in bovine retinal pericytes. Biochem Biophys Res Commun. 2002;290(3):973–8.
221. Whittier F, Spinowitz B, Wuerth JP, et al. Pimagedine safety profile in patients wity Type 1 diabetes. J Am Soc Nephrol. 1999;10:184A.
222. Nilsson BO. Biological effects of aminoguanidine: an update. Inflamm Res. 1999;48:509–15.
223. Picard S, Parthasarathy S, Fruebis J, Witztum JL. Aminoguanidine inhibits oxidative modification of low density lipoprotein protein and the subsequent increase in uptake by macrophage scavenger receptors. Proc Natl Acad Sci USA. 1992;89(15): 6876–80.
224. Jedidi I, Thérond P, Zarev S, Cosson C, Couturier M, Massot C, Jore D, Gardès-Albert M, Legrand A,

Bonnefont-Rousselot D. Paradoxical protective effect of aminoguanidine toward low-density lipoprotein oxidation: inhibition of apolipoprotein B fragmentation without preventing its carbonylation. Mechanism of action of aminoguanidine. Biochemistry. 2003;42(38):11356–65.
225. Oak JH, Youn JY, Cai H. Aminoguanidine inhibits aortic hydrogen peroxide production. VSMC NOX activity and hypercontractility in diabetic mice. Cardiovasc Diabetol. 2009;8:65.
226. Misko TP, Moore WM, Kasten TP, Nickols GA, Corbett JA, Tilton RG, McDaniel ML, Williamson JR, Currie MG. Selective inhibition of the inducible nitric oxide synthase by aminoguanidine. Eur J Pharmacol. 1993;233(1):119–25.
227. Wu G. Nitric oxide synthesis and the effect of aminoguanidine and NG-monomethyl-L-arginine on the onset of diabetes in the spontaneously diabetic BB rat. Diabetes. 1995;44(3):360–4.
228. Khalifah RG, Baynes JW, Hudson BG. Amadorins: novel post-Amadori inhibitors of advanced glycation reactions. Biochem Biophys Res Commun. 1999;257(2):251–8.
229. Onorato JM, Jenkins AJ, Thorpe SR, Baynes JW. Pyridoxamine, an inhibitor of advanced glycation reactions, also inhibits advanced lipoxidation reactions. Mechanism of action of pyridoxamine. J Biol Chem. 2000;275(28):21177–84.
230. Metz TO, Alderson NL, Thorpe SR, Baynes JW. Pyridoxamine, an inhibitor of advanced glycation and lipoxidation reactions: a novel therapy for treatment of diabetic complications. Arch Biochem Biophys. 2003;419(1):41–9.
231. Alkhalaf A, Klooster A, van Oeveren W, Achenbach U, Kleefstra N, Slingerland RJ, Mijnhout GS, Bilo HJ, Gans RO, Navis GJ, Bakker SJ. A double-blind, randomized, placebo-controlled clinical trial on benfotiamine treatment in patients with diabetic nephropathy. Diabetes Care. 2010;33(7):1598–601.
232. Karachalias N, Babaei-Jadidi R, Rabbani N, Thornalley PJ. Increased protein damage in renal glomeruli, retina, nerve, plasma and urine and its prevention by thiamine and benfotiamine therapy in a rat model of diabetes. Diabetologia. 2010;53(7): 1506–16.
233. Balakumar P, Rohilla A, Krishan P, Solairaj P, Thangathirupathi A. The multifaceted therapeutic potential of benfotiamine. Pharmacol Res. 2010; 61(6):482–8.
234. Katare RG, Caporali A, Oikawa A, Meloni M, Emanueli C, Madeddu P. Vitamin B1 analog benfotiamine prevents diabetes-induced diastolic dysfunction and heart failure through Akt/Pim-1-mediated survival pathway. Circ Heart Fail. 2010;3(2): 294–305.
235. Du X, Edelstein D, Brownlee M. Oral benfotiamine plus alpha-lipoic acid normalises complication-causing pathways in type 1 diabetes. Diabetologia. 2008;51(10):1930–2.
236. Beltramo E, Berrone E, Tarallo S, Porta M. Effects of thiamine and benfotiamine on intracellular glucose metabolism and relevance in the prevention of diabetic complications. Acta Diabetol. 2008;45(3): 131–41.
237. Waanders F, van den Berg E, Nagai R, van Veen I, Navis G, van Goor H. Renoprotective effects of the AGE-inhibitor pyridoxamine in experimental chronic allograft nephropathy in rats. Nephrol Dial Transplant. 2008;23(2):518–24.
238. Degenhardt TP, Alderson NL, Arrington DD, Beattie RJ, Basgen JM, Steffes MW, Thorpe SR, Baynes JW. Pyridoxamine inhibits early renal disease and dyslipidemia in the streptozotocin-diabetic rat. Kidney Int. 2002;61(3):939–50.
239. Stitt A, Gardiner TA, Alderson NL, Canning P, Frizzell N, Duffy N, Boyle C, Januszewski AS, Chachich M, Baynes JW, Thorpe SR. The AGE inhibitor pyridoxamine inhibits development of retinopathy in experimental diabetes. Diabetes. 2002;51(9):2826–32.
240. Alderson NL, Chachich ME, Youssef NN, Beattie RJ, Nachtigal M, Thorpe SR, Baynes JW. The AGE inhibitor pyridoxamine inhibits lipemia and development of renal and vascular disease in Zucker obese rats. Kidney Int. 2003;63(6):2123–33.
241. Jenkins AJ, Best JD, Klein RL, Lyons TJ. Lipoproteins, glycoxidation and diabetic angiopathy. Diabet Metab Res Rev. 2004;20(5):349–68.
242. Lyons TJ, Jenkins AJ. Glycation, oxidation, and lipoxidation in the development of the complications of diabetes: a carbonyl stress hypothesis. Diabet Rev. 1997;5:365–91.
243. Stitt AW, Jenkins AJ, Cooper ME. Advanced glycation end products and diabetic complications. Expert Opin Investig Drugs. 2002;11(9):1205–23.
244. Brown SM, Smith DM, Alt N, Thorpe SR, Baynes JW. Tissue-specific variation in glycation of proteins in diabetes: evidence for a functional role of amadoriase enzymes. Ann N Y Acad Sci. 2005;1043: 817–23.
245. Monnier VM, Wu X. Enzymatic deglycation with amadoriase enzymes from Aspergillus sp. as a potential strategy against the complications of diabetes and aging. Biochem Soc Trans. 2003;31: 1349–53.
246. Monnier VM, Sell DR. Prevention and repair of protein damage by the Maillard reaction in vivo. Rejuvenation Res. 2006;9(2):264–73.
247. Cohen MP, Sharma K, Jin Y, Hud E, Wu VY, Tomaszewski J, Ziyadeh FN. Prevention of diabetic nephropathy in db/db mice with glycated albumin antagonists. A novel treatment strategy. J Clin Invest. 1995;95(5):2338–45.
248. Mitsuhashi T, Li YM, Fishbane S, Vlassara H. Depletion of reactive advanced glycation endproducts from diabetic uremic sera by a lysozyme-linked matrix. J Clin Invest. 1997;100:847–54.
249. Zheng F, Cai W, Mitsuhashi T, Vlassara H. Lysozyme enhances renal excretion of advanced glycation endproducts in vivo and suppresses adverse age-mediated cellular effects in vitro: a potential AGE

sequestration therapy for diabetic nephropathy? Mol Med. 2001;7(11):737–47.
250. Li YM, Tan AX, Vlassara H. Antibacterial activity of lysozyme and lactoferrin is inhibited by binding of advanced glycation-modified proteins to a conserved motif. Nat Med. 1995;1:1057–61.
251. Wautier JL, Zoukourian C, Chappey O, Wautier MP, Guillausseau PJ, Cao R, Hori O, Stern D, Schmidt AM. Receptor-mediated endothelial cell dysfunction in diabetic vasculopathy. Soluble receptor for advanced glycation end products blocks hyperpermeability in diabetic rats. J Clin Invest. 1996;97(1):238–43.
252. Bucciarelli LG, Wendt T, Qu W, Lu Y, Lalla E, Rong LL, Goova MT, Moser B, Kislinger T, Lee DC, Kashyap Y, Stern DM, Schmidt AM. RAGE blockade stabilizes established atherosclerosis in diabetic apolipoprotein E-null mice. Circulation. 2002;106(22):2827–35.
253. Santilli F, Vazzana N, Bucciarelli LG, Davì G. Soluble forms of RAGE in human diseases: clinical and therapeutical implications. Curr Med Chem. 2009;16(8):940–52.
254. Yan SF, Ramasamy R, Schmidt AM. Soluble RAGE: therapy and biomarker in unraveling the RAGE axis in chronic disease and aging. Biochem Pharmacol. 2010;79(10):1379–86.
255. Zhang H, Tasaka S, Shiraishi Y, Fukunaga K, Yamada W, Seki H, Ogawa Y, Miyamoto K, Nakano Y, Hasegawa N, Miyasho T, Maruyama I, Ishizaka A. Role of soluble receptor for advanced glycation end products on endotoxin-induced lung injury. Am J Respir Crit Care Med. 2008;178(4):356–62.
256. Zieman SJ, Melenovsky V, Clattenburg L, Corretti MC, Capriotti A, Gerstenblith G, Kass DA. Advanced glycation endproduct crosslink breaker (alagebrium) improves endothelial function in patients with isolated systolic hypertension. J Hypertens. 2007;25(3):577–83.
257. Steppan J, Tran H, Benjo AM, Pellakuru L, Barodka V, Ryoo S, Nyhan SM, Lussman C, Gupta G, White AR, Daher JP, Shoukas AA, Levine BD, Berkowitz DE. Alagebrium in combination with exercise ameliorates age-associated ventricular and vascular stiffness. Exp Gerontol. 2012;47(8): 565–72.
258. Gurbuz N, Sagdic G, Sanli A, Ciftcioglu A, Bassorgun I, Baykal A, Usta MF. Therapeutic effect of combination of alagebrium (ALT-711) and sildenafil on erectile function in diabetic rats. Int J Impot Res. 2012;24(3):114–21.
259. Hartog JW, Willemsen S, van Veldhuisen DJ, Posma JL, van Wijk LM, Hummel YM, Hillege HL, Voors AA, BENEFICIAL investigators. Effects of alagebrium, an advanced glycation endproduct breaker, on exercise tolerance and cardiac function in patients with chronic heart failure. Eur J Heart Fail. 2011;13(8):899–908.
260. Kiland JA, Gabelt BT, Tezel G, Lütjen-Drecoll E, Kaufman PL. Effect of the age cross-link breaker alagebrium on anterior segment physiology, morphology, and ocular age and rage. Trans Am Ophthalmol Soc. 2009;107:146–58.
261. Coughlan MT, Thallas-Bonke V, Pete J, Long DM, Gasser A, Tong DC, Arnstein M, Thorpe SR, Cooper ME, Forbes JM. Combination therapy with the advanced glycation end product cross-link breaker, alagebrium, and angiotensin converting enzyme inhibitors in diabetes: synergy or redundancy? Endocrinology. 2007;148(2):886–95.
262. Freidja ML, Tarhouni K, Toutain B, Fassot C, Loufrani L, Henrion D. The AGE-breaker ALT-711 restores high blood flow-dependent remodeling in mesenteric resistance arteries in a rat model of type 2 diabetes. Diabetes. 2012;61(6):1562–72.
263. Krautwald M, Leech D, Horne S, Steele ML, Forbes J, Rahmadi A, Griffith R, Münch G. The advanced glycation end product-lowering agent ALT-711 is a low-affinity inhibitor of thiamine diphosphokinase. Rejuvenation Res. 2011;14(4):383–91.

# Lipoprotein (LDL and HDL) Oxidation in Diabetes Mellitus

9

Marielle Kaplan, Michael Aviram, and Tony Hayek

## Introduction

Diabetes mellitus (DM) is associated with premature and accelerated atherosclerosis. The precise mechanisms underlying the accelerated progression of atherosclerosis development in DM are poorly understood, but hyperglycemia and its associated metabolic changes accelerate diabetes complications and atherosclerosis development.

A critical event during the early stages of atherogenesis is the formation and accumulation of lipid-laden macrophage foam cells. Conversion of macrophages into foam cells involves several mechanisms including increased cellular lipid peroxidation (through activation of the NADPH oxidase complex), increased oxidized-LDL uptake by macrophages (via scavengers receptors SRA and CD36), decreased HDL-mediated cholesterol efflux from the foam cells, and increased rate of cellular cholesterol biosynthesis.

Several studies have shown that diabetes is associated with increased oxidative stress which is considered to be one of the major mechanisms for the induction of atherosclerosis in diabetes. Accelerated atherosclerosis development in diabetic animal models is associated with enhanced lipid peroxidation and cholesterol accumulation. Moreover, glucose uptake by macrophages increases cellular oxidative stress and the formation of atherogenic AGE (advanced glycation end products), and this effect is linked to increased activity of macrophage NADPH oxidase, following cell incubation with glucose.

Numerous studies have attempted to evaluate the role of hyperglycemia on cells of the artery wall, including endothelial cells, smooth muscle cells, and monocyte-derived macrophages. Glucose might contribute to increased oxidative stress directly, or indirectly, via the generation of AGEs or of reactive oxygen/nitrogen species (ROS/RNS). High glucose concentrations have been shown to lead to diacylglycerol (DAG) accumulation and protein kinase C (PKC) activation in vascular cells, as well as to increased glucose flux through the aldose reductase pathway. Diabetes is also associated with reduced levels of antioxidants such as the glutathione (GSH) system, including glutathione peroxidase and reductase, vitamin C and vitamin E. During early diabetes-induced atherogenesis, the extent of LDL oxidation by macrophages is increased due to activation of several pro-oxidant systems. Indeed, supplementation of antioxidants such as vitamin E or moderate consumption of polyphenol-rich pomegranate juice or red wine by diabetic patients was shown to significantly reduce their serum and cellular oxidative stress. However, large-scale

M. Kaplan
The Laboratory of Clinical Biochemistry, Rappaport Family Institute for Research in the Medical Sciences, Rambam Medical Center, Haifa, Israel

M. Aviram • T. Hayek, M.D. (✉)
The Lipid Research Laboratory, Technion Faculty of Medicine, Rappaport Family Institute for Research in the Medical Sciences and Rambam Medical Center, Haifa, Israel
e-mail: t_hayek@rambam.health.gov.il

A.J. Jenkins et al. (eds.), *Lipoproteins in Diabetes Mellitus*, Contemporary Diabetes,
DOI 10.1007/978-1-4614-7554-5_9, © Springer Science+Business Media New York 2014

trials of antioxidant supplementation to the general population and also to diabetic patients were negative regarding vascular endpoints, probably because of population inclusion/exclusion criteria, as well as dosages used.

The paraoxonases (PON) which include PON1, PON2, and PON3, possess lactonase activity and antioxidant properties. HDL-bound PON1 in serum is decreased in blood harvested from diabetic patients. Recent studies have shown that PON1 activity decreases in parallel to the duration of DM, and this is associated with the acceleration of cardiovascular disease (CVD) development in DM patients. PON1 in HDL from type 2 diabetic patients is heavily glycated, and as a result, have decreased ability to metabolize cellular lipid peroxides. Similarly, in vitro studies demonstrate that glucose inactivates PON1, and glycated PON1 has reduced antioxidative capacity. In a recent publication, we have shown that PON1 through its antioxidant activity towards macrophages and serum has a protective role against diabetes development. PON1 stimulates production of insulin and glucose transport protein 4 (Glut 4). PON1 administration to streptozotocin (STZ)-induced diabetic mice substantially attenuates diabetes development via its unique anti oxidative properties and its ability to stimulate pancreatic β-cell insulin production and secretion.

Understanding the mechanisms involved in diabetes-induced lipoproteins and arterial macrophages abnormalities may allow us to find effective tools to delay diabetes development and its associated atherosclerosis complications.

## Diabetes Mellitus (DM) and Atherosclerosis

The incidence of diabetes mellitus (DM) is increasing worldwide and is a major public health problem. In fact it is estimated that 210 million people were diagnosed with diabetes worldwide in 2010. These numbers will increase by 50 % in the next 20 years with a tremendous burden on health care systems throughout the world [1].

Diabetes is a complex metabolic disorder characterized by defects in the body's ability to control glucose and insulin homeostasis. There are two types of diabetes: type 1 and type 2. Type 1 is linked mostly to genetics and to the production of antibodies that destroy the pancreatic β cells [2, 3]. Type 2 diabetes, which accounts for more than 90 % of individuals diagnosed with diabetes, results primarily from insulin resistance and has been linked to different factors including age, obesity, and environmental factors [3].

DM is known to be associated with premature and accelerated atherosclerosis. Patients with diabetes are at 2–4 times increased risk for coronary artery disease (CAD), stroke, and peripheral artery disease [4]. Atherosclerosis and its complications are the major cause of death in these patients. More than 30 % of patients hospitalized for acute myocardial infarction have diabetes and another 30 % have impaired glucose tolerance [5]

The relation between diabetes and premature vascular disease is well-established [6] and prospective studies indicate that long-term glycemic control is an important predictor not only of microvascular disease, but also of macrovascular complications [7], further correlating diabetic complications with hyperglycemic levels and length of exposure to hyperglycemia. Vascular complications can be caused by macro- and micro-angiopathy. Macroangiopathy in diabetes consists mainly of an accelerated form of atherosclerosis and affects the coronary, carotid and peripheral arteries, thus increasing the risk of myocardial infarction, stroke and diabetic foot disease [8]. On the other hand, microangiopathy in diabetes is responsible for retinopathy, nephropathy, and neuropathy. Both type 1 and 2 diabetes are associated with accelerated atherosclerosis. Strong epidemiological evidence supports an association between glycemic control and CVD risk [9, 10]. Results from The United Kingdom Prospective Diabetes Study (UKPDS) indicate a linear relationship between HbA1c and CVD endpoints, particularly myocardial infarction [11].

The precise mechanisms underlying the acceleration and progression of atherosclerosis in DM are poorly understood, but it is postulated that hyperglycemia accelerates atherosclerosis by inducing endothelial dysfunction, increased inflammatory burden, increased formation of advanced glycation and products (AGEs), and increased lipid peroxidation of lipoproteins leading to enhanced macrophage foam cell formation, the hallmark of atherosclerosis [12].

Atherosclerosis is initiated by the adhesion of monocytes to arterial endothelial cells, followed by their migration into the subendothelial space in response to chemotactic activation processes. Monocytes then differentiate into intimal macrophages, which take up oxidized lipids. As lipid uptake progresses, the cells form lipid inclusion bodies and take on the appearance of a "foam cell." Foam cells can undergo apoptosis. Apoptotic cells and cellular debris can coalesce to form fatty streak lesions. High glucose levels affect several mechanisms along this process, including activation of nuclear factor kappa B (NFκB) [13], which facilitates monocyte adhesion to endothelial cells, differentiation of monocytes into macrophages and increased expression of pro-inflammatory cytokines [14] associated with induction of protein kinase C [15]. It has been proposed that glucose might act directly or indirectly via the generation of advanced glycation end products (AGEs) to foster the progression of atherogenesis [16].

The treatment of hyperglycemia in diabetic patients does not always prevent vascular complications, possibly because high oxidative stress in DM patients is not therapeutically addressed. Therefore, antioxidant therapy may be of great interest in these patients, and it has recently been suggested that diabetic subjects with complications may have defective cellular antioxidant responses against the oxidative stress generated by hyperglycemia.

## Lipid Abnormalities in Diabetes Mellitus

Lipid abnormalities in patients with type 2 DM play an important role in the development of atherosclerosis. The lipid derangements in DM are not only quantitative but also qualitative abnormalities of lipoproteins which are atherogenic. The main quantitative abnormalities are increased triglyceride levels and low HDL-C levels [17].

Hypertriglyceridemia in the patient with insulin resistance is attributable to: (1) hepatic overproduction of VLDL-Tg and (2) reduced catabolism of VLDL particles of lipoprotein lipase (LPL) which is responsible for the degradation of triglycerides in the VLDL particles [18]. The main qualitative abnormality induced by diabetes in triglycerides is the overproduction of large VLDL particles, which are relatively richer in triglycerides compared to smaller VLDL particles. The large VLDL particles are easily taken up by scavenger receptors in macrophages leading to foam cell formation [19].

Although plasma LDL-C levels are usually normal in type 2 diabetes, it has some qualitative abnormalities which potentially make it more atherogenic. The LDL particles in diabetics tend to be small and dense [20]. the LDL particles in diabetic subjects also appear to have reduced affinity for the LDL receptor and are more easily oxidized.

Another lipoprotein abnormality in diabetes is decreased HDL cholesterol levels, mainly due to increased catabolism of HDL particles. This effect on HDL-C is related mainly to insulin resistance, since the same effect on HDL catabolism is observed also in obese insulin resistant non-diabetic patients [20]. As triglyceride rich VLDL particles accumulate in serum secondary to reduced clearance by lipoprotein lipase, CETP catalyzes a 1:1 stoichiometric exchange of cholesterol ester out of HDL for triglyceride in VLDL. As the HDL particle becomes progressively more enriched with triglyceride, it becomes a better substrate for lipolysis and degradation by hepatic lipase.

Finally, AGE-modified albumin can inhibit SR-B1-mediated efflux of cholesterol to HDL [21]. These findings suggest that AGE proteins in the circulation also might interfere with the functions of SR-BI in reverse cholesterol transport by inhibiting the selective uptake of HDL-cholesteryl ester, as well as cholesterol efflux from peripheral cells to HDL. Thus, alterations in the delivery and removal of lipid from macrophages by lipoproteins and other proteins that have been modified by prolonged exposure to high glucose conditions might lead to lipid accumulation and foam cell formation.

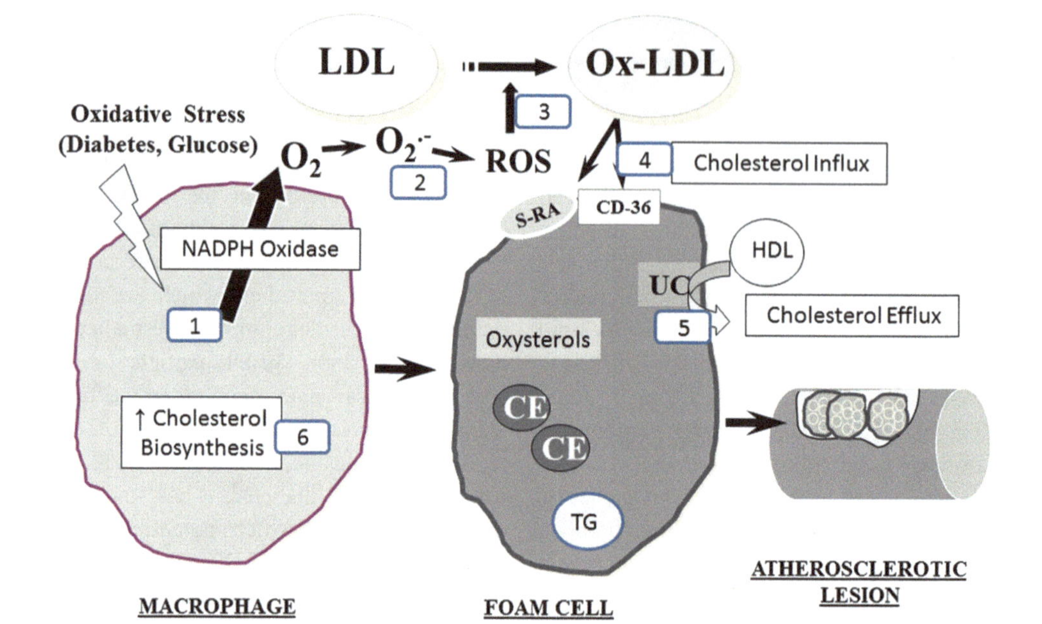


**Fig. 9.1** Macrophages foam cell formation. Under oxidative stress, macrophages generate reactive oxygen species and through activation of NADPH oxidase complex (1) increase the production and release of superoxide ions (2), thus leading to extensive LDL oxidation (3) increased oxidized LDL (OX-LDL) uptake by macrophages via their scavenges receptors SRA and CD36 (4) thus leading to foam cell formation. Conversion of macrophages into foam cells also involves decreased HDL-mediated cholesterol efflux (5) and increased cellular cholesterol biosynthesis (6)

## Lipoprotein Oxidation in Atherogenesis

A critical event in the early stages of atherosclerosis is the accumulation of lipid-laden macrophage foam cells [22]. Conversion of macrophages into foam cells involves several mechanisms including increased cellular and lipoprotein lipid peroxidation, increased oxidized-LDL uptake, decreased HDL-mediated cholesterol efflux, and increased cellular cholesterol biosynthesis. Under oxidative stress, macrophages can generate reactive oxygen species (ROS) and, through activation of NADPH oxidase complex, increase the production and release of superoxide ions, thus leading to extensive LDL oxidation and increased oxidized LDL (OX-LDL) uptake by macrophages via their scavenger receptors SRA and CD36, resulting in foam cell formation [23] (Fig. 9.1).

It was shown in previous studies that LDL is oxidized in vivo under certain atherogenic conditions and, indeed, circulating OX-LDL exist in human plasma of patients with CAD and their levels correlate positively with the severity of CAD [24]. OX-LDL is present in atherosclerotic lesions from human and animal models [25]. Unlike the LDL receptor, OX-LDL receptors are not regulated by cellular cholesterol levels. The uptake of OX-LDL occurs via the scavenger receptors CD36 and scavenger receptor A (SRA), which leads to cholesterol accumulation and foam cell formation [23].

The process of LDL oxidation is unlikely to occur in plasma because of the high concentrations of antioxidants and metal cation chelation agents. LDL oxidation is more likely to occur within the artery wall, an environment depleted of antioxidants [26]. It is not clear which cells in the arterial wall are responsible for LDL oxidation, but it is postulated that endothelial cells [27] and smooth muscle cells (SMC) [28] could contribute to LDL oxidation, a process which requires the presence of transition metal ions such as copper and iron ions. LDL oxidation by macrophages also has a major role during early stage of atherosclerosis [29].

Cell mediated oxidation of LDL depends on the balance between cellular pro-oxidants such as NADPH oxidase, lipoxygenase, or myeloperoxidase and cellular antioxidants such as the glutathione system and superoxide dismutase, as well as the balance between pro-oxidants and antioxidants in the lipoprotein particles themselves [23].

LDL oxidation starts with the consumption of its antioxidants. After depleting LDL of its antioxidants, transition metal ions catalyze propagation reactions, which include the breakdown of lipid hydroperoxides and the formation of aldehydes. These reactions are responsible for the oxidative modification of Apo B 100, which alter the charge and three-dimensional configuration of this apoprotein. Affinity for the LDL receptor decreases and the LDL particles are taken up by macrophages [30].

Several biological and biochemical mechanisms were suggested to be involved in macrophage mediated oxidation of LDL including transition metal cations, superoxide anions, NADPH oxidase, lipoxygenase, myeloperoxidase, and reactive nitrogen species [23, 30].

Cellular LDL oxidation requires the presence of iron or copper ions. Several mechanisms are involved in this process but the most important is the ability of macrophages to reduce those metals which then rapidly react with lipid hydroperoxides, leading to the formation of reactive lipid radicals and to the conversion of reduced metal back to its oxidized form [31]. Superoxide ions are required for the initiation of LDL oxidation. In macrophages the predominant source of superoxide is the NADPH oxidase system [32]. We have demonstrated that LDL in the presence of copper ions activates the NADPH oxidase complex. Further evidence for the role of superoxide anions in the oxidation of LDL by macrophages was demonstrated in cells from patients with chronic granulomatous disease, who lack NADPH oxidase and do not generate superoxide anions or oxidized LDL [33]. Previous studies with an in-vitro knockout mouse model of P47 phox (one of the cytosolic subunits of NADPH oxidase) showed that both superoxide anion and LDL oxidation are inhibited [34]. Thus, superoxide and other free radicals derived from NADPH oxidase activation contribute to lipid peroxidation.

Another oxygenase that may participate in oxidation of LDL is myeloperoxidase (MPO). MPO is a heme protein released by activated neutrophils and monocytes and is present in tissue macrophages such as those in atherosclerotic plaques. MPO may play a role in monocyte-macrophage oxidation of LDL by several pathways, such as amplifying the oxidizing potential of H2O2 to reactive oxygen species (ROS), aldehydes, and nitrating agents [35, 36]. MPO-mediated oxidation reactions occur in the absence of metal ions.

Nitric oxide (NO) is formed by multiple vascular cells including monocytes and macrophages [37], and the expression of NO synthase was demonstrated in human coronary atherosclerotic plaques. NO may have both anti and pro-oxidant effects. NO exerts an antioxidant effect, attenuating the extent of cell-mediated oxidation of LDL [38], but NO could also be a pro-oxidant as evidenced by the observation that, when tissue oxidant defense mechanisms become depleted, NO can initiate lipoprotein lipid peroxidation [38].

The paraoxonase gene family includes PON1, PON2, and PON3 which are lactonase enzymes [39]. In humans, PON1 and low levels of PON3 (but not PON2) are found in serum in association with HDL. In humans, PON1 mRNA expression is limited mainly to the liver. In contrast, PON2 is more widely expressed in a variety of tissues, including human and mouse macrophages [40]. All PON proteins were shown to protect from atherosclerosis development, but their mechanism of action is currently unknown. All PONs also have the capacity to protect cells from oxidative stress [41]. PON2, unlike PON1, is not present in the circulation but rather found in cells including macrophages. PON2 like PON1 possesses antioxidant and anti-atherosclerotic properties [41]. The balance between cellular pro oxidants (such as NADPH oxidase) and antioxidants (such as PON2) in arterial wall macrophages determines the extent of LDL oxidation. Macrophage PON2 was shown to be increased under oxidative stress, probably as a compensation mechanism.

## Lipoprotein Oxidation in Diabetes Mellitus

Several studies have shown that diabetes is associated with increased oxidative stress which is considered to be one of the major mechanisms for induction of atherosclerosis in diabetes [42]. The increased oxidative stress is accompanied by increased ROS generation, oxidative stress markers, and decrement of antioxidants. Diabetic patients are highly prone to oxidative stress because hyperglycemia depletes natural antioxidants and facilitates the production of oxygen and nitrogen free radicals [43].

A consequence of diabetes is hyperglycemia, which in turn contributes to the progression and maintenance of an overall oxidative environment. Macrovascular and microvascular complications are the leading cause of morbidity and mortality in diabetic patients, but the complications are tissue specific and result from similar mechanisms with many being linked to oxidative stress.

Oxidative stress is thought to be a major risk factor in the onset and progression of diabetes. Many of the common risk factors such as obesity, increased age, and unhealthy eating habits all contribute to an oxidative environment that may alter insulin sensitivity either by increasing insulin resistance or impairing glucose tolerance. The mechanisms by which this occurs are multifactorial. The mechanism by which oxidative stress may induce diabetes includes increased insulin resistance, increased β cell dysfunction, impaired glucose tolerance, and increased mitochondrial dysfunction [44].

In our studies we have examined the relationship between diabetes, increased lipid peroxidation, and enhanced atherosclerosis by using the Apo E knockout mouse model which develop severe hypercholesterolemia and extensive atherosclerosis on a chow diet [45]. We have shown previously that accelerated atherosclerosis in this animal model is associated with enhanced lipid peroxidation [46]. Diabetic induction in APO E knockout ($E^{\circ}$) mice for three months using streptozotocin (STZ) injection led to an increase of their atherosclerosis lesion area. This phenomenon was associated with a significant increment of macrophage oxidative stress (Fig. 9.2a, b).

Numerous studies have attempted to evaluate the role of high glucose conditions on cells of the artery wall, including endothelial cells, smooth muscle cells, and macrophages. It has been proposed that glucose might act directly via the generation of advanced glycation end-products (AGEs) or reactive oxygen species. Thus, hyperglycemia, one factor shared by both type 1 and type 2 diabetes, is a major contributor to oxidative stress [47, 48]. Cellular glucose could be toxic and directly linked to increased cellular lipid peroxidation, since in vitro studies showed that pre-culture of endothelial cells or smooth muscle cells in glucose-enriched media, increased the cells ability to oxidize LDL which was accompanied by enhanced secretion of superoxide anion. This could be the result of direct generation of ROS or by altering the redox balance. This is thought to occur via several well-studied mechanisms, including activation of protein kinase C [6] and overproduction of superoxide by the mitochondrial electron transport chain [49], increased intracellular formation of advanced glycation end-products (AGEs), and increased flux through the polyol pathway [50]. Hyperglycemia specifically induces cellular oxidative stress by the following pathways:

1. Glucose auto oxidation leads to an overproduction of NADPH, which increases the production of superoxide radicals and leads to the formation of several reactive oxygen species such as superoxide anion, which can facilitate LDL oxidation in vitro [51].
2. Glucose induces the formation of advanced glycation end products (AGEs) which activates the receptor for AGE (RAGE) present on many vascular cells [52]. Stimulation of RAGE causes the production of reactive oxygen species (ROS) [53]. Scavenger receptors on arterial macrophages can take up modified lipoproteins, including LDL that have become oxidized as a result of glucose-mediated oxidative stress [24], or modified by AGEs [54].
3. Activation of the polyol pathway reduces the availability of NADPH, which in turn

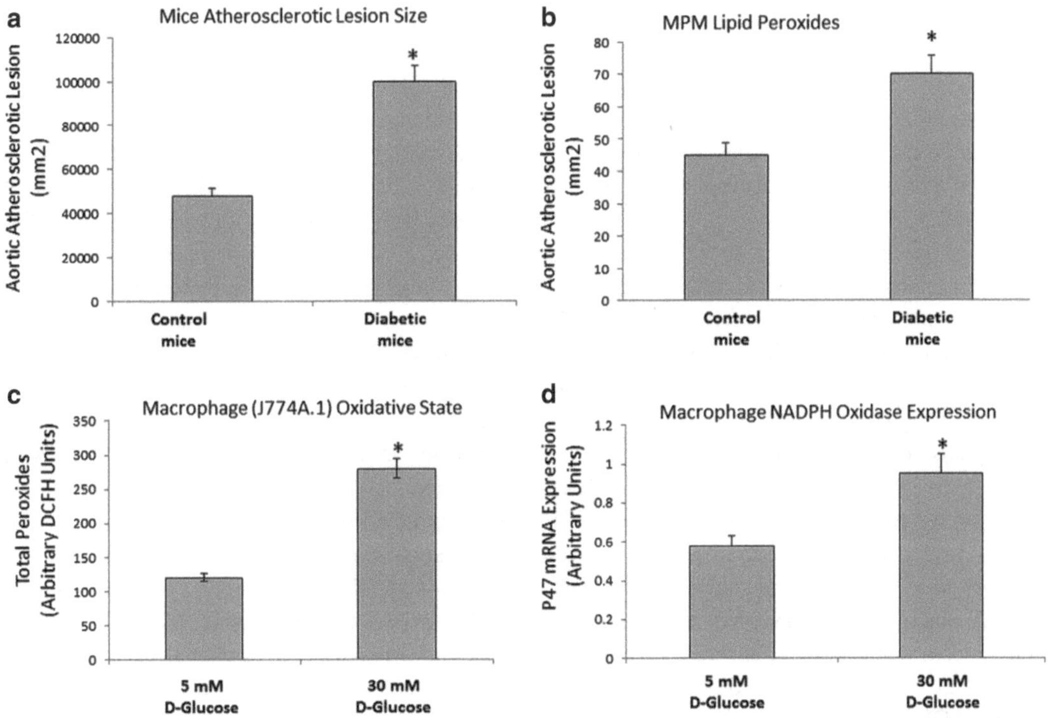


**Fig. 9.2** Increased atherosclerotic lesion area and macrophage lipid peroxidation in diabetic mice and increased macrophage lipid peroxidation and NADPH oxidase expression in glucose-enriched macrophages. Aortic segments from STZ-induced diabetic mice for 3 months and age-matched untreated E0 mice were analyzed for their aortic atherosclerotic lesion area (**a**), $n=10$,$^*p<0.01$. Peritoneal macrophages (MPM) from STZ-induced diabetic mice for 3 months were analyzed for their lipid peroxides content (**b**). J-774 A.1 macrophages were grown for 7–10 days in glucose-enriched media (5–30 mM) and analyzed for their lipid Peroxides content (**c**), and NADPH Oxidase expression (**d**), $n=4$,$^*p<0.01$

reduces glutathione regeneration and increases oxidation [50].

4. Activation of Protein Kinase C resulting from enhanced de novo synthesis of diacylglycerol from glucose via triose phosphate, whose availability is increased because increased ROS inhibit activity of glycolytic enzymes [55]. The enhanced activity of PKC isoforms could also result from the interaction between AGEs and their cell-surface receptors [56].

All these mechanisms are activated by a single upstream event: mitochondrial overproduction of reactive oxygen species (ROS) [57].

It is known that multiple pathways contribute to accelerated atherosclerosis in diabetes including endothelial dysfunction, increased plasma lipoprotein oxidation and our studies demonstrate another possible mechanism related to increased macrophage lipid oxidation in STZ-induced diabetic mice [45]. These data, however, do not establish a causal relationship between glucose and cellular lipid peroxidation since additional factors associated with diabetes might have been involved in increased macrophage lipid peroxidation. In order to examine whether the effect of glucose on macrophage lipid peroxidation is a direct effect, in vitro studies were performed using the J774 cell line. Glucose enrichment of macrophages after exposure to high glucose concentrations was shown to induce oxidative stress (macrophage oxidative state and macrophage NADPH oxidase expression) in a dose-dependent way (Fig. 9.2c, d). In this study, increased cellular lipid peroxidation was associated with increased ability to take up OX-LDL, increased macrophage CD36 mRNA expression and increased macrophage cholesterol content. A glucose upregulating effect on OX-LDL uptake was specific for the modified LDL since glucose enrichment did not affect the macrophage uptake of native LDL [58].

The above results for the direct effect of glucose on macrophages in vitro was demonstrated only by using D-Glucose which is taken up by cells and not L-glucose which cannot penetrate the surface membrane of cells. Thus glucose uptake by macrophages is needed in order to increase macrophage oxidation and this effect could be linked to previously reported data that diabetes induction led to an increased activity of NADPH oxidase [59]. These results are in accordance with previous data showing that human monocyte derived macrophages (HMDM) incubated with high glucose concentrations increased the expression of CD36. Some evidence demonstrates also a role for AGE and RAGE in the induction of CD36 mRNA expression in macrophages [60].

## Antioxidants in DM

Cells and tissues contain antioxidant defense mechanisms, which help prevent ROS production and maintain the redox balance of the cell or tissue [61]. Epidemiological studies suggest that low levels of antioxidants are associated with increased risk for cardiovascular disease (CVD), and that increased intakes appear to be protective. Several antioxidants such as vitamin E and flavonoids such as glabridin, tannins, and red wine were all shown to substantially inhibit macrophage-mediated oxidation of LDL by increasing cellular GSH [62]. During early atherogenesis, the extent of LDL oxidation by macrophages is determined by the balance between antioxidants in cells [23]. We have previously found that GSH content and glutathione peroxidase activity are both inversely related to macrophage-mediated oxidation of LDL. We have shown that MPM from E° mice contain decreased GSH levels and a profound increase of lipid peroxide content compared to MPM from controls. The E° MPM also demonstrated increased ability to reduce superoxide anions and to oxidize LDL [63].

Flavonoids are powerful antioxidants that act against LDL oxidation, and their antioxidant capacity is related to their localization in the LDL particle, as well as to their chemical structures [64]. Flavonoids, which are mostly hydrophilic and thus not LDL-bound, can act as potent inhibitors of LDL oxidation via several mechanisms, which include: (1) scavenging of free radicals by acting as reducing agents, as hydrogen atom donating molecules, and as singlet oxygen quenchers; (2) chelation of transition metal ions, thereby reducing the metal's capacity to generate free radicals; (3) sparing of vitamin E and of carotenoids ([beta]-carotene, lycopene) in the LDL particle, thus protecting LDL from oxidation; and (4) preserving or increasing serum paraoxonase activity, thus promoting hydrolysis of LDL-associated lipid peroxides.

Diabetes is associated with reduced levels of antioxidants such as GSH, vitamin C, and vitamin E [65, 66]. Glycation of antioxidant enzymes during hyperglycemia can impair cellular defense mechanism, leading to the development of oxidative stress and the progression of diabetes with its complications [67]. Glycation of superoxide dismutase and esterases can inhibit their enzymatic activity. Glycation of thioredoxin inhibits its antioxidant activity. Thus, a reduction in antioxidative enzymes and inhibition of enzymatic activity due to glycation in diabetes significantly contributes to the oxidative environment in diabetes.

Diabetic patients are highly prone to oxidative stress. Consequently, antioxidant treatment in diabetes could be beneficial. Indeed it was shown that vitamin E or red wine supplementation to diabetic patients significantly reduced their serum oxidative stress [68, 69]. In addition to vitamin E and red wine, other types of antioxidants were shown to be effective in diabetes such as vitamin C, *N*-acetyl cysteine, garlic, and aged garlic [70].

In spite of these reports, recent trials of supplementation of antioxidants to the general population and also diabetic patients were all negative regarding vascular disease endpoints [71]. These studies have reduced the interest for antioxidant supplementation in general including in diabetics. The current American Diabetes Association recommendations do not encourage vitamin supplementation to diabetic patients unless a deficiency state is evident [72].

The potent antioxidant pomegranate juice (PJ) possesses impressive antioxidative properties due to its polyphenols, and consumption of PJ in humans for a period of one year significantly reduced LDL oxidation [73]. We have shown that PJ consumption in patients (non-diabetics) with carotid artery stenosis for three years caused a significant reduction of oxidative stress in their blood and significant reduction of carotid atherosclerotic lesions as measured by B-mode ultrasonography [74].

In a short term study we have shown that consumption of PJ by diabetic patients for three months did not change glycemic indices (glucose and HgbA1C) nor the levels of cholesterol and triglycerides in these patients, but it resulted in a significant reduction of serum lipid peroxidation and TBARS (that were high before PJ treatment in diabetics vs. healthy volunteers), whereas PON1 activity was significantly increased [75]. In diabetic patients the amount of macrophage cellular lipid peroxidation was significantly increased compared to controls. PJ consumption for three months significantly reduced cellular peroxides to levels lower than those observed in healthy volunteers. These effects of PJ on both serum and macrophages in diabetics could contribute to the accelerated atherogenesis in these patients. The PJ antioxidative effect could be related to its potent tannins which scavenge a wide spectrum of free radicals [76], as well as PJ-induced increment of PON1 in the serum of diabetic patients that can also contribute to the antioxidative effect of PJ in diabetics [77]. The increased uptake of OX-LDL by macrophages in diabetic subjects could be related to the increased expression of the scavenger receptor CD36 which is induced by glucose and/or the high oxidative state. In vitro incubation of PJ with the macrophages of diabetic patients resulted in a significant reduction of OX-LDL uptake [75]. Similar observations were seen when PJ was administrated to STZ-diabetic mice and also when J774 macrophages were incubated with PJ [78].

We have also shown by using different models with low vs. high oxidative states that in STZ-injected mice, the development of hyperglycemia and the severity of oxidative stress are both significantly reduced [79]. Vitamin E supplementation of APO E knockout ($E^0$) mice with enhanced atherosclerosis and increased oxidative stress reduced serum oxidative stress and significantly reduced diabetes development, 12 days after STZ injection (Fig. 9.3a, b).

Similar findings were shown by using P47 knockout mice lacking NADPH oxidase activity and characterized by a very low oxidative state compared to control mice. In this model, glucose levels were much lower after STZ injection compared to controls and only 25 % of the mice developed diabetes (Fig. 9.3c, d). Thus, it seems that enhanced oxidative stress could be responsible for the development of processes that lead to hyperglycemia and consequent diabetic development. On the other hand decreased oxidative stress in mice could be responsible for the reduction in new-onset diabetes mellitus.

## Paraoxonase 1 (PON1) in Diabetes Mellitus

PON1 is an HDL-associated esterase/lactonase, found mainly in serum and it protects against lipid peroxidation in lipoproteins, macrophages, and atherosclerotic lesions. The activity of PON1 is inversely correlated to the risk of CAD [41]. Diabetes is associated with increased oxidative stress and low serum PON1 activity [80].

PON1 activity has been shown to be reduced in patients with DM. These patients also appear to be predisposed to the development of severe multivessel CAD [81]. PON1 activity was found to decrease in parallel to the DM duration, and

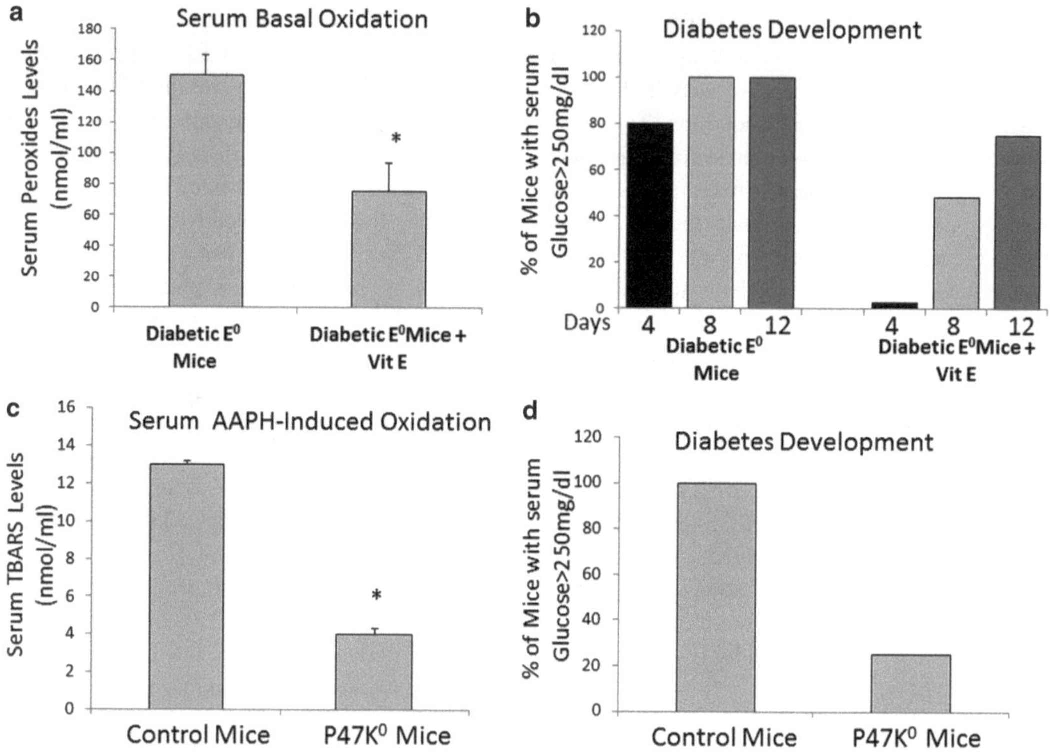


**Fig. 9.3** Decreased serum oxidative state and diabetes development in atherosclerotic (E0) mice treated with vitamin E and in NADPH oxidase knockout mice. Blood drawn from fasting Vit E-treated diabetic mice were analyzed for their serum basal oxidation (**a**) as well as for their glucose levels in order to assess diabetes development (**b**) in comparison to untreated diabetic E0 mice. Blood drawn from fasting NADPH oxidase knockout mice diabetic mice were analyzed for their serum basal oxidation (**c**) as well as for their glucose levels in order to assess diabetes development (**d**) in comparison to diabetic control mice

this phenomenon may be related to acceleration of CHD in DM patients. We have shown that in diabetes, a significant amount of serum PON1 is dissociated from HDL to the lipoprotein deficient serum (LPDS) fraction (as a free PON1). PON1 in LPDS, unlike PON1 in HDL, is less able to protect against lipid peroxidation [82]. PON1 in HDL from type 2 diabetic patients is glycated and, as a result, has decreased ability to metabolize membrane lipid hydroperoxides [83, 84]. Similarly, in vitro studies demonstrated that glucose inactivates PON1, and glycated PON1 has reduced ability to hydrolyze membrane hydroperoxides [83].

In order to examine the effect of PON1 on the development of diabetes we used mice with different PON1 expression levels:

- Mice lacking expression of PON1: PON1 knockout ($K^0$) mice.
- Mice expressing mouse PON1: C57Bl control mice.
- Mice expressing human PON1 in addition to mouse PON1: PON1 Transgenic (Tg) mice.

In order to study the effect of PON1 on the development of diabetes half of the three groups of mice were injected with STZ, whereas the second half served as controls. In the non-diabetic mice macrophage superoxide ion release was

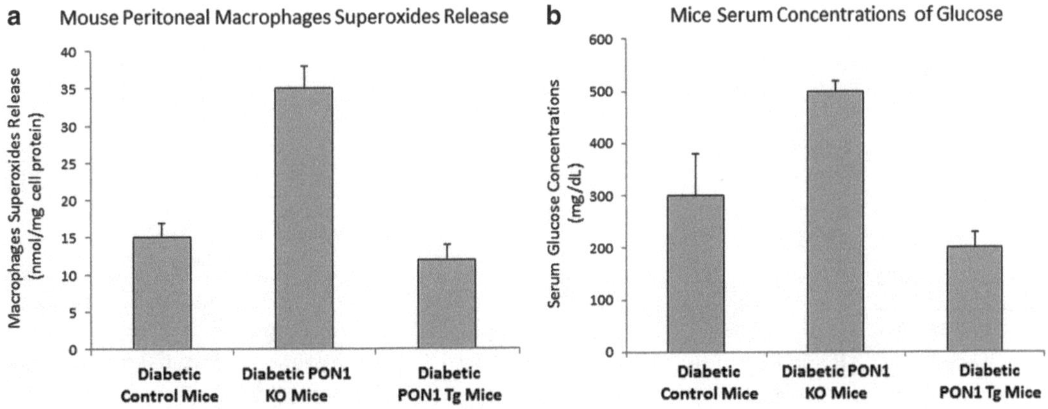


**Fig. 9.4** Modulation of PON1 expression in mice affects macrophages superoxide release and serum glucose levels of diabetic mice: Macrophages from PON1 Knockout (KO) diabetic mice and PON1 Transgenic (Tg) diabetic mice were analyzed for their superoxide anion release in comparison to diabetic control mice (**a**). Serum from PON1 KO diabetic mice and PON1 Tg diabetic mice were analyzed for their glucose levels in comparison to diabetic control mice (**b**)

increased in PON1 K° mice and decreased in PON1 Tg mice vs. controls. These effects were similar after STZ injection but more pronounced, showing a direct inhibitory effect of PON1 on cellular oxidation (Fig. 9.4a). Regarding the effect of PON1 on diabetes development, we have shown that following induction of diabetes, levels of glucose significantly increased in PON1 K° mice, whereas they remained significantly lower in PON1 Tg mice in comparison to control diabetic mice (Fig. 9.4b). After 45 days of STZ injections diabetes developed in all control and PON1 K° mice but only in 67 % of PON1 Tg mice. Moreover, the rate of mortality in controls was significantly lower than in PON1 K° mice after 45 days whereas in the PON1 Tg mice there was no mortality. Interestingly the insulin levels in PON1 K° mice were decreased significantly after STZ injection compared to controls. These studies in PON1 K° mice and PON1 Tg mice suggest indirectly that PON1 has a protective role against diabetes development secondary to its unique antioxidant properties [79].

Recently, we examined the direct ability of PON1 administration to STZ mice to reduce the development of diabetes. In this study more than one third of STZ injected mice did not develop diabetes when pretreated with recombinant PON1. Moreover, the serum glucose levels were lower in the PON1 pretreated mice compared to vehicle-treated mice following STZ administration [85].

Since diabetes is characterized by increased oxidative stress and PON1 possesses antioxidative properties, we next examined the possible relationship between the antioxidative effect of PON1 and serum lipid peroxidation. In serum from diabetic mice, lipid peroxides were increased by 90-fold vs. serum from controls. PON1 administration to controls did not affect the very low serum oxidative stress. However, PON1 administration to diabetic mice reduced serum lipid peroxides by 30-fold compared to diabetic mice injected with PBS [85].

A similar trend was shown in MPM from diabetic mice where superoxide anion release was increased by 150 % compared to MPM from controls. However, in diabetic mice injected with PON1 the MPM superoxide anion release was reduced by 22 % compared to MPM derived from diabetic mice injected with PBS.

Thus, PON1, an enzyme that attenuates oxidative stress in macrophages and serum, has a protective role against STZ-induced diabetes development probably via its antioxidative properties (Fig. 9.5).

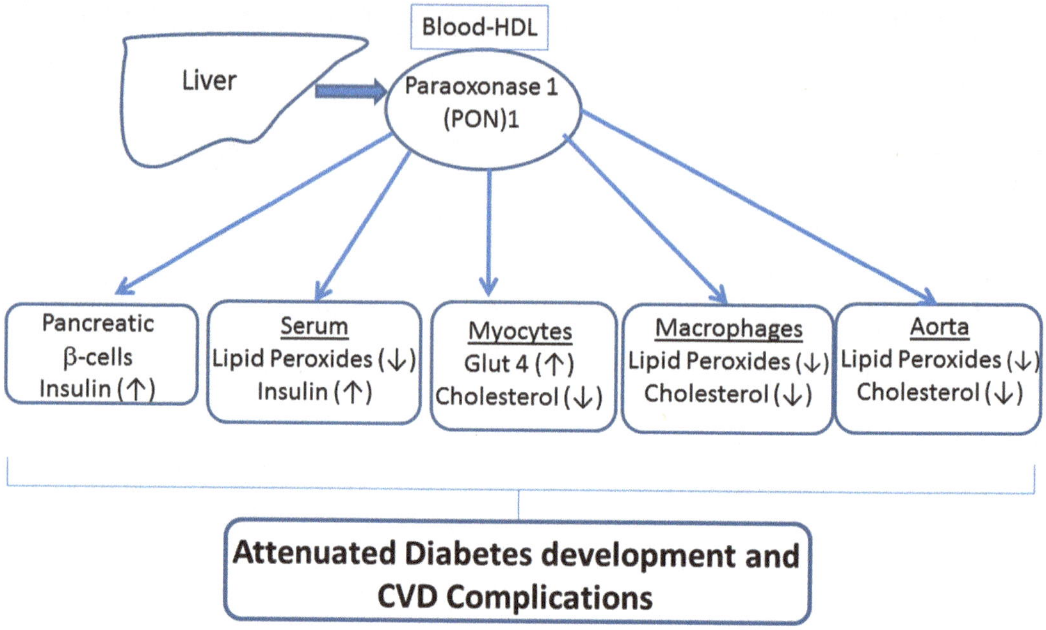


**Fig. 9.5** Effect of PON1 on diabetes. PON1 administration to mice protects against diabetes development, via beneficial effects on insulin content, Glut4 transporter, lipid peroxidation, and cholesterol levels in blood, pancreatic β cells, myocytes, macrophages, and aorta

Oxidation characteristics were also studied in β cells that were incubated with low and high glucose concentrations in the presence of PBS or PON1 as well as other antioxidants including PJ, vitamin E, and punicalagin, and it was shown that total cellular peroxides were significantly reduced in PON1, PJ, vitamin E, punicalagin-treated cells vs. PBS-treated cells [85].

## Conclusions

As diabetes becomes a pandemic disease, much effort is involved in elucidating the mechanisms involved in atherogenesis induced by diabetes. It is well-documented that hyperglycemia directly contributes to accelerated atherosclerosis development in diabetes, by increasing macrophage glucose association and glucose metabolic products (such as Advanced Glycosylation End products) accumulation, leading to macrophage foam cell formation. Diabetes, in general, and, specifically, hyperglycemia, are associated with increased lipid peroxidation both in lipoproteins and in cells of the arterial wall such as macrophages. Diabetes is also associated with lipid abnormalities such as increased serum triglyceride levels and low serum HDL concentration.

Diabetes is associated with reduced levels of antioxidants, including antioxidative enzymes, partly due to accelerated glycation processes. The reduced availability of antioxidants contributes significantly to the increased oxidative stress in diabetes. Moreover, the paraoxonase enzymes (humoral PON1 and cellular PON2) are inactivated in severe diabetic patients. Treatment of diabetic mice with PON1 significantly and substantially delayed the development of diabetes.

Understanding the mechanisms involved in diabetes-induced oxidative stress, as well as of the involvement of antioxidants (such as the glutathione system and paraoxonases) in diabetes-induced atherosclerosis complications (such as retinopathy, nephropathy, neuropathy, and cardiovascular diseases), is imperative in order to prevent such diabetes complications and to offer diabetic patients appropriate novel therapeutic options.

## References


1. Matthews DR, Matthews PC. Banting Memorial Lecture 2010^. Type 2 diabetes as an 'infectious' disease: is this the Black Death of the 21st century? Diabet Med. 2011;28(1):2–9.
2. Daneman D. Type 1 diabetes. Lancet. 2006;367(9513): 847–58.
3. Nolan CJ, Damm P, Prentki M. Type 2 diabetes across generations: from pathophysiology to prevention and management. Lancet. 2011;378(9786):169–81.
4. Fisher M. Diabetes and atherogenesis. Heart. 2004; 90(3):336–40.
5. Norhammar A, Tenerz A, Nilsson G, Hamsten A, Efendíc S, Rydén L, Malmberg K. Glucose metabolism in patients with acute myocardial infarction and no previous diagnosis of diabetes mellitus: a prospective study. Lancet. 2002;359(9324):2140–4.
6. Brownlee M. The pathobiology of diabetic complications: a unifying mechanism. Diabetes. 2005;54: 1615–25.
7. Diabetes Control and Complications Trial Research Group. The effect of intensive treatment of diabetes on the development and progression of long-term complications in insulin-dependent diabetes mellitus. N Engl J Med. 1993;329:977–86.
8. Creager MA, Luscher TF, Cosentino F, Beckman JA. Diabetes and vascular disease: pathophysiology, clinical consequences, and medical therapy: part I. Circulation. 2003;108(12):1527–32.
9. Kannel WB, McGee DL. Diabetes and glucose tolerance as risk factors for cardiovascular disease: the Framingham study. Diabetes Care. 1979;2:120–6.
10. Prince CT, Becker DJ, Costacou T, Miller RG, Orchard TJ. Changes in glycaemic control and risk of coronary artery disease in type 1 diabetes mellitus: findings from the Pittsburgh Epidemiology of Diabetes Complications Study (EDC). Diabetologia. 2007;50:2280–8.
11. Turner RC, Millns H, Neil HA, Stratton IM, Manley SE, Matthews DR, Holman RR. Risk factors for coronary artery disease in non-insulin dependent diabetes mellitus: United Kingdom Prospective Diabetes Study (UKPDS: 23). BMJ. 1998;316:823–8.
12. Mazzone T, Chait A, Plutzky J. Cardiovascular disease risk in type 2 diabetes mellitus: insights from mechanistic studies. Lancet. 2008;371:1800–9.
13. Piga R, Naito Y, Kokura S, Handa O, Yoshikawa T. Short-term high glucose exposure induces monocyte-endothelial cells adhesion and transmigration by increasing VCAM-1 and MCP-1 expression in human aortic endothelial cells. Atherosclerosis. 2007;193: 328–34.
14. Dasu MR, Devaraj S, Jialal I. High glucose induces IL-1beta expression in human monocytes: mechanistic insights. Am J Physiol Endocrinol Metab. 2007;293:E337–46.
15. Srivastava AK. High glucose-induced activation of protein kinase signaling pathways in vascular smooth muscle cells: a potential role in the pathogenesis of vascular dysfunction in diabetes. Int J Mol Med. 2002;9(1):85–9.
16. Chait A, Bornfeldt KE. Diabetes and atherosclerosis: is there a role for hyperglycemia? J Lipid Res. 2009;50:S335–9.
17. Tomkin GH. Atherosclerosis, diabetes and lipoproteins. Expert Rev Cardiovasc Ther. 2010;8(7): 1015–29.
18. Brunzell JD, Deeb SS. Familial lipoprotein lipase deficiency, Apo C-II deficiency, and hepatic lipase deficiency. In: Scriver CR, Beaudet AL, Sly WS, Valle D, editors. The metabolic & molecular bases of inherited disease. 8th ed. New York: McGraw-Hill; 2001. p. 2789–816.
19. Bos G, Dekker JM, Nijpels G, et al. A combination of high concentrations of serum triglyceride and non-high-density-lipoprotein-cholesterol is a risk factor for cardiovascular disease in subjects with abnormal glucose metabolism—the Hoorn Study. Diabetologia. 2003;46:910–6.
20. Jenkins AJ, Rowley KG, Lyons TJ, Best JD, Hill MA, Klein RL. Lipoproteins and diabetic microvascular complications. Curr Pharm Des. 2004;10(27): 3395–418.
21. Ohgami N, Miyazaki A, Sakai M, Kuniyasu A, Nakayama H, Horiuchi S. Advanced glycation end products (AGE) inhibit scavenger receptor class B type I-mediated reverse cholesterol transport: a new crossroad of AGE to cholesterol metabolism. J Atheroscler Thromb. 2003;10:1–6.
22. Berliner JA, Navab M, Fogelman AM, Frank JS, Demer LL, Edwards PA, Watson AD, Lusis AJ. Atherosclerosis: basic mechanisms: oxidation. Inflammation and genetics. Circulation. 1995;91: 2488–96.
23. Aviram M. Macrophage foam cell formation during early atherogenesis is determined by the balance between pro-oxidants and anti-oxidants in arterial cells and blood lipoproteins. Antioxid Redox Signal. 1999;1(4):585–94.
24. Kaplan M, Aviram M. Ox-LDL atherogenic and proinflammatory characteristics during macrophage foam cell formation: an inhibitory role for nutritional antioxidants and serum paraoxonase. Clin Chem Lab Med. 1999;37:777–87.
25. Ylä-Herttuala S, Rosenfeld ME, Parthasarathy S, Glass CK, Sigal E, Witztum JL, Steinberg D. Colocalization of 15-lipoxygenase mRNA and protein with epitopes of oxidized low density lipoprotein in macrophage-rich areas of atherosclerotic lesions. Proc Natl Acad Sci USA. 1990;87(18):6959–63.
26. Steinberg D, Parthasarathy S, Carew TE, Khoo JC, Witztum JL. Beyond cholesterol. Modifications of low-density lipoprotein that increase its atherogenicity. N Engl J Med. 1989;320:915–24.
27. Parthasarathy S, Wieland E, Steinberg D. A role for endothelial cell lipoxygenase in the oxidative modification of low density lipoprotein. Proc Natl Acad Sci USA. 1989;86:1046–50.

28. Stocker R, Keaney JF. Role of oxidative modifications in atherosclerosis. Physiol Rev. 2004;84:1381–478.
29. Steinberg D. The LDL modification hypothesis of atherogenesis: an update. J Lipid Res. 2009;50: S376–81.
30. Yoshida H, Kisugi R. Mechanisms of LDL oxidation. Clin Chim Acta. 2010;411(23–24):1875–82.
31. Parthasarathy S, Steinberg D. Cell-induced oxidation of LDL. Curr Opin Lipidol. 1992;3:313–7.
32. Aviram M. Interaction of oxidized low density lipoprotein with macrophages in atherosclerosis, and the antiatherogenicity of antioxidants. Eur J Clin Chem Clin Biochem. 1996;34(8):599–608.
33. Aviram M, Rosenblat M, Etzioni A, Levy R. Activation of NADPH oxidase required for macrophage-mediated oxidation of low-density lipoprotein. Metabolism. 1996;45(9):1069–79.
34. Bey EA, Cathcart MK. In vitro knockout of human p47phox blocks superoxide anion production and LDL oxidation by activated human monocytes. J Lipid Res. 2000;41(3):489–95.
35. Carr AC, Myzak MC, Stocker R, McCall MR, Frei B. Myeloperoxidase binds to low-density lipoprotein: potential implications for atherosclerosis. FEBS Lett. 2000;487:176–80.
36. Klebanoff SJ. Myeloperoxidase: friend or foe. J Leukoc Biol. 2005;77:598–625.
37. Beckman JS, Koppenol WH. Nitric oxide, superoxide, and peroxynitrite: the good, the bad, and the ugly. Am J Physiol. 1996;271:C1424–37; Cell Physiol 40.
38. Hogg N, Struck A, Goss SP, et al. Inhibition of macrophage-dependent low density lipoprotein oxidation by nitric-oxide donors. J Lipid Res. 1995; 36:1756–62.
39. Ng CJ, Shih DM, Hama SY, Villa N, Navab M, Reddy ST. The paraoxonase gene family and atherosclerosis. Free Radic Biol Med. 2005;38:153–63.
40. Ng CJ, Wadleigh DJ, Gangopadhyay A, Hama S, Grijalva VR, Navab M, Fogelman AM, Reddy ST. Paraoxonase-2 is an ubiquitously expressed protein with antioxidant properties, and is capable of preventing cell-mediated oxidative modification of low-density lipoprotein. J Biol Chem. 2001;276:44444–9.
41. Rosenblat M. M. Aviram. Paraoxonases role in the prevention of cardiovascular diseases. Biofactors. 2009;35(1):98–104.
42. Maritim AC, Sanders RA, Watkins III JB. Diabetes, oxidative stress, and antioxidants: a review. J Biochem Mol Toxicol. 2003;17(1):24–38.
43. Gökkusu C, Palanduz S, Ademoğlu E, Tamer S. Oxidant and antioxidant systems in niddm patients: influence of vitamin E supplementation. Endocr Res. 2001;27(3):377–86.
44. Ceriello A. Oxidative stress and glycemic regulation. Metabolism. 2000;49(2, Suppl 1):27–9.
45. Hayek T, Hussein K, Aviram M, Coleman R, Keidar S, Pavoltzky E, Kaplan M. Macrophage-foam cell formation in streptozotocin-induced diabetic mice: stimulatory effect of glucose. Atherosclerosis. 2005; 183: 25–33.
46. Coleman R, Hayek T, Keidar S, Aviram M. A mouse model for human atherosclerosis: long-term histopathological study of lesion development in the aortic arch of apolipoprotein E-deficient (E0) mice. Acta Histochem. 2006;108(6):415–24.
47. Giugliano D, Ceriello A, Paolisso G. Oxidative stress and diabetic vascular complications. Diabetes Care. 1996;19:257–67.
48. Folli F, Corradi D, Fanti P, Davalli A, Paez A, Giaccari A, Perego C, Muscogiuri G. The role of oxidative stress in the pathogenesis of type 2 diabetes mellitus micro- and macrovascular complications: avenues for a mechanistic-based therapeutic approach. Curr Diabetes Rev. 2011;7(5):313–24.
49. Koya D, King GL. Protein kinase C activation and the development of diabetic complications. Diabetes. 1998;47:859–66.
50. Lee AY, Chung SS. Contributions of polyol pathway to oxidative stress in diabetic cataract. FASEB J. 1999;13:23–30.
51. Hunt JV, Dean RT, Wolff SP. Hydroxyl radical production and autooxidative glycosylation. Biochem J. 1988;256:205–12.
52. Yao D, Brownlee M. Hyperglycemia-induced reactive oxygen species increase expression of the receptor for advanced glycation end products (RAGE) and RAGE ligands. Diabetes. 2010;59(1):249–55.
53. Goldin A, Beckman JA, Schmidt AM, Creager MA. Advanced glycation end products: sparking the development of diabetic vascular injury. Circulation. 2006;114:597–605.
54. Stitt AW, Jenkins AJ, Cooper ME. Advanced glycation end products and diabetic complications. Expert Opin Investig Drugs. 2002;11(9):1205–23.
55. Inoguchi T, Battan R, Handler E, Sportsman JR, Heath W, King GL. Preferential elevation of protein kinase C isoform beta II and diacylglycerol levels in the aorta and heart of diabetic rats: differential reversibility to glycemic control by islet cell transplantation. Proc Natl Acad Sci USA. 1992;89:11059–63.
56. Scivittaro V, Ganz MB, Weiss MF. AGEs induce oxidative stress and activate protein kinase C-beta (II) in neonatal mesangial cells. Am J Physiol. 2000;278:F676–83.
57. Nishikawa T, Edelstein D, Du XL, Yamagishi S, Matsumura T, Kaneda Y, Yorek MA, Beebe D, Oates PJ, Hammes HP, Giardino I, Brownlee M. Normalizing mitochondrial superoxide production blocks three pathways of hyperglycaemic damage. Nature. 2000; 404:787–90.
58. Hayek T, Kaplan M, Kerry R, Aviram M. Macrophage NADPH oxidase activation, impaired cholesterol fluxes, and increased cholesterol biosynthesis in diabetic mice: a stimulatory role for D-glucose. Atherosclerosis. 2007;195(2):277–86.
59. Sonta T, Inoguchi T, Tsubouchi H, Sekiguchi N, Kobayashi K, Matsumoto S, Utsumi H, Nawata H. Evidence for contribution of vascular NAD(P)H oxidase to increased oxidative stress in animal models of diabetes and obesity. Free Radic Biol Med. 2004; 37(1):115–23.

60. Iwashima Y, Eto M, Hata A, Kaku K, Horiuchi S, Ushikubi F, Sano H. Advanced glycation end products-induced gene expression of scavenger receptors in cultured human monocyte-derived macrophages. Biochem Biophys Res Commun. 2000;277(2): 368–80.
61. Aviram M. Review of human studies on oxidative damage and antioxidant protection related to cardiovascular diseases. Free Radic Res. 2000;33(Suppl): S85–97.
62. Aviram M, Kaplan M, Rosenblat M, Fuhrman B. Dietary antioxidants and paraoxonases against LDL oxidation and atherosclerosis development. Handb Exp Pharmacol. 2005;170:263–300.
63. Rosenblat M, Aviram M. Macrophage glutathione content and glutathione peroxidase activity are inversely related to cell-mediated oxidation of LDL: in vitro and in vivo studies. Free Radic Biol Med. 1998;24(2):305–17.
64. Fuhrman B, Aviram M. Flavonoids protect LDL from oxidation and attenuate atherosclerosis. Curr Opin Lipidol. 2001;12(1):41–8.
65. Chertow B. Advances in diabetes for the millennium: vitamins and oxidant stress in diabetes and its complications. MedGenMed. 2004;6(3 Suppl):4.
66. Dagenais GR, Marchioli R, Yusuf S, Tognoni G. Beta-carotene, vitamin C, and vitamin E and cardiovascular diseases. Curr Cardiol Rep. 2000;2:293–9.
67. Arai K, Iizuka S, Tada Y, Oikawa K, Taniguchi N. Increase in the glycosylated form of erythrocyte Cu-Zn-superoxide dismutase in diabetes and close association of the nonenzymatic glucosylation with the enzyme activity. Biochim Biophys Acta. 1987;924:292–6.
68. Aviram M, Fuhrman B. Wine flavonoids protect against LDL oxidation and atherosclerosis. Ann N Y Acad Sci. 2002;957:146–61.
69. Suksomboon N, Poolsup N, Sinprasert S. Effects of vitamin E supplementation on glycaemic control in type 2 diabetes: systematic review of randomized controlled trials. J Clin Pharm Ther. 2011;36(1): 53–63.
70. Golbidi S, Ebadi SA, Laher I. Antioxidants in the treatment of diabetes. Curr Diabetes Rev. 2011;7(2):106–25.
71. Yusuf S, Dagenais G, Pogue J, Bosch J, Sleight P. Vitamin E supplementation and cardiovascular events in high-risk patients. The Heart Outcomes Prevention Evaluation Study Investigators. N Engl J Med. 2000;342:154–60.
72. American Diabetes Association. Nutrition principles and recommendations in diabetes. Diabetes Care. 2004;27 suppl 1:s36.
73. Aviram M, Dornfeld L, Kaplan M, Coleman R, Gaitini D, Nitecki S, Hofman A, Rosenblat M, Volkova N, Presser D, Attias J, Hayek T, Fuhrman B. Pomegranate juice flavonoids inhibit low-density lipoprotein oxidation and cardiovascular diseases: studies in atherosclerotic mice and in humans. Drugs Exp Clin Res. 2002;28(2–3):49–62.
74. Aviram M, Rosenblat M, Gaitini D, Nitecki S, Hoffman A, Dornfeld L, Volkova N, Presser D, Attias J, Liker H, Hayek T. Pomegranate juice consumption for 3 years by patients with carotid artery stenosis reduces common carotid intima-media thickness, blood pressure and LDL oxidation. Clin Nutr. 2004;23(3):423–33.
75. Rosenblat M, Hayek T, Aviram M. Anti-oxidative effects of pomegranate juice (PJ) consumption by diabetic patients on serum and on macrophages. Atherosclerosis. 2006;187(2):363–71.
76. Tzulker R, Glazer I, Bar-Ilan I, Holland D, Aviram M, Amir R. Antioxidant activity, polyphenol content, and related compounds in different fruit juices and homogenates prepared from 29 different pomegranate accessions. J Agric Food Chem. 2007;55(23): 9559–70.
77. Rock W, Rosenblat M, Miller-Lotan R, Levy AP, Elias M, Aviram M. Consumption of wonderful variety pomegranate juice and extract by diabetic patients increases paraoxonase 1 association with high-density lipoprotein and stimulates its catalytic activities. J Agric Food Chem. 2008;56(18):8704–13.
78. Rosenblat M, Volkova N, Coleman R, Aviram M. Pomegranate byproduct administration to apolipoprotein e-deficient mice attenuates atherosclerosis development as a result of decreased macrophage oxidative stress and reduced cellular uptake of oxidized low-density lipoprotein. J Agric Food Chem. 2006;54(5): 1928–35.
79. Rozenberg O, Shiner M, Aviram M, Hayek T. Paraoxonase 1 (PON1) attenuates diabetes development in mice through its antioxidative properties. Free Radic Biol Med. 2008;44(11):1951–9.
80. Mackness MI, Durrington PN. Paraoxonase: another factor in NIDDM cardiovascular disease (letter). Lancet. 1995;346:856.
81. Abbott CA, Mackness MI, Kumar S, Boulton AJ, Durrington PN. Serum paraoxonase activity, concentration and phenotype distribution in diabetes mellitus and its relationship to serum lipids and lipoprotein. Arterioscler Thromb Vasc Biol. 1995;11:1812–8.
82. Rosenblat M, Karry R, Aviram M. Paraoxonase 1 (PON1) is a more potent antioxidant and stimulant of macrophage cholesterol efflux, when present in HDL than in lipoprotein-deficient serum: relevance to diabetes. Atherosclerosis. 2006;187:74–81.
83. Mastorikou M, Mackness B, Liu Y, Mackness M. Glycation of paraoxonase 1 inhibits its activity and impairs the ability of high-density lipoprotein to metabolize membrane lipid hydroperoxides. Diabet Med. 2008;25:1049–55.
84. Mastorikou M, Mackness M, Mackness B. Defective metabolism of oxidized phospholipid by HDL from people with type 2 diabetes. Diabetes. 2006;55: 3099–103.
85. Koren-Gluzer M, Aviram M, Meilin E, Hayek T. The antioxidant HDL-associated paraoxonase-1 (PON1) attenuates diabetes development and stimulates β-cell insulin release. Atherosclerosis. 2011;219(2):510–8.

# 10 The Role of Modified Forms of LDL and Corresponding Autoantibodies in the Development of Complications in Diabetes

Maria F. Lopes-Virella and Gabriel Virella

Oxidative stress is believed to be a critical factor in the initiation of pathogenic pathways that lead to the development of complications in diabetes mellitus [1]. Hyperglycemia plays a key role by inducing mitochondrial overproduction of reactive oxygen species (e.g., superoxide anion, hydrogen peroxide, and others), which, in turn, will lead to a variety of modifications of proteins, enzymes, and other substrates, including the formation of advanced glycation end-products (AGE) and oxidation [1, 2].

Lipoproteins are polymolecular assemblies that can be modified as a consequence of oxidation and glycation. Endothelial cells, monocytes/macrophages, lymphocytes, and smooth muscle cells (SMC) are all able to enhance the rate of oxidation of low-density lipoprotein (LDL). Reactive oxygen species and sulfur-centered radicals initiate metal ion-dependent lipid peroxidation resulting in the generation of aldehydes that interact with lysine residues in ApoB-100. Myeloperoxidase, a heme enzyme secreted by activated macrophages, is able to catalyze lipid peroxidation independent of free metal ions. Oxidation of arachidonic acid, usually secondary to oxidative stress, prostaglandin synthesis by endothelial cells (EC) and platelet activation, leads to the formation of aldehydes that interact with the lysine residues of ApoB100 causing its aggregation, and the resulting modification is generally referred to as malondialdehyde (MDA)-modified LDL [3].

## The Pathogenic Role of Modified LDL

The pathogenic role of modified LDL in the progression of atherosclerosis is well-established. It has been investigated from two different angles: the direct pro-atherogenic effect of modified forms of LDL [2, 4] and the consequences of the immune response directed against neoepitopes resulting from lipoprotein modification [5]. Both types of effects have been extensively characterized in the case of oxidized LDL (oxLDL). Oxidized LDL is taken up by macrophages via receptor-mediated pathways involving primarily CD36 [2, 6, 7] and it induces cholesteryl ester (CE) accumulation and the transformation of macrophages into foam cells [8, 9]. In addition, high concentrations of oxLDL are cytotoxic and experimental data suggests that oxLDL can injure vascular cells, both endothelial and smooth muscle cells (SMC) [10, 11]. Furthermore, oxLDL induces enhanced synthesis of growth factors

M.F. Lopes-Virella, M.D., Ph.D. (✉)
Department of Medicine, Medical University of South Carolina, 114 Doughty Street, Charleston, SC 29425, USA

Ralph A. Johnson VA Medical Center, Charleston, SC, USA
e-mail: virellam@musc.edu

G. Virella
Department of Microbiology and Immunology, Medical University of South Carolina, Charleston, SC, USA

A.J. Jenkins et al. (eds.), *Lipoproteins in Diabetes Mellitus*, Contemporary Diabetes, DOI 10.1007/978-1-4614-7554-5_10, including platelet-derived growth factor-AA (PDGF-AA) and PDGF receptor in SMC, as well as of granulocyte-monocyte colony stimulating factor, macrophage colony stimulating factor (M-CSF) and granulocyte-colony stimulating factor in aortic endothelial cells from humans and rabbits [12]. In addition, oxidized LDL may affect fibrinolysis by inhibiting the secretion of tissue plasminogen activator (tPA) by human endothelial cells [13] and stimulating the secretion of plasminogen activator inhibitor (PAI)-1 [13]. Thus, oxLDL is unable to stimulate the endothelium-dependent activation of fibrinolysis and may promote a chronic prothrombotic state. The cell-mediated immune system is also activated by the presentation of oxLDL oligopeptides by antigen presenting cells, activating T helper 1 cells (Th1) cells in the vascular wall. As a consequence of their activation, Th-1 cells release interferon-γ that activates macrophages and induces the release chemokines that attract more T cells to the area. The process becomes self-perpetuating, resulting in a chronic inflammatory reaction [14, 15].

Oxidized LDL has also been found to have pro-inflammatory effects relevant to the atherosclerotic process. It has chemotactic effects on monocytes [16], enhances monocyte adhesion to EC in culture [17, 18], enhances the expression of vascular cell adhesion molecule 1 (VCAM 1) and intercellular adhesion molecule 1 (ICAM 1) by human aortic endothelial cells induced by tumor necrosis factor-alpha (TNF alpha) [19] and of ICAM-1 in resting human endothelial vein cells [20]. These proinflammatory effects are the result of the activation of a variety of functional pathways. Oxidized LDL has been shown to activate a variety of cell types expressing CD36 and other scavenger receptors and contribute to the generation of reactive oxygen species (ROS) [21]. On macrophages, the interaction of oxLDL and CD36 (mediated by oxidized phospholipids) results in activation of the src family members Fyn/Lyn, and of several components of the MAP kinase pathway, including MKKK, MKK, FAK, and MAPK (JNK) [7]. The activation of these kinases and associated proteins such as Vav are associated with foam cell formation as well as with unregulated actin polymerization and loss of cell polarity causing a migration defect and the trapping of activated cells in the atheromatous lesions [7]. In platelets the same signaling events lead to enhanced platelet reactivity and enhanced formation of thrombi [22]. Recently it has been reported that ligation of CD36 by oxLDL leads to the formation of a toll-like receptor heterodimer (TLR-4-TLR-6) that, in turn, will activate MyD88 and nuclear factor kappa B (NFkB), a critical step in inducing the synthesis and release of proinflammatory cytokines [23].

The advanced glycation end-products (AGE) LDL (as well as other AGE-modified proteins) have also been shown to have pro-inflammatory properties [24, 25]. AGE-modified proteins will impact endothelial cells eliciting increased permeability and pro-coagulant activity [26] as well as overexpression of VCAM-1 [27]. AGE also contributes to fibroblast proliferation and T lymphocyte activation, which results in the release of increased amounts of interferon-γ that will activate monocytes and macrophages, inducing in turn the release of pro-inflammatory cytokines and chemokines [26], thus creating the conditions for a chronic inflammatory reaction in the arterial wall. The impact of AGE in the atherosclerotic process associated with diabetes was confirmed in streptomycin-induced diabetic ApoE −/− mice. Administration of soluble forms of AGE receptors (RAGE) resulted in reduction of vascular permeability and reduced the progression of atheromatous lesions [28].

## The Adaptive Immune Response Elicited by Modified LDL

The pro-inflammatory properties of modified LDL appear to be considerably enhanced as a consequence of their immunogenicity. The immunogenicity of modified LDL was first reported by Steinbrecher et al. based on the immunization of laboratory animals with modified lipoproteins [29]. Of all the modified forms of LDL, oxLDL has been studied in greatest detail from the immunological point of view. Steinbrecher as well as Palinski et al. characterized its immunogenic epitopes [30, 31]. Furthermore, human autoantibodies to oxLDL were the first to be purified and characterized [32–34]. Immune complexes (IC) containing modified LDL have been isolated from the peripheral blood of patients with diabetes, cardiovascular disease, and healthy individuals [35, 36]. Both oxidized LDL and corresponding antibodies have been isolated from atheromatous human tissue [32, 37]. Thus, it seems reasonable to use circulating IC as a sampling of the IC that are deposited in the vessel wall. The formation of LDL-IC in circulation is likely to be inconsequential, but those IC formed in the vessel wall will result in enhanced phagocytosis and increased presentation of peptides derived from modified LDL to T helper cells, which are a critical step in the perpetuation vascular inflammation, as described above.

In several studies we have consistently found that the predominant isotype of modified LDL antibodies is IgG [33, 34, 38–40]. This is a significant finding because IgG antibodies are pro-inflammatory [33, 34, 38–40]. As reported by our group, predominance of circulating IgG antibodies with higher avidity over IgM antibodies in isolated oxLDL-IC is associated with parameters indicative of deteriorating renal function in the DCCT/EDIC cohort [40, 41]. Several groups have reported data suggesting that IgM antibodies to oxidized phospholipids and oxidized LDL have protective effects with relation to the development of atherosclerosis [42–47], although whether this protective effect extends to antibodies recognizing modified peptides seems questionable based on data published by Fredrickson and co-workers [48]. We have carried out two studies on the correlation between the levels of IgG and IgM antibodies to oxLDL contained in isolated IC from patients with type 1 diabetes and the development of nephropathy. In one of the studies we found that the predominance of immune complexes containing IgG antibodies to oxLDL with relatively high avidity was associated with abnormal albuminuria [40, 41]. In a more recent study we found significant positive associations of IgG oxLDL antibody concentration in isolated IC with serum creatinine and albumin excretion rate, as well as a negative correlation with estimated glomerular filtration rate were observed. IgM oxLDL antibody concentrations did not show any correlation with those parameters [40]. Both studies, however, were based on small groups of patients (33 and 34 patients, respectively). We have studied a much larger population of 932 patients with type 2 diabetes, and while the study confirms the predominance of IgG over IgM oxLDL antibodies in isolated immune complexes (Table 10.1), 28 patients had IgG/IgM ratios ≤2 and 9 had ratios <1. That subpopulation may be relatively protected against development of atherosclerosis but the data analysis of that study is still in progress, and it can become complicated by the relatively small number of patients with low IgG/IgM antibody ratio. In conclusion, at this point a solid conclusion about the protective role of IgM modified LDL antibodies in humans is not warranted. If a predominant IgM response has protective effects against the development of atherosclerosis, it is difficult to see how that information can be translated into the clinical setting.

**Table 10.1** Quantitative distribution of IgG- and IgM-oxidized LDL antibodies contained in immune complexes isolated from the serum of 929 patients with type 2 diabetes

| | IgG[a] | IgM[a] | IgG/IgM ratio |
|---|---|---|---|
| Mean | 84.2 | 4.5 | 34.0 |
| S.D. | 82.8 | 7.1 | 43.6 |
| Median | 60.2 | 2.6 | 19.7 |
| Range | 0.2–588 | 0–135 | 0.2–482 |

[a]Values in μg/mL

## The Composition of Circulating Modified LDL Immune Complexes and Diabetic Complications

Besides studying the pathogenic role of modified LDL antibodies [40, 49–51], we developed methodology that allows the measurement of modified forms of LDL and the corresponding antibodies involved in IC formation through the isolation and fractionation of circulating IC [36, 40, 41, 52]. This is an important methodological improvement over the direct assay of modified

LDL or their corresponding antibodies in serum or plasma samples because most modified LDL in circulation is associated with the corresponding antibodies, and the measurements of either component of the circulating complexes is inaccurate due to the mutual saturation of antigen and antibody binding sites [36, 39, 52].

In contrast with the conflicting data generated by studies of modified LDL or antibodies to modified LDL [39, 53], data generated in clinical studies carried out on the DCCT/EDIC cohort (type 1 diabetes) with our assay have shown that high levels of oxLDL and AGE-LDL in isolated and fractionated IC are associated with increased risk for developing diabetic nephropathy [54]. Using coronary artery calcification (CAC) indices and carotid intima-media thickness (IMT) as endpoints indicative of cardiovascular disease progression we also found that increased levels of oxLDL and of AGE-LDL in circulating IC are associated in the DCCT/EDIC cohort with the development of coronary calcification and with increased levels and progression of carotid IMT. The levels of MDA-LDL in isolated IC show a significant but weaker correlation with increased carotid IMT [55, 56]. In contrast, in patients with type 2 diabetes (VADT cohort), the levels of oxLDL and AGE-LDL in circulating IC are not significantly associated with the occurrence of acute events, but high concentrations of MDA-LDL in IC are strong predictors of acute events, especially myocardial infarction (MI) [57]. In agreement with our data, Holvoet et al. reported in two separate studies a link between high levels of oxLDL and established CAD and between elevated plasma MDA-LDL levels and plaque instability [58, 59].

The correlation between MDA-LDL levels and plaque instability is particularly significant because it has been well-established that atherosclerotic plaque rupture is a critical event triggering thrombus formation, arterial luminal obstruction, and subsequent acute coronary syndromes [60]. Plaques that are prone to rupture consist of a larger intimal lesion with abundant macrophages and foam cells and a thinned fibrous cap [61]. Necropsy studies have demonstrated that atherosclerosis in diabetic patients is more extensive and accelerated than that in non-diabetic patients [62]. Furthermore, studies have also shown that atherosclerotic lesions in diabetic patients were more vulnerable as they had larger intimal lesions and more macrophage infiltration as compared to those in non-diabetic patients [63]. Analysis of gene expression in atherosclerotic plaques showed that when compared to stable plaques, vulnerable plaques have higher expression of matrix metalloproteinases (MMP) with collagenase activity, which contribute to the thinning of the fibrous cap, causing plaque instability and rupture [64]. Among the metalloproteinases, MMP-9 has been the object of considerable interest in recent years and according to some studies is an independent risk factor for atherothrombotic events [65, 66]. MMP-9 synthesis and release can be induced through TLR-4 stimulation, usually involving bacterial endotoxins [67] but also by minimally modified LDL [68]. The association of circulating MDA-LDL and IC-associated MDA-LDL specifically with plaque instability/acute CV events raises interesting questions such as whether IC containing different modified forms of LDL may lead to distinct gene regulation and in the case of MDA-LDL lead to plaque instability by inducing macrophage apoptosis and/or increased synthesis of matrix metalloproteinases, such as MMP-9 [69]. OxLDL-IC, in contrast, induce the release of proinflammatory cytokines [50] and promote collagen synthesis by smooth muscle cells [70], and therefore are more likely to contribute to atheroma progression without a significant effect on plaque stability (Fig. 10.1).

Considerable interest has been raised by the accumulation of apoptotic macrophages around the necrotic core of vulnerable plaques [69]. A variety of pro-apoptotic insults has been proposed to play a significant role in the evolution of atheromas, including oxidative stress, endoplasmic reticulum (ER) stress, accumulation of non-esterified (free) cholesterol, and effects of pro-inflammatory cytokines released by activated macrophages [69]. Accumulation of free cholesterol in macrophages in combination with signals delivered through scavenger receptors or with interferon-γ, known to be released by activated T lymphocytes in atheromas [15, 71], leads to serine phosphorylation of STAT-1 which is a critical element in the induction

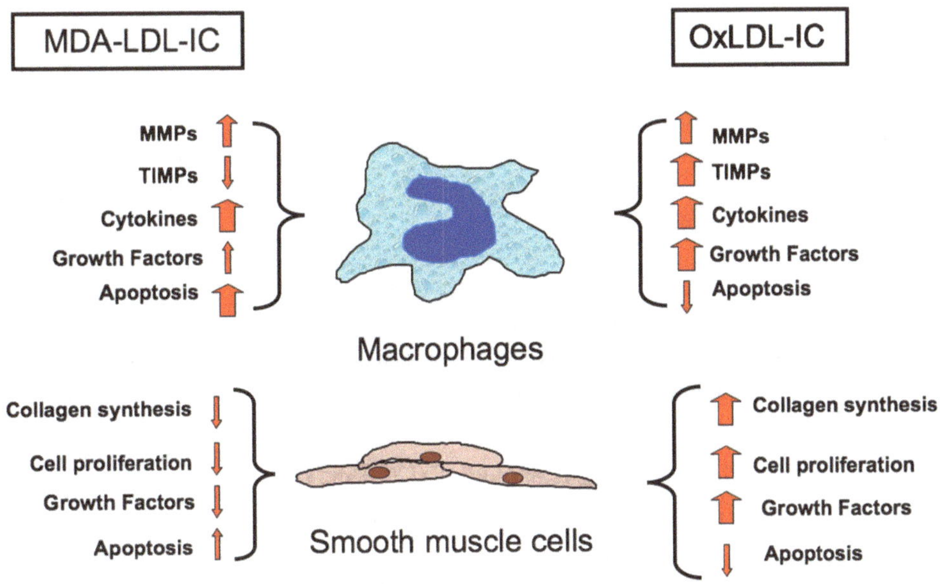


**Fig. 10.1** Diagrammatic representation of the different effects of immune complexes prepared with human copper-oxidized malondialdehyde-modified LDL and the corresponding human antibodies reported by several groups (see text). While both types of immune complexes induce the release of pro-inflammatory cytokines, MDA-LDL-IC are pro-apoptotic while oxLDL-IC are anti-apoptotic and induce the release of proliferation and growth factors by macrophages and smooth muscle cells, and only oxLDL-IC induce collagen synthesis by smooth muscle cells

of apoptosis secondary to ER stress [72]. The apoptotic macrophages in atheromas are ingested by functional macrophages (efferocytosis). Efferocytosis in early lesions seems to result in suppression of inflammation, while in advanced lesions is associated with enhanced inflammation [69]. This evolution appears to be a result of defective efferocytosis, allowing the apoptotic cells to undergo necrosis, resulting in the accumulation of cell fragments that promote inflammation and plaque instability [69].

## Pathogenic Mechanisms of Modified LDL IC

We have published extensive data proving that oxLDL-IC are more potent activators of human macrophages than oxLDL [50, 51, 73, 74]. The uptake of IC prepared with native or copper-oxidized LDL by human monocyte-derived macrophages is primarily mediated by Fcγ receptors, primarily FcγRI [75–77] and it has been shown that the binding of oxLDL antibody blocks the interaction of oxLDL with CD36 [78], so scavenger receptors are not involved in the process. The dependency of the vascular inflammatory process on the activation of phagocytic cells via Fcγ receptors has been demonstrated in double-knockout (DKO) mice generated by crossing apolipoprotein E-deficient mice (apoE(−/−)) with FcγR γ-chain-deficient mice (gamma(−/−)) [79]. The progression of atherosclerosis in the DKO mice is significantly reduced in comparison with apoE(−/−) mice. For MDA-LDL IC and AGE-LDL-IC FcγRI is also involved but possible involvement of scavenger receptors or receptors for AGE-modified proteins has not been excluded.

One fundamental property of LDL-IC is their ability to deliver large concentrations of free and esterified cholesterol to macrophages [51, 75, 80]. The intracellular accumulation of free cholesterol is a known inducer of ER stress, which is believed to be the prime stimulus for the chain of events that results in modification of LDL and atheroma formation. However, experimental studies have shown that ER stress usually protects against apoptosis [69]. In fact, both oxLDL at concentrations not exceeding 75 μg/mL and oxLDL-IC prevent macrophage apoptosis [77, 81]. Whether the anti-apoptotic effect of oxLDL is a consequence of the induction of ER stress is not clear, because in addition to enhanced generation of reactive oxygen and nitrogen species [82], several other mechanisms seem to be involved, including the release of M-CSF mediated by the activation of a PI3K-dependent pathway, upregulation of the anti-apoptotic Bcl-XL gene by NFkB activation, activation of sphingosine kinase, which causes the levels of anti-apoptotic sphingosine-1-phosphate to increase, and inhibition of acid sphingomyelinase, which prevents pro-apoptotic ceramide generation [81, 83]. The anti-apoptotic effect is more pronounced with oxLDL-IC [77, 84] and is not unique to oxLDL-IC, because it has also been reproduced with KLH-anti-KLH IC [77]. However, there are significant differences between oxLDL-IC and other IgG-containing IC. Only oxLDL-IC can induce foam cell formation and the magnitude of the pro-inflammatory response induced in human macrophages is greater with oxLDL-IC than with KLH-IC, for example [50].

While oxLDL cell signaling is mediated by scavenger receptors, oxLDL-IC deliver activating signals via Fcγ receptors. The cross-linking of Fcγ receptors by IC induces phosphorylation of immunoreceptor tyrosine-based activation motifs (ITAMs) by kinases of the Src family, and consequent activation of the Syk pathway [85, 86]. Activation of Syk triggers the mitogen-activated protein kinase (MAPK) signaling cascade, which includes ERK1/2, p38 MAPK, and c-Jun N-terminal kinase (JNK). MAPK activation is also essential for Fc-mediated activation of NFκB [87]. Following the general rule, oxLDL-IC primarily engage FcγRI and induce the activation of the MAPK pathway [88], which is responsible for the expression of pro-inflammatory gene products. In addition, cross-linking of FcγRs by oxLDL-IC activates PI3K and c-Akt [77]. Activated c-Akt promotes cell survival by at least four different mechanisms: (1) phosphorylating the Bad component of the Bad/Bcl-$X_L$ complex which results in its dissociation and cell survival, (2) caspase 9 inactivation, (3) regulation of the expression of transcription factors, and (4) activating IKK kinases which phosphorylate IκB and, as a consequence, release the active form of NFkB, which induces the expression of genes favoring cell survival [89] (Fig. 10.2). The repertoire of oxLDL-IC-induced pro-survival genes is much wider than that induced by oxLDL alone [74]. Also, oxLDL-IC induce HSP70B expression in macrophages. This protein binds to the internalized lipid moiety of oxLDL-IC and prevents its degradation, while at the same time inducing sphingokinase-1 [82, 90].

In contrast to oxLDL, there is no published information concerning pathways of cell activation triggered by MDA-LDL or MDA-LDL-IC. The association of MDA-LDL with acute coronary syndromes [3, 59] and the association of high levels of MDA-LDL in the circulating IC isolated from patients with type 2 diabetes who had acute CVD events, mainly MI [57], strongly suggest that MDA-LDL and MDA-LDL-IC have proapoptotic activity. The different effects of cellular uptake of oxLDL-IC and MDA-LDL-IC (Fig. 10.1) could be a result of structural differences between MDA-LDL and oxLDL. The extent of MDA-lysine modification is much greater in laboratory produced MDA-LDL than in copper-oxidized LDL [52]. This difference results in the generation of epitopes unique to MDA-LDL, and the fact that MDA-LDL antibodies obtained by immunization of rabbits with laboratory-prepared MDA-LDL react with LDL isolated from IC proves that MDA-LDL with identical epitopes and, therefore, with similar structural characteristics, is generated in vivo. Also, while copper oxidation predominantly results in ApoB fragmentation, MDA modification is associated with ApoB aggregation [91]. Obviously, these differences in ApoB could determine different biological properties of the two forms of modified LDL. For example, it has been reported that the processing of heavily oxidized and aggregated LDL by macrophages is defective [92]. Thus, the uptake of MDA-LDL IC could result in a variety of conditions that could promote apoptosis, including: (1) the release of much higher concentrations of free cholesterol in the cell, (2) intracellular accumulation of aggregated LDL, (3) cytoplasmic release of lipoprotein degradation

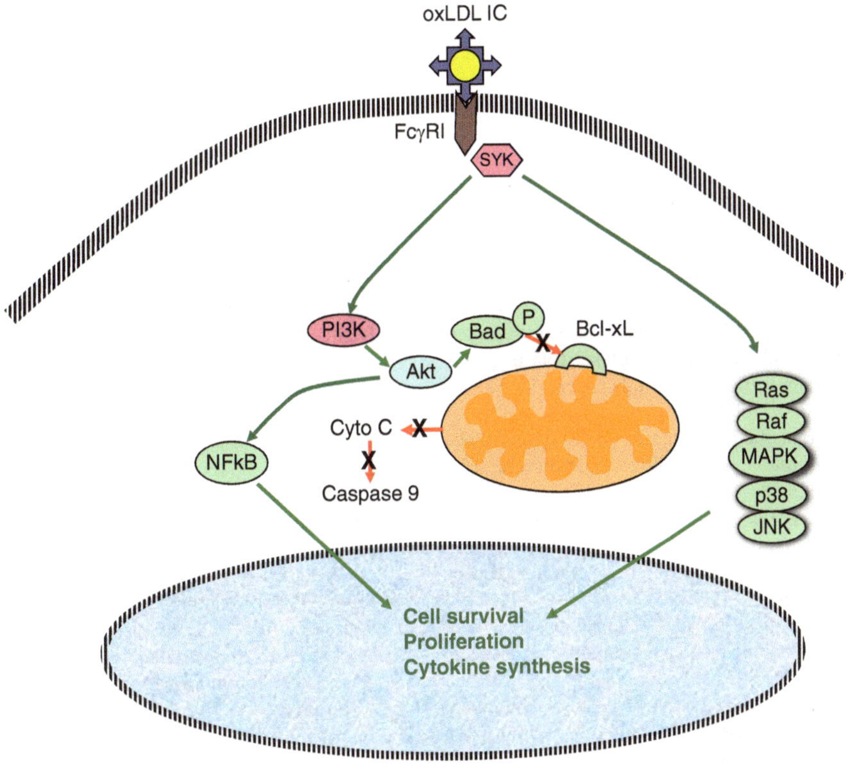


**Fig. 10.2** Diagrammatic representation of the activation pathways triggered by oxLDL-IC through the engagement of FcγRI. Two main pathways are activated, the MAPK pathway which is important for the activation of cell proliferation and cytokine synthesis, and the Akt pathway, which also contributes to the induction of cell proliferation and cytokine synthesis through NFκB activation and also promotes cell survival through the dissociation of the Bad/ $Bcl\text{-}X_L$ complex, blocking the pathway that leads to the activation of caspase 9

products and oxidized phosphatidylcholine, which could be transported to the extracellular compartment and then react with scavenger receptors and/or TLRs, delivering signals that would favor the activation of pro-apoptotic pathways.

There is considerable interest in identifying biomarkers indicative of plaque instability. A variety of proteins and enzymes have been proposed as candidates, as reviewed recently by Koenig. [93] Besides MMPs, reactive proteins (CRP), cytokines (IL-6, IL-18), enzymes (glutathione peroxidase, lipoprotein-associated phospholipase A-2 (Lp-PLA2)), myeloperoxidase, chemotactic proteins (monocyte chemotactic protein-1), and modified lipoproteins have been proposed as indicators of plaque instability [3, 58, 59, 66, 94, 95]. Our data suggest that modified forms of LDL can also be useful biomarkers for cardiovascular disease [54–56] and plaque vulnerability risk [57].

In conclusion, modified LDL plays a key role as a persistent insult leading to chronic vascular inflammation. The pro-inflammatory effects of modified LDL are significantly enhanced as a consequence of the formation of immune complexes as a consequence of the reactivity of different LDL modification with specific antibodies. In general, modified LDL IC have proinflammatory properties, but both clinical and experimental data suggest that there are differences in the consequences of cellular uptake of IC depending on the predominant type of LDL modification. This novel finding opens a variety of basic and clinical research perspectives, ranging from the investigation of the molecular mechanisms that are responsible for the different cellular effects of different LDL modifications to the definition of specific LDL modifications as risk factors able to discriminate between patients with different types or degrees of diabetes-associated complications.

## References


1. Giacco F, Brownlee M. Oxidative stress and diabetic complications. Circ Res. 2010;107:1058–70.
2. Miller YI, Choi SH, Fang L, Tsimikas S. Lipoprotein modification and macrophage uptake: role of pathologic cholesterol transport in atherogenesis. Subcell Biochem. 2010;51:229–51.
3. Holvoet P. Endothelial dysfunction, oxidation of low-density lipoprotein, and cardiovascular disease. Ther Apher. 1999;3:287–93.
4. Lopes-Virella MF, Virella G. The role of immune and inflammatory processes in the development of macrovascular disease in diabetes. Front Biosci. 2003;8:s750–68.
5. Lopes-Virella MF, Virella G. Clinical significance of the humoral immune response to modified LDL. Clin Immunol. 2010;134:55–65.
6. Parthasarathy S, Printz DJ, Boyd D, Joy L, Steinberg D. Macrophage oxidation of low-density lipoprotein generates a modified form recognized by the scavenger receptor. Arteriosclerosis. 1986;6:505–10.
7. Silverstein RL, Li W, Park YM, Rahaman SO. Mechanisms of cell signaling by the scavenger receptor CD36: implications in atherosclerosis and thrombosis. Trans Am Clin Climatol Assoc. 2010;121: 206–20.
8. Hoff HF, O'Neil J, Chisolm GM, Cole TB, Quehenberger O, Esterbauer H, Jurgens G. Modification of low density lipoprotein with 4-hydroxynonenal induces uptake by macrophages. Arteriosclerosis. 1989;9:538–49.
9. Fogelman AM, Schechter I, Seager J, Hokom M, Child JS, Edwards PA. Malondialdehyde alteration of low density lipoproteins leads to cholesterol ester accumula-tion in human monocytes/macrophages. Proc Natl Acad Sci USA. 1980;77:2214–8.
10. Hessler JR, Morel DW, Lewis LJ, Chisolm GM. Lipoprotein oxidation and lipoprotein-induced cytotoxicity. Arteriosclerosis. 1983;3:215–22.
11. Henriksen T, Evensen SA, Carlander B. Injury to human endothelial cells in culture induced by LDL. Scand J Clin Lab Invest. 1979;39:361–4.
12. Rajavashisth TB, Andalibi A, Territo MC. Induction of endothelial cell expression of granulocyte and macrophage colony-stimulating factors by modified LDL. Nature. 1990;344:254–7.
13. Kugiyama K, Sakamoto T, Musumi I, Sugiyama S, Ohgushi M, Ogawa H, Horiguchi M, Yasue H. Transferrable lipids in oxidized LDL stimulate PAI-1 and inhibt tPA release from endothelial cells. Circulation Res. 1993;73:335–43.
14. Andersson J, Libby P, Hansson GK. Adaptive immunity and atherosclerosis. Clin Immunol. 2010;134: 33–46.
15. De Boer OJ, van der Wal AC, Verhagen CE, Becker AE. Cytokin secretion profiles of cloned T cells from human aortic atherosclerotic plaques. J Pathol. 1999;188:174–9.
16. Quinn MT, Parthasarathy S, Fong LG, Steinberg D. Oxidatively modified low density lipoproteins: a potential role in recruitment and retention of monocyte/macrophages during atherogenesis. Proc Nat Acad Sci USA. 1987;84:2995–8.
17. Berliner JA, Territo MC, Sevanian A, Raimin S, Kim JA, Bamshad B, Ester-son M, Fogelman AM. Minimally modified low density lipoprotein stimulates monocyte endothelial interactions. J Clin Invest. 1990;85:1260–6.
18. Kume N, Cybulsky MI, Gimbrone MAJ. Lysophosphatidyl-choline, a component of atherogenic lipoproteins, induces mononuclear leukocyte adhesion molecules in cultured human and rabbit arterial endothelial cells. J Clin Invest. 1992;90:1138–44.
19. Kahn BV, Parthasarathy SS, Alexander RW, Medford RM. Modified LDL and its constituents augment cytokine-activated vascular cell adhesion molecule -1 gene expression in human vascular endothelial cells. J Clin Invest. 1995;95:1262–70.
20. Takei A, Huang Y, Lopes-Virella MF. Expression of adhesion molecules by human endothelial cells exposed to oxidized low density lipoprotein. Influences of degree of oxidation and location of oxidized LDL. Atherosclerosis. 2001;154:79–86.
21. Li W, Febbraio M, Reddy SP, Yu DY, Yamamoto M, Silverstein RL. CD36 participates in a signaling pathway that regulates ROS formation in murine VSMCs. J Clin Invest. 2010;120:3996–4006.
22. Silverstein RL. Type 2 scavenger receptor CD36 in platelet activation: the role of hyperlipemia and oxidative stress. Clin Lipidol. 2009;4:767.
23. Stewart CR, Stuart LM, Wilkinson K, van Gils JM, Deng J, Halle A, Rayner KJ, Boyer L, Zhong R, Frazier WA, Lacy-Hulbert A, El Khoury J, Golenbock DT, Moore KJ. CD36 ligands promote sterile inflammation through assembly of a Toll-like receptor 4 and 6 heterodimer. Nat Immunol. 2010;1:155–61.
24. Vlassara H, Cai W, Crandall J, Goldberg T, Oberstein R, Dardaine V, Peppa M, Rayfield EJ. Inflammatory mediators are induced by dietary glycotoxins, a major risk factor for diabetic angiopathy. Proc Natl Acad Sci USA. 2002;99:15596–601.
25. Wendt T, Bucciarelli L, Qu W, Lu Y, Yan SF, Stern DM, Schmidt AM. Receptor for advanced glycation endproducts (RAGE) and vascular inflammation: insights into the pathogenesis of macrovascular complications in diabetes. Curr Atheroscler Rep. 2002;4:228–37.
26. Vlassara H, Bucala R, Striker L. Pathogenic effects of advanced glycosylation: biochemical, biologic, and clinical implications for diabetes and aging. Lab Invest. 1994;70:138–51.

27. Schmidt AM, Hori O, Chen JX, Li JF, Crandall J, Zhang J, Cao R, Yan SD, Brett J, Stern D. Advanced glycation endproducts interacting with their endothelial receptor induce expression of vascular cell adhesion molecule-1 (VCAM-1) in cultured human endothelial cells and in mice. A potential mechanism for the accelerated vasculopathy of diabetes. J Clin Invest. 1995;96:1395–403.
28. Bucciarelli LG, Wendt T, Qu W, Lu Y, Lalla E, Rong LL, Goova MT, Moser B, Kislinger T, Lee DC, Kashyap Y, Stern DM, Schmidt AM. RAGE blockade stabilizes established atherosclerosis in diabetic apolipoprotein E-null mice. Circulation. 2002;106(22):2827–35.
29. Steinbrecher UP, Fisher M, Witztum JL, Curtiss LK. Immunogenicity of homologous low density lipoprotein after methylation, ethylation, acetylation, or carbamylation: generation of antibodies specific for derivatized lysine. J Lipid Res. 1984;25:1109–16.
30. Steinbrecher UP. Oxidation of human low density lipoprotein results in derivatization of lysine residues of apolipoprotein B by lipid peroxide decomposition products. J Biol Chem. 1987;262:3603–8.
31. Palinski W, Yla-Herttuala S, Rosenfeld ME, Butler SW, Socher SA, Parthasarathy S, Curtiss LK, Witztum JL. Antisera and monoclonal antibodies specific for epitopes generated during oxidative modification of low density lipoprotein. Arteriosclerosis. 1990;10: 325–35.
32. Yla-Herttuala S, Palinski W, Butler S, Picard S, Steinberg D, Witztum JL. Rabbit and human atherosclerotic lesions contain IgG that recognizes epitopes of oxidized LDL. Arterioscler Thromb. 1994;14:32–40.
33. Mironova M, Virella G, Lopes-Virella MF. Isolation and characterization of human antioxidized LDL autoantibodies. Arterioscler Thromb Vasc Biol. 1996;16:222–9.
34. Virella G, Koskinen S, Krings G, Onorato JM, Thorpe SR, Lopes-Virella M. Immunochemical characterization of purified human oxidized low-density lipoprotein antibodies. Clin Immunol. 2000;95:135–44.
35. Mironova MA, Klein RL, Virella GT, Lopes-Virella MF. Anti-modified LDL antibodies, LDL-containing immune complexes, and susceptibility of LDL to in vitro oxidation in patients with type 2 diabetes. Diabetes. 2000;49:1033–41.
36. Virella G, Thorpe S, Alderson NL, Derrick MB, Chassereau C, Rhett JM, Lopes-Virella MF. Definition of the immunogenic forms of modified human LDL recognized by human autoantibodies and by rabbit hyperimmune antibodies. J Lipid Res. 2004;45: 1859–67.
37. Yla-Herttuala S. Macrophages and oxidized low density lipoproteins in the pathogenesis of atherosclerosis. Ann Med. 1991;2:561–7.
38. Virella G, Thorpe SR, Alderson NL, Stephan EM, Atchley DH, Wagner F, Lopes-Virella MF, Group DER. Autoimmune response to advanced glycosylation end-products of human low density lipoprotein. J Lipid Res. 2003;443:487–93.
39. Virella G, Lopes-Virella MF. Lipoprotein autoantibodies: measurement and significance. Clin Diagn Lab Immunol. 2003;10:499–505.
40. Virella G, Carter RE, Saad A, Crosswell EG, Game BA, Lopes-Virella MF. Distribution of IgM and IgG antibodies to oxidized LDL in immune complexes isolated from patients with type 1 diabetes and its relationship with nephropathy. Clin Immunol. 2008;127:394–400.
41. Atchley DH, Lopes-Virella MF, Zheng D, Virella G. Oxidized LDL-anti-oxidized LDL immune complexes and diabetic nephropathy. Diabetologia. 2002;45:1562–71.
42. Tsimikas S, Brilakis ES, Lennon RJ, Miller ER, Witztum JL, McConnell JP, Kornman KS, Berger PB. Relationship of IgG and IgM autoantibodies to oxidized low density lipoprotein with coronary artery disease and cardiovascular events. J Lipid Res. 2007;48:425–33.
43. Frostegard J. Low level natural antibodies against phosphorylcholine: a novel risk marker and potential mechanism in atherosclerosis and cardiovascular disease. Clin Immunol. 2010;134:47–54.
44. Yamashita T, Freigang S, Eberle C, Pattison J, Gupta S, Napoli C, Palinski W. Maternal immunization programs postnatal immune responses and reduces atherosclerosis in offspring. Circ Res. 2006;99:e51–64.
45. Su J, Georgiades A, Wu R, Thulin T, de Faire U, Frostegard J. Antibodies of IgM subclass to phosphorylcholine and oxidized LDL are protective factors for atherosclerosis in patients with hypertension. Atherosclerosis. 2006;188:160–6.
46. Faria-Neto JR, Chyu KY, Li X, Dimayuga PC, Ferreira C, Yano J, Cercek B, Shah PK. Passive immunization with monoclonal IgM antibodies against phosphorylcholine reduces accelerated vein graft atherosclerosis in apolipoprotein E-null mice. Atherosclerosis. 2006;189:83–90.
47. Karvonen J, Paivansalo M, Kesaniemi YA, Horkko S. Immunoglobulin M type of autoantibodies to oxidized low-density lipoprotein has an inverse relation to carotid artery atherosclerosis. Circulation. 2003; 108(17):2107–12.
48. Fredrikson GN, Hedblad B, Berglund G, Alm R, Nilsson JA, Schiopu A, Shah PK, Nilsson J. Association between IgM against an aldehyde-modified peptide in apolipoprotein B-100 and progression of carotid disease. Stroke. 2007;38:1495–500.
49. Lopes-Virella MF, McHenry MB, Lipsitz S, Yim E, Wilson PF, Lackland DT, Lyons T, Jenkins AJ, Virella G. Immune complexes containing modified lipoproteins are related to the progression of internal carotid intima-media thickness in patients with type 1 diabetes. Atherosclerosis. 2007;190:359–69.
50. Saad AF, Virella G, Chassereau C, Boackle RJ, Lopes-Virella MF. OxLDL immune complexes activate complement and induce cytokine production by MonoMac 6 cells and human macrophages. J Lipid Res. 2006;47:1975–83.

51. Virella G, Atchley DH, Koskinen S, Zheng D, Lopes-Virella M. Pro-atherogenic and pro-inflammatory properties of immune complexes prepared with purified human oxLDL antibodies and human oxLDL. Clin Immunol. 2002;105:81–92.
52. Virella G, Derrick MB, Pate V, Chassereau C, Thorpe SR, Lopes-Virella MF. Development of capture assays for different modifications of human low-density lipoprotein. Clin Diagn Lab Immunol. 2005;12:68–75.
53. Lopes-Virella MF, Virella G, Orchard TJ, Koskinen S, Evans RW, Becker DJ, Forrest KY. Antibodies to oxidized LDL and LDL-containing immune complexes as risk factors for coronary artery disease in diabetes mellitus. Clin Immunol. 1999;90:165–72.
54. Lopes-Virella MF, Carter RE, Baker NL, Lachin J, Virella G, Group DER. High levels of oxidized LDL in circulating immune complexes are associated with increased odds of developing abnormal albuminuria in Type 1 diabetes. Nephrol Dial Transplant. [Epub ahead of print] (doi: 10.1093/ndt/gfr454. Accessed 19 Aug 2011; PMID: 21856760).
55. Lopes-Virella MF, Baker NL, Hunt KJ, Lachin J, Nathan D, Virella G. Oxidized LDL immune complexes and coronary artery calcification in type 1 diabetes. Atherosclerosis. 2011;214:462–7.
56. Lopes-Virella MF, Hunt KJ, Baker NL, Lachin J, Nathan DM, Virella G. The Levels of Oxidized LDL and AGE- LDL in Circulating Immune Complexes are strongly associated with increased levels of Carotid Intima-Media Thickness and its progression in Type 1 Diabetes. Diabetes. 2011;60:582–9.
57. Lopes-Virella MF, Hunt KJ, Baker NL, Moritz T, Virella G, Investigators TVGo. Levels of MDA—LDL in circulating immune complexes predict myocardial infarction in the VADT study in the veterans affairs diabetes trial (VADT) ATVB. 2012;224:526–31.
58. Holvoet P, Perez G, Zhao Z, Brouwers E, Bernar H, Collen D. Malondialdehyde-modified low density lipoproteins in patients with atherosclerotic disease. J Clin Invest. 1995;95:2611–9.
59. Holvoet P, Vanhaecke J, Janssens S, Van de Werf F, Collen D. Oxidized LDL and malondialdehyde-modified LDL in patients with acute coronary syndromes and stable coronary artery disease. Circulation. 1998;98:1487–94.
60. Libby P, Theroux P. Pathophysiology of coronary artery disease. Circulation. 2005;111:3481–8.
61. Shah PK. Pathophysiology of coronary thrombosis: role of plaque rupture and plaque erosion. Prog Cardiovasc Dis. 2002;44:357–68.
62. Jarrett RJ. Atherosclerosis, diabetes and obesity. Proc Nutr Soc. 1981;40:209–12.
63. Moreno PR, Murcia AM, Palacios IF, Leon MN, Bernardi VH, Fuster V, Fallon JT. Coronary composition and macrophage infiltration in atherectomy specimens from patients with diabetes mellitus. Circulation. 2000;102:2180–4.
64. Galis ZS, Sukhova GK, Lark MW, Libby P. Increased expression of matrix metalloproteinases and matrix degrading activity in vulnerable regions of human atherosclerotic plaques. J Clin Invest. 1994;94:2493–503.
65. Blankenberg S, Rupprecht HJ, Poirier O, Bickel C, Smieja M, Hafner G, Meyer J, Cambien F, Tiret L. Plasma concentrations and genetic variation of matrix metalloproteinase 9 and prognosis of patients with cardiovascular disease. Circulation. 2003;107:1579–85.
66. Loftus IM, Naylor AR, Bell PR, Thompson MM. Plasma MMP-9—a marker of carotid plaque instability. Eur J Vasc Endovasc Surg. 2001;21:17–21.
67. Lundberg AM, Hansson GK. Innate immune signals in atherosclerosis. Clin Immunol. 2010;134(1):5–24.
68. Choi SH, Harkewicz R, Lee JH, Boullier A, Almazan F, Li AC, Witztum JL, Bae YS, Miller YI. Lipoprotein accumulation in macrophages via toll-like receptor-4-dependent fluid phase uptake. Circ Res. 2009;104:1355–63.
69. Seimon T, Tabas I. Mechanisms and consequences of macrophage apoptosis in atherosclerosis. J Lipid Res. 2009;50(Suppl):S382–7.
70. Abdelsamie SA, Li Y, Huang Y, Lee M-H, Klein RL, Virella G, Lopes-Virella MF. Oxidized LDL immune complexes stimulate collagen IV production in mesangial cells via Fc gamma receptor I. Clin Immunol. 2011;139:258–66.
71. de Boer OJ, van der Wal AC, Houtkamp MA, Ossewaarde JM, Teeling P, Becker AE. Unstable atherosclerotic plaques contain T-cells that respond to Chlamydia pneumoniae. Cardiovasc Res. 2000;48:402–8.
72. Lim WS, Timmins JM, Seimon TA, Sadler A, Kolodgie FD, Virmani R, Tabas I. Signal transducer and activator of transcription-1 is critical for apoptosis in macrophages subjected to endoplasmic reticulum stress in vitro and in advanced atherosclerotic lesions in vivo. Circulation. 2008;117:940–51.
73. Virella G, Munoz JF, Galbraith GM, Gissinger C, Chassereau C, Lopes-Virella MF. Activation of human monocyte-derived macrophages by immune complexes containing low-density lipoprotein. Clin Immunol Immunopath. 1995;75:179–89.
74. Hammad SM, Twal WO, Barth JL, Smith KJ, Saad AF, Virella G, Argraves WS, Lopes-Virella MF. Oxidized LDL immune complexes and oxidized LDL differentially affect the expression of genes involved with inflammation and survival in human U937 monocytic cells. Atherosclerosis. 2009;202(2):394–404.
75. Lopes-Virella MF, Griffith RL, Shunk KA, Virella GT. Enhanced uptake and impaired intracellular metabolism of low density lipoprotein complexed with anti-low density lipoprotein antibodies. Arterioscl Thromb. 1991;11:1356–67.
76. Lopes-Virella MF, Binzafar N, Rackley S, Takei A, La Via M, Virella G. The uptake of LDL-IC by human macrophages: predominant involvement of the Fc gamma RI receptor. Atherosclerosis. 1997;135:161–70.
77. Oksjoki R, Kovanen PT, Lindstedt KA, Jansson B, Pentikainen MO. OxLDL-IgG immune complexes induce survival of human monocytes. Arterioscler Thromb Vasc Biol. 2006;26:576–83.

78. Nagarajan S. Anti-OxLDL IgG blocks OxLDL interaction with CD36, but promotes FcgammaR, CD32A-dependent inflammatory cell adhesion. Immunol Lett. 2007;108:52–61.
79. Hernandez-Vargas P, Ortiz-Munoz G, Lopez-Franco O, Suzuki Y, Gallego-Delgado J, Sanjuan G, Lazaro A, Lopez-Parra V, Ortega L, Egido J, Gomez-Guerrero C. Fcgamma receptor deficiency confers protection against atherosclerosis in apolipoprotein E knockout mice. Circ Res. 2006;99:1188–96.
80. Griffith RL, Virella GT, Stevenson HC, Lopes-Virella MF. Low density lipoprotein metabolism by human macrophages activated with low density lipoprotein immune complexes. A possible mechanism of foam cell formation. J Exp Med. 1988;168:1041–59.
81. Hundal RS, Gomez-Munoz A, Kong JY, Salh BS, Marotta A, Duronio V, Steinbrecher UP. Oxidized low density lipoprotein inhibits macrophage apoptosis by blocking ceramide generation, thereby maintaining protein kinase B activation and Bcl-XL levels. J Biol Chem. 2003;278:24399–408.
82. Al Gadban MM, Smith KJ, Soodavar F, Piansay C, Chassereau C, Twal WO, Klein RL, Virella G, Lopes-Virella MF, Hammad SM. Differential trafficking of oxidized LDL and oxidized LDL immune complexes in macrophages: impact on oxidative stress. PLoS One. 2010;5(9):e12534.
83. Chen JH, Riazy M, Wang SW, Dai JM, Duronio V, Steinbrecher UP. Sphingosine kinase regulates oxidized low density lipoprotein-mediated calcium oscillations and macrophage survival. J Lipid Res. 2010;51:991–8.
84. Hammad SM, Taha TA, Nareika A, Johnson KR, Lopes-Virella MF, Obeid LM. Oxidized LDL immune complexes induce release of sphingosine kinase in human U937 monocytic cells. Prostaglandins Other Lipid Mediat. 2006;79:126–40.
85. Tohyama Y, Yamamura H. Protein tyrosine kinase, syk: a key player in phagocytic cells. J Biochem. 2009;145:267–73.
86. Crowley MT, Costello PS, Fitzer-Attas CJ, Turner M, Meng F, Lowell C, Tybulewicz VL, DeFranco AL. A critical role for Syk in signal transduction and phagocytosis mediated by Fcgamma receptors on macrophages. J Exp Med. 1997;186:1027–39.
87. Luo Y, Pollard JW, Casadevall A. Fcgamma receptor cross-linking stimulates cell proliferation of macrophages via the ERK pathway. J Biol Chem. 2010;285:4232–42.
88. Huang Y, Jaffa A, Koskinen S, Takei A, Lopes-Virella MF. Oxidized LDL-containing immune complexes induce Fc gamma receptor I-mediated mitogen-activated protein kinase activation in THP-1 macrophages. Arterioscler Thromb Vasc Biol. 1999;19:1600–7.
89. Datta SR, Brunet A, Greenberg ME. Cellular survival: a play in three Akts. Genes Dev. 1999;13:2905–27.
90. Smith KJ, Twal WO, Soodavar F, Virella G, Lopes-Virella MF, Hammad SM. Heat shock protein 70B′ (HSP70B′) expression and release in response to human oxidized low density lipoprotein immune complexes in macrophages. J Biol Chem. 2010;285: 15985–93.
91. Viita H, Narvanen O, Yla-Herttuala S. Different apolipoprotein B breakdown patterns in models of oxidized low density lipoprotein. Life Sci. 1999;65: 783–93.
92. Hoff HF, Zyromski N, Armstrong D, O'Neil J. Aggregation as well as chemical modification of LDL during oxidation is responsible for poor processing in macrophages. J Lipid Res. 1993;34:1919–29.
93. Koenig W, Khuseyinova N. Biomarkers of atherosclerotic plaque instability and rupture. Arterioscler Thromb Vasc Biol. Jan 2007;27:15–26.
94. Colley KJ, Wolfert RL, Cobble ME. Lipoprotein associated phospholipase A(2): role in atherosclerosis and utility as a biomarker for cardiovascular risk. EPMA J. 2011;2:27–38.
95. Pelisek J, Rudelius M, Zepper P, Poppert H, Reeps C, Schuster T, Eckstein HH. Multiple biological predictors for vulnerable carotid lesions. Cerebrovasc Dis. 2009;28:601–10.

# Lipid: Extracellular Matrix Interactions as Therapeutic Targets in the Atherosclerosis of Diabetes

11

Narin Osman and Peter J. Little

## Introduction

Cardiovascular disease is the largest single cause of premature mortality in developed nations and it is increasing as such in developing and emerging countries. Cardiovascular disease is the commonest cause of death of adults with diabetes [1]. Cardiovascular disease is manifest as myocardial infarctions (MIs) and strokes and their sequelae of heart failure and severe neurological conditions, respectively. Historical predications for cardiovascular disease are likely to be underestimates because they have been based on predictions of the rate of development of obesity in the population and these in term have been seriously underestimated. Obesity rates have increased rapidly due to poor nutrition, mostly excessive energy intake, and low levels of physical activity and independently increasing amounts of sedentary time [2]. Obesity causes insulin resistance and perturbed metabolic profile leading to hyperglycemia and type 2 diabetes mellitus [3], and unfortunately excess body fat is now also common in people with type 1 diabetes [4]. Although it has been quite controversial, there is a very solid link between hyperglycemia and the development of cardiovascular disease [5]. Vascular disease in diabetes is usually categorized into microvascular disease affecting the eyes, kidneys, and nerves and macrovascular disease causing MIs, strokes, and peripheral vascular disease including erectile dysfunction. The association of hyperglycemia is stronger with microvascular than macrovascular disease [6]. What has been controversial is the impact of medically treating hyperglycemia on the reduction of macrovascular disease, and this matter remains unresolved [6].

Cardiovascular disease is the most prominent cause of mortality and morbidity with some 40 % of people without diabetes dying prematurely of cardiovascular disease and this rises to above 50 % in people with diabetes [7]. Notwithstanding these facts, there have been substantial reductions in the rates of cardiovascular disease in developed countries in the last decade [8]. In decreasing order of risk severity, the modifiable factors driving cardiovascular disease are smoking, state of well-being, blood pressure, hyperlipidemia, and hyperglycemia [8]. The abovementioned reductions in the rate of cardiovascular disease have occurred due to reduced rates of smoking and better treatment of blood pressure [8], i.e., public health and medical policies have correctly and successfully addressed the two major drivers of cardiovascular disease.

One of the biggest issues is the role of the factors such as the metabolic milieu and blood pressure in causing diabetes to be associated with

N. Osman
RMIT University, Melbourne, VIC, Australia

P.J. Little, B.Pharm., Ph.D. (✉)
Department of Pharmacy, RMIT University, Plenty Road, P.O. Box 71, Bundoora, VIC 3083, Australia

Monash University, Melbourne, VIC, Australia
e-mail: peter.little@rmit.edu.au

A.J. Jenkins et al. (eds.), *Lipoproteins in Diabetes Mellitus*, Contemporary Diabetes,
DOI 10.1007/978-1-4614-7554-5_11, 

higher rates of cardiovascular disease. There has been a large amount of research directed at identifying the factors associated with diabetes that cause increased rates of cardiovascular disease in this population. Much work has been directed at the impact of hyperglycemia or elevated glucose levels at molecular, cellular, animal, and clinical levels [7, 9–11]. The epidemiological data indicates that although the rates of cardiovascular disease are higher in people with diabetes [7] and the rates have fallen over the last few decades, the relative deleterious impact of diabetes (an approximately two-fold change) remains about the same [12]. This leads to the conclusion that the factors, diabetes-specific factors, through which diabetes increases cardiovascular disease, have not been identified. Active research on the mechanism of diabetes might also yield information on the relationship between the factors causing diabetes and thus driving cardiovascular disease. Much information has arisen from the investigation of drugs to treat hyperglycemia, for example, thiazolidinediones (TZDs) [10, 13, 14]. Notwithstanding that several toxic effects led to the demise of TZDs as major drugs for the treatment of insulin resistance and hyperglycemia, the multiple studies generated by the availability of these agents [15, 16] have greatly increased our knowledge and understanding of diabetes. This pathway of increased understanding of the underlying mechanisms is continuing through the investigation of new classes of antihyperglycemic agents with novel mechanisms of action, including sodium glucose transporter inhibitors [17] and agents such as dipeptidyl peptidase-4 (DPP-4) inhibitor "gliptins" targeted at the incretin system [18].

There has been intensive research for many years on the factors causing the initiation and development of atherosclerosis [19–22]. Very detailed histological studies have shown that atherosclerosis in humans commences with the deposition of lipids in the vessel wall and that this occurs due to trapping and retention of lipoproteins in the subendothelial space by modified matrix molecules, most prominently proteoglycans [23–27]. These proteoglycans are biochemically structurally modified by the actions of growth factors and hormones on cells in the vessel wall which synthesize and secrete lipid-binding proteoglycans. The most prominent change is an increase in the size of the glycosaminoglycan (GAG) chains on chondroitin sulfate/dermatan sulfate proteoglycans such as biglycan and decorin [28–32] and these in turn show increased binding to lipoproteins [28, 33, 34]. There are also other biochemical changes which increase the atherogenicity of GAG chains [24]. Following the retention of lipoproteins by proteoglycans in the vessel wall and modifications such as glycation and oxidation, discussed elsewhere in this book, there is a long slow inflammatory process which generates atherosclerotic plaques [35–37]. Plaques may be stable or labile, and the sudden unpredictable rupture of a labile atherosclerotic plaque in, for example, a coronary artery can generate a life-threatening clinical event [38, 39]. This description relates to human atherosclerosis. In animal models of high-fat-fed genetically modified and atherosclerosis-prone mice, the process is artificially driven more rapidly and the latter inflammatory stage in humans becomes the predominant mechanism in animal models [27]. There are no really good animal models that reflect the two-stage development of human atherosclerosis, as described above [27]. Due to the focus on the inflammatory stage by the weight of research in animal models, it has been convenient for us to refer to the lipid-matrix interaction stage as the pre-inflammatory stage [40].

Appreciating the ongoing role of cardiovascular disease as a major cause of premature mortality in both the presence and absence of diabetes, the general factors driving the initiation, development, and potentially the regression of atherosclerosis are the focus of this chapter. The factors causing the inflammatory stage of atherosclerosis and their role as potential targets for therapeutic agents have recently been reviewed by us [37]. The initiation of human atherosclerosis depends on matrix lipoprotein interactions, and that is the main subject of this chapter [26, 27]. Although there is little information on the specific role of factors associated with diabetes, those factors are raised when information is available. The aim is to identify possible targets for the generation of agents to prevent the initiation or progression or to mediate regression of atherosclerosis in individuals both with and without the added confounding factors associated with diabetes. Lipoprotein matrix interactions are discussed in the context of atherosclerosis, but it is recognized that similar processes may contribute to lipoprotein-related microvascular injury, such as in the kidney and eye, and discussed elsewhere in this book.

## Biochemical and Cellular Mechanisms of Atherosclerosis

Atherosclerosis is a disease of lipid retention and inflammation at specific locations in the vessel wall determined by blood flow [23, 26, 36, 41], and it manifests as the formation of complex biochemical and morphological entities known as plaques. Raised circulating levels of cholesterol are a prerequisite for the initiation and development of atherosclerosis, but they are not sufficient on their own. A neointima develops in the blood vessel wall below the endothelium of an atherosclerosis-prone blood vessel. The cellular arrangement of predominantly vascular smooth muscle cells is somewhat random compared to the ordered arrangement in the normal vessel wall where the cells are oriented circumferentially in the interest of maintaining vascular tone and blood pressure. Not only are the vascular smooth muscle cells in a deranged distribution but they are also phenotypically modulated from the "contractile" to the "synthetic" state as described by Campbell and Campbell [42]. Phenotypic change is driven by growth factors and modifications to the extracellular matrix specifically the withdrawal of a normal matrix which suppresses phenotypic modulation. The growth factors also determine that the cells produce increased amounts of extracellular matrix. A quantitatively relatively small but functionally and, in this case, pathologically important component is the protein carbohydrate complexes known as proteoglycans [43]. Glycosaminoglycan (GAG) chains on proteoglycans are long, linear, highly negatively charged (sulfated and carboxylated) entities which bind strongly to positively charged amino acids on the apolipoproteins on low-density lipoprotein (LDL) [24, 44, 45]. Considerable evidence supports the further involvement of growth factors through their action to modify the structure, particularly to elongate the GAG chains, which increases their binding to lipoproteins [26, 28]. The binding of lipoproteins to matrix molecules is associated with biochemical modifications to the trapped lipids and lipoproteins, and principally the oxidation of these species produces agents which are highly inflammatory [46]. Specific induction of monocyte chemotactic protein-1 (MCP-1) on endothelial cells leads to the attraction, migration, and penetration of the vessel wall by pro-inflammatory monocytes and T cells [37, 47]. T cells perform a normal immune role by recognizing local antigens which then initiates an immune response and local inflammation [37]. Regulatory immune processes oppose the inflammatory response but in most circumstances, and particularly in the presence of high levels of circulating lipids and other pro-inflammatory stimuli, these restorative processes are slowly overwhelmed. The developing plaque is an active entity which expands and contracts and expands over time. Microrupture with homeostasis and thrombosis, local ischemia, apoptosis, and cell rupture all contribute to plaque development [48]. Plaques may be stable or labile, although the factors determining this critical outcome are not understood due to the present lack of a suitable animal model [49]. The diseased vessel initially undergoes outward remodeling to compensate for the luminal encroachment of the developing plaque, but subsequently this is decompensated and the developing plaque will encroach upon the lumen of the vessel wall [38]. Luminal encroachment will restrict blood flow leading to clinically significant myocardial ischemia and pain. It is currently believed that it is the nature of the plaque—stable versus labile—that determines the life-threatening nature of atherosclerosis, where the acute rupture of a labile plaque with overlying thrombosis can very acutely lead to myocardial infarction, ventricular arrhythmia, and death.

## Extracellular Matrix in Atherosclerosis

Histological studies show that human atherosclerosis commences with the deposition of lipids in the vessel wall and that this occurs due to trapping and retention by atherogenic matrix molecules, most prominently proteoglycans [50–52]. Following the retention by proteoglycans and chemical modification of lipoproteins in the vessel wall, there is a long slow inflammatory process which generates atherosclerotic plaques. Plaques may be stable or labile, and the sudden unpredictable rupture of a labile atherosclerotic plaque, in, for example, a coronary artery, generates the life-threatening clinical event. Numerous factors determine the stability of plaques with collagens increasing stability and matrix metalloproteinases (MMPs) destabilizing plaques [53]. Thus, extracellular matrix is a major determinant of the initiation, progression, and potentially regression of atherosclerotic plaques.

## Role of Collagens in Atherosclerosis

In the healthy blood vessel wall, fibrillar types I and III collagens are most prevalent. Vascular smooth muscle cells stabilize the vessel wall by secreting soluble collagen that polymerizes into insoluble fibrils that confers structural and tensile strength to plaque structure [54]. In addition, collagens are active components of the matrix, interacting with a variety of cell types and molecules. As atherosclerosis develops, smooth muscle cells transition from a contractile to synthetic phenotype [42]. Concomitantly there is a significant increase in non-fibrillar network-forming type VIII collagen by endothelial cells, smooth muscle cells, and macrophages in the early stages of atherosclerosis. Collagen VIII is seen in the subendothelial intimal extracellular matrix and is usually only seen in small amounts in normal vessels [55]. Collagens I, III, and V together comprise up to 60 % of atherosclerotic plaque protein and contribute appreciably to the narrowing of arterial lumens in atherosclerosis [54]. They are synthesized by smooth muscle cells to facilitate migration but also by endothelial cells, adventitial fibroblasts, and macrophages [55]. Collagens influence cell behavior and phenotype via feedback mechanisms through integrins $\alpha_1\beta_1$, $\alpha_2\beta_1$, and $\alpha_{10}\beta_1$ and tyrosine kinase discoidin domain (DDR1 and DDR2) receptor-mediated signaling. The integrins bind directly to collagen sequences GFOGER, GLOGER, and GASGER [56]. The DDRs bind to triple helical collagens and DDR2 binds to collagens I–III peptide sequence GVMGFO [57]. Types I and III collagen synthesis is observed in the vessel intima [58] with the precursor protein type I procollagen only demonstrated in aortic lesions, not in normal human arteries [55]. In advanced plaques type I collagen predominates in the fibrous cap and in the vicinity of microvessels [54]. Type V collagen has been demonstrated immunohistochemically in the media of atherosclerotic plaques [59].

Collagens have the capacity to influence the extent of smooth muscle cell proliferation in atherosclerosis. In vivo, following injury of porcine coronary arteries, polymerized fibrillar type I collagen deposition initiates upregulation of cyclin-dependent kinase inhibitor p27kip1 and decreased smooth muscle cell proliferation [60]. mRNA levels of collagen types I and III are elevated in human diabetic atherosclerotic coronary arteries [61]. In vitro soluble type I collagen has been demonstrated to stimulate smooth muscle cell proliferation via activation of phospholipase C and phosphatidylinositol 3-kinase (PI3K) pathways and via integrin $\alpha_2\beta_1$-binding and platelet-derived growth factor receptor cross talk [62]. Injured rat carotid arteries showing intimal hyperplasia have increased collagen VIII expression with smooth muscle cell migration [63]. Smooth muscle cell spreading and migration is considered to be facilitated by an increased expression and activity of MMPs and a weak adherence of these cells to collagen type VIII [64].

A key event in the development of atherosclerosis is the recruitment, migration differentiation, and cytokine production by monocytes from the circulation into the ECM of the blood vessel wall. Collagen interacts with monocyte/macrophages in atherosclerotic plaques via integrins and DDRs mediate numerous atherogenic effects. Monocytes adherent to collagen specifically induce at least 316 genes [65]. Adhesion of monocytes on type I collagen increases cell spreading, phagocytic activity and uptake of LDL, and matrix metalloproteinase 9 expression [66]. Collagen can also serve as a store of pro-atherogenic molecules including modified lipoproteins, via lipoprotein lipase bound to decorin, which in turn binds directly to collagen [67], growth factors, and advanced glycation end products (AGEs). AGEs form irreversible cross-links with collagen backbones and in diabetic apoE KO mice collagen types III and IV are increased significantly and total collagen content is increased tenfold in atherosclerotic plaques [68].

The fibrous cap of atherosclerotic plaques consists of fibrillar collagens and elastin providing protection against rupture and potential thrombosis. Overexpression of MMPs in human and experimental atheromatous plaques provides conditions where cleavage of collagen monomers into fragments via cleavage of the Gly-Ile bond by MMPs 1, 8, and 13 [69] allows further degradation of collagen content, especially at the shoulder region of plaques [54]. Excessive collagen may lead to vessel stenosis and a lack of collagen can result in architectural instability and rupture of the fibrous cap.

## Role of Matrix Metalloproteinases in Atherosclerosis

Matrix metalloproteinases (MMPs) play a key role in degradation and turnover of the extracellular matrix. Over 25 MMPs have been described: collagenases, stromelysins, matrilysins, metalloelastases, and membrane-type MMPs [70]. They are zinc-dependent proteases classified according to their substrate specificity and structure. Endothelial cells, smooth muscle cells, and monocytes synthesize and secrete the latent proforms of the enzymes, and activation mediators include plasmin, thrombin, angiotensin, nitric oxide and reactive oxygen species, hyperglycemia, and other MMPs. Matrix composition is a regulated balance between cytokine and growth factor-mediated matrix formation and MMP-driven degradation. Experimental and clinical data demonstrate the involvement of MMPs and their inhibiting factors, tissue inhibitors of metalloproteinases (TIMPs), in vascular remodeling such as in the formation and progression of atherosclerotic plaques [71, 72]. Experimental animal studies using balloon angioplasty or ligature have demonstrated MMP upregulation and resultant intimal expansion, collagen accumulation, and increased atheroma formation. Changes are associated with smooth muscle cell migration, activation of macrophages, and disturbed MMP/TIMP equilibrium [71, 72].

In vitro studies of vascular endothelial cells treated with high glucose concentrations modeling diabetes show increased expression of some MMPs and TIMPs, not others [73, 74]. In type 1 and type 2 diabetes, altered plasma concentrations of MMP-2, MMP-9, and TIMP-1 have also been reported and exacerbate the progress of atherosclerosis [75].

## Role of Proteoglycans in Atherosclerosis

Proteoglycans are large complex macromolecules which are synthesized and secreted by cells of the normal and atherosclerotic vessel wall [76]. Proteoglycans are found predominantly in the extracellular matrix and on the cell surface of most eukaryotic cells. Proteoglycans are comprised of a polypeptide core protein of defined molecular weight and one or more covalently attached glycosaminoglycan (GAG) chains of variable molecular weight. The molecular weight of the GAG chains, and thus the proteoglycans, varies because of the less specific nature of the synthetic process for GAGs occurring in the Golgi apparatus. Notably growth factors and phenotypic alterations can stimulate the increased expression of proteoglycan core proteins but also activate Golgi processes, resulting in an increase in the mean molecular weight of the GAG chains and thus the proteoglycans [24]. The cloning of the genes that encode proteoglycan core proteins [76] provided the opportunity to name the molecules based on their actual core proteins, and hence decorin, biglycan, versican, and perlecan can also be categorized by the chemical structure of the GAG chains and hence chondroitin sulfate, dermatan sulfate, heparan sulfate, or keratin sulfate. The disaccharide components of GAG chains are carboxylated and can be further enzymatically sulfated and thus are negatively charged at physiological pH. The diversity of the structures of proteoglycans is enormous due to the variety of GAG chains and their attachment to different core proteins [77]. Different GAG chains on the same core protein, particularly the linkages between monosaccharides, produce marked differences in structure and properties of these molecules [77]. The most highly expressed proteoglycans are chondroitin sulfate (CS) proteoglycans [78]. CS proteoglycans are synthesized by the sequential alternative addition of monosaccharide (glucuronic acid and N-acetylglucosamine) and the subsequent epimerization of any of the glucuronic acid residues to iduronic acid, by convention, alters the description of the GAG from CS to dermatan sulfate (DS) [79]. The array of proteoglycans occurring in the vessel wall includes CS proteoglycan, versican, the CS/DS proteoglycans, biglycan and decorin, the heparan sulfate (HS) proteoglycan, perlecan and the keratan sulfate (KS) proteoglycan, and mimecan. Proteoglycans represent only a small component, a few percent, by mass of the vessel wall extracellular matrix [80, 81], but they are considerably more important because of their diverse functionality and their role in pathological processes. Proteoglycans represent up to 20 % of total protein synthesis in vascular smooth muscle [82, 83]. The active degradation of proteoglycans by proteases and GAG-degrading enzymes means there is a high turnover of proteoglycans in the vessel wall, which renders them as a therapeutic target relative, for example, to elastin components which are very long-lived. Proteoglycans are not only space-occupying extracellular molecules (a property which is greatly exaggerated by the attraction of water molecules) [76] but highly functional, being involved in matrix-growth factor interaction and indirectly controlling cellular functions, including proliferation and secretion [78].

The major structural property related to atherosclerosis is the ability of certain proteoglycans, particularly biglycan and specifically its CS/DS GAG chains, to bind to the apolipoprotein B (apoB) on LDL. Although the binding and trapping of lipid in the vessel wall as a contributing factor to atherosclerosis has been known for many years [50], the involvement of extracellular matrix molecules, including proteoglycans, led to the response to retention hypothesis [23, 25]. The hypothesis states that the subendothelial retention of lipid by matrix molecules including proteoglycans is the initiating step in atherosclerosis.

*Decorin* is a small leucine-rich proteoglycan with a small core protein and one DS GAG chain and a molecular weight of approximately 100 kD. Decorin is a cellular or pericellular proteoglycan closely related in structure and function to biglycan with which it is often closely co-localized [51]. Decorin binds to numerous molecules and its name arises because it binds to or "decorates" type 1 collagen fibrils, and thus plays a role in fibrillogenesis. Decorin also interacts with transforming growth factor-beta (TGF-β), and it can modify TGF-β signaling and responses and serve as a reservoir of TGF-β in tissues such as the blood vessel wall [84]. TGF-β is implicated in many vascular complications of diabetes, in particular renal damage [9].

*Biglycan* is a small leucine-rich proteoglycan found in multiple tissues including the vessel wall, bone, and tendon. Biglycan has two DS GAG chains and a molecular weight of approximately 200 kD. As for most proteoglycans, forms can be found with one and with no GAG chains, although the implications of these forms are unclear. Biglycan, as decorin, binds to collagen, and indeed in some systems the two can apparently compete for binding to collagen. Biglycan is the most highly secreted proteoglycan by human vascular smooth muscle cells and it is prominently expressed in blood vessels and its expression is increased in diseased vessels.

*Versican* is a very large multi-domain protein with multiple covalently attached GAG chains and a molecular weight of some 100 kD. Versican is prominently expressed in blood vessels and also in cartilage. Versican is poly-functional secondary to its diverse structural elements. Human vascular smooth muscle cells secrete very little versican, but its expression is increased by growth factor such as platelet-derived growth factor (PDGF) [83]; however, primate vascular smooth muscle cells secrete large amounts of versican, and the level is also increased by PDGF [85]. The core protein has an N-terminal, C-terminal, and GAG-binding domain. The protein occurs in four isoforms known as V0, V1, V2, and V3, where V3 has no GAG attachment sites [86]. Versican is associated with cell adhesion, migration, and proliferation [87]. The N-terminal of versican interacts with the nonprotein-containing nonsulfated GAG, hyaluronan, indicating the extent to which proteoglycan and GAGs and the molecules with which they interact can control normal and pathogenic vascular functions.

*Perlecan* is a heparan sulfate proteoglycan thus having GAG chains with distinct properties. Perlecan is produced in small amounts by vascular smooth muscle cells (in comparison to decorin and biglycan), but it is present in substantial amounts in the vessel wall, suggesting that it may be more stable and have a lower turnover rate than the CS/DS proteoglycans. Perlecan heparan sulfate chains are proatherogenic in mice, possibly through increased lipoprotein retention, altered vascular permeability, and the ability to inhibit smooth muscle cell growth [88].

## Role of Hyaluronan in Atherosclerosis

Hyaluronan (HA), a glycosaminoglycan composed of repeating N-acetylglucosamine and glucuronic acid linked together by alternating β-1,3 and β-1,4 linkages, is upregulated and accumulates in developing atherosclerotic lesions with the highest expression in the media and a negative concentration gradient towards the plaque [89]. HA is synthesized by smooth muscle cells, endothelial cells, and adventitial fibroblasts. Experimental animal studies have demonstrated that HA deposition coincides with smooth muscle cell proliferation and migration [90–92] and is related to increased levels of associated molecules HA receptor CD44, hyaladherin TSG-6, and versican [93]. HA anchored to the surface of endothelial cells by its receptors CD44 or RHAMM assists monocyte and lymphocyte movement into the vessel wall at the early stages of atherosclerosis [90]. HA degradation products, from the effects of hyaluronidase and reactive oxygen species, induce the release of pro-inflammatory cytokines interleukin-1 (IL-1) and tumor necrosis factor-alpha (TNF-α) [94]. In vivo studies with transgenic ApoE knockout mice overexpressing HA synthase 2 demonstrated an increased progression of atherosclerosis in the aorta [95], while CD44-null ApoE knockout mice have less atherosclerosis due to the failure of macrophage recruitment to atherosclerotic lesions [91]. HA is known to be elevated in atherosclerotic vessels of animal models of diabetes and also in the plasma of diabetic patients [96]. HA is associated with increased atherosclerotic lesion instability and lipoprotein retention, leading to accelerated atherogenesis [97].

## Extracellular Matrix as a Therapeutic Target

### Collagens as Targets for Atherosclerosis Therapy

Early theories suggested that increased collagen production in atheroma added to the burden of luminal stenosis; however more recent clinical findings point to the involvement of thrombi from ruptured plaques as the culprit in acute coronary episodes, rather than stenoses. The state of the dynamic remodeling of the atherosclerotic plaque fibrous cap may determine the clinical fate of a given lesion [20]. Plaque rupture may result from low levels of collagen, which may result from increased collagen catabolism (as described earlier) by matrix metalloproteinases or decreased and/or altered collagen synthesis. Accumulation of non-fibrillar collagen or defective collagen results in plaques with vulnerable caps and the likelihood of clinical sequelae [98]. Thus the balance of synthesis and degradation of collagen is of utmost importance in treatment strategies for the prevention of atherosclerosis. To date there are no therapies targeted directly at collagen production, assembly, or catabolism; however current therapies have resulted in some interesting effects on collagen. Statin treatment has proved to have clinical benefit in reducing plaque size by limiting plaque lipid load and thereby stabilizing atherosclerotic plaques [99]. Dietary lipid lowering in rabbits decreased macrophage accumulation, as well as endothelial cell and smooth muscle cell activation, which decreased the collagenase MMP 1 expression and increased collagen levels [100]. A clinical study demonstrated that pravastatin treatment to lower lipids increased collagen content and decreased matrix metalloproteinases in human carotid plaques [101]. Blocking formation of AGEs in diabetic ApoE knockout mice attenuates aortic plaque collagen I accumulation and may affect plaque stability [68]. Viable collagen-directed therapies for the prevention or treatment of atherosclerosis are yet to be discovered.

## MMPs as a Therapeutic Target in Atherosclerosis

The use of MMP inhibitors (MMPI) as therapeutic agents aims to reduce ECM degradation, thereby stabilizing plaques. This does present an opportunity for an imbalance in ECM expansion. MMPI drugs, including batimastat, ilomastat, marimastat, and tanomastat, have existed for more than 25 years. Unfortunately numerous failed clinical trials have lowered interest in this approach. The majority of MMPI drugs are broad spectrum synthetic MMP inhibitors, like the tetracycline antibiotic doxycycline [102], which has been shown to limit intimal remodeling both in vitro [103] and in vivo [104]. An alternative inhibitory method is to overexpress TIMPs to alter the balance between MMPs and TIMPs. Overexpression of TIMPs has produced differing results such as either decreased neointimal thickening [105–107] or no change in aortic plaque size [108]. Targeted deletion of TIMP-1 in ApoE-null mice also gave contradictory results, either unchanged [109] or decreased plaque formation [110]. More recently, rosuvastatin treatment has been demonstrated to inhibit the expression of MMP-2 and MMP-9 and limit the progression of atherosclerosis in LDL-receptor-deficient mice [111]. Overall, targeting MMPs for therapeutic purposes in atherosclerosis is complex, partly because of the redundancy of MMPs in the ECM and partly because of the precise balance between MMPs and TIMPs in the vessel wall. Currently there are no suitable drug candidates for direct MMP targeting in atherosclerosis.

## Proteoglycans as Therapeutic Targets

Lipids bind to GAG chains, and the role of the growth-factor-mediated hyperelongation of GAG chains has been hypothesized to be a substantial contributing factor to the ability of vessel wall proteoglycans to bind and retain lipid and thus represents a therapeutic target [26, 34, 112]. The GAG chain properties which determine the strength of their interaction with lipids are the length of the chains, the sulfation pattern, and the degree of epimerization [24]. Each of these properties is under specific cellular regulation.

Many enzymes have been discovered which mediate the synthesis of proteoglycans and specifically GAG chains, but the extent to which the mechanism of assembly is known varies from type to type [52]. Furthermore, the widespread expression of proteoglycans suggests that these synthetic enzymes will not represent therapeutic targets. Growth factors and hormones can regulate the synthesis of proteoglycan core proteins and GAG chains (*see* Fig. 11.1), often via highly specific signaling pathways, and it is more likely that these signaling pathways, which may be tissue specific, will represent therapeutic targets [28, 32, 113–116].

Biglycan expression in vascular smooth muscle cells is increased by TGF-β, which also markedly increases the size of the GAG chains on the biglycan, and accordingly there is a strong

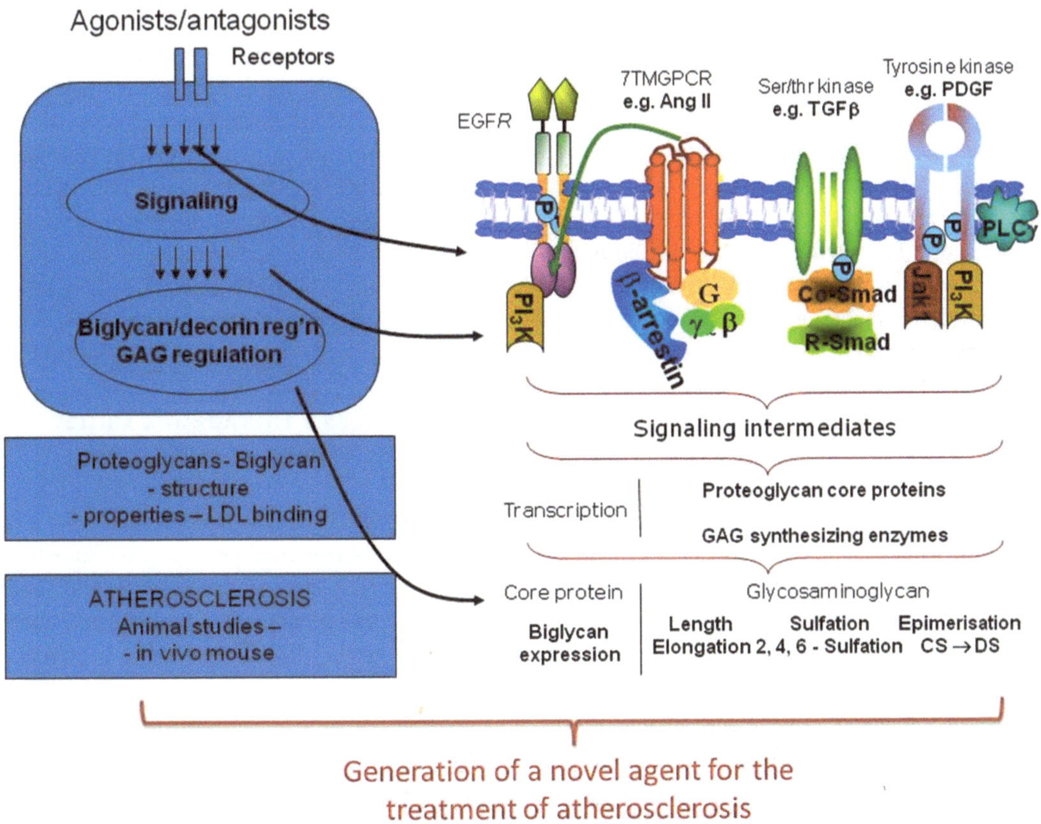


**Fig. 11.1** Process involved in the generation of an inhibitor of proteoglycan synthesis for the prevention of atherosclerosis. An inhibitor of growth factor-mediated elongation of glycosaminoglycan chains on proteoglycans, such as biglycan, secreted by vascular smooth muscle cells has the potential to inhibit the matrix lipoprotein interaction which results in the deposition of lipid in the vessel wall as the initiating step in atherosclerosis. Such a product would be used jointly with a statin drug (see text for details)

association with biglycan, TGF-β, and lipid as a causal step in the development of atherosclerosis, and this is a therapeutic target [28, 115, 116].

The most investigated area of the potential of therapeutic agents directed at proteoglycan synthesis is the signaling pathways that mediate elongation of CS/DS GAG chains on biglycan because of the direct association with increased lipid binding [26]. Many growth factors and hormones stimulate vascular smooth muscle cells to synthesize and secrete biglycan with increased GAG length [117], a phenomenon that we have termed hyperelongation, because it represents a further elongation of GAG than that seen under basal conditions [26]. Vasoactive factors that stimulate GAG elongation include seven-transmembrane G protein-coupled receptor agonists, such as angiotensin II, endothelin-1, and thrombin; protein tyrosine kinase receptor agonists such as PDGF and epidermal growth factor (EGF); and serine/threonine kinase agonists such as TGF-β (Fig. 11.1) [117]. Taking the serine/threonine kinase receptor for TGF-β, transforming growth factor-β receptor I (TβRI), as an example, there has been considerable progress in characterizing the pathways through which this receptor leads to GAG hyperelongation and in distinguishing these pathways from those that mediate increased expression of the proteoglycan core protein [32, 118]. TGF-β also stimulates a pathway, known as non-Smad, which involves the activation of the MAP kinase pathway leading to stimulation of Erk1/2 and phosphorylation of Smad in the linker region. The linker region is located between receptor Smads

Mad homology domains 1 and 2. Although phosphorylation in the linker region was originally shown to inhibit Smad function [119, 120], most recent studies show that linker region phosphorylation is a positive driver of Smad responses [116, 121, 122]. There is a small group of serine and threonine residues in the linker region of Smad transcription factors, and these are linked to specific downstream pathways that regulate gene transcription, including that controlling the expression of genes which mediate GAG elongation [121]. For vasoactive agents which are mitogens, such as PDGF, which also stimulate proteoglycan core protein expression, the core protein expression and mitogenic pathways appear to be common or at least similar, including PI3K and Akt, whereas GAG elongation pathways are mediated via MAP kinases, especially Erk1/2 [32]. The highly specific biochemical targets that have been identified in this work have the potential to be used for the development of drugs to prevent GAG elongation and lipid deposition in atherogenesis.

The potential for inhibiting GAG elongation and preventing lipid deposition and atherosclerosis has been demonstrated in animal models [32, 34]. The antitumor agent imatinib (STI 571, Gleevec, Glivec) was developed for the inhibition of Abl tyrosine kinase in chronic myeloid leukemia, in which this kinase is constitutively activated [123]. Imatinib has been characterized as a tyrosine kinase inhibitor and it inhibits only a small number of kinases. In the vascular context, imatinib inhibits Abl as well as Kit and PDGF receptor kinase [124]. Imatinib is a potent inhibitor of PDGF-stimulated GAG elongation [32, 34]. GAG chains isolated from vascular smooth muscle cells treated with imatinib show reduced binding to normal human LDL, and high-fat-fed atherosclerosis-prone mice treated with imatinib show reduce lipid deposition ex vivo and in vivo [32, 34]. Atherosclerosis is associated with many growth factors and hormones, and intriguingly we have found that imatinib inhibits the GAG elongation action of not only tyrosine kinase agonists but also of seven-transmembrane G protein-coupled receptor and serine/threonine kinase agonists (Little, unpublished observation). These latter agonists have distinct signaling pathways (Fig. 11.1), so identifying the precise target of the action of imatinib might produce a therapeutically useful GAG inhibitor. Such a drug would be used in combination with a HMG CoA reductase inhibitor (statin), such that the statin would reduce circulating levels of atherogenic lipoproteins and the GAG inhibitor would render the vessel wall less sticky, with the overall effect of a reduced rate of progression of atherosclerosis [125].

## Hyaluronan as a Therapeutic Target in Atherosclerosis

HA is a potential target for the prevention of atherosclerosis as evidenced by its involvement in the multiple early changes in the vessel wall, both structurally and as an inflammatory component [126]. To date very little progress has been made on specifically targeting components of the ECM, including HA. There are however examples of drugs influencing HA metabolism, such as anti-inflammatory steroids prednisolone, hydrocortisone, dexamethasone, and betamethasone, significantly inhibiting HA synthesis and not sulfated glycosaminoglycan synthesis [127]. The nonsteroidal anti-inflammatory drug etoricoxib, a cyclooxygenase enzyme COX2 inhibitor, blocks HAS2 production of HA [128]. The immunosuppressive drug sirolimus causes a significant reduction in HAS1-3 mRNA levels and hyaluronan synthesis [129], and the statin lovastatin reduces HA accumulation in Watanabe heritable hyperlipidemic rabbits [130]. These examples demonstrate potential beneficial therapeutic effects in the acute inflammatory phase of atherosclerosis where HA production is elevated.

## Conclusions

It is very surprising that all of the research over the last two decades has not led to more novel agents for the treatment of atherosclerosis. Nevertheless this chapter on lipid-matrix interactions and other bodies of work focused on the role of inflammation in the development of atherosclerosis [37] clearly demonstrate that there are many preclinical targets which have not been fully explored for their potential as therapeutic targets. Work in these areas has been impeded by the lack of animal models which reproduce the human disease with high fidelity, so new models are urgently required. Although diabetes drives an almost two-fold increase in the rate of development of atherosclerosis and of cardiovascular disease [7], the factors that are specific to diabetes have not been identified [12], and that is an area requiring more research and new insights.

The early pre-inflammatory phase of the development of atherosclerosis occurs due to the interaction of extracellular matrix molecules in the vessel wall with circulating lipid species, which enter the vessel wall and are retained. Although the area of circulating lipids has received considerable attention, the properties of the extracellular matrix of the vessel wall and the interaction of the matrix with circulating lipids which enter the wall has been less appreciated and investigated. Perhaps therein lies the pathway to a new therapeutic agent, to work alone or more likely in combination with a lipid-lowering agent, to retard the development of atherosclerosis and cardiovascular disease. Even in the absence of knowledge of the diabetes-specific factors that accelerate atherosclerosis, such therapies will likely also be beneficial to people with diabetes.

**Acknowledgements** Work described in this report was supported by a National Health and Medical Research Council Australia Project Grant (#1022800 Little and Osman) and National Heart Foundation of Australia grant-in-aid (#G10M5211 Little and Osman).

## References

1. Fowler MJ. Microvascular and macrovascular complications of diabetes. Clin Diabetes. 2011;26(2).
2. Thorp AA, et al. Sedentary behaviors and subsequent health outcomes in adults a systematic review of longitudinal studies, 1996–2011. Am J Prev Med. 2011;41(2):207–15.
3. Weyer C, et al. Hypoadiponectinemia in obesity and type 2 diabetes: close association with insulin resistance and hyperinsulinemia. J Clin Endocrinol Metab. 2001;86(5):1930–5.
4. Couper JJ, et al. Weight gain in early life predicts risk of islet autoimmunity in children with a first-degree relative with type 1 diabetes. Diabetes Care. 2009;32(1):94–9.
5. Reusch JE, Wang CC. Cardiovascular disease in diabetes: where does glucose fit in? J Clin Endocrinol Metab. 2011;96(8):2367–76.
6. Stratton IM, et al. Association of glycaemia with macrovascular and microvascular complications of type 2 diabetes (UKPDS 35): prospective observational study. BMJ. 2000;321(7258):405–12.
7. Haffner SJ, Cassells H. Hyperglycemia as a cardiovascular risk factor. Am J Med. 2003;115 (Suppl 8A):6S–11.
8. Roger VL, et al. Heart disease and stroke statistics-2011 update: a report from the American Heart Association. Circulation. 2011;123(4):e18–209.
9. Brownlee M. Biochemistry and molecular cell biology of diabetic complications. Nature. 2001; 414(6865):813–20.
10. Fruchart JC, Staels B, Duriez P. PPARS, metabolic disease and atherosclerosis. Pharmacol Res. 2001; 44(5):345–52.
11. Cooper ME, et al. Mechanisms of diabetic vasculopathy: an overview. Am J Hypertens. 2001;14(5 Pt 1):475–86.
12. Preis SR, et al. Trends in cardiovascular disease risk factors in individuals with and without diabetes mellitus in the Framingham Heart Study. Circulation. 2009;120(3):212–20.
13. Hannan KM, et al. Troglitazone stimulates repair of the endothelium and inhibits neointimal formation in denuded rat aorta. Arterioscler Thromb Vasc Biol. 2003;23(5):762–8.
14. de Dios ST, et al. Inhibitory activity of clinical thiazolidinedione peroxisome proliferator activating receptor-gamma ligands toward internal mammary artery, radial artery, and saphenous vein smooth muscle cell proliferation. Circulation. 2003;107(20): 2548–50.
15. Nissen SE, Wolski K. Effect of rosiglitazone on the risk of myocardial infarction and death from cardiovascular causes. N Engl J Med. 2007;356(24): 2457–71.
16. Diamond GA, Bax L, Kaul S. Uncertain effects of rosiglitazone on the risk for myocardial infarction and cardiovascular death. Ann Intern Med. 2007; 147(8):578–81.
17. Ghosh RK, et al. SGLT2 inhibitors: a new emerging therapeutic class in the treatment of type 2 diabetes mellitus. J Clin Pharmacol. 2012;52(4):457–63.
18. Drucker DJ, Nauck MA. The incretin system: glucagon-like peptide-1 receptor agonists and dipeptidyl peptidase-4 inhibitors in type 2 diabetes. Lancet. 2006;368(9548):1696–705.
19. Ross R. The pathogenesis of atherosclerosis. N Engl J Med. 1986;314:488–500.
20. Libby P. Inflammation in atherosclerosis. Nature. 2002;420(6917):868–74.

21. Kolodgie FD, et al. Differential accumulation of proteoglycans and hyaluronan in culprit lesions: insights into plaque erosion. Arterioscler Thromb Vasc Biol. 2002;22(10):1642–8.
22. Konstantinov IE, Mejevoi N, Anichkov NM. Nikolai N. Anichkov and his theory of atherosclerosis. Tex Heart Inst J. 2006;33(4):417–23.
23. Williams KJ, Tabas I. The response-to-retention hypothesis of early atherogenesis. Arterioscler Thromb Vasc Biol. 1995;15(5):551–61.
24. Ballinger ML, et al. Regulation of glycosaminoglycan structure and atherogenesis. Cell Mol Life Sci. 2004;61(11):1296–306.
25. Tabas I, Williams KJ, Boren J. Subendothelial lipoprotein retention as the initiating process in atherosclerosis: update and therapeutic implications. Circulation. 2007;116(16):1832–44.
26. Little PJ, Osman N, O'Brien KD. Hyperelongated biglycan: the surreptitious initiator of atherosclerosis. Curr Opin Lipidol. 2008;19:448–54.
27. Finn AV, et al. Pharmacotherapy of coronary atherosclerosis. Expert Opin Pharmacother. 2009;10(10): 1587–603.
28. Little PJ, et al. Proteoglycans synthesized by arterial smooth muscle cells in the presence of transforming growth factor-beta1 exhibit increased binding to LDLs. Arterioscler Thromb Vasc Biol. 2002;22(1): 55–60.
29. Gustafsson M, Boren J. Mechanism of lipoprotein retention by the extracellular matrix. Curr Opin Lipidol. 2004;15(5):505–14.
30. Hashimura K, et al. Androgens stimulate human vascular smooth muscle cell proteoglycan biosynthesis and increase lipoprotein binding. Endocrinology. 2005;146(4):2085–90.
31. Ivey ME, Osman N, Little PJ. Endothelin-1 signalling in vascular smooth muscle: pathways controlling cellular functions associated with atherosclerosis. Atherosclerosis. 2008;199(2):237–47.
32. Getachew R, et al. PDGF beta-receptor kinase activity and ERK1/2 mediate glycosaminoglycan elongation on biglycan and increases binding to LDL. Endocrinology. 2010;151(9):4356–67.
33. Camejo G, et al. Association of apo B lipoproteins with arterial proteoglycans: pathological significance and molecular basis. Atherosclerosis. 1998; 139(2):205–22.
34. Ballinger ML, et al. Imatinib inhibits vascular smooth muscle proteoglycan synthesis and reduces LDL binding in vitro and aortic lipid deposition in vivo. J Cell Mol Med. 2010;14:1408–18.
35. Ross R. Atherosclerosis—an inflammatory disease. N Engl J Med. 1999;340(2):115–26.
36. Libby P. Inflammation and cardiovascular disease mechanisms. Am J Clin Nutr. 2006;83(2):456S–60.
37. Little PJ, Chait A, Bobik A. Cellular and cytokine-based inflammatory processes as novel therapeutic targets for the prevention and treatment of atherosclerosis. Pharmacol Ther. 2011;131(3): 255–68.
38. Davies MJ. Stability and instability: two faces of coronary atherosclerosis. The Paul Dudley White Lecture 1995. Circulation. 1996;94(8):2013–20.
39. Falk E, Fernandez-Ortiz A. Role of thrombosis in atherosclerosis and its complications. Am J Cardiol. 1995;75(6):3B–11.
40. Burch ML, et al. G protein coupled receptor transactivation: extending the paradigm to include serine/threonine kinase receptors. Int J Biochem Cell Biol. 2012;44(5):722–7.
41. Pasterkamp G, de Kleijn DP, Borst C. Arterial remodeling in atherosclerosis, restenosis and after alteration of blood flow: potential mechanisms and clinical implications. Cardiovasc Res. 2000;45(4): 843–52.
42. Campbell JH, Campbell GR. The role of smooth muscle cells in atherosclerosis. Curr Opin Lipidol. 1994;5(5):323–30.
43. Wight TN. Cell biology of arterial proteoglycans. Arteriosclerosis. 1989;9(1):1–20.
44. Camejo G, et al. Identification of Apo B-100 segments mediating the interaction of low density lipoproteins with arterial proteoglycans. Arteriosclerosis. 1988;8(4):368–77.
45. Williams KJ, Tabas I. The response-to-retention hypothesis of atherogenesis reinforced. Curr Opin Lipidol. 1998;9(5):471–4.
46. Steinberg D. The LDL modification hypothesis of atherogenesis: an update. J Lipid Res. 2009; 50(Suppl):S376–81.
47. Moore KJ, Tabas I. Macrophages in the pathogenesis of atherosclerosis. Cell. 2011;145(3):341–55.
48. Libby P. Vascular biology of atherosclerosis: overview and state of the art. Am J Cardiol. 2003; 91(3A):3A–6.
49. Schwartz SM, et al. Plaque rupture in humans and mice. Arterioscler Thromb Vasc Biol. 2007;27(4): 705–13.
50. Skalen K, et al. Subendothelial retention of atherogenic lipoproteins in early atherosclerosis. Nature. 2002;417(6890):750–4.
51. Nakashima Y, et al. Early human atherosclerosis: accumulation of lipid and proteoglycans in intimal thickenings followed by macrophage infiltration. Arterioscler Thromb Vasc Biol. 2007;27(5): 1159–65.
52. Anggraeni VY, et al. Correlation of C4ST-1 and ChGn-2 expression with chondroitin sulfate chain elongation in atherosclerosis. Biochem Biophys Res Commun. 2011;406(1):36–41.
53. Newby AC, Southgate KM, Davies M. Extracellular matrix degrading metalloproteinases in the pathogenesis of arteriosclerosis. Basic Res Cardiol. 1994;89 Suppl 1:59–70.
54. Rekhter MD. Collagen synthesis in atherosclerosis: too much and not enough. Cardiovasc Res. 1999; 41(2):376–84.
55. Plenz GA, et al. Vascular collagens: spotlight on the role of type VIII collagen in atherogenesis. Atherosclerosis. 2003;166(1):1–11.

56. Siljander PR, et al. Integrin activation state determines selectivity for novel recognition sites in fibrillar collagens. J Biol Chem. 2004;279(46):47763–72.
57. Adiguzel E, et al. Collagens in the progression and complications of atherosclerosis. Vasc Med. 2009;14(1):73–89.
58. Jaeger E, et al. Joint occurrence of collagen mRNA containing cells and macrophages in human atherosclerotic vessels. Atherosclerosis. 1991;86(1):55–68.
59. Schuppan D, et al. Immunofluorescent localization of type-V collagen as a fibrillar component of the interstitial connective tissue of human oral mucosa, artery and liver. Cell Tissue Res. 1986;243(3):535–43.
60. Tanner FC, et al. Expression of cyclin-dependent kinase inhibitors in vascular disease. Circ Res. 1998;82(3):396–403.
61. Chung AW, et al. Enhanced cell cycle entry and mitogen-activated protein kinase-signaling and downregulation of matrix metalloproteinase-1 and -3 in human diabetic arterial vasculature. Atherosclerosis. 2007;195(1):e1–8.
62. Hollenbeck ST, et al. Type I collagen synergistically enhances PDGF-induced smooth muscle cell proliferation through pp60src-dependent crosstalk between the alpha2beta1 integrin and PDGFbeta receptor. Biochem Biophys Res Commun. 2004; 325(1):328–37.
63. Bendeck MP, et al. Differential expression of alpha 1 type VIII collagen in injured platelet-derived growth factor-BB-stimulated rat carotid arteries. Circ Res. 1996;79(3):524–31.
64. Adiguzel E, et al. Migration and growth are attenuated in vascular smooth muscle cells with type VIII collagen-null alleles. Arterioscler Thromb Vasc Biol. 2006;26(1):56–61.
65. de Fougerolles AR, et al. Global expression analysis of extracellular matrix-integrin interactions in monocytes. Immunity. 2000;13(6):749–58.
66. Wesley 2nd RB, et al. Extracellular matrix modulates macrophage functions characteristic to atheroma: collagen type I enhances acquisition of resident macrophage traits by human peripheral blood monocytes in vitro. Arterioscler Thromb Vasc Biol. 1998;18(3):432–40.
67. Pentikainen MO, et al. Lipoprotein lipase in the arterial wall: linking LDL to the arterial extracellular matrix and much more. Arterioscler Thromb Vasc Biol. 2002;22(2):211–7.
68. Forbes JM, et al. Advanced glycation end product interventions reduce diabetes-accelerated atherosclerosis. Diabetes. 2004;53(7):1813–23.
69. Newby AC. Dual role of matrix metalloproteinases (matrixins) in intimal thickening and atherosclerotic plaque rupture. Physiol Rev. 2005;85(1):1–31.
70. Visse R, Nagase H. Matrix metalloproteinases and tissue inhibitors of metalloproteinases: structure, function, and biochemistry. Circ Res. 2003;92(8):827–39.
71. Back M, Ketelhuth DF, Agewall S. Matrix metalloproteinases in atherothrombosis. Prog Cardiovasc Dis. 2010;52(5):410–28.
72. Raffetto JD, Khalil RA. Matrix metalloproteinases and their inhibitors in vascular remodeling and vascular disease. Biochem Pharmacol. 2008;75(2):346–59.
73. Death AK, et al. High glucose alters matrix metalloproteinase expression in two key vascular cells: potential impact on atherosclerosis in diabetes. Atherosclerosis. 2003;168(2):263–9.
74. Ho FM, et al. Opposite effects of high glucose on MMP-2 and TIMP-2 in human endothelial cells. J Cell Biochem. 2007;101(2):442–50.
75. Hopps E, Caimi G. Matrix metalloproteinases in metabolic syndrome. Eur J Intern Med. 2012;23(2): 99–104.
76. Iozzo RV. Matrix proteoglycans: from molecular design to cellular function. Annu Rev Biochem. 1998;67:609–52.
77. Sugahara K, Kitagawa H. Recent advances in the study of the biosynthesis and functions of sulfated glycosaminoglycans. Curr Opin Struct Biol. 2000; 10(5):518–27.
78. Hynes RO, Naba A. Overview of the matrisome—an inventory of extracellular matrix constituents and functions. Cold Spring Harb Perspect Biol. 2012; 4(1):a004903.
79. Prydz K, Dalen KT. Synthesis and sorting of proteoglycans. J Cell Sci. 2000;113(Pt 2):193–205.
80. Wight T. In: Fuster V, Ross R, Topol EJ editors. The vascular extracellular matrix, in Atherosclerosis and coronary artery disease. Philadelphia: Lippincott-Raven; 1996. p. 421–440
81. Hascall VC, Heinegard DK, Wight TN. In: Hay ED editor. Proteoglycans: metabolism and pathology, in cell biology of extracellular matrix. New York: Plenum Press; 1991. p. 149–175.
82. de Dios ST, et al. Regulation of the atherogenic properties of vascular smooth muscle proteoglycans by oral anti-hyperglycemic agents. J Diabetes Complications. 2007;21(2):108–17.
83. Little PJ, et al. Genistein inhibits PDGF-stimulated proteoglycan synthesis in vascular smooth muscle without blocking PDGFbeta receptor phosphorylation. Arch Biochem Biophys. 2012;525(1):25–31.
84. Schaefer L, Schaefer RM. Proteoglycans: from structural compounds to signaling molecules. Cell Tissue Res. 2010;339(1):237–46.
85. Cardoso LE, et al. Platelet-derived growth factor differentially regulates the expression and post-translational modification of versican by arterial smooth muscle cells through distinct protein kinase C and extracellular signal-regulated kinase pathways. J Biol Chem. 2010;285(10):6987–95.
86. Merrilees MJ, et al. Retrovirally mediated overexpression of versican v3 by arterial smooth muscle cells induces tropoelastin synthesis and elastic fiber formation in vitro and in neointima after vascular injury. Circ Res. 2002;90(4):481–7.
87. Raines EW. The extracellular matrix can regulate vascular cell migration, proliferation, and survival: relationships to vascular disease. Int J Exp Pathol. 2000;81(3):173–82.

88. Tran-Lundmark K, et al. Heparan sulfate in perlecan promotes mouse atherosclerosis: roles in lipid permeability, lipid retention, and smooth muscle cell proliferation. Circ Res. 2008;103(1):43–52.
89. Papakonstantinou E, et al. The differential distribution of hyaluronic acid in the layers of human atheromatic aortas is associated with vascular smooth muscle cell proliferation and migration. Atherosclerosis. 1998;138(1):79–89.
90. Evanko SP, Angello JC, Wight TN. Formation of hyaluronan- and versican-rich pericellular matrix is required for proliferation and migration of vascular smooth muscle cells. Arterioscler Thromb Vasc Biol. 1999;19(4):1004–13.
91. Cuff CA, et al. The adhesion receptor CD44 promotes atherosclerosis by mediating inflammatory cell recruitment and vascular cell activation. J Clin Invest. 2001;108(7):1031–40.
92. Wight TN, Merrilees MJ. Proteoglycans in atherosclerosis and restenosis: key roles for versican. Circ Res. 2004;94(9):1158–67.
93. Lesley J, et al. TSG-6 modulates the interaction between hyaluronan and cell surface CD44. J Biol Chem. 2004;279(24):25745–54.
94. Bot PT, et al. Hyaluronic acid: targeting immune modulatory components of the extracellular matrix in atherosclerosis. Curr Med Chem. 2008;15(8): 786–91.
95. Chai S, et al. Overexpression of hyaluronan in the tunica media promotes the development of atherosclerosis. Circ Res. 2005;96(5):583–91.
96. Jiang D, Liang J, Noble PW. Hyaluronan as an immune regulator in human diseases. Physiol Rev. 2011;91(1):221–64.
97. McDonald TO, et al. Diabetes and arterial extracellular matrix changes in a porcine model of atherosclerosis. J Histochem Cytochem. 2007;55(11):1149–57.
98. Finn AV, et al. Concept of vulnerable/unstable plaque. Arterioscler Thromb Vasc Biol. 2010;30(7): 1282–92.
99. Libby P, Aikawa M. Mechanisms of plaque stabilization with statins. Am J Cardiol. 2003;91(4A): 4B–8.
100. Aikawa M, et al. Lipid lowering by diet reduces matrix metalloproteinase activity and increases collagen content of rabbit atheroma: a potential mechanism of lesion stabilization. Circulation. 1998; 97(24):2433–44.
101. Crisby M, et al. Pravastatin treatment increases collagen content and decreases lipid content, inflammation, metalloproteinases, and cell death in human carotid plaques: implications for plaque stabilization. Circulation. 2001;103(7):926–33.
102. Lim CS, et al. Matrix metalloproteinases in vascular disease—a potential therapeutic target? Curr Vasc Pharmacol. 2010;8(1):75–85.
103. Franco C, et al. Doxycycline alters vascular smooth muscle cell adhesion, migration, and reorganization of fibrillar collagen matrices. Am J Pathol. 2006; 168(5):1697–709.
104. Courtman DW, et al. Inward remodeling of the rabbit aorta is blocked by the matrix metalloproteinase inhibitor doxycycline. J Vasc Res. 2004;41(2): 157–65.
105. Forough R, et al. Metalloproteinase blockade by local overexpression of TIMP-1 increases elastin accumulation in rat carotid artery intima. Arterioscler Thromb Vasc Biol. 1998;18(5):803–7.
106. Baker AH, et al. Divergent effects of tissue inhibitor of metalloproteinase-1, -2, or -3 overexpression on rat vascular smooth muscle cell invasion, proliferation, and death in vitro. TIMP-3 promotes apoptosis. J Clin Invest. 1998;101(6):1478–87.
107. George SJ, et al. Adenovirus-mediated gene transfer of the human TIMP-1 gene inhibits smooth muscle cell migration and neointimal formation in human saphenous vein. Hum Gene Ther. 1998;9(6):867–77.
108. Johnson JL, et al. Suppression of atherosclerotic plaque progression and instability by tissue inhibitor of metalloproteinase-2: involvement of macrophage migration and apoptosis. Circulation. 2006;113(20): 2435–44.
109. Lemaitre V, Soloway PD, D'Armiento J. Increased medial degradation with pseudo-aneurysm formation in apolipoprotein E-knockout mice deficient in tissue inhibitor of metalloproteinases-1. Circulation. 2003;107(2):333–8.
110. Silence J, Collen D, Lijnen HR. Reduced atherosclerotic plaque but enhanced aneurysm formation in mice with inactivation of the tissue inhibitor of metalloproteinase-1 (TIMP-1) gene. Circ Res. 2002;90(8):897–903.
111. Guo H, et al. Rosuvastatin inhibits MMP-2 expression and limits the progression of atherosclerosis in LDLR-deficient mice. Arch Med Res. 2009; 40(5):345–51.
112. Little PJ, Ballinger ML, Osman N. Vascular wall proteoglycan synthesis and structure as a target for the prevention of atherosclerosis. Vasc Health Risk Manag. 2007;3:1–8.
113. Ivey ME, Little PJ. Thrombin regulates vascular smooth muscle cell proteoglycan synthesis via PAR-1 and multiple downstream signalling pathways. Thromb Res. 2008;123:288–97.
114. Ballinger ML, et al. Endothelin-1 activates ETA receptors on human vascular smooth muscle cells to yield proteoglycans with increased binding to LDL. Atherosclerosis. 2009;205(2):451–7.
115. Dadlani H, et al. Smad and p38 MAP kinase-mediated signaling of proteoglycan synthesis in vascular smooth muscle. J Biol Chem. 2008;283(12): 7844–52.
116. Burch ML, et al. TGF-beta stimulates biglycan synthesis via p38 and ERK phosphorylation of the linker region of Smad2. Cell Mol Life Sci. 2010; 67(12):2077–90.
117. Yang SN, et al. Growth factor-mediated hyper-elongation of glycosaminoglycan chains on biglycan requires transcription and translation. Arch Physiol Biochem. 2009;115(3):147–54.

118. Osman N, et al. TGF-beta stimulates biglycan core protein synthesis but not glycosaminoglycan chain elongation via Akt phosphorylation in vascular smooth muscle. Growth Factors. 2011;29(5):203–10.
119. Kretzschmar M, et al. A mechanism of repression of TGFbeta/Smad signaling by oncogenic Ras. Genes Dev. 1999;13(7):804–16.
120. Massague J. Integration of Smad and MAPK pathways: a link and a linker revisited. Genes Dev. 2003;17(24):2993–7.
121. Burch ML, Zheng W, Little PJ. Smad linker region phosphorylation in the regulation of extracellular matrix synthesis. Cell Mol Life Sci. 2011;68(1):97–107.
122. Matsuzaki K. Smad phosphoisoform signaling specificity: the right place at the right time. Carcinogenesis. 2011;32(11):1578–88.
123. Bartram CR, et al. Translocation of c-abl oncogene correlates with the presence of a Philadelphia chromosome in chronic myelocytic leukaemia. Nature. 1983;306(5940):277–80.
124. Buchdunger E, et al. Abl protein-tyrosine kinase inhibitor STI571 inhibits in vitro signal transduction mediated by c-kit and platelet-derived growth factor receptors. J Pharmacol Exp Ther. 2000;295(1):139–45.
125. Boren J, et al. Role of extracellular retention of low density lipoproteins in atherosclerosis. Curr Opin Lipidol. 2000;11(5):451–6.
126. Toole BP, Wight TN, Tammi MI. Hyaluronan-cell interactions in cancer and vascular disease. J Biol Chem. 2002;277(7):4593–6.
127. Saarni H, Tammi M, Doherty NS. Decreased hyaluronic acid synthesis, a sensitive indicator of cortisol action on fibroblast. J Pharm Pharmacol. 1978;30(3):200–1.
128. Sussmann M, et al. Induction of hyaluronic acid synthase 2 (HAS2) in human vascular smooth muscle cells by vasodilatory prostaglandins. Circ Res. 2004;94(5):592–600.
129. Goueffic Y et al. Sirolimus blocks the accumulation of hyaluronan (HA) by arterial smooth muscle cells and reduces monocyte adhesion to the ECM. Atherosclerosis. 2007;195:23–30.
130. Sakr SW, et al. Hyaluronan accumulation is elevated in cultures of low density lipoprotein receptor-deficient cells and is altered by manipulation of cell cholesterol content. J Biol Chem. 2008;283(52):36195–204.

# Tools for Assessing Lipoprotein Metabolism in Diabetes Mellitus

12

Richard L. Klein

## Introduction

Understanding the whole body (systemic) and cellular metabolism of lipoproteins, including that of the modified lipoproteins that occur in diabetes mellitus, has potential to improve the quantitative and qualitative changes in lipoproteins that contribute to the macrovascular and microvascular complications of type 1 and type 2 diabetes [1, 2] and facilitate development of therapeutics that can improve clinical outcomes. An excellent example of how understanding lipoprotein metabolism has improved clinical outcomes is that an understanding of the LDL receptor, intracellular cholesterol metabolism, and the central role of HMG-CoA reductase led to the development of HMG-CoA reductase inhibitors (statins), which substantially reduce cardiovascular events in both diabetic and nondiabetic people [3–5].

Cell culture, animal, and human kinetic lipoprotein studies can contribute knowledge as to lipoprotein metabolism and the effects of clinical factors such as diabetes, renal damage, and of genetic effects (such as via usage of gene knockout or transfection and silencing RNA), and of drugs. In this chapter we will describe the general principles of commonly used techniques for in vivo studies of lipoprotein kinetics which can be applied to human subjects and to animals and for the assessment of lipoprotein metabolism in cultured cells, using examples from our research.

R.L. Klein, Ph.D. (✉)
Division of Endocrinology, Diabetes, and Medical Genetics, Medical University of South Carolina, Clinical Science Building, 8th Floor, 96 Jonathan Lucas Street, Charleston, SC 29425, USA
e-mail: kleinrl@musc.edu

## Lipoprotein Kinetic Studies

In clinical practice and in many clinical research studies, lipid or apolipoprotein levels are commonly measured (as described in another chapter in this book) and reported, including often as the study endpoint. While these static measures are very useful and are valuable in clinical practice, studies of lipoprotein metabolism are important research tools, akin to looking at a movie (a lipoprotein kinetics study) rather than at a photo or an individual frame of the movie (a traditional lipid panel). Such kinetic studies are complex and require specific skill sets and instrumentation and, due to their high cost, are also usually conducted in small numbers of subjects.

Alterations in lipid levels may relate to differences in lipoprotein production or lipoprotein clearance, or both, and even in the absence of altered lipid levels, there may be changes in lipoprotein production and the rates and pathways of lipoprotein clearance.

While kinetic studies have been undertaken in animals, apart from nonhuman primates [6], the lipoprotein metabolic pathways of animals, particularly rodents, differ substantially from that of

A.J. Jenkins et al. (eds.), *Lipoproteins in Diabetes Mellitus*, Contemporary Diabetes,
DOI 10.1007/978-1-4614-7554-5_12, © Springer Science+Business Media New York 2014

humans. For example, in man most circulating cholesterol is present in Low-Density Lipoprotein (LDL), while in rodents most circulating cholesterol is carried in High-Density Lipoproteins (HDL) [7].

As LDL is the major circulating lipoprotein and as apoB100 is present in Very-Low-Density Lipoprotein (VLDL) and its metabolic products of Intermediate Density Lipoprotein (IDL) and LDL, most kinetic studies relate to apoB-containing lipoproteins.

## Apolipoprotein B Turnover Studies

Two general approaches to apoB kinetic studies are taken. The first and earlier technique utilizes radiation and the more modern technique uses stable isotopes.

### Radiation-Based Studies

The study of apoB metabolism has been approached in a number of ways in both normal as well as hyperlipidemic states in human subjects. The most widely used technique to measure clearance of apoB employs radioiodination of purified VLDL or LDL, usually obtained by ultracentrifugation, which is then reinjected into the study subjects. The decrease in lipoprotein radioactivity is monitored in sequential blood samples collected from each subject.

Another approach has utilized intravenous administration of a radioactively labeled amino acid precursor, such as $^{75}$Se-labeled methionine, or [$^{3}$H]leucine, with subsequent determination of its appearance in, and disappearance from, the lipoprotein fraction(s) of interest. Both of these approaches use radioactive isotopes and require extensive computerized mathematical modeling to properly estimate lipoprotein residence time in plasma using stochastic or multicompartmental analysis of plasma radioactivity decay curves.

Radioiodination of LDL has been used successfully to monitor LDL turnover because it has been extensively documented that apolipoprotein B (apoB) is unique among the apoproteins in that it is not exchangeable between lipoprotein classes [8] while it is also the major protein component of LDL. In contrast, apoB in VLDL represents only approximately 40 % of the total protein mass, and radioiodination of VLDL results in labeling of other apoprotein components. In addition, a larger proportion of the radiolabel may be found in the lipid moiety of the particle than with LDL and may result in less than 50 % of total radioactivity being localized in apoB [9]. Therefore, studies of apoB metabolism after injection of radiolabeled VLDL require the isolation of apoB from the other labeled components to permit accurate specific activity measurements. This led to the development of methods to rapidly and quantitatively isolate apoB from other radiolabeled apolipoproteins and lipids, and which permit multiple apoB specific activity determinations on lipoproteins isolated from limited volume plasma samples. One frequently utilized method uses 1,1′,3,3′-tetramethylurea (TMU) to solubilize VLDL apoproteins and leave behind precipitated apoB [10], while another uses butanol-isopropyl ether [11].

To circumvent lipid contamination, other investigators have endogenously labeled VLDL with $^{75}$Se-labeled methionine or $^{3}$H-labeled lysine. However, interpretation of data from this type of experiments conducted in humans is difficult to analyze mathematically because of the inherent complexity of endogenous labeling. These experiments also do not allow complete analysis of the source of apoB input into the higher density lipoprotein classes; thus, precursor-product relationships between VLDL apoB and apoB in the other lipoprotein density classes cannot be easily studied [12–14]. A general organization and method of conduct of these types of investigations are shown in the schematic presented in Fig. 12.1.

The methods described above rely on radioactively labeled lipoproteins or infusions of radioactivity. This approach, however, is considered by some to be non-ideal for several reasons:

(a) Lipoproteins and apolipoproteins potentially can be modified, such as by oxidation or aggregation, during isolation and radioiodination which may influence their metabolic behavior in vivo.
(b) A steady-state condition where production and clearance rates are taken to be constant is difficult or impossible to document and, therefore, must be assumed, an assumption that may not always be physiologically accurate.

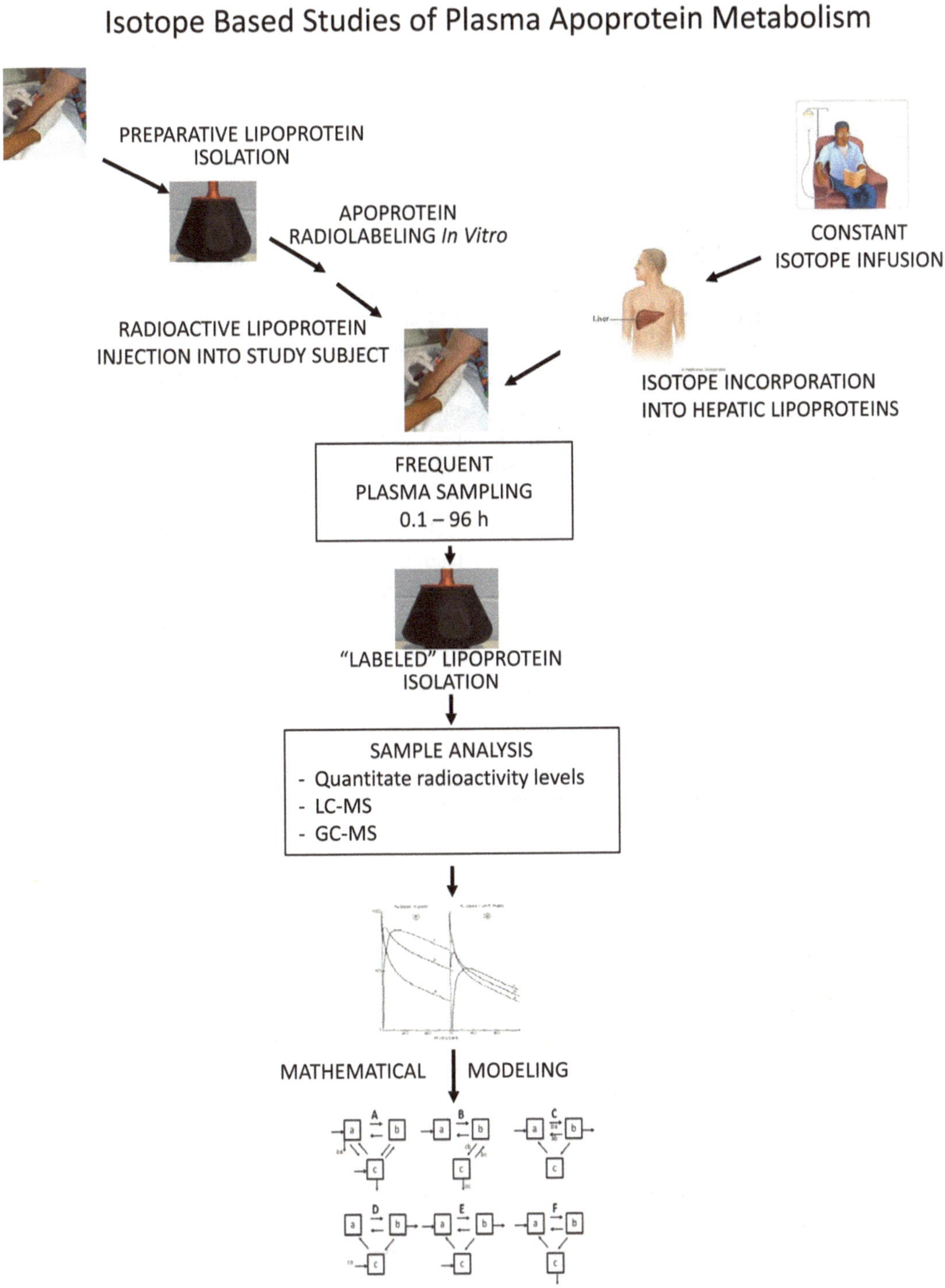


**Fig. 12.1** The design and general method of conduct of investigations of lipoprotein and apoprotein metabolism which employ isotopes. Studies investigating lipoprotein metabolism in plasma frequently employ isotopic labeling of the apoprotein moiety of the particles. Both radioisotopes and nonradioactive, stable nuclides (e.g., $^{2}H$, $^{15}N$) are frequently used to label lipoprotein protein. Studies of lipoprotein metabolism fall into one of two general classes: studies in which lipoproteins are initially isolated and the apoprotein radiolabeled before the lipoprotein is injected back into the study subject and studies in which isotopes are infused at a constant rate until they are absorbed into the liver and subsequently incorporated into lipoprotein proteins. In the latter type of study, the lipoprotein particles which are secreted de novo by the liver contain the stable nuclides which permit these lipoproteins to be distinguished from those already present in the circulation. Both approaches require frequent sampling of plasma from the study subject. Lipoprotein metabolism may be studied using whole plasma but more often individual

(c) Studies cannot be undertaken in young children or in pregnant women, nor can multiple studies be undertaken in the same volunteer due to exposure to potentially hazardous levels of radioactivity.

## Stable Isotope-Based Studies

A new experimental approach to investigations of apoB metabolism has been developed which relies on modern instrumentation and which eliminates complications associated with the administration of radioactivity to humans. This method uses intravenous infusion of stable isotope-labeled amino acids after a priming dose that achieves and maintains an isotopic steady state [15, 16] that is necessary for the successful conduct of this type of study. The intricacies and advantages or disadvantages associated with each of these three types of lipoprotein, or lipoprotein precursor, tracer infusion studies have been discussed at length in other excellent articles [17].

## Dual Radiolabel Studies

As discussed in the chapter on lipoprotein glycation, the incubation of human LDL with glucose results in a nonenzymatic formation of a Schiff base between the monosaccharide and lysyl residues in apoB. As a greater percentage of the lysyl residues of apoB in LDL become modified by glycation, the fractional catabolic rate of the glycated LDL decreases in in vivo studies [18]. The rates of catabolism of glycated LDL by cultured human skin fibroblasts are also decreased suggesting that glycated LDL is catabolized primarily via a receptor-independent process. Thus, radiolabeled LDL which has been extensively glycated is frequently injected concomitantly with native LDL radiolabeled using another isotope, and the rates of LDL metabolism via receptor-independent and receptor-dependent pathways, respectively, estimated from the ratio of the fractional catabolic rates determined using each uniquely radiolabeled lipoprotein preparation [18].

## HDL-Related Turnover Studies

Studies investigating the synthesis and catabolism of HDL apolipoproteins, primarily apoA-I and apoA-II, are conducted in a manner similar to those described above for apoB. Lipoproteins containing radiolabeled apolipoproteins(s) are injected into each study subject, and the lipoprotein fraction of interest is isolated from serially collected blood samples to monitor radioactivity decay patterns. Investigating the metabolism of HDL apolipoproteins using this type of study technique is inherently more difficult because it has been documented that protein in HDL is freely exchangeable between HDL particles and lipoproteins in other density classes [19, 20].

It is these types of kinetic studies that have led to the knowledge regarding changes in VLDL, LDL, and HDL production and clearance in people with vs. without diabetes as is described in the chapter on lipoprotein metabolism in diabetes.

## Lipoprotein Metabolism in Cultured Cells

Investigations of lipoprotein metabolism in cultured cells generally focus on three distinct stages of cell-lipoprotein interaction:

(a) Lipoprotein binding to cell surface lipoprotein receptors
(b) Internalization of the lipoprotein from the cell surface in preparation for subsequent metabolism by the cell (if binding of the lipoprotein to the receptor results in receptor internalization)
(c) Degradation of the internalized lipoprotein in the cell lysosomal compartment

**Fig. 12.1** (continued) lipoprotein classes are separated and purified using ultracentrifugation or other methodology. Lipoprotein metabolism or "turnover" is quantitated as the appearance/disappearance of radioactivity in plasma and isolated lipoprotein fractions when radioactive tracers have been employed. When stable nuclides are infused, plasma and lipoprotein samples must be extensively processed to enable detection and quantitation of the stable isotopes using gas chromatography (GC) or liquid chromatography (LC) in combination with mass spectroscopy (MS). Both approaches ultimately require sophisticated, computer-aided, mathematical modeling to convert the patterns of isotope appearance/disappearance in plasma/lipoproteins into intuitive metabolic pathways

## Lipoprotein Binding to Cells

The Nobel Prize in Physiology or Medicine in 1985 was awarded to Joseph L. Goldstein and Michael S. Brown. Their Nobel prize-winning research not only elucidated the molecular mechanism whereby exogenous cholesterol in VLDL and LDL downregulates cellular 3-hydroxy-3-methylglutaryl coenzyme A reductase enzymatic activity (HMG-CoA reductase), the rate-limiting step of cellular endogenous cholesterol biosynthesis, but it also developed many of the techniques necessary for the study of lipoprotein metabolism in cultured cells. Many of these research techniques remain in use today. Their earliest studies demonstrated that LDL radiolabeled with tracer $^{125}$I-iodine can be taken up by cultured fibroblasts from normal subjects in a temperature dependent process that is highly specific, reaches equilibrium with time, and is saturable at low levels of LDL [21].

These studies clearly demonstrated for the first time that the amount of $^{125}$I-LDL bound to the cells was reduced by the addition of a 50-fold excess of non-radiolabeled, native LDL, which suggested that the radiolabeled LDL and native LDL were competing for a limited number of specific binding sites. Furthermore, these studies introduced the concept of "specific" lipoprotein binding to cells, which would be reported from this juncture as the difference between the lipoprotein radioactivity bound to cells in the absence and presence of excess native LDL. The development of techniques to measure both "specific" lipoprotein binding as well as "nonspecific" binding (defined as the level of $^{125}$I-LDL radioactivity bound in the presence of a 50-fold excess of native LDL) enabled these investigators to conduct Scatchard analyses of the LDL binding to fibroblast receptors. These study results suggested the presence of a specific LDL binding site of high affinity which could be saturated at relatively low LDL concentrations (20 μg/ml). Most importantly, these studies demonstrated that specific LDL binding appeared to be required in the process by which LDL normally suppressed HMG-CoA reductase activity and further, the binding of LDL to fibroblasts from patients homozygous for familial hypercholesterolemia was defective and appeared to explain the previously reported failure of LDL to suppress the synthesis of this enzyme in fibroblasts isolated from these patients [21].

## Lipoprotein Degradation by Cells

While studying the binding of $^{125}$I-LDL to normal fibroblasts, Brown and Goldstein noted that the $^{125}$I-LDL bound to cells was ultimately degraded to form a product that was dialyzable and which could no longer be precipitated with trichloracetic acid (TCA) [22]. In subsequent studies [23] they refined this technique to include an additional step in which the acid-soluble material appearing in the culture media harvested after cells were incubated with $^{125}$I-LDL at 37 °C for several hours was oxidized with hydrogen peroxide and then extracted with chloroform. This step eliminated the artifactual contamination of the small amount of radioactive free iodide that persisted in the $^{125}$I-LDL preparation despite extensive dialysis. Control studies conducted by incubating the $^{125}$I-LDL preparation at 37 °C in culture media without cells revealed that the formation of this iodide-free, acid-soluble degradative product of LDL was absolutely dependent on the presence of cells and, furthermore, was linear with time up to at least 30 h. The use of this cell-free, spontaneous degradation control became routine for all subsequent studies of lipoprotein metabolism by cells. Most of the TCA-soluble material secreted into the culture medium was identified to be $^{125}$I-tyrosine. Uptake of LDL by both the specific, high-affinity process and also the nonspecific, lower-affinity process results in degradation of the lipoprotein, and the degradation processes appear to be similar [22].

## Lipoprotein Accumulation by Cells

To demonstrate the conversion of bound $^{125}$I-LDL to acid-soluble material, cultured human fibroblast cells were first preincubated at 4 °C with $^{125}$I-LDL. These conditions permit the LDL to bind to cell surface receptors as demonstrated by continued LDL susceptibility to protease degradation [21, 22] even after 4 h incubation, but without appearance of $^{125}$I-acid-soluble material in the media. Cells which had been preincubated at 4 °C with $^{125}$I-LDL were then transferred to medium without $^{125}$I-LDL and were additionally incubated at either 4° or 37 °C. At the beginning of this second incubation, all radioactivity bound to the cells was precipitable with TCA. When the cells were incubated at 37 °C, nearly all this bound radioactivity was released into the cell culture medium within 3 h, and approximately two thirds had been converted to acid-soluble material. In contrast, when the cells were incubated at 4 °C, only about one third of the $^{125}$I bound to the cells was released, and all the radioactivity was precipitable by TCA. The difference in the amounts of radioactivity localized to cells incubated at 37 °C (bound and internalized, but not degraded LDL) compared to that found in cells incubated at 4° (bound LDL only) is considered to be accumulated LDL. These types of studies are not conducted as often as those measuring lipoprotein binding or degradation.

## Studies of Glycated LDL Metabolism by Human Macrophages

We have used the techniques described above to investigate the metabolism of in vivo glycated LDL by cultured human macrophages. Using sequential ultracentrifugation we isolated LDL ($1.019 < d < 1.063$ g/ml) from 10 adult patients with type 1 diabetes and from 10 age-, sex-, and race-matched non-diabetic subjects to serve as controls [24]. The HbA1c level in the diabetic patients and in the nondiabetic, control subjects averaged 8.2±0.6 and 5.6±0.1 %, respectively. We incubated human monocyte-derived macrophages with increasing concentrations of $^{125}$I-LDL from each diabetic patient and matched control subject for 20 h at 37 °C and then determined the amount of $^{125}$I-TCA-soluble (non-iodide) material formed by the cells and secreted into the culture medium. We calculated the rates of high-affinity, receptor-mediated degradation of the LDL as the difference between LDL degradation levels in cells incubated with only $^{125}$I-LDL and parallel incubations containing $^{125}$I-LDL plus a 25-fold excess of non-radiolabeled LDL. Corrections were made for the small amounts of $^{125}$I-acid-soluble material that was found in parallel incubations without cells. We determined there was no significant difference between the receptor-mediated degradation of LDL isolated from control subjects and diabetic patients. Unexpectedly, we observed a significant increase ($p < 0.05$) in the rates of total and non-high-affinity receptor-mediated degradation of LDL from diabetic patients compared to that isolated from control subjects. We determined that there were no statistically significant differences in the lipid composition of LDL isolated from the two groups, and therefore, we investigated whether abnormalities in apoB could be responsible for the altered pattern of degradation.

ApoB can also be covalently modified by incubation with glucose in vitro and is similar to the LDL from diabetic patients (modified in vivo). We determined that the level of glycation in LDL from the diabetic patients was increased four-fold over that determined in LDL from the control subjects. This was a critical observation because these results suggested the presence of an abnormality in LDL apoproteins that could alter LDL metabolism by macrophages even in patients who were in relatively good glycemic control (HbA1c 8.2±0.6 %) and whose LDL lipid composition was normal. We pursued additional studies to determine the mechanism responsible for the enhanced degradation of LDL from diabetic patients by human macrophages.

To further investigate the interaction of glycated LDL with human macrophages, we modified LDL in vitro by incubating LDL isolated from plasma pooled from young, healthy, euglycemic donors with glucose for seven days at 37 °C, which we have shown will increase the fructoselysine content of the LDL to levels observed in LDL isolated from diabetic patients [25]. As reviewed in the chapter on lipoprotein glycation, fructoselysine is an early glycation product. We incubated $^{125}$I-labeled native and in vitro glycated LDL (glc-LDL) with human macrophages and determined the rates of LDL degradation [26]. We determined that the rates of total degradation of glc-LDL were greater than those of control LDL, particularly at high LDL concentrations. More significantly, the degradation of glc-LDL by the classic LDL receptor pathway was slightly less than that of control LDL. This suggested that the increase in degradation of glc-LDL was mediated by a pathway independent of the classic LDL receptor [26]. Additional studies in our laboratory demonstrated that the increased degradation of glc-LDL by human macrophages was not mediated by the scavenger receptor or by carbohydrate receptors known to be expressed on human macrophages. This series of studies suggested that in human macrophages, there exists a low-affinity, high-capacity pathway that enhances the uptake and degradation of glc-LDL.

### Cellular Metabolism of Lipoprotein Cholesterol

The early seminal studies conducted by Brown and Goldstein [27] clearly demonstrated that LDL, but not VLDL or HDL, could significantly reduce the activity of HMG-CoA reductase in fibroblasts. Subsequent studies further revealed that when LDL was incubated with cultured fibroblasts, there was a 30- to 40-fold increase in the rate of incorporation of $^{14}$C-oleate into the fatty acid fraction of cellular cholesteryl esters [28]. Most importantly, the stimulation of cholesteryl ester formation by LDL occurred despite the fact that endogenous synthesis of unesterified cholesterol was completely suppressed by the lipoprotein. That is, exogenous cholesterol in the LDL rather than endogenous cholesterol synthesized by the cell appeared to provide the cholesterol substrate for cellular cholesterol esterification.

Using this same approach, we determined that LDL isolated from hyperglycemic, normolipidemic diabetic patients stimulated cholesteryl ester synthesis rates in human macrophages significantly more than LDL isolated from nondiabetic, control subjects [24]. We further determined that the increase in cellular cholesteryl ester synthesis in cells incubated with LDL from diabetic patients did not result from increases in cholesterol content in the LDL compared to LDL from the control subjects but rather resulted from enhanced catabolism of the LDL particles by the glycated LDL receptor present on human macrophages as detailed above. We further demonstrated that the enhancement in cholesteryl ester synthesis by macrophages exposed to glc-LDL was paralleled by intracellular accumulation of cholesteryl ester [26].

Lastly, these findings clearly demonstrate the importance of glycation of apoprotein B in LDL on inducing abnormal LDL-macrophage interaction. They are also of interest because they suggest the presence of abnormal lipoprotein metabolism in diabetes even in patients who are in relatively good glycemic control and whose plasma lipid and lipoprotein levels are normal.

## Future Directions

It is expected that these or related tools to study lipoprotein metabolism will continue to be of use in the assessment of systemic and cellular lipoprotein metabolism. They have contributed to our understanding of lipoprotein metabolism in diabetes (and in health and other disease states) and of the effects of lipoprotein modifications, such as by glycation. Other clinical, animal, and cell culture research has demonstrated that changes in lipoproteins levels and composition can promote atherosclerosis and the retinal and renal complications of diabetes. Moderately effective treatments have been developed to reduce the lipid-related vascular damage, but unfortunately such complications still occur. Residual risk may reside within alterations in lipoprotein metabolism, including the cellular handling (and responses to) lipoproteins. The tools described herein, most likely used with other cell biology, molecular techniques, and drug development tools, may facilitate the development of treatments to tightly control dyslipoproteinemia and reduce the vascular complications of diabetes.

**Acknowledgements** This work was supported in part by the Biomedical Laboratory Research and Development Program of the Department of Veterans Affairs. The contents of this document do not represent the views of the Department of Veterans Affairs or the United States Government. The author also acknowledges the contributions of his collaborators Professors John Baynes and Susan Thorpe, Timothy Lyons, Maria Lopes-Virella, Ms. Andrea Semler, and the DCCT/EDIC Research Group.

## References

1. Jenkins AJ, Rowley KG, Lyons TJ, Best JD, Hill MA, Klein RL. Lipoproteins and diabetic microvascular complications. Curr Pharm Des. 2004;10(27):3395–418.
2. Jenkins AJ, Best JD, Klein RL, Lyons TJ. Lipoproteins, glycoxidation and diabetic angiopathy. Diabetes Metab Res Rev. 2004;20(5):349–68.

3. Baigent C, Blackwell L, Emberson J, Holland LE, Reith C, Bhala N, Peto R, Barnes EH, Keech A, Simes J, Collins R, Cholesterol Treatment Trialists' (CTT) Collaboration. Efficacy and safety of more intensive lowering of LDL cholesterol: a meta-analysis of data from 170,000 participants in 26 randomised trials. Lancet. 2010;376(9753):1670–81.
4. Mihaylova B, Emberson J, Blackwell L, Keech A, Simes J, Barnes EH, Voysey M, Gray A, Collins R, Baigent C, Cholesterol Treatment Trialists' (CTT) Collaborators. The effects of lowering LDL cholesterol with statin therapy in people at low risk of vascular disease: meta-analysis of individual data from 27 randomised trials. Lancet. 2012;380(9841):581–90.
5. Kearney PM, Blackwell L, Collins R, Keech A, Simes J, Peto R, Armitage J, Baigent C, Cholesterol Treatment Trialists' (CTT) Collaborators. Efficacy of cholesterol-lowering therapy in 18,686 people with diabetes in 14 randomised trials of statins: a meta-analysis. Lancet. 2008;371(9607):117–25.
6. Marzetta CA, Johnson FL, Zech LA, Foster DM, Rudel LL. Metabolic behavior of hepatic VLDL and plasma LDL apoB-100 in African green monkeys. J Lipid Res. 1989;30(3):357–70.
7. Chapman JM. Comparative analysis of mammalian lipoproteins. In: Segrest JP, Albers JJ, editors. Methods in Enzymology. Plasma lipoproteins Part A: Preparation, Structure and Molecular Biology. 1986;Vol 128:70–143.
8. Sigurdsson G, Nicoll A, Lewis B. Conversion of very low density lipoprotein to low density lipoprotein. J Clin Invest. 1971;56:1481–90.
9. Bilheimer DW, Eisenberg S, Levy RI. The metabolism of very low density lipoprotein proteins. 1. Preliminary in vitro and in vivo observations. Biochim Biophys Acta. 1972;260:212–21.
10. Kane JP. A rapid electrophoretic technique for identification of subunit species of apoproteins in serum lipoproteins. Anal Biochem. 1973;53:350–64.
11. Klein RL, Zilversmit BD. Direct determination of human and rabbit apolipoprotein B selectively precipitated with butanol-isopropyl ether. J Lipid Res. 1984;25:1380–6.
12. Eaton RP. Incorporation of $^{75}$Se-selenomethionine into human apoproteins. I. Characterization of specificity in very low density and low density lipoproteins. Diabetes. 1975;25:32–43.
13. Eaton RP, Crespin S, Kipnis DM. Incorporation of $^{75}$Se-selenomethionine into human apoproteins. II. Characterization of metabolism of very low density and low density lipoproteins in vivo and in vitro. Diabetes. 1975;25:44–50.
14. Eaton RP. Incorporation of $^{75}$Se-selenomethionine into human apoproteins. III. Kinetic behavior of isotopically labeled plasma apoprotein in man. Diabetes. 1976;25:679–90.
15. Cryer DR, Matsushima T, Marsh JB, Yudkoff M, Coates PM, Cortner JA. Direct measurement of apolipoprotein B synthesis in human low density lipoprotein using stable isotopes and mass spectrometry. J Lipid Res. 1986;27:508–16.
16. Cohn JS, Wagner DA, Cohn SD, Millar JS, Schaefer EJ. Measurement of very low density and low density lipoprotein apolipoprotein (apo) B-100 and high density lipoprotein apo A-I production in human subjects using deuterated leucine. Effect of fasting and feeding. J Clin Invest. 1990;85:804–11.
17. Shipley RA, Clark RE. Tracer methods for in vivo kinetics. Theory and applications. New York, NY: Academic Press; 1972. p. 239.
18. Sasaki J, Okamura T, Cottam GL. Measurement of receptor-independent metabolism of low-density lipoprotein. An application of glycosylated low-density lipoprotein. Eur J Biochem. 1983;131:535–8.
19. Sodhi HS, Gould RG. Interaction of apoHDL with HDL and other lipoproteins. Atherosclerosis. 1970; 12:439–50.
20. Shepherd J, Patsch JR, Packard CJ, Gotto Jr AM, Taunton OD. Dynamic properties of human high density lipoprotein apoproteins. J Lipid Res. 1978;19: 383–9.
21. Brown MS, Goldstein JL. Familial hypercholesterolemia: defective binding of lipoproteins to cultured fibroblasts associated with impaired regulation of 3-hydroxy-3-methylglutaryl coenzyme A reductase activity. Proc Nat Acad Sci. 1974;71(3):788–92.
22. Goldstein JL, Brown MS. Familial hypercholesterolemia: identification of a defect in the regulation of 3-hydroxy-3-methylglutaryl coenzyme A reductase activity associated with overproduction of cholesterol. Proc Natl Acad Sci. 1973;70(10):2804–8.
23. Goldstein JL, Brown MS. Binding and degradation of low density lipoproteins by cultured human fibroblasts. Comparison of cells from a normal subject and from a patient with homozygous familial hypercholesterolemia. J Biol Chem. 1974;249(16): 5153–62.
24. Lyons TJ, Klein RL, Baynes JW, Stevenson HC, Lopes-Virella MF. Stimulation of cholesteryl ester synthesis in human monocytes-derived macrophages by low density lipoproteins from Type 1 (insulin-dependent) diabetic patients: the influence of non-enzymatic glycosylation of low-density lipoproteins. Diabetologia. 1987;30:916–23.
25. Lyons TJ, Baynes JW, Patrick JS, Colwell JA, Lopes-Virella MF. Glycosylation of LDL in patients with Type 1 (insulin dependent) diabetes: correlations with other parameters of glycaemic control. Diabetologia. 1986;29:685–9.
26. Lopes-Virella MF, Klein RL, Lyons TJ, Stevenson HC, Witztum JL. Glycosylation of low-density lipoprotein enhances cholesteryl ester synthesis in human monocyte-derived macrophages. Diabetes. 1988;37:550–7.
27. Brown MS, Goldstein JL. Regulation of 3-hydroxy-3-methylglutaryl coenzyme A reductase activity in human fibroblasts by lipoproteins. Proc Natl Acad Sci USA. 1973;70(7):2162–6.
28. Goldstein JL, Dana SE, Brown MS. Esterification of low density lipoprotein cholesterol in human fibroblasts and its absence in homozygous familial hypercholesterolemia. Proc Natl Acad Sci USA. 1974; 70(11):4288–92.

# Endothelial Dysfunction and Dyslipidemia in Type 2 Diabetes: Pathogenesis, Significance and Therapy

13

Sandra J. Hamilton and Gerald F. Watts

## Introduction

Type 2 diabetes mellitus (T2DM) markedly increases the risk of all forms of cardiovascular disease [1, 2]. Endothelial dysfunction (ED), or endotheliopathy, is an early indicator of diabetic vascular disease and independently predicts cardiovascular risk [3]. Major factors that contribute to ED include dyslipoproteinemia [4], oxidative stress and inflammation [5–7]. Dysglycemia, hypertension and insulin resistance are clearly important, but probably chiefly operate through oxidative stress and pro-inflammatory pathways [5, 8, 9]. Both invasive and non-invasive methods for assessing endothelial function have generated a wealth of knowledge concerning the pathogenesis and therapeutic regulation of endotheliopathy in T2DM [3, 10]. We review this area with a focus on dyslipoproteinemia.

S.J. Hamilton, R.N., Ph.D.
Combined Universities Centre for Rural Health, University of Western Australia, Geraldton, Australia

G.F. Watts, D.Sc., Ph.D., M.D., F.R.A.C.P., F.R.C.P (✉)
Cardiometabolic Research Centre, School of Medicine and Pharmacology, Royal Perth Hospital Unit, University of Western Australia, MRF Building, G Block, Wellington Street, Perth, WA 6000, Australia
e-mail: gerald.watts@uwa.edu.au

## Endothelial Function

### Normal Endothelial Function and Nitric Oxide

The endothelium maintains vascular homeostasis through multiple regulatory functions, including the release of several vasoactive factors that maintain vessel wall tone and blood fluidity, while limiting smooth muscle cell proliferation and inflammation [10–12]. Arguably, the most important of the endothelium derived molecules is nitric oxide (NO), although maintenance of endothelial function also involves endothelin-1 (ET-1), angiotensin II, prostacyclin and endothelial-derived hyperpolarizing factor (EDHF) [3].

In response to shear stress or activation of muscarinic receptors by the G-protein signalling pathway, endothelial NO synthase (eNOS) is activated. This generates, in a tightly coupled process, NO and citrulline from L-arginine, molecular oxygen and reduced nicotinamide adenine dinucleotide phosphate (NADPH) [3, 11]. NO released by this process stimulates soluble guanylate cyclise (Fig. 13.1a). The production of cyclic guanosine 3′,5′-monophosphate (cGMP) results in vasodilation and inhibits chemotaxis and platelet aggregation [13].

A.J. Jenkins et al. (eds.), *Lipoproteins in Diabetes Mellitus*, Contemporary Diabetes,
DOI 10.1007/978-1-4614-7554-5_13, © Springer Science+Business Media New York 2014

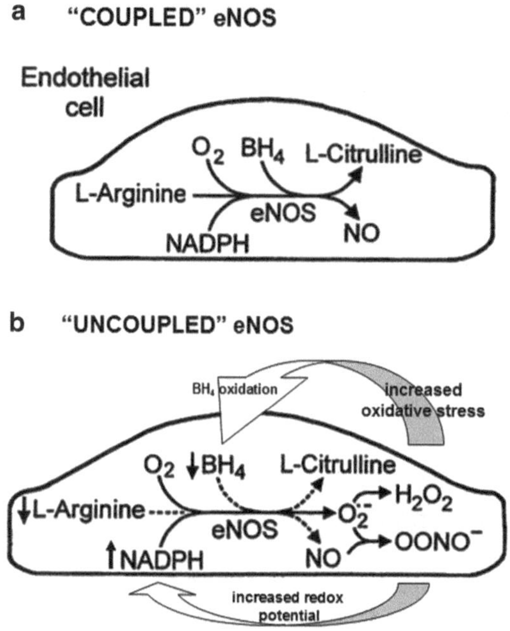


**Fig. 13.1** (**a**) Nitric oxide (NO) is produced from L-arginine and molecular oxygen ($O_2$) by endothelial nitric oxide synthase (eNOS) in a tightly "coupled" process involving tetrahydrobiopterin ($BH_4$) and NADPH. (**b**) In diabetes, increased redox imbalance (due to increased NADH/NADPH) and decreased availability of $BH_4$ (due to oxidation) leads to "uncoupling" of NO production. This results in transfer of electrons to $O_2$ to form superoxide ($O_2^{\cdot-}$). Superoxide in turn reacts with and consumes NO, forming the oxidant species peroxynitrite ($OONO^-$). Hence, oxidative stress and endothelial dysfunction are further increased [14]. Adapted from Katusic ZS [15]

## In Vivo Measurement of Endothelial Function

Endothelial function may be measured indirectly in the peripheral circulation by assessing the vasodilatory responses of conduit and resistance arteries to stimuli that increase NO release (Table 13.1) [3, 13, 16]. In the brachial artery, shear stress is generated by hyperemia following an induced period of local ischemia, and flow-mediated dilatation (FMD) is measured using high-resolution ultrasonography or even magnetic resonance imaging [17, 18]. Blood flow changes in the forearm microcirculation following hyperemia, or intra-arterial infusion of muscarinic receptor agonists such as acetylcholine, can be measured using venous occlusion strain-gauge plethysmography [19, 20]. An emerging non-invasive clinical tool to assess ED is digital peripheral arterial tonometry (PAT) (Endo-PAT, Itamar Medical) [21, 22].

Endothelial function in coronary arteries may also be assessed, in response to pharmacological agonist or shear stress stimuli, using quantitative angiography to measure vessel diameter changes [23]. Non-invasive methods, such as positron emission tomography, may also be undertaken, but are costly [13].

Circulating biomarkers may be measured as indirect indices of endothelial cell damage, activation and inflammation (Table 13.1) [24–30]. Impaired mobilization or depletion of endothelial progenitor cells derived from bone marrow are involved in the pathogenesis of ED, and their circulating levels can also be used as a marker of ED [31–34]. Recently, a relationship between progenitor cells and cell-derived microparticles has been demonstrated [33]. Microparticles (MP) are small membrane-shed vesicles derived from cell surfaces under conditions of cellular activation or injury/apoptosis [33, 35]. Thus, endothelial-derived microparticles (EMP) may be potential markers of ED [33, 35]. Vascular extracellular superoxide dismutase (ecSOD) activity, the major antioxidant enzyme system of the vessel wall, was substantially reduced in patients with CAD and closely associated with NO-mediated vasodilation, suggesting that reduced ecSOD activity contributes to the reduced bioavailability of NO [36]. However, measurement of ecSOD requires the intravenous injection of heparin; therefore, its utility as a surrogate marker of ED in the clinical setting is less practicable.

## Endothelial Dysfunction

### Endothelial Dysfunction: Uncoupling of eNOS

Endothelial dysfunction reflects an imbalance between release of vasodilator and vasoconstrictor endothelial-derived factors. A decrease in the bioavailability of NO, involves either a decrease in NO synthesis or inactivation of NO due to increased endothelial production of reactive oxygen species (ROS) [37]. With increased oxi-

**Table 13.1** Techniques and methods for assessing endothelial function in humans

| Coronary circulation | Peripheral circulation | Circulating biomarkers |
|---|---|---|
| QC Angiography | Ultrasonography: FMD | ADMA, NO |
| PE Tomography | Plethysmography: FABF | ET-1 |
| | Endo-PAT | hs-CRP |
| | | vWF |
| *Vasodilatory Stimuli* | | PAI-1 |
| Acetylcholine | | ICAM, VCAM |
| Shear Stress | | Selectins |
| Nitrates | | EP Cells |
| NOS inhibitors | | EMP |

Key: *QC Angiography* quantitative coronary angiography, *PE Tomography* positron emission tomography, *FMD* flow-mediated dilation, *FABF* forearm blood flow, *Endo-PAT* non-invasive peripheral artery tonometry, *NOS* nitric oxide synthase, *ADMA* asymmetric dimethylarginine, *NO* nitric oxide, *ET-1* endothelin-1, *hs-CRP* high sensitivity C-reactive protein, *vWF* von Willebrand factor, *PAI-1* plasminogen activator inhibitor-1, *ICAM* intercellular adhesion molecule, *VCAM* vascular cell adhesion molecule, *EP Cells* endothelial progenitor cells, *EMP* endothelial-derived microparticles

dative stress, tetrahydrobiopterin ($BH_4$), a cofactor that tightly regulates NO production, is oxidized resulting in the uncoupling of eNOS and reduced NO production [14]. Elevated levels of asymmetric dimethylarginine (ADMA), an endogenous inhibitor of eNOS through competition with L-arginine, may further reduce NO production [13]. This perpetuates a cycle of vascular oxidative stress through the transfer of electrons to molecular oxygen, forming oxidant species such as superoxide and peroxynitrite, which further consumes NO and increases oxidative stress (Fig. 13.1b) [14, 38].

Endothelial dysfunction may also involve altered levels of vasoconstrictors, such as endothelin-1 and angiotensin II, and other vasodilators such as endothelial-derived hyperpolarizing factor (EDHF) and prostacyclin [3, 37].

## Predictive Value of Endothelial Dysfunction

Several studies in diverse groups of subjects have shown that ED measured by the aforementioned techniques in different vascular beds is predictive of clinical events [39–54]. The principal studies are shown in Table 13.2. Some of these studies included type 2 diabetic patients. In type 2 diabetic patients with normal coronary arteries, coronary artery dysfunction, as assessed by cold-pressor test, was found to predict long-term cardiovascular outcomes, with a relative risk of 4.9 [49]. In a study of asymptomatic type 2 diabetic patients who underwent myocardial perfusion imaging, normal endothelial function had a 93 % negative predictive value in excluding CAD [50]. In patients with newly diagnosed CAD and impaired brachial artery FMD (40 % with diabetes), a persistently impaired FMD was an independent predictor of future cardiovascular events after six months of optimized lifestyle changes and pharmacotherapy [52]. A community based study in 1,016 older adults (72 % with diabetes) demonstrated that impaired forearm endothelial-dependent vasodilation was associated with a five year risk of major adverse cardiovascular events [54]. A recent meta-analysis of 14 observational studies and a recent review, both concluded that FMD is predictive of cardiovascular events and provides prognostic information that is at least equal to the information gained from conventional cardiovascular risk factors; however, future research is required to confirm FMD's efficacy in the assessment of CVD risk [55, 56].

## Pathogenesis of Endothelial Dysfunction in Type 2 Diabetes Mellitus

Endothelial dysfunction has been demonstrated in T2DM in both the resistance and conduit vessels of the peripheral circulation [57–61], as well as in the coronary circulation [62, 63]. Plasma levels of the soluble adhesion molecules

**Table 13.2** Selected studies evaluating endothelial dysfunction as a predictor of cardiovascular events

| Study (year) | *n* | Patient population | Arterial bed | Technique(s) | Endpoints | Mean follow-up (months) | Endothelial dysfunction as an independent predictor | Estimated RR of CV events |
|---|---|---|---|---|---|---|---|---|
| Papaioannou et al. [50] | 75 | T2DM patients without CAD | Brachial | FMD, NMD, MPI | CAD | 60 | No association | na |
| Nitenberg et al. [49] | 124 | Patients with HT or T2DM and normal coronary arteries | Coronary | CPT | CAD,CVD | 112 | Yes | 4.9 |
| Nitenberg et al. [48] | 72 | T2DM patients without CAD | Coronary | CPT | CAD,CVD | 45 | Yes | 2.8 |
| Chan et al. [46] | 152 | Patients with CAD | Brachial | FMD | CAD, CVD | 34 | Yes | 4.7[a] |
| | | | Carotid | IMT | | | | |
| Halcox et al. [44] | 308 | Patients with and without CAD | Coronary | Acetylcholine response | CAD,CVD | 46 | Yes | 1.4 |
| Perticone et al. [43] | 225 | Patients with untreated hypertension | Forearm | FABF | CAD,CVD, PVD | 32 | Yes | 2.1 |
| Schachinger et al. [41] | 147 | Patients with chest pain or SVD | Coronary | Acetylcholine response, CPT, FMD, NMD | CAD,CVD, PVD | 80 | Yes | na |
| Al Suwaidi et al. [39] | 157 | Patients with mild CAD | Coronary | Acetylcholine, adenosine, and nitroglycerin responses | CAD | 28 | na | na |
| Muiesan et al. [51] | 172 | Patients with uncomplicated hypertension (28 % with diabetes) | Brachial | FMD | CV events | 109 | Yes | 2.5[b] |
| Yeboah et al. [53] | 3,026 | Population based cohort of without known CVD | Brachial | FMD | CV event | 60 | Yes | na |
| Kitta et al. [52] | 251 | Patients with CAD and optimized therapy (40 % with diabetes) | Brachial | FMD | CVD | 36 | Yes | 1.8[c] |
| Lind et al. [54] | 1,016 | Community based study of older adults (>70 years), 72 % with diabetes | Forearm, Brachial, Radial, Carotid | Acetylcholine and sodium nitroprusside, FMD, PWA, IMT | CV disease (MI or stroke | 60 | Yes, Forearm EDV only | na |

Key: *RR* relative risk, *CV* cardiovascular, *T2DM* type 2 diabetes mellitus, *CAD* coronary artery disease, *EDV* endothelial-dependent vasodilation, *FMD* Flow-mediated dilation of Brachial Artery, *NMD* nitroglycerin-mediated dilation, *MPI* myocardial perfusion imaging, *na* not assessed, *HT* hypertension, *CPT* cold-pressor test, *CVD* cerebrovascular disease, *IMT* intima medial thickness, *FABF* forearm blood flow, *PVD* peripheral vascular disease, *PWA* pulse wave –based method, *SVD* single vessel disease

[a]Approximation for patients with high IMT plaque burden

[b]Estimated for patients with impaired FMD compared to those with preserved FMD

[c]Estimated for patients with persistently impaired FMD compared to those with improved FMD

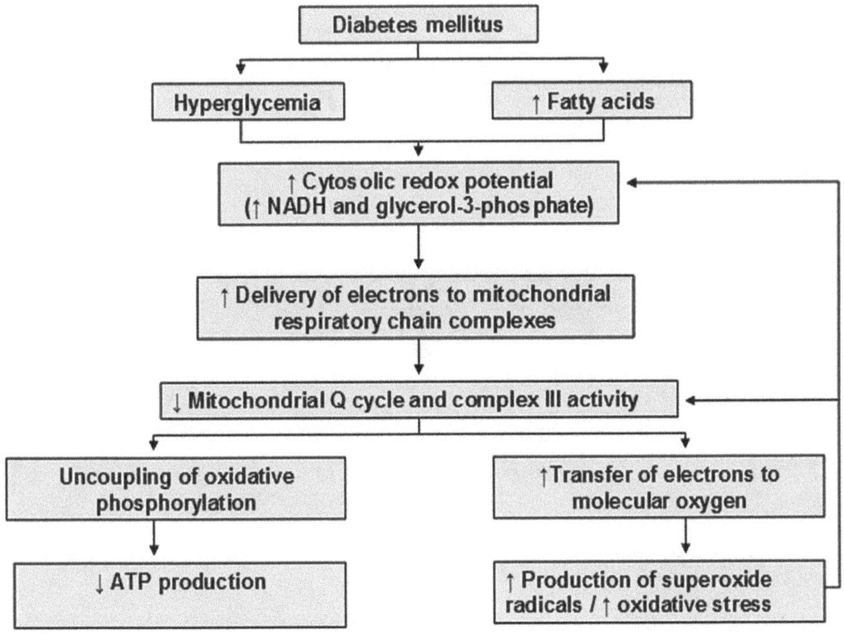


**Fig. 13.2** Mechanism whereby hyperglycemia and elevated fatty acids induce uncoupling of mitochondrial oxidative phosphorylation and increased oxidative stress in diabetes. *ATP* adenosine triphosphate, *NADH* reduced nicotinamide adenine dinucleotide

E-selectin, vascular cellular adhesion molecule (VCAM)-1 and intercellular adhesion molecule (ICAM)-1 are elevated in subjects with T2DM [3, 29, 30, 64]. Similarly, increased plasma levels of von Willebrand factor (vWF), a measure of endothelial cell damage and activation, are found in diabetes [3, 30, 64]. Microalbuminuria is an independent predictor of ED and may indicate widespread vascular dysfunction in diabetes [3, 65].

The precise pathogenetic mechanisms underlying the development of ED in T2DM remain unclear, but at inception they probably involve uncoupling of both eNOS activity (Fig. 13.1b), and mitochondrial oxidative phosphorylation (Fig. 13.2), as well as the activation of vascular NAD(P)H oxidase. These three mechanisms essentially result in increased generation of superoxide ($O_2^{\bullet-}$) radicals, eNOS uncoupling, and the overproduction of peroxynitrite. The main factors that combine to cause these biochemical disturbances are dyslipoproteinemia, oxidative stress [4], and inflammation [5–7]. Additional clinical factors that may contribute, either individually or synergistically, to ED in T2DM include hypertension [66], visceral obesity [67], insulin resistance [5, 68, 69], postprandial hyperlipidemia [70–72], fasting and postprandial hyperglycemia [73–75] and elevated levels of ADMA [37, 76].

The impact of insulin resistance in T2DM operates at an insulin signalling level in endothelial cells and in adipose tissue and skeletal muscle [5]. Impaired insulin receptor substrate-1 (IRS-1) and phosphatidylinositol (PI) 3-kinase insulin signalling results in decreased production of NO and ED on the one hand, and decreased glucose transporter (GLUT4) translocation and peripheral insulin resistance on the other. Insulin resistance also increases fatty acid availability which uncouples mitochondrial function in endothelial cells. This generates ROS by increasing advanced glycation end-products (AGES), protein kinase C (PKC) and *N*-acetylglucosamine (glcNAC), impairing eNOS activity and inducing ED. Inflammation, lipotoxicity and glucotoxicity are all increased in diabetes and collectively contribute to insulin resistance and ED [5]. Figure 13.3 suggests that the pathogenesis of ED in T2DM has oxidative stress as the central pathway for a wide spectrum of risk factors [3].

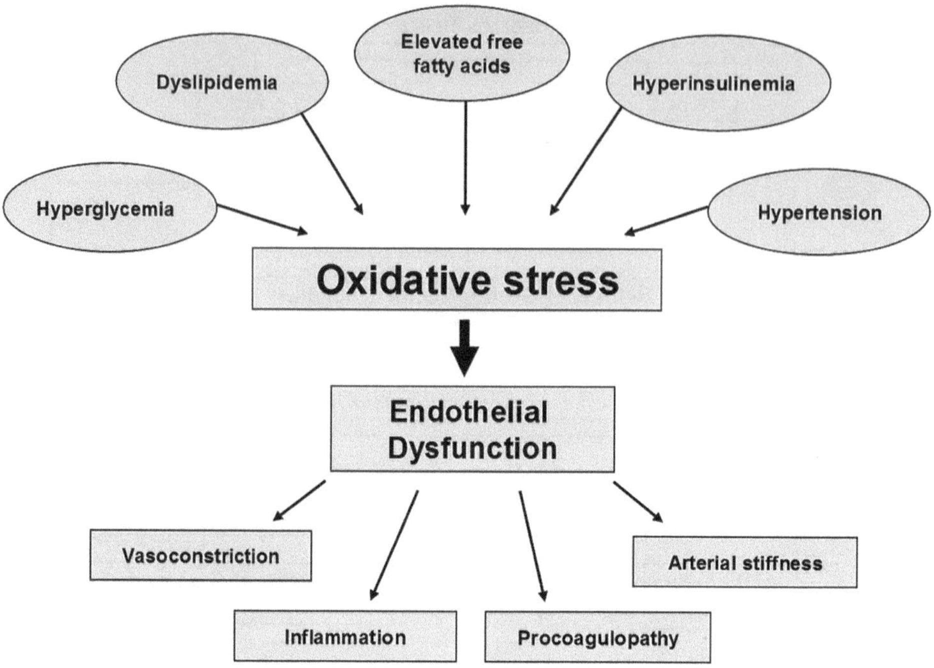


**Fig. 13.3** Pathogenesis and consequences of endothelial dysfunction in type 2 diabetes mellitus. Oxidative stress also contributes to endothelial dysfunction by activating protein kinase C, polyol, hexosamine and NFkappa B pathways, as well as by increasing asymmetric dimethylarginine and advanced glycation end-products

## Treating Endothelial Dysfunction in Type 2 Diabetes

Strategies for treating ED in T2DM will necessarily target the pathophysiological factors that underlie endotheliopathy, such as hyperglycemia, insulin resistance, dyslipidemia, increased oxidative stress, inflammation and hypertension [77, 78]. Treatment options range from lifestyle interventions to nutritional supplements and specific pharmacological therapies. The results of selected intervention studies are summarized in Table 13.3.

### Lifestyle Interventions

Diet and exercise programs aimed at achieving weight loss improve many of the metabolic abnormalities in T2DM that contribute to ED, such as hyperglycemia, insulin resistance, visceral obesity, hypertension and dyslipidemia. Weight loss and increased physical activity have been shown to improve ED in type 2 diabetic patients. In an uncontrolled study, obese insulin resistant subjects (including subjects with T2DM), who underwent a six month lifestyle modification programme of caloric restriction and regular supervised exercise, achieved a 7 % mean reduction in body weight, with improvement in brachial artery FMD and reduction in markers of endothelial activation and coagulation [79]. Insulin sensitivity, glycemic control and HDL-cholesterol levels also improved.

A randomized, crossover study of combined aerobic and resistance exercise training for eight weeks demonstrated an increase in brachial artery FMD and acetylcholine (ACh)-stimulated forearm blood flow (FABF) in T2DM subjects [80]. Although glycemic control also improved, reductions in HbA1c and fasting glucose were not correlated with changes in endothelial function. Indeed, it appears that the benefits of exercise in improving ED are not necessarily dependent on improvement in traditional cardiovascular risk factors [81], suggesting that repeated exercise may also act directly on the vasculature via a shear stress-related mechanism,

**Table 13.3** Randomized controlled trials investigating the therapeutic regulation of endothelial function in patients with type 2 diabetes mellitus

| Study (year) | *n* | Treatment | Treatment duration (months) | Endpoint | Treatment effect |
|---|---|---|---|---|---|
| Lifestyle interventions | | | | | |
| Maiorana et al. [80] | 16 | Aerobic and resistance exercise | 2 | FMD, ACh stimulated FABF | + |
| Antiglycaemic agents and insulin sensitizers | | | | | |
| Bagg et al. [91] | 43 | Improved glycemic control/usual gylcaemic control | 5 | FMD | ns |
| Rask-Madsen et al. [97] | 28 | Insulin therapy/no hypoglycaemic drug theapy | 2 | Insulin stimulated FABF response to Ach | + |
| Sundaresan et al. [98] | 14 | Metformin/glibenclamide | 1 | FABF response to diazoxide, ACh, SNP, norepinephrine | ns |
| Williams et al. [99] | 14 | Glibenclamide/placebo | 1 | FABF response to Ach | ns |
| Spallarossa et al. [100] | 20 | Glibenclamide/glimepriride/diet | 2 | FMD | ns |
| Wascher et al. [101] | 15 | Gliclazide/glibenclamide | 1 | FABF response to hyperaemia | |
| Abbink et al. [102] | 24 | Glibenclamide/glimepiride or metformin | 2 | FABF response to diazoxide, ACh, dipyridamole, forearm ischaemia | ns |
| Manzella et al. [103] | 16 | Rapaglinide/glibenclamide | 2 | FMD | +[a] |
| Schmoelzer et al. [104] | 12 | Rapaglinide/control | 2 h | FMD | + |
| Mather et al. [105] | 43 | Metfromin/placebo | 3 | FABF response to Ach | + |
| Natali et al. [106] | 74 | Rosiglitazone, Metformin, or placebo | 4 | FABF response to Ach | +[b] |
| Caballero et al. [108] | 87 | Troglitazone/placebo | 3 | FMD | +[c] |
| Martens et a l [110] | 20 | Pioglitazone/Placebo | 1 | FMD | + |
| Pistrosch et al. [111] | 12 | Rosiglitazone/nateglinide | 3 | FABF response to Ach | +[b] |
| Shimabukuro et al. [112] | 14 | Acarbose/placebo prior to a test meal | 1 week | FABF response to hyperemia | + |
| Nystrom et al. [114] | 12 | Recombinant glucagon-like peptide-1/saline | 1 week | FMD | + |
| Koska et al. [113] | 28 | Exenatide/placebo | Single dose | PAT | + |
| Antihypertensive agents | | | | | |
| O'Driscoll et al. [126] | 10 | Enalapril/placebo | 1 | FABF response to Ach | + |
| Cheetham et al. [128] | 9 | Losartan/placebo | 1 | FABF response to Ach | + |
| Cheetham et al. [129] | 12 | Losatan/placebo | 1 | FMD | + |
| Ceriello et al. [127] | 20 | Atorvastatin/irbesartan/placebo | 1 week | FMD | + |
| Flammer et al. [130] | 13 | Losartan/atenolol | 1 | FMD | +[d] |
| Davies et al. [131] | 42 | Spironolactone/placebo | 1 | FABF response to Ach | – |
| Yilmaz et al. [136] | 108 | Valsartin/amlodipine/valsartin + amlodipine | 3 | FMD | +[e] |

(continued)

**Table 13.3** (continued)

| Study (year) | *n* | Treatment | Treatment duration (months) | Endpoint | Treatment effect |
|---|---|---|---|---|---|
| Antioxidants and nutritional supplements | | | | | |
| Watts et al. [139] | 40 | $CoQ_{10}$/placebo | 3 | FMD | + |
| Playford et al. [140] | 20 | $CoQ_{10}$/placebo | 3 | FABF response to ACh, BK, SNP | ns |
| Lim et al. [141] | 80 | $CoQ_{10}$/placebo | 3 | Microcirculatory function | ns |
| Anderson et al. [144] | 20 | Vitamin C/placebo | 2 week | FMD | + |
| Paolisso et al. [146] | 40 | Vitamin E/placebo | 2 | FMD | + |
| Darko et al. [150] | 35 | Vitamin C/placebo | 3 week | FABF response to Ach | ns |
| Tousoulis et al. [149] | 41 | Vitamin C/atorvastatin/placebo | 4 week | FABF response to hyperaemia | +[f] |
| Chen et al. [151] | 32 | Vitamin C/placebo | 1 | FABF response to ACh, SNP or insulin | ns |
| Gazis et al. [152] | 48 | α-tocopherol/placebo | 2 | FABF response to ACh, BK, SNP | ns |
| Beckman et al. [153] | 23 | Vitamin E and C/placebo | 6 | FMD | ns |
| Mangoni et al. [160] | 26 | Folic acid/placebo | 1 | FABF response to Ach | + |
| Title et al. [161] | 19 | Folic acid/placebo | 2 week | FMD | + |
| Miscellaneous therapies | | | | | |
| Desouza et al. [162] | 14 | Sildenafil/placebo | 2 week | FMD | + |
| Koh et al. [167] | 20 | Conjugated equine oestrogen/placebo | 2 | FMD | ns |
| Silvestri et al. [168] | 30 | HRT/Tibolone/DHEAS | 1 | FMD | +[g] |
| Howes et al. [169] | 16 | Red clover derived isoflavones/placebo | 1 | FABF response to Ach | ns |
| Kwang et al. [177] | 35 | Testosterone/Placebo | 3 | FMD | + |
| Bilsborough et al. [178] | 13 | Pentoxifylline/placebo | 2 | FABF response to ACh, FMD | ns |
| Butler et al. [179] | 11 | Allopurinol | 1 | FABF response to Ach | + |

Key: *FMD* Flow-mediated dilation of Brachial Artery, *ACh* acetylcholine, *FABF* forearm blood flow, + indicates improved endothelial function, *ns* no significant effect, *SNP* sodium nitroprusside, *BK* bradykinin, – indicates a decreased response, *PAT* peripheral arterial tonometry, *HRT* hormone replacement therapy, *DHEAS* dehydroepiandrosterone-sulphate

[a]+ in rapaglinide only

[b]+ in rosiglitazone only

[c]in recently diagnosed diabetics (<3 years) without microvascular disease

[d]+ in losartan only

[e]+ in all three treatment groups

[f]+ in Atorvastatin only

[g]+ in HRT only

possibly involving endothelial nitric oxide synthase (eNOS) up-regulation or reduced nitric oxide (NO) degradation by free radicals [82].

Epidemiological studies provide a large body of evidence supporting the association between cigarette smoking and cardiovascular events [83]. Cigarette smoking is also associated with the premature development of macrovascular and microvascular complications in patients with T2DM [84]. Cigarette smoke increases inflammation, thrombosis and oxidation of LDL-cholesterol, with experimental and clinical evidence supporting the notion that increased oxidative stress results in vascular dysfunction [83]. Both active and passive cigarette smoking are associated with a dose-related impairment of endothelial function [85–87]. Brachial artery FMD was assessed in current and former healthy young adult smokers [85]. Former male smokers, but not former female smokers, had higher FMD than current smokers, suggesting that endothelial function may improve with smoking cessation [85]. A larger randomized, placebo controlled study investigated the effects of five smoking cessation pharmacotherapies on brachial artery FMD in 1,504 subjects [88]. Despite a greater weight gain, FMD significantly improved in subjects who quit and remained abstinent at one year, but did not change in those who continued to smoke [88]. Studies assessing the effects of smoking cessation in T2DM patients are warranted.

### Lipid-Regulating Therapy

Lipid regulating therapies improve diabetic dyslipidaemia; however, the various agents work via differing mechanisms, targeting to a greater or lesser degree the various aspects of the dyslipoproteinaemia. These therapies, through both lipid lowering effects and direct effects on the vasculature may improve ED. The mechanisms and vascular benefits of statins, fibric acid derivatives, nicotinic Antiglycemic acid (niacin) and omega-3 fatty acids are reviewed in more detail in a subsequent section.

### Antiglycaemic Agents and Insulin Sensitizers

Hyperglycemia contributes to ED by multiple mechanisms, many of which result in increased oxidative stress [89, 90]. The effect of short-term blood glucose control on endothelial function was examined in poorly controlled T2DM subjects, who were randomized to improved glycaemic control (multi-agent therapy, including insulin, to achieve and maintain glycaemic targets) or usual treatment for 20 weeks: no difference in brachial artery FMD was found between the treatment groups [9].

#### Insulin Therapy

Insulin treatment not only reduces glycemia, but may also directly increase endothelial NO production through 1-phosphotidylinositol 3-kinase signalling [92]. In an uncontrolled study in T2DM subjects on oral hypoglycemic therapy, switching to pre-meal insulin lispro at a dose to maintain equivalent glycemic control, improved fasting and postprandial brachial artery FMD, an effect that was further augmented by concomitant vitamin C therapy [93].

In uncontrolled studies in T2DM patients treated with oral hypoglycemic therapy, the addition of insulin treatment improved glycemia control and brachial artery FMD [94] or forearm vascular reactivity [95, 96]. A randomized, controlled trial in T2DM subjects with ischemic heart disease showed that insulin therapy reduced HbA1c levels and improved insulin-stimulated, but not unstimulated, FABF response to ACh [97].

#### Sulphonylureas and Insulin Secretagogues

Sulphonylureas reduce glycemia by binding to specific (SUR1) receptors, resulting in closure of pancreatic beta-cell potassium-dependent ATP channels and stimulation of endogenous insulin secretion. However, controlled, crossover studies of glibenclamide therapy in T2DM subjects did not show any change in acetylcholine-stimulated FABF response compared with metformin or placebo [98, 99], and treatment with either glibenclamide or glimepiride did not alter brachial artery FMD compared with diet treatment alone [100]. One double-blind, randomized, crossover trial in T2DM subjects suggested that gliclazide reduced FABF responses to hyperemia compared with glibenclamide, possibly due to differential binding of these agents to sulphonylurea receptors

[101]. However, another study did not show any difference between these two agents on ACh-stimulated FABF [102]. In a randomized crossover study, treatment with repaglinide (a short-acting insulin secretagogue), but not glibenclamide, increased brachial artery FMD in diet-treated T2DM subjects; improvement in endothelial function was correlated with changes in postprandial glycemia [103]. In subjects with impaired glucose tolerance, ED following a glucose challenge was related to the level of hyperglycemia. Reduction in the glycaemic response following a single dose of repaglinide, ameliorated ED in a glucose dependent manner [104].

### Metformin

Although its main anti-hyperglycemic action is to suppress hepatic gluconeogenesis, possibly by stimulation of AMP-activated kinase pathways, metformin may also increase insulin sensitivity in peripheral tissues. In a placebo-controlled trial, metformin treatment increased ACh-stimulated FABF and insulin sensitivity in diet-treated T2DM patients [105]. However, another randomized, double-blind, placebo-controlled trial in T2DM patients failed to show improvement in insulin sensitivity or ACh-stimulated FABF with metformin therapy, despite improved glycemic control [106].

### Thiazolidinediones

Thiazolidinediones improve insulin sensitivity and reduce glycemia via PPAR-gamma receptor-mediated effects on adipocytes resulting in decreased hepatic glucose output and increased peripheral glucose uptake by skeletal muscle [107]. In addition, as PPAR-gamma receptors are also present in the endothelium, vascular smooth muscle cells and macrophages, these agents may also have direct anti-inflammatory and anti-atherogenic effects on the vasculature.

In a randomized, double-blind, placebo-controlled trial, troglitazone increased brachial artery FMD in recently diagnosed T2DM subjects without macrovascular disease, but not in subjects with more long-standing disease or macrovascular complications [108]. In a small uncontrolled trial, pioglitazone-treated T2DM subjects showed improvement in brachial artery FMD, with a significant association between changes in FMD and insulin sensitivity [109]. In a randomized, double-blind, placebo-controlled, crossover study in T2DM subjects, pioglitazone was also shown to increase brachial artery FMD, but improvement in endothelial function was not correlated with favourable changes in plasma insulin, free fatty acids, adiponectin or C-reactive protein (CRP) [110]. In double-blind, crossover trials, rosiglitazone was shown to increase ACh-stimulated FABF in T2DM patients [106, 111].

### Alpha-Glucosidase Inhibitors

Administration of a single dose of Acarbose, an alpha-glucosidase inhibitor that targets postprandial hyperglycemia, has been shown to attenuate postprandial impairment of hyperemic FABF response in diet-treated T2DM patients [112].

### Incretins

Glucagon-like peptide (GLP)-1 is an incretin that reduces glycemia by stimulating insulin secretion, suppressing glucagon secretion and slowing gastrointestinal motility. Gliptins inhibit dipeptidyl peptidase-4, thereby increasing incretin levels which in turn increases insulin secretion and decreases glycemia, predominantly through postprandial mechanisms [113]. In a randomized crossover study, infusion of recombinant GLP-1 was shown to increase brachial artery FMD in T2DM subjects, without any change in insulin resistance [114]. In a randomized crossover study, improved postprandial endothelial function following a single subcutaneous injection of exenatide (a DPP4 inhibitor) in T2DM patients was associated with decreased triglyceride but not glucose concentrations [113].

### Amylin Agonists

Pramlintide, a synthetic amylin agonist, is associated with modest improvements in HbA1c levels and weight loss in insulin requiring T2DM patients. [115, 116] Pramlintide has also been shown to improve cardiovascular risk factors in T2DM patients: modest reductions in triglyceride levels [117] and improvement in markers of inflammation and oxidation have been reported [116, 117].

### Other Emerging Therapies for T2DM

Type 2 sodium-glucose cotransporter inhibitors (SGLT2) have been shown to normalize glycemia by promoting renal glucose excretion in animal models [118]. Evidence suggests that succinobucol, a probucol analogue, has protective effects in diabetes via antiatherosclerotic, anti-inflammatory, antioxidant and potential antidiabetic activities [119].

Future longer-term cardiovascular outcome studies and postprandial arterial function studies, investigating the effects of incretins, gliptins, alpha-glucosidase inhibitors, amylin agonists, and succinobucol in statin-treated T2DM patients are warranted to establish if their effects translate to improved cardiovascular outcomes.

### Antihypertensive Agents

In hypertension, increased oxidative stress and release of endothelial-derived constricting factors result in ED [8]. The coexistence of diabetes and hypertension has been shown to have an additive deleterious effect on endothelial function in the forearm resistance arteries [120]. Hyperglycemia increases the production of angiotensin II (Ang II) in the vessel wall [121]. Ang II stimulates vascular NAPH oxidase, increasing oxidative stress [122] and NF-kappaB activity, thereby activating inflammatory cytokines and vascular expression of cell adhesion molecules [9]. Hence, renin-angiotensin system (RAS) inhibition may improve endothelial function by reducing vascular oxidative stress and inflammation. Ang II may also promote release and production of vasoconstrictors such as endothelin-1 and prostaglandin-H2, which contribute to ED and hypertension.

### Angiotensin-Converting Enzyme (ACE) Inhibitors

In a small uncontrolled study in hypertensive T2DM subjects, treatment with perindopril reduced blood pressure but did not improve methacholine-stimulated FABF [123]. However, a randomized, open parallel group study showed that quinapril treatment increased serotonin-stimulated FABF in T2DM subjects, perhaps by increasing vascular adiponectin expression [124]. In T2DM patients with proteinuria, improvement in brachial artery FMD following short term ramipril treatment was associated with a reduction in serum hsCRP and plasma long pentraxin 3 (PTX3) [125]. Furthermore, a double-blind, placebo-controlled crossover study showed that enalapril lowered blood pressure and improved ACh-stimulated FABF in T2DM subjects without vascular disease [126].

### Angiotensin Receptor Antagonists

In randomized, controlled crossover trials, angiotensin type 1 receptor antagonists were shown to improve both FABF response to ACh and brachial artery FMD in subjects with T2DM [127–130]. Improvement in endothelial function occurred despite no significant change in blood pressure, and may relate to other treatment effects on oxidative stress, inflammation and endothelial cell activation.

### Aldosterone Antagonists

On a cautious note, a randomized, double-blind, placebo-controlled trial showed that treatment with spironolactone worsened ACh-stimulated FABF in T2DM subjects, possibly due to worsening of glycemic control and increase in plasma Ang II [131].

### Calcium Channel Blockers

Evidence for the effects of calcium channel blockade (CCB) on endothelial dysfunction is inconsistent. In a comparative study of antihypertensive agents, CCB (amlodipine) did not improve brachial artery FMD in patients with CAD [132]. In contrast, amlodipine improved endothelial function in hypertensive patients [133]. A study examining the effects CCB on endothelial function in hypertensive patients suggests a divergent effect for different types of these agents: efonidipine, a T- and L-type CCB, but not nifedipine, an L-type CCB, improved endothelial function and markers of oxidative stress [134]. Further, in patients with stable angina pectoris, combination CCB and ACE inhibition improved endothelial function, arterial stiffness and urinary albumin excretion more effectively than CCB alone [135]. However, in hypertensive T2DM patients with proteinuria, treatment with amlodipine, valsartan (an angiotensin II receptor blocker) or a combination of both, improved brachial artery FMD and proteinuria. Improvement in endothelial function was associated with reductions in PTX3 and soluble TNF-like weak inducer of apoptosis (sTWEAK) [136].

## Antioxidants and Nutritional Supplements

Supplementation with antioxidants and/or factors essential to NO production may potentially improve ED in T2DM by re-coupling eNOS and mitochondrial function, as well as decreasing vascular NAD(P)H oxidase activity.

Increased oxidative stress in T2DM may disrupt coenzyme $Q_{10}$ ($CoQ_{10}$) composition and levels, resulting in defective antioxidant defences and further exacerbating oxidative stress and increasing membrane fluidity [14, 137, 138]. In endothelial cells this may lead to uncoupling of eNOS and a reduction in the release and subsequent activity of NO. $CoQ_{10}$ as a potent antioxidant may decrease oxidative stress by not only quenching reactive oxidant species, but also by "recoupling" mitochondrial oxidative phosphorylation, thereby reducing superoxide production [14]. $CoQ_{10}$ supplementation improved brachial artery FMD in treatment naive diabetic patients with dyslipidemia, but there was no change in glyceryl-trinitrate mediated endothelial-independent response, forearm vascular reactivity or plasma $F_2$-isoprostanes [139, 140]. However, $CoQ_{10}$ supplementation did not improve microcirculatory endothelial function in type 2 diabetic patients, despite repleted plasma $CoQ_{10}$ concentrations [141].

Vascular responses to several other antioxidants and nutritional supplements have been examined, with inconsistent results being reported. Vitamin C (ascorbic acid) and vitamin E (tocopherol) have well-described antioxidant properties. However, studies examining their effect on ED in T2DM patients have yielded mixed results, some demonstrating benefit [142–148], while others have failed to show an effect [149–153]. Alpha-lipoic acid, another compound with free radical-scavenging activity, was shown to improve ACh-stimulated FABF [143]. Despite the potential for vascular benefit with the polyphenolic antioxidants present in red wine [154, 155], benefit has not been demonstrated in T2DM patients [156]. Supplementation with L-arginine, a principal substrate for eNOS, improved both brachial artery FMD and post-ischaemic forearm hyperaemia in T2DM women [148]. Oxidation of tetrahydrobiopterin ($BH_4$) may lead to uncoupling of eNOS, reducing NO production and further generating oxidant species. Intra-arterial $BH_4$ infusion was shown to improve FABF response to ACh in T2DM subjects [157]. Folic acid, a strong peroxynitrite scavenger, may also protect $BH_4$ from oxidation, reversing eNOS uncoupling [158]. Folic acid has been shown to improve FABF and brachial artery FMD in T2DM patients [159–161].

## Miscellaneous Therapies

### Phosphodiesterase Inhibitors

The vasorelaxation effect of NO on vascular smooth muscle is mediated by cyclic GMP (cGMP), which is catabolised by phosphodiesterase (PDE). PDE inhibitors, which are used to treat erectile dysfunction, increase the bioavailability of cGMP, which activates protein kinase G thereby promoting vasodilatation and a penile erection. Sildenafil, a selective PDE-5 inhibitor, has been shown to increase brachial artery FMD in a double-blind, placebo-controlled, cross-over study in T2DM men with erectile dysfunction [162].

### Estrogen Therapy

Epidemiological studies have suggested a protective effect of estrogen on cardiovascular risk, but intervention trials of sex hormone replacement in post-menopausal women have reported no benefit, and even a possible initial adverse effect, on cardiovascular outcomes [163, 164]. Although estrogen therapy may protect endothelial function by up-regulating endothelial NO production, reducing the formation of cyclooxygenase (COX) derived endothelium-derived contracting factors and have favorable effects on lipids and blood pressure, it may also have adverse effects in increasing vascular inflammation and cell adhesion [8, 165]. The effect of hormone replacement therapy on endothelial function in postmenopausal T2DM women has been inconsistent [166–169].

#### Testosterone Therapy

In men with testosterone deficiency brachial artery FMD has been reported to be both increased [170, 171] and impaired [172–174]. Testosterone deficiency is associated with elevated triglyceride and low HDL-cholesterol concentrations [175] and this could explain its association with impaired endothelial function. Evidence for the effect of testosterone replacement on endothelial function is inconsistent, however. Testosterone replacement for 12 weeks reduced FMD in hypogonadal men [171]. In a small study, hypogonadal men were found to develop impaired FMD four weeks following testosterone pellet implantation [176]. In contrast, in a randomized, placebo-controlled study, 12 weeks of testosterone replacement improved brachial artery reactivity in men with CAD [177]. Studies of the effect of testosterone replacement on endothelial function in diabetic men with androgen deficiency are warranted.

#### Tumour Necrosis Factor (TNF)-Alpha Inhibitors

The pro-inflammatory cytokine tumour necrosis factor (TNF)-alpha may contribute to ED by stimulating vascular NADPH oxidase and increasing superoxide production and oxidative stress. However, in a randomized crossover study, pentoxifylline, an inhibitor of TNF-alpha production, did not alter ACh-stimulated FABF in T2DM subjects, despite reduction in serum TNF-alpha levels [178].

#### Xanthine Oxidase Inhibitors

Xanthine oxidase is an enzyme present in endothelial cells that when activated increases oxidative stress. In a small randomized placebo-controlled trial allopurinol, an inhibitor of xanthine oxidase, was shown to improve ACh-stimulated FABF, and hence resistance artery function in mildly hypertensive T2DM subjects. There was no reduction in blood pressure, however [179].

## Diabetic Dyslipidemia

### Pathogenesis of Diabetic Dyslipidemia in Type 2 Diabetes

Dyslipidemia is a common risk factor and a strong predictor of CVD in T2DM patients [180]. Elevated plasma concentrations of triglycerides and reduced high-density lipoprotein (HDL)-cholesterol, in both the fasting and postprandial states, are the major lipoprotein abnormalities in diabetic dyslipidemia. The accumulation of small dense low-density lipoprotein (sdLDL) particles and triglyceride-rich lipoproteins (TRLs), including chylomicron remnants and very-low density lipoprotein (VLDL) remnants, are also characteristic of the atherogenic lipid profile [181–184]. These abnormalities are reflected by increased plasma concentrations of non-HDL cholesterol and apolipoprotein B-100 (apoB) [182]. In the postprandial state there is an increase in plasma TRLs and their remnants and qualitative changes in low-density lipoprotein (LDL) and HDL particles [181]. Therefore, hypertriglyceridemia is a marker of a range of lipoprotein abnormalities not routinely measured in clinical practice [182].

The aetiology of diabetic dyslipidemia is complex [185, 186]. It relates collectively to hyperglycemia [187], insulin resistance [187], hyperinsulinemia [187, 188], abdominal visceral adipose disposition and increased liver fat content [188], and dysregulated fatty acid metabolism [188]. Insulin resistance increases fatty acid flux from visceral adipose tissue to the liver, inducing increased liver fat content, over production of $VLDL_1$ particles [181, 188] and a reduction in the inhibitory effect of insulin on hepatic apoB secretion [189–191]. Hyperglycemia further aggravates the overproduction of $VLDL_1$, in particular increased $VLDL_1$ triglyceride production rate [187]. Collectively, plasma glucose, insulin and free fatty acids explain approximately half of the variation in $VLDL_1$ production rate [187].

Impaired chylomicron clearance in T2DM results from the reduced activity of lipoprotein lipase (LPL), an endothelial bound enzyme, and decreased receptor-mediated endocytosis in the liver [181, 192, 193]. $VLDL_1$ particles compete with chylomicrons and its remnants for clearance by saturating the lipolytic capacity of LPL and the activity of hepatic receptors [181, 192]. Hepatic secretion of apolipoprotein CIII (apo-CIII) is also increased in insulin resistance. This small protein, which is attached to VLDL, contributes to the delayed clearance of TRLs by inhibiting LPL and the binding of remnant TRLs to hepatic clearance receptors [192]. These mechanisms collectively account for postprandial lipaemia [181, 192] and may be an important causal mechanism of ED in T2DM and treatment targets for reducing residual cardiovascular risk.

Important compositional and atherogenic changes in lipoproteins are seen in T2DM [181]. An increased VLDL triglyceride pool leads to cholesterol depletion and triglyceride enrichment of LDL and HDL, mediated via the action of cholesteryl ester transfer protein (CETP) [181, 182]. Increased phospholipid transfer protein (PLTP) activity may contribute to hypertriglyceridemia and compositional changes in HDL. Further, the over activity of hepatic lipase, commonly increased in T2DM, increases the lipolysis of triglyceride enriched LDL and HDL particles [3, 4]. Compositional changes in HDL are also mediated by the actions of lipoprotein lipase (LPL) [181]. Collectively, these compositional changes produce smaller and denser lipoprotein particles that are potentially more atherogenic. Small dense LDL particles more easily penetrate the arterial wall and have a higher binding affinity to intimal proteoglycans than more buoyant larger LDL particles [3, 181, 194, 195]. In the intima, retained LDL particles are modified when exposed to oxidative stress, with sdLDL having an increased sensitivity to oxidation; glycation of LDL further increases this susceptibility to oxidation [181]. A predominant feature of diabetic dyslipidemia is low HDL-cholesterol concentrations with greater reductions in $HDL_2$ than $HDL_3$ [181]. In parallel to these reductions in HDL particles are reductions in plasma levels of apolipoprotein A-I (apoA-I) and apoA-II and HDL lipoproteins containing both Apo A-I and Apo A-II (LpA-I:A-II) [3, 181, 196]. These compositional changes in HDL particles are important in respect to ED and atherogenicity, as they are associated with a reduction in rates of reverse cholesterol transport and a decrease in the direct anti-atherogenic effects of HDL, including its anti-oxidant, anti-inflammatory and anti-thrombotic effects [3, 197–199]. These lipoprotein abnormalities and the associated risk of ED and cardiovascular disease in T2DM may be determined by various genes that regulate lipid and lipoprotein functionality, for example, LPL [200], apolipoprotein E [201], apoC-III [202, 203] and CETP [204]. This suggests a connection for the genetic control of ED in T2DM [3].

## Treatment of Diabetic Dyslipidemia

Current clinical guidelines emphasize lifestyle modifications and pharmacotherapy for the reduction of dyslipidemia and CVD risk in T2DM patients [205, 206].

### Lifestyle Interventions

Initial management should include an individualized lifestyle modification programme to optimize weight loss and glcyemic control. Benefits of weight reduction in T2DM increase steadily with increasing weight loss and include reductions in waist circumference, blood pressure, fasting glucose, $HbA_{1c}$ and serum triglycerides, resulting in improved metabolic control and CVD risk factor reduction [207, 208]. In the Look AHEAD (Action for Health in Diabetes) study, weight loss and improved physical fitness in type 2 diabetic patients was associated with improved glcyemic control and CVD risk factor reduction [208, 209]. In type 2 diabetic patients, a reduction in insulin resistance and fat mass following prolonged aerobic exercise resulted in improvements in lipoprotein metabolism [210].

### Lipid Regulating Therapy

Should dyslipidemia persist following a trial of intensified lifestyle changes, the next approach is pharmacotherapy, either an intensification of statin therapy or the addition of a second lipid regulating agent.

### Hydroxymethylglutaryl (HMG)-CoA Reductase Inhibitors (Statins)

Patients with an increasing number of metabolic syndrome components, with or without diabetes, have a progressive risk of CVD, and derive greater incremental benefit from higher dose statin therapy [211]. Statin therapy in hypertriglyceridemic patients, with and without T2DM, reduces triglyceride concentrations by up to 45 % [212–216], in a dose dependent manner and proportional to LDL-cholesterol lowering [215, 216]. Statin-treated patients with combined low LDL-cholesterol (<1.8 mmol/L) and low triglyceride (<1.7 mmol/L) levels had the lowest CHD event rate in the PROVE IT-TIMI 22 trial [217]. Evidence suggests that statins may mediate triglyceride lowering in T2DM by increasing the catabolism of TRL- triglyceride [213] and the TRL's VLDL1-ApoB, VLDL2-ApoB and IDL-ApoB [218]. Statins may further mediate triglyceride lowering by reducing the production rate and secretion of VLDL1-ApoB [218].

### Fibric Acid Derivatives

A recent meta-analysis concluded that fibrates are effective in reducing CVD events, primarily by prevention of coronary events [219]. The lipid-regulating effects of fibrates, mediated via PPAR-alpha receptor, are predominantly to promote fatty acid catabolism and reverse cholesterol transport, resulting in triglyceride lowering and increase in HDL-cholesterol and LDL particle size [107]. In a subgroup analysis of the Helsinki Heart Study, diabetic patients when compared with non-diabetic subjects were more dyslipidemic, at higher CVD risk and achieved a modest but non-significant reduction in CVD risk with gemfibrozil therapy [220]. The Fenofibrate Intervention and Event Lowering in Diabetes (FIELD) study demonstrated that fenofibrate reduced CVD events in hypertriglyceridemic T2DM patients with or without low HDL-cholesterol [221]. Indeed, in FIELD a post hoc analysis showed that the greatest benefit of fenofibrate therapy was seen in patients with triglycerides ≥2.3 mmol/L and reduced HDL-cholesterol; a relative risk reduction of 27 % was demonstrated [221].

The benefits of combined fibrate and statin therapy was examined in the Action to Control Cardiovascular Risk in Diabetes (ACCORD)-Lipid study. In ACCORD-Lipid, 5,518 simvastatin-treated patients with diabetes were randomized to receive either fenofibrate or placebo. Compared to simvastatin alone, 4.7 years of combination therapy did not reduce the rate of major fatal or nonfatal cardiovascular events [222]. However, in a valid pre-specified analysis of patients with triglycerides >2.3 mmol/L and HDL-cholesterol <0.9 mmol/L (approximately 17 % of the ACCORD-Lipid population), combined therapy achieved an additional 31 % reduction in cardiovascular risk, though this did not achieve statistical significance [222]. ACCORD Lipid did not support the use of combined statin and fenofibrate therapy in the majority of T2DM patients [222], but in those who have hypertriglyceridemia with or without low HDL-cholesterol, despite intensification of statin therapy, adding a fibrate may be beneficial in reducing residual CVD risk.

### Nicotinic Acid (Niacin)

Niacin is one of the oldest lipid regulating therapies and remains the most potent therapy available for increasing HDL-cholesterol [223, 224]. Many of niacin's effects are thought to derive from its action on adipose tissue [225]. However, the cellular mechanism for Niacin's lipid-lowering effects were not fully elucidated until the identification in 2003 of a G protein-coupled receptor GPR109A (HM74A), which is highly expressed in adipose tissue and acts as a high affinity receptor for nicotinic acid and mediates it antilipolytic effects [223, 226–229]. By binding to GPR109A, niacin inhibits hormone-sensitive lipase activity, resulting in decreased free fatty acid (FFA) release from adipose tissues. This results in a decreased flux of FFA to the liver that may reduce triglyceride production and subsequent hepatic VLDL production [226, 230, 231]. Niacin may also directly and non-competitively inhibit hepatic diacylglycerol acyl transferase (DGAT-2), the key enzyme in triglyceride synthesis [231, 232]. Although niacin increases HDL-cholesterol by up to 30 % (at therapeutic doses), a mechanism for this HDL raising effect remains to be fully elucidated but it may involve the down-regulation of the HDL-catabolism receptor [224, 230, 233, 234]. The lipid-regulating effects of niacin may be further mediated through PPAR-mediated transcriptional regulation and may involve all three PPAR isoforms, alpha (α), gamma (γ) and delta (δ) [225].

Niacin has been shown to be effective in lowering cardiovascular risk when used as monotherapy [182, 235–237], with recent post hoc analyses of the Coronary Drug Project demonstrating that the benefits were independent of hyperglycemia, metabolic syndrome and diabetes [182, 237–239]. Combination therapy with a stain and niacin is associated with regression of coronary atherosclerosis and carotid intima–media thickness (CIMT) in patients at high cardiovascular risk with low HDL-cholesterol levels, including those with diabetes [240–243]. These beneficial effects may reflect the reduction in triglycerides and increase in HDL-cholesterol seen with ER Niacin [182].

However, the question of whether adding niacin to statin therapy translates to improved cardiovascular outcomes in T2DM remains unanswered. The Atherothrombosis Intervention in Metabolic Syndrome with Low HDL-cholesterol/High Triglyceride and Impact on Global Health Outcomes (AIM-HIGH) study was discontinued after 36 months of follow-up due to lack of clinical benefit from the addition of ER Niacin to statin (± ezetimibe) therapy, despite significant improvements in HDL-cholesterol and triglycerides [244]. The Heart Protection Study-2 and the Treatment of HDL to reduce the incidence of vascular events (HPS2-THRIVE), due to report in 2013, will address if adding ER Niacin to statin therapy reduces CVD events in high-risk patients with prior vascular disease, a significant proportion having the metabolic syndrome or diabetes [245].

### Omega-3 Fatty Acids

Supplementation with omega-3 fatty acid ethyl esters (eicosapentaenoic acid (EPA) and docosahexaenoic acid (DHA)), at doses of 3–4 g daily, lower plasma triglycerides particularly in patients with hypertriglyceridemia [182, 192]. Evidence suggests combined statin and omega-3 fatty acid therapy may reduce cardiovascular events. In the Gruppo Italian per lo Studio della Sopravvivenza nell'Infarto Miocardio GISSI-Prevenzione (GISSI-Prevenzione) study, combination EPA/DHA dosed at 1 g daily reduced all cause mortality and sudden death in subjects with previous myocardial infarction [246]. The Japan Eicosapentaenoic Acid Lipid Intervention Study (JELIS) demonstrated a reduction in major cardiovascular events with combined omega-3 fatty acids (EPA 1,800 mg daily) and low dose statin (pravastatin 10 mg or simvastatin 5 mg daily) compared to statin alone [247]. However, this cardiovascular benefit may relate in part to the anti-arrhythmic effects of omega-3 fatty acids and is independent of minor changes in plasma triglycerides [182, 192]. A comprehensive review of the cardiovascular effects of omega-3 fatty acids has recently been published [248]. Importantly, there is no published outcome evidence demonstrating the beneficial effects of treating residual hypertriglyceridemia with omega-3 fatty acid therapy in statin-treated T2DM patients [182].

### Cholesteryl Ester Transfer Protein (CETP) Inhibition

Cholesteryl ester transfer protein (CETP) inhibitors have the potential to correct diabetic dyslipidemia by inhibiting the heteroexchange of neutral lipids among lipoproteins in both fasting and postprandial states. In subjects with low HDL-cholesterol concentrations, 4 weeks of torcetrapib treatment, alone or in combination with atorvastatin, resulted in a dose-related increase in plasma HDL-cholesterol and reductions in triglyceride and LDL-cholesterol concentrations [249, 250]. The off-target effects of torcetrapib on blood pressure are not seen with other CETP inhibitors, such as anacetrapib, dalcetrapib and evacetrapib, so that this class of agents may still have a role as second line agents in the management of diabetic dyslipidemia [251]. However, the preliminary results from the Dal-VESSEL study were reported as showing no effect of dalcetrapib on FMD, but the Dal-PLAQUE study [252] suggested a small trend to improvement in plaque volume; diabetic subjects were not specifically studied and the effect on clinical endpoints must await publication of the Dal-OUTCOMES study. The effect of CETP inhibitors on endothelial function in diabetes warrants investigation, however.

## Evidence That Lipid Regulation Improves Endothelial Function in Diabetes

The rationale for lipid regulation of diabetic dyslipidemia is well supported by studies showing correction of endothelial dysfunction. The results of selected intervention studies utilizing lipid regulating therapy are reviewed below and summarized in Table 13.4.

### Hydroxymethylglutaryl (HMG)-CoA Reductase Inhibitors (Statins)

Statins, inhibitors of hydroxymethylglutaryl (HMG)-CoA reductase, have been proven in large clinical trials to reduce cardiovascular mortality in a wide range of population subgroups, including subjects with diabetes [253]. Apart from their main effect in lowering LDL-cholesterol, statins may also have direct anti-inflammatory and antioxidant effects on the vasculature [77]. Statins have been shown to improve endothelial function in non-diabetic subjects with dyslipidaemia [254, 255], but results in T2DM subjects have been inconsistent and contradictory. Uncontrolled studies have not shown any benefit of statin therapy on serotonin-stimulated forearm blood flow (FABF) or brachial artery FMD in T2DM subjects [256–259]. One trial suggested improvement in endothelial function in a subgroup who achieved greater LDL-lowering [259], but another showed no benefit despite intensive lipid-lowering [257].

A number of randomized, placebo-controlled studies have shown a beneficial effect of statins on brachial artery FMD in T2DM subjects: [127, 260–262] on treatment improvement in endothelial function occurred within days, prior to any plasma lipid changes and was correlated with a reduction in oxidative stress, inflammation and endothelial cell activation [127, 260, 262]. Compared with placebo, atorvastatin was associated with a reduction in vascular cell adhesion molecules (VCAM1) and E-selectin, suggesting an improvement in endothelial function in T2DM patients that was independent of the lipid-regulating effects of atorvastatin [263]. In male subjects with stable atherosclerosis (30 % with diabetes), treatment with rosuvastatin or atorvastatin inhibited Rho/Rho kinase pathway activity and this inhibition was associated with improvement in brachial artery FMD in the absence of a reduction in plasma LDL-cholesterol level [264]. In statin-naïve, hypertriglyceridemic T2DM patients who had no history of CVD, atorvastatin or rosuvastatin significantly improved FMD and plasma levels of CRP, but associations between FMD and CRP or triglycerides were not reported [265]. In a recent study in normocholesterolemic T2DM patients with no evidence of CAD, four weeks of low dose atrovastatin (10 mg/day) significantly improved brachial artery FMD compared with placebo. A third of the patients in this study were reported to have had dyslipidemia at baseline, but on-treatment lipids were not reported [266].

However, there are randomized, double-blind, placebo-controlled studies that have shown no effect of statin therapy on brachial artery FMD in subjects with T2DM [267, 268], despite improvements in dyslipidaemia [269–271]. Studies examining the effect of statin therapy on forearm vascular reactivity in T2DM subjects have shown improvement with atorvastatin [149], but not with cerivastatin [272]. However, in the latter study, ACh-stimulated FABF increased with co-infusion of L-NMMA (inhibitor of NOS), suggesting an effect of treatment on non-NO vasoactive mediators, such as EDHF.

### Emerging LDL-Cholesterol Lowering Therapies

Emerging LDL-cholesterol lowering therapies merit investigation of their vascular effects in T2DM patients. Inhibition of proprotein convertase

**Table 13.4** Randomized controlled trials investigating the therapeutic regulation of endothelial function in patients with type 2 diabetes mellitus: Lipid regulating therapies

| Study (year) | *n* | Treatment | Treatment duration (months) | Endpoint | Treatment effect |
|---|---|---|---|---|---|
| Lipid regulating agents | | | | | |
| *Statins* | | | | | |
| Tsunekawa et al. [260] | 27 | Cerivastatin/Placebo | 3 days | FMD | + |
| Tan et al. [261] | 80 | Atorvastatin/Placebo | 6 | FMD | + |
| Ceriello et al. [262] | 30 | Simvastatin/Placebo | 3–6 days + 3 | FMD | + |
| Ceriello et al. [127] | 20 | Atorvastatin/irbesartan/placebo | 1 week | FMD | + |
| Dalla et al. [263] | 25 | Atorvastatin/placebo | 12 | VCAMI and E-selectin | + |
| Brunetti et al. [265] | 22 | Atorvastatin/rosuvastatin | 3 | FMD | + |
| Adel et al. [266] | 60 | Atorvastatin/placebo | 4 week | FMD | + |
| Economides et al. [267] | 40 | Atorvastatin/placebo | 3 | FMD | ns |
| Beishuizen et al. [268] | 250 | Cerivastatin replaced by simvastatin | 24 | FMD | ns |
| Van Venrooij et al. [269] | 133 | Atorvastatin 10 mg/Atorvastatin 80 mg | 7.5 | FMD | ns |
| Tantikosoom et al. [271] | 42 | Atorvastatin/placebo | 7.5 | FMD | ns |
| Tousoulis et al. [149] | 41 | Atorvastatin/Vitamin C/No treatment | 1 | FABF response to post-ischaemic hyperemia | +[a] |
| Tran et al. [272] | 11 | Cerivastatin/placebo | 2 | FABF response to ACh and L-NMMA | ns |
| *Fibrates* | | | | | |
| Playford et al. [281] | 40 | Fenofibrate/placebo | 3 | FMD | + |
| Playford et al. [140] | 20 | Fenofibrate/placebo | 3 | FABF response to ACh, BK, SNP | ns |
| Evans et al. [283] | 20 | Ciprofibrate/placebo | 3 | FMD | + |
| Avogaro et al. [284] | 10 | Gemfibrozil/placebo | 3 | FMD | + |
| Fegan et al. [285] | 10 | Fenofibrate/placebo | 3 | Blood flow responses to iontophoresis of ACh | ns |
| Hiukka et al. [286] | 170 | Fenofibrate/placebo | 60 | IMT, AIx, biomarkers of endothelial activation | ns |

| | | | | | |
|---|---|---|---|---|---|
| *Niacin* | | | | | |
| No studies identified in T2DM patients | | | | | |
| *Omega-3 fatty acids* | | | | | |
| McVeigh et al. [294] | 23 | Fish oil/placebo | 1.5 | FABF response to ACh | + |
| Woodman et al. [295] | 51 | EPA/DHA/placebo | 1.5 | FMD | ns |
| West et al. [296] | 18 | MUFA ± omega-3 FA | Three test meals over 3 week | FMD | + |
| Combination therapies | | | | | |
| Hamilton et al. [310] | 15 | Statin + fenofibrate/statin + placebo | 3 | FMD + forearm microcirculatory function | + |
| Fegan et al. [285] | 11 | Cerivastatin + fenofibrate | 3 | Skin blood flow response to iontophoresis and skin maximum hyperaemia | ns |
| Lee et al. [315] | 71[b] | Statin + Niacin/statin/placebo | 12 | Carotid MRI, aortic distensibility, MRI brachial artery FMD | +[c] |
| Hamilton et al. [316] | 15 | Statin + Niacin/statin alone | 5 | Small artery vasodilation and compliance | + |
| Hamilton et al. [320] | 23 | Statin+ $CoQ_{10}$/statin + placebo | 3 | FMD | + |
| Koh et al. [322] | 50 | Simvastatin + ramipril | 2 | FMD | ++ |
| Ceriello et al. [127] | 20 | Atorvastatin + irbesartan | 1 week | FMD | ++ |
| Playford et al. [140] | 20 | Fenofibrate + $CoQ_{10}$ | 3 | FABF response to ACh, BK, SNP | + |
| Luescher et al. [331] | 476[d] | Dalcetrapib + statin/placebo + statin | 9 | FMD | ns |

Key: *FMD* Flow-mediated dilation of Brachial Artery, *ACh* acetylcholine, *FABF* forearm blood flow; + indicates improved endothelial function, *ns* no significant effect, *SNP* sodium nitroprusside, *BK* bradykinin, *L-NMMA* L-nitro-mono-methyl arginine, *EPA* eicosapentaenoic acid, *DHA* docosahexaenoic acid, *T2DM* type 2 diabetes mellitus, ++ indicates combination therapy improved FMD more than monotherapy alone, *AIx* augmentation index, *IMT* intima–media thickness, *MUFA* monounsaturated fatty acids, ± with or without, *omega-3 FA* omega-3 fatty acids, $CoQ_{10}$ coenzyme $Q_{10}$, *VCAM1* vascular cell adhesion molecules 1

[a]+ in atorvastatin only

[b]Only 65 % of the patients T2DM

[c]+ in Carotid MRI only

[d]Only 45 % of patients T2DM

subtilisin/kexin type 9 (PCSK9), an important regulator of the LDL receptor, exerts beneficial effects on LDL and VLDL metabolism, but its role in humans is still to be elucidated [273]. Colesevelam, a more tolerable and potent bile acid sequestrant, is effective at lowering LDL-cholesterol either as monotherapy or in combination with a statin [274]. It has also been demonstrated to improve glycemic control in T2DM patients [274, 275] and could potentially improve endothelial function by reducing lipotoxicity and glucotoxicity, but no studies reporting its effects on endothelial function are available. Mipomersen, an apoB synthesis inhibitor, has been shown to reduce apoB, LDL-cholesterol and lipoprotein (a) in patients with familial hypercholesterolemia on maximally tolerated lipid-lowering therapy and in healthy volunteers and patients with mild to moderate hypercholesterolemia [276–278]. Studies in T2DM patients are required.

### Fibric Acid Derivatives

In addition to their lipid-regulating effects, fibrates may also reduce vascular inflammation and endothelial cell activation. In randomized controlled studies fenofibrate and related drugs appear to have a reasonably consistent beneficial effect on endothelial function in both non-diabetic and T2DM subjects. Fenofibrate has been shown to improve brachial artery FMD in non-diabetic subjects with mixed hyperlipidemia or primary hypertriglyceridemia [279, 280]. Fenofibrate improved brachial artery FMD in statin-naïve T2DM patients with dyslipidemia [281]. However, fenofibrate alone did not significantly improve forearm microcirculatory function in such patients [140]. Moreover, Chew et al. recently demonstrated that fenofibrate and $CoQ_{10}$ independently and interactively lowered 24-h ambulatory blood pressure [282] consistent with their beneficial effects on endothelial function in resistance arterioles. Ciprofibrate and gemfibrozil have been shown to improve brachial artery FMD in type 2 diabetic subjects in fasting and postprandial states [283, 284]. However, 12 weeks of fenofibrate therapy in T2DM patients did not improve microvascular endothelial-dependent function when assessed by skin blood flow response to the iontophoresis of acetylcholine [285]. In these studies, the effects of fenofibrate on markers of oxidative stress and insulin sensitivity were also inconsistent [140, 281, 283].

Although short-term fenofibrate therapy may improve endothelial function [279–281], a substudy of the longer-term FIELD study showed no such treatment effect on carotid intima–media thickness, augmentation index or biomarkers of endothelial function in T2DM patients [286]. However, the FIELD study subjects were mostly low risk (as evidenced by the low CVD event rate) and had not been selected for having ED at baseline.

Fenofibrate also has beneficial microvascular effects. In FIELD, monotherapy with fenofibrate, when compared with placebo, significantly reduced the need for laser therapy for diabetic retinopathy [287] and may delay albuminuria progression and impairment of renal function [288]. Recent reports from ACCORD show that both the addition of fenofibrate to simvastatin and intensive glycemic therapy reduced progression of diabetic retinopathy [289, 290]. In T2DM patients with hypertriglyceridemia and retinopathy, adding a fibrate to statin therapy and weight loss, may be safe and effective treatment options for cardiovascular and retinopathy risk reduction compared with intensification of hypoglycemic and/or statin therapy.

### Nicotinic Acid (Niacin)

Niacin may also improve endothelial function and reduce CVD events through direct effects on the vasculature [225]. Two studies have reported on niacin monotherapy: In a controlled study in 22 healthy men with low HDL-cholesterol (<1.04 mmol/L) no-flush niacin 1.5 g/day for 12 weeks significantly improved FMD but no change was demonstrated in plasma lipids or chylomicron remnants suggesting a direct vascular effect by niacin [291]. In metabolic syndrome patients allocated to ER niacin (1,000 mg/day) or placebo for 52 weeks, niacin improved FMD by 22 % ($p<0.001$), significantly regressed CIMT, decreased high sensitivity C-reactive protein (hsCRP) by 20 % ($p=0.013$) and significantly improved plasma lipids (HDL-cholesterol, LDL-cholesterol and triglycerides) [292]. No studies have reported on patients with T2DM. Collectively, these studies demonstrate that niacin is effective in improving endothelial function in subjects with low HDL-cholesterol. Further, improvements in both lipids and inflammatory markers suggest that both lipid-mediated and direct mechanisms are involved in the beneficial vascular effects of niacin.

### Omega-3 Fatty Acids

Omega-3 fatty acids derived from marine fish oil predominantly lower triglycerides, but may also have beneficial effects on HDL subfractions and LDL-particle size, as well as direct actions on the vasculature to reduce inflammation and endothelial cell activation [293]. Randomized, double-blind, controlled trials of omega-3 fatty acid supplementation in T2DM subjects have shown improvement in ACh-stimulated FABF [294], but no change in brachial artery FMD [295]. In hypertriglyceridaemic T2DM subjects, inclusion of omega-3 fatty acids in a meal containing predominantly unsaturated fatty acids reduced postprandial lipaemia and improved brachial artery FMD [296], possibly by attenuating the postprandial rise in lipoprotein subclass containing apolipoproteins B and C (LpB:C) [297]. In subjects with metabolic syndrome it is possible that improvement in forearm vasodilator response is attributable to docosahexaenoic acid (DHA) and not the eicosapentaenoic acid (EPA) component of fish oils [298].

### Probucol

Experimental evidence suggests that probucol may limit oxidative LDL modification and reduce atherogenesis [299]. Probucol reduced coronary restenosis rates following percutaneous transluminal coronary angioplasty [300] and CIMT in patients with hypercholesterolaemia [301]. In T2DM patients, administration of probucol or atorvastatin decreased urinary 8-hydroxy-2′-deoxyguanosine, a biomarker of overall systemic oxidative stress in vivo, probucol having a greater effect in patients with higher oxidative stress at baseline [302]. Whether probucol improves endothelial function and decreases cardiovascular (CV) events in diabetes have not been examined.

In summary, the lipid regulating agents discussed above (statins, fibrates, niacins and omega-3 fatty acids) all correct diabetic dyslipidemia, improving lipid and lipoprotein composition and concentrations to varying degrees and by different mechanisms (Table 13.5). Collectively, these agents have been demonstrated to improve ED, but not all the findings are consistent. Endothelial dysfunction is a complex condition with multiple factors contributing to its pathogenesis. A multifactorial strategy that combines lipid regulating drug therapy with other interventions, such as lifestyle changes, insulin sensitizers and antioxidant and cofactor supplementation, is likely to achieve the best cardiovascular outcome.

### Combination Therapies

In large prospective clinical outcome trials (HPS, CARDS, TNT and CTT meta-analysis) the residual risk of CVD events in T2DM remains high, despite achievement of optimal or near optimal LDL-cholesterol levels with statin therapy [253, 303–305]. Studies examining the effects of statins on ED have demonstrated inconsistent and contradictory results (Table 13.4) [127, 149, 260–272]. It is possible that in T2DM, treatment with a single therapeutic agent may not adequately improve endothelial function. Several complementary treatment options are possible.

#### Statins and Fibrates

In T2DM combination statin and fibrate therapy can significantly benefit dyslipidemia and cardiovascular risk status [306–309]. However, there is limited evidence investigating the effects of combined statin/fibrate therapy on ED in T2DM patients. In a randomized, double-blind, crossover study, fenofibrate significantly improved brachial artery FMD and forearm microcirculatory function in statin-treated T2DM patients with LDL-Cholesterol <2.6 mmol/L and ED [310]. Improvement in FMD was inversely associated with on-treatment LDL-cholesterol and apoB concentrations, indicating that the improvement in endothelial function may in part relate to enhanced reduction in LDL-cholesterol and apoB

**Table 13.5** Possible mechanisms of action of four lipid-regulating agents that improve endothelial function, Adapted from Woodman et al. 2005

| Parameter | Statins | Fibrates | Niacins | Omega-3 fatty acids |
|---|---|---|---|---|
| ↓ LDL-cholesterol | ++ | ± | + | ± |
| ↑ LDL particle size | + | ++ | ++ | + |
| ↓ Triglyceride | + | +++ | ++ | ++ |
| ↓ Chylomicron remnants | ++ | ± | ± | ± |
| ↑ HDL-cholesterol | + | ++ | +++ | ± |
| ↑ PPAR activation/expression | + | +++ | ++ | + |
| ↓ Vascular inflammation | + | + | + | + |
| ↑ NO production | + | + | + | ± |
| ↓ Endothelin-1 synthesis/expression | + | + | ± | ± |
| ↓ Oxidative stress | + | + | + | + |

*LDL* low density lipoprotein, *NO* nitric oxide, *PPAR* peroxisome proliferator-activated receptor, *statin* HMG-CoA reductase inhibitor, ↓ indicates decreased, ↑ indicates increased, + indicates minor effect, ++ indicates moderate effect, +++ indicates major effect, ± indicates equivocal effect

concentrations [310]. In contrast, microvascular endothelial function, assessed by skin blood flow response to iontophoresis of acetylcholine and sodium nitroprusside and skin maximum hyperaemia to local heating, was not improved in T2DM subjects treated with combination cerivastatin and fenofibrate therapy [285].

Both statin and fibrate therapies have been shown to improve biomarkers of inflammation in subjects with T2DM. In 300 subjects with diabetic dyslipidaemia, simvastatin or fenofibrate alone or in combination, lowered levels of plasma hsCRP and lipoprotein-associated phospholipase $A_2$ (Lp-$PLA_2$). However, there was no additive effect from the combination therapy [311].

## Statins and Niacins

Nicotinic acid effectively raises HDL-cholesterol, lowers triglycerides and increases LDL particle size [224]. In diabetic subjects combination niacin and atorvastatin therapy improves the atherogenic lipid profile more effectively than monotherapy [312]. Combined statin and niacin therapy has been shown to reduce the progression of coronary and carotid artherosclerosis [240–243]. Two studies have reported on the effects of combined statin/niacin therapy on endothelial function in patients with CAD [313, 314]. In these studies, the addition of niacin significantly improved endothelial function in patients with low HDL-cholesterol levels [313, 314]. In the Oxford Niaspan Study, the effect of modified-release nicotinic acid (Niaspan) on atherosclerosis and endothelial function was assessed in statin-treated patients with low HDL-cholesterol, together with either (1) T2DM and CAD, (2) carotid atherosclerosis or (3) peripheral atherosclerosis; 65 % of the patients had T2DM. Compared with placebo, 12 months of niacin treatment significantly reduced carotid atherosclerosis, but did not alter either aortic distensibility or brachial artery FMD [315]. In a parallel group study, 15 statin-treated T2DM with LDL-cholesterol <2.5 mmol/L and ED were randomized to niacin (nicotinic acid prolonged release) or no additional therapy [316]. Niacin significantly improved small artery vasodilatory function and compliance and reduced serum triglycerides by 47 %. An inverse association between maximal forearm post-ischemic blood flow and change in serum triglycerides, suggests that a reduction in triglycerides may in part explain the improvement in endothelial function [316].

## Statins and Antioxidants

In patients with ischemic cardiomyopathy (40 % with diabetes), atorvastatin (10 mg/day) significantly improved post-ischemic FABF. However, the co-administration of vitamin E (400 IU/day) with atorvastatin blunted the effect of atorvastatin on post ischemic FABF, although the effect remained significant [317].

Given the potential for statins to inhibit the cellular synthesis of plasma $CoQ_{10}$, a by-product of isoprenoid metabolism, their full benefit on improving endothelial function may be blunted [318, 319]. In a randomized, double-blind, crossover study, $CoQ_{10}$ supplementation significantly improved FMD in statin-treated T2DM patients with LDL-cholesterol <2.5 mmol/L and ED [320]. $CoQ_{10}$ supplementation has been shown to improve ecSOD levels and endothelial relaxation of the brachial artery in patients with CAD (20 % with diabetes and 80 % statin-treated) [321], indicating that the beneficial effects of $CoQ_{10}$ on endothelial function are in part related to improvements in local vascular oxidative stress.

### Statins and Antihypertensive Agents

Statins and antihypertensive agents such as ACE inhibitors, angiotensin II receptor antagonist, or calcium channel blockers, have differing mechanisms of action on the arterial wall. Therefore it is conceivable that in combination they will have an additive and synergistic effect on endothelial function [127, 322–324]. In hypercholesterolemia T2DM patients, ramipril combined with simvastatin significantly improved FMD and reduced malondialdehyde (MDA) and hs-CRP levels compared to ramipril or simvastatin alone [322]. Both ramipril alone and combination therapy improved adiponectin levels and insulin sensitivity, but there was no additive effect with combination therapy [322]. In T2DM, postprandial hyperglycemia and hypertriglyceridemia independently and cumulatively decreased FMD and increased biomarkers of inflammation. Short-term treatment (one week) with atorvastatin and irbesartan, alone or in combination counterbalanced these detrimental effects, combination therapy being more effective than either monotherapy [127]. Longer-term studies utilizing combined statin and ARB therapy in T2DM are required. In patients with hypercholesterolemia and hypertension, evidence supports the anti-atherosclerotic effects of combined statin and calcium channel blocker therapy, particularly the combination of amlodipine and atorvastatin [323, 325–327].

### Fibrates and Antioxidants

In dyslipidemic type 2 diabetic patients with ED, combination fenofibrate and $CoQ_{10}$ significantly improved endothelium-dependent and -independent forearm blood flow response to intra-arterial vasodilator infusions [140]. Moreover, it has recently been demonstrated that fenofibrate and $CoQ_{10}$ independently and interactively lowered 24-h ambulatory blood pressure [282], consistent with their beneficial effects on endothelial function in resistance arterioles. This synergistic effect of fenofibrate and $CoQ_{10}$ in improving endothelial function may involve co-activation of PPAR-α in endothelial and smooth muscle cells, improving the production and action of NO and decreasing the synthesis of endothelin-1.

### Other Combinations: Ezetimibe, Omega-3 Fatty Acids, CETP Inhibitors

In subjects with T2DM, co-administration of ezetimibe on background statin therapy significantly lowered CRP to a greater extent than that of statin alone [328]. In the Stop Atherosclerosis in Native Diabetics Study (SANDS), aggressive LDL-cholesterol lowering with statins alone or statins plus ezetimibe resulted in similar regression of CIMT in those patients who achieved equivalent LDL-cholesterol reductions [329], but the comparative therapeutic effects on endothelial function were not studied. Omega-3 fatty acid supplementation has been consistently shown to improve endothelial function in T2DM [294, 296, 298], but whether it enhances the effect of statins and other agents reviewed above remains to be demonstrated.

Dalcetrapib, a CETP inhibitor, was investigated in the dal-VESSEL study for its efficacy and safety on endothelial function, blood pressure, lipids and clinical outcomes in patients with CHD or CHD risk equivalent and below average HDL-cholesterol; 45 % of patients had T2DM. Patients were also treated with a statin and/or other cholesterol lowering agents to a LDL-cholesterol <2.6 mmol/L [330]. In this randomized, double-blinded, placebo controlled study, 36 weeks of dalcetrapib reduced CETP activity by almost 50 % and HDL-cholesterol by 30 %, but brachial artery FMD, ambulatory blood pressure

**Table 13.6** Recommended treatment targets for diabetic dyslipidemia

| | | NCEP ATP III [206, 332] | ADA [205, 333] | NHFA [334] | European guidelines [335–337] |
|---|---|---|---|---|---|
| LDL-cholesterol (mmol/L) | Very high risk | <1.8 | <1.8 | <2.0 | <1.8 |
| | High risk | <2.6 | <2.6 | <2.5 | <2.5 |
| Triglycerides (mmol/L) | | | <1.7 | <1.5 | <1.7 |
| HDL-cholesterol (mmol/L) | Male | | >1.0 | >1.0 | >1.0 |
| | Female | | >1.3 | >1.0 | >1.2 |
| Non-HDL cholesterol (mmol/L) | Very high risk | <2.6 | <2.6 | | <2.6 |
| | High risk | <3.4 | <3.4 | | <3.3 |
| ApoB (g/L) [3, 7] | Very high risk | | <0.8 | | <0.8 |
| | High risk | | <0.9 | | <1.0 |

and biomarkers of inflammation, oxidative stress and coagulation did not alter with either dalcetrapib or placebo [331].

## Guidelines for the Management of Diabetic Dyslipidemia

Several guidelines provide evidence-based recommendations for addressing diabetic dyslipidemia [205, 206, 332–336] and two recent reports focus more specifically on elevated triglycerides and low HDL-cholesterol [337, 338]. Table 13.6 summarizes the recommended treatment targets for diabetic dyslipidemia.

In patients with T2DM, lowering of LDL-cholesterol remains the primary focus of therapeutic interventions [205, 206, 332, 333]. In T2DM patients with overt CVD or in those at high risk (over the age of 40 years with one or more other major CVD risk factor) statin therapy and therapeutic lifestyle changes (TLCs) should be initiated regardless of baseline lipid levels. In lower risk patients, statin therapy should be initiated if LDL-cholesterol levels remain above 2.6 mmol/L following TLC efforts or in those with several CVD risk factors [205]. These recommendations are supported by evidence of CVD reduction in diabetic patients in large outcome-based clinical trials and of improvement in endothelial function with statin therapy [127, 253, 260–262, 303–305]. If LDL-cholesterol target levels are not achieved with a maximum tolerated statin dose, then adding a second therapeutic agent (ezetimibe, fibrate, or niacin) may be required [205]. For patients with elevated triglycerides (>2.3 mmol/L) the use of non-HDL cholesterol as a secondary treatment target (a non-HDL cholesterol goal of 0.78 mmol/L above the patients LDL-cholesterol goal) is recommended [206, 332]. ApoB, a measure of LDL particle number is also a recommended treatment target in patients at cardiometabolic risk [333, 336]. In these patients, combination therapy with a second lipid regulating agent (fibrate, niacin, or Omega 3 fatty acids) or intensification of LDL-cholesterol lowering is recommended [206, 333, 337]. Evidence from ACCORD supports the use of combined statin and fenofibrate therapy in hypertriglyceridemic T2DM patients (ACCORD-lipid 2010). There is also limited evidence suggesting improvement in endothelial function with combination therapy; statin and fibrate in T2DM patients [310], or statin and niacin in patients with and without T2DM [313, 314, 316]. However, with combination therapy the risk of myopathy is increased requiring patient education and monitoring. Patients with severely elevated triglycerides (>5.5 mmol/L) are at risk of pancreatitis and the treatment priority is to reduce triglycerides by dietary modifications and pharmacotherapy [333]. To mitigate this risk the FDA has approved the use of omega-3 fatty acid ethyl esters as an adjunct to dietary interventions [182, 192].

## Conclusion

T2DM patients are at markedly increased risk of CVD events. Endothelial dysfunction (ED) is the earliest manifestation of vascular involvement in diabetes and heralds the increased risk of CVD. ED can be examined indirectly in the peripheral circulation by several non-invasive methods. Studies of ED serve two useful purposes in cardiovascular research. First, they can help identify agents that could be tested as monotherapy or combination therapy in clinical endpoint trials. Second, they can provide mechanisms for the cardiovascular benefits of these treatments. Clinical trials of interventions on ED may be hampered by subject selection bias, statistical underpowering and technical imprecision in measurements. These factors may account for variation in findings among some of the studies reviewed. As methodologies are refined, measurement of endothelial function could in time provide a practical clinical tool for risk stratifying patients and guiding the intensity of treatments to reverse or prevent progression of cardiovascular disease in diabetes.

Therapeutic interventions, including lifestyle changes and lipid-regulating agents, correct diabetic dyslipidaemia via several mechanisms. They have also been shown to improve ED, but not all studies demonstrate a consistent benefit. Together with dyslipoproteinemia, increased oxidative stress is a major factor involved in the pathogenesis of ED in T2DM. Supplementation with antioxidants may also potentially improve endothelial dysfunction in T2DM, but the reported effects on endothelial function have again not always been consistent. Other interventions, including L-arginine and folate supplementation and PDE-5 inhibitors, have been demonstrated to improve ED in diabetes, but there is no consistent evidence that they reduce cardiovascular events in clinical trials. These and other new and emerging therapies require investigation in longer term clinical outcome studies.

Therapeutic guidelines recommend a multifactorial lifestyle and pharmacotherapy approach for the management of CVD risk in T2DM. Treatment targets have been specified for LDL-cholesterol, non-HDL cholesterol (or apoB), glycated hemoglobin and blood pressure. Interventions, such as lipid regulating therapy, ACE inhibitors, metformin and fish oils, have been shown to reduce cardiovascular events in large clinical endpoint trials. However, in these trials residual risk of CVD events (i.e. the risk of cardiovascular events which persists in many patients despite the intervention being tested) in statin-treated patients remains high, despite the achievement of optimal or near optimal plasma LDL-cholesterol concentrations.

There are reasonable data suggesting that residual diabetic dyslipidemia and CV risk in diabetics on a statin may be targeted with fenofibrate, there being no clinical endpoint trials at present supporting adding niacin or marine-derived n-3 polyunsaturated fatty acids. High residual CV risk is seen with a spectrum of interventions (e.g. anti-glycemic, anti-hypertensive, anti-dyslipidemic treatments) tested in trials and employed in the standard care of the patient with diabetes. Well-designed studies of endothelial function in appropriately selected volunteers afford a good opportunity to test new therapeutic interventions and their eventual utilization in the care of the diabetic patient.

## References

1. Haffner S, Lehto S, Ronnemaa T, Pyorala K, Laakso M. Mortality from coronary heart disease in subjects with type 2 diabetes and in nondiabetic subjects with and without prior myocardial infarction. N Engl J Med. 1998;339(4):229–34.
2. Kim J, Koh KK, Quon MJ. The union of vascular and metabolic actions of insulin in sickness and in health. Arterioscler Thromb Vasc Biol. 2005;25(5):889–91.
3. Woodman RJ, Chew GT, Watts GF. Mechanisms, significance and treatment of vascular dysfunction in type 2 diabetes mellitus: focus on lipid-regulating therapy. Drugs. 2005;65(1):31–74.
4. Watts GF, Playford DA. Dyslipoproteinaemia and hyperoxidative stress in the pathogenesis of endothelial dysfunction in non-insulin dependent diabetes mellitus: an hypothesis. Atherosclerosis. 1998;141(1):17–30.
5. Kim J, Montagnani M, Koh KK, Quon MJ. Reciprocal relationships between insulin resistance

and endothelial dysfunction: molecular and pathophysiological mechanisms. Circulation. 2006; 113(15):1888–904.
6. Nesto R. C-reactive protein, its role in inflammation, Type 2 diabetes and cardiovascular disease, and the effects of insulin-sensitizing treatment with thiazolidinediones. Diabet Med. 2004;21(8):810–7.
7. Dandona P, Aljada A, Chaudhuri A, Mohanty P. Endothelial dysfunction, inflammation and diabetes. Rev Endocr Metab Disord. 2004;5:189–97.
8. Versari D, Daghini E, Virdis A. Endothelium-dependent contractions and endothelial dysfunction in human hypertension. Brit J Pharmacol. 2009;157: 527–36.
9. Leiter LA, Lewanczuk RZ. Of the renin-angiotensin system and reactive oxygen species: Type 2 diabetes and angiotensin II inhibition. Am J Hypertens. 2005;18(1):121–8.
10. Widlansky ME, Gokce N, Keaney J, Vita JA. The clinical implications of endothelial dysfunction. J Am Coll Cardiol. 2003;42:1149–60.
11. Esper R, Nordaby R, Vilarino J, Paragano A, Cacharron J, Machado RA. Endothelial dysfunction: a comprehensive appraisal. Cardiovasc Diabetol. 2006;5(1):1–18.
12. Vita JA, Keaney Jr JF. Endothelial function: a barometer for cardiovascular risk? Circulation. 2002;106(6):640–2.
13. Levine TB, Levine AB. The endothelium and nitric oxide. *Metabolic syndrome and cardiovascular disease*. Philadelphia PA: Saunders Elsevier; 2006. p. 173–210.
14. Chew GT, Watts GF. Coenzyme $Q_{10}$ and diabetic endotheliopathy: oxidative stress and the 'recoupling hypothesis'. QJM. 2004;97(8):537–48.
15. Katusic ZS. Vascular endothelial dysfunction: does tetrahydrobiopterin play a role? Am J Physiol Heart Circ Physiol. 2001;281(3):H981–6.
16. Corretti MC, Anderson TJ, Benjamin EJ, Celermajer D, Charvonneau F, Creager MA, Deanfield J, Drexler H, Gerhard-Herman M, Herrington D, Vallance P, Vita J, Vogel R. Guidelines for the ultrasound assessment of endothelial-dependent flow-mediated vasodilation of the brachial artery: a report of the international brachial artery reactivity task force. J Am Coll Cardiol. 2002;39(2):257–65.
17. Pyke KE, Tschakovsky ME. The relationship between shear stress and flow-mediated dilatation: implications for the assessment of endothelial function. J Physiol. 2005;568(2):357–69.
18. Al-Qaisi M, Kharbanda RK, Mittal TK, Donald AE. Measurement of endothelial funciton and its clinical utility for cardiovascular risk. Vasc Health Risk Manag. 2008;4:647–52.
19. Higashi Y, Sasaki S, Nakagawa K, Matsuura H, Kajiyama G, Oshima T. A noninvasive measurement of reactive hyperemia that can be used to assess resistance artery endothelial function in humans. Am J Cardiol. 2001;87(1):121–5.
20. Benjamin N, Calver A, Collier J, Robinson B, Vallance P, Webb D. Measuring forearm blood flow and interpreting the responses to drugs and mediators. Hypertension. 1995;25(5):918–23.
21. Rubinshtein R, Kuvin JT, Soffler M, Lennon RJ, Lavi S, Nelson RE, Pumper GM, Lerman LO, Lerman A. Assessment of endothelial function by non-invasive peripheral arterial tonometry predicts late cardiovascular adverse events. Eur Heart J. 2010;31(9):1142–8.
22. Fitch KV, Stavrou E, Looby SE, Hemphill L, Jaff MR, Grinsopon SK. Associations of cardiovascular risk factors with two surrogate markers of subclinical atherosclerosis: Endothelial function and carotid intima media thickness. Atherosclerosis. 2011; 217(2):437–40.
23. Kato MD, Shiode MD, Yamagata MD, Matsuura MD, Kajiyama MD. Coronary segmental responses to acetylcholine and bradykinin in patients with atherosclerotic risk factors. Am J Cardiol. 1997;80(6): 751–5.
24. Stehouwer CD, Stroes ES, Hackeng WH, Mulder PG, Den Ottolander GJ. von Willebrand factor and development of diabetic nephropathy in IDDM. Diabetes. 1991;40(8):971–6.
25. Jensen T, Bjerre-Knudsen J, Feldt-Rasmussen B, Deckert T. Features of endothelial dysfunction in early diabetic nephropathy. Lancet. 1989;1(8636): 461–3.
26. Gearing AJH, Newman W. Circulating adhesion molecules in disease. Immunol Today. 1993;14(10): 506–12.
27. Albertini JP, Valensi P, Lormeau B, Aurousseau MH, Ferriere F, Attali JR, Gattegno L. Elevated concentrations of soluble E-selectin and vascular cell adhesion molecule-1 in NIDDM. Effect of intensive insulin treatment. Diabetes Care. 1998;21(6): 1008–13.
28. Hwang SJP, Ballantyne CMM, Sharrett AR, Smith SCP, Davis CE, Gotto AMJ, Boerwinkle E. Circulating Adhesion Molecules VCAM-1, ICAM-1, and E-selectin in Carotid Atherosclerosis and Incident Coronary Heart Disease Cases: The Atherosclerosis Risk In Communities (ARIC) Study. Circulation. 1997;96(12):4219–25.
29. Thorand B, Baumert J, Chambless L, Meisinger C, Kolb H, Doring A, Lowel H, Koenig W, for the MONICA/KORA Study Group. Elevated markers of endothelial dysfunction predict type 2 diabetes mellitus in middle-aged Men and women from the general population. Arterioscler Thromb Vasc Biol. 2006;26(2):398–405.
30. Lim SC, Caballero AE, Smakowski P, LoGerfo FW, Horton ES, Veves A. Soluble intercellular adhesion molecule, vascular cell adhesion molecule, and impaired microvascular reactivity are early markers of vasculopathy in type 2 diabetic individuals without microalbuminuria. Diabetes Care. 1999;22(11): 1865–70.

31. Hill JM, Zalos G, Halcox JPJ, Schenke WH, Waclawiw MA, Quyyumi AA, Finkel T. Circulating endothelial progenitor cells, vascular function, and cardiovascular risk. N Engl J Med. 2003;348(7): 593–600.
32. Giannotti G, Doerries C, Mocharla PS, Mueller MF, Bahlmann FH, Horvath T, Jiang H, Sorrentino SA, Steenken N, Manes C, Marzilli M, Rudolph KL, Luscher TF, Drexler H, Landmesser U. Impaired endothelial repair capacity of early endothelial progenitor cells in prehypertension: relation to endothelial dysfunction. Hypertension. 2010;55(6): 1389–97.
33. Curtis AM, Zhang L, Medenilla E, Gui M, Wiolkinson PF, Hu E, Giri J, Doraiswamy V, Gunda S, Burgert ME, Moore JS, Edelberg JM, Mohler ER. Relationship of microparticles to progenitor cells as a measure of vascular health in a diabetic population. Cytometry. 2010;78B(5):329–37.
34. Avogaro A, Albiero M, Menegazzo L, de Kreutzenberg S, Fadini GP. Endothelial dysfunction in diabetes. Diabetes Care. 2011;34(Supplement 2): S285–90.
35. Nozaki T, Sugiyama S, Koga H, Sugamura K, Ohba K, Matsuzawa Y, Sumida H, Matsui K, Jinnouchi H, Ogawa H. Significance of a multiple biomarkers strategy including endothelial dysfunction to improve risk stratification for cardiovascular events in patients at high risk for coronary heart disease. J Am Coll Cardiol. 2009;54(7):601–8.
36. Landmesser U, Merten R, Spiekermann S, Buttner K, Drexler HB. Vascular extracellular superoxide dismutase activity in patients with coronary artery disease: relation to endothelium-dependent vasodilation. Circulation. 2000;101(19):2264–70.
37. Russo G, Leopold JA, Loscalzo J. Vasoactive substances: nitric oxide and endothelial dysfunction in atherosclerosis. Vasc Pharmacol. 2002;38(5): 259–69.
38. Alp NJ, Channon KM. Regulation of endothelial nitric oxide synthase by tetrahydrobiopterin in vascular disease. Arterioscler Thromb Vasc Biol. 2004;24(3):413–20.
39. Suwaidi JA, Hamasaki S, Higano ST, Nishimura RA, Holmes Jr DR, Lerman A. Long-term follow-Up of patients with mild coronary artery disease and endothelial dysfunction. Circulation. 2000; 101(9):948–54.
40. Neunteufl T, Heher S, Katzenschlager R, Wolfl G, Kostner K, Maurer G, Weidinger F. Late prognostic value of flow-mediated dilation in the brachial artery of patients with chest pain. Am J Cardiol. 2000; 86(2):207–10.
41. Schachinger VM, Britten MBM, Zeiher AMM. Prognostic impact of coronary vasodilator dysfunction on adverse long-term outcome of coronary heart disease. Circulation. 2000;101(16):1899–906.
42. Kuvin JT, Patel AR, Sliney KA, Pandian NG, Rand WM, Udelson JE, Karas RH. Peripheral vascular endothelial function testing as a noninvasive indicator of coronary artery disease. J Am Coll Cardiol. 2001;38(7):1843–9.
43. Perticone F, Ceravolo R, Pujia A, Ventura G, Iacopino S, Scozzafava A, Ferraro A, Chello M, Mastroroberto P, Verdecchia P, Schillaci G. Prognostic significance of endothelial dysfunction in hypertensive patients. Circulation. 2001;104(2): 191–6.
44. Halcox JPJ, Schenke WHB, Zalos GRN, Mincemoyer RRN, Prasad AMB, Waclawiw MAP, Nour KRA, Quyyumi AAM. Prognostic value of coronary vascular endothelial dysfunction. Circulation. 2002;106(6):653–8.
45. Kuvin JTM, Karas RHM. Clinical utility of endothelial function testing: ready for prime time? Circulation. 2003;107(25):3243–7.
46. Chan SY, Mancini GBJ, Kuramoto L, Schulzer M, Frohlich J, Ignasezewski A. The prognostic importance of endothelial dysfunction and carotid atheromaburden in patients with coronary artery disease. J Am Coll Cardiol. 2003;42(6):1037–43.
47. Quyyumi AA. Prognostic value of endothelial function. Am J Cardiol. 2003;91(12, Supplement 1): 19–24.
48. Nitenberg A, Valensi P, Sachs R, Cosson E, Attali JR, Antony I. Prognostic value of epicardial coronary artery constriction to the cold pressor test in type 2 diabetic patients with angiographically normal coronary arteries and No other major coronary risk factors. Diabetes Care. 2004;27(1):208–15.
49. Nitenberg A, Pham I, Antony I, Valensi P, Attali JR, Denis C. Cardiovascular outcome of patients with abnormal coronary vasomotion and normal coronary arteriography is worse in type 2 diabetes mellitus than in arterial hypertension: A 10 year follow-up study. Atherosclerosis. 2005;183(1):113–20.
50. Papaioannou GI, Kasapis C, Seip RL, Grey NJ, Katten D, Wackers FJT, Inzucchi SE, Engel S, Taylor A, Young LH, Chyun D, Davey JA, Iskandrian AE, Ratner RE, Robinson EC, Carolan S, Heller GV. Value of peripheral vascular endothelial function in the detection of relative myocardial ischemia in asymptomatic type 2 diabetic patients who underwent myocardial perfusion imaging. J Nucl Cardiol. 2006;13(3):362–8.
51. Muiesan ML, Salvetti M, Paini A, Monteduro C, Galbassini G, Poisa P, Porteri E, Agabiti-Rosei C, Paderno V, Belotti E, Rizzoni D, Castellano M, Agabiti-Rosei E. Prognostic role of flow-mediated dilatation of the brachial artery in hypertensive patients. J Hypertens. 2008;26(8):1612–8.
52. Kitta Y, Obata JE, Nakamura T, Hirano M, Kodama Y, Fujioka D, Saito Y, Kawabata K, Sano K, Kobayashi T, Yano T, Nakamura K, Kagiyama K. Persistent impairment of endothelial vasomotor function Has a negative impact on outcome in patients with coronary artery disease. J Am Coll Cardiol. 2009;53(4):323–30.

53. Yeboah JM, Folsom ARM, Burke GLM, Johnson C, Polak JF, Post W, Lima JA, Crouse JR, Herrington DM. Predictive value of brachial flow-mediated dilation for incident cardiovascular events in a population-based study: the multi-ethnic study of atherosclerosis. Circulation. 2009;120(6):502–9.
54. Lind LM, Berglund LP, Larsson AM, Sundstrom JM. Endothelial function in resistance and conduit arteries and 5-year risk of cardiovascular disease. Circulation. 2011;123(14):1545–51.
55. Inaba Y, Chen J, Bergmann S. Prediction of future cardiovascular outcomes by flow-mediated vasodilatation of brachial artery: a meta-analysis. Int J Card Imaging. 2010;26(6):631–40.
56. Green DJ, Jones H, Thijssen D, Cable NT, Atkinson G. Flow-mediated dilation and cardiovascular event prediction: does nitric oxide matter? Hypertension. 2011;57(3):363–9.
57. McVeigh GE, Brennan GM, Johnston GD, McDermott BJ, McGrath LT, Henry WR, Andrews JW, Hayes JR. Impaired endothelium-dependent and independent vasodilation in patients with type 2 (non-insulin-dependent) diabetes mellitus. Diabetologia. 1992;35(8):771–6.
58. Watts GF, O'Brien SF, Silvester W, Millar JA. Impaired endothelium-dependent and independent dilatation of forearm resistance arteries in men with diet-treated non-insulin-dependent diabetes: role of dyslipidaemia. Clin Sci. 1996;91(5):567–73.
59. Williams SB, Cusco JA, Roddy MA, Johnstone MT, Creager MA. Impaired nitric oxide-mediated vasodilation in patients with non-insulin-dependent diabetes mellitus. J Am Coll Cardiol. 1996;27(3):567–74.
60. Enderle MD, Benda N, Schmuelling RM, Haering HU, Pfohl M. Preserved endothelial function in IDDM patients, but not in NIDDM patients, compared with healthy subjects. Diabetes Care. 1998;21(2):271–7.
61. Henry RMA, Ferreira I, Kostense PJ, Dekker JM, Nijpels G, Heine RJ, Kamp O, Bouter LM, Stehouwer CDA. Type 2 diabetes is associated with impaired endothelium-dependent, flow-mediated dilation, but impaired glucose metabolism is not: the Hoorn study. Atherosclerosis. 2004;174(1):49–56.
62. Nitenberg A, Valensi P, Sachs R, Dali M, Aptecar E, Attali JR. Impairment of coronary vascular reserve and ACh-induced coronary vasodilation in diabetic patients with angiographically normal coronary arteries and normal left ventricular systolic function. Diabetes. 1993;42(7):1017–25.
63. Prior JO, Quinones MJ, Hernandez-Pampaloni M, Facta AD, Schindlr TH, Sayre JW, Hsueh WA, Schelbert HR. Coronary circulatory dysfunction in insulin resistance, impaired glucose tolerance, and type 2 diabetes mellitus. Circulation. 2005;111(18):2291–8.
64. Guerci B, Kearney-Schwartz A, Bohme P, Zannad F, Drouin P. Endothelial dysfunction and type 2 diabetes. Part 1: physiology and methods for exploring the endothelial function. Diabetes Metab. 2001;27 (4 Pt 1):425–34.
65. Papaioannou GI, Seip RL, Grey NJ, Katten D, Taylolr A, Inzucchi SE, Young LH, Chyun DA, Davey JA, Wackers FJT, Iskandrian AE, Ratner RE, Robinson EC, Carolan S, Engel S, Heller GV. Brachial artery reactivity in asymptomatic patients with type 2 diabetes mellitus and microalbuminuria (from the Detection of Ischemia in Asymptomatic Diabetics-Brachial Artery Reactivity study). Am J Cardiol. 2004;94(3):294–9.
66. Iiyama K, Nagano M, Yo Y, Nagano N, Kamide K, Higaki J, Mikami H, Ogihara T. Impaired endothelial function with essential hypertension assessed by ultrasonography. Am Heart J. 1996;132(4):779–82.
67. Arcaro G, Zamboni M, Rossi L, Turcato E, Covi G, Armellini F, Bosello O, Lechi A. Body fat distribution predicts the degree of endothelial dysfunction in uncomplicated obesity. Int J Obes. 1999;23(9):936–42.
68. Cleland SJ, Petrie JR, Small M, Elliott HL, Connell JMC. Insulin Action Is Associated With Endothelial Function in Hypertension and Type 2 Diabetes. Hypertension. 2000;35(1):507–11.
69. Petrie JR, Ueda S, Webb DJ, Elliott HL, Connell JMC. Endothelial nitric oxide production and insulin sensitivity : a physiological link with implications for pathogenesis of cardiovascular disease. Circulation. 1996;93(7):1331–3.
70. Nappo F, Esposito K, Cioffi M, Giugliano G, Molinari AM, Paolisso G, Marfella R, Giugliano D. Postprandial endothelial activation in healthy subjects and in type 2 diabetic patients: Role of fat and carbohydrate meals. J Am Coll Cardiol. 2002;39(7):1145–50.
71. Anderson RA, Evans ML, Ellis GR, Graham J, Morris K, Jackson SK, Lewis MJ, Rees A, Frenneaux MP. The relationships between post-prandial lipaemia, endothelial function and oxidative stress in healthy individuals and patients with type 2 diabetes. Atherosclerosis. 2001;154(2):475–83.
72. Anderson RA, Jones CJH, Goodfellow J. Is the fatty meal a trigger for acute coronary syndromes. Atherosclerosis. 2001;159(1):9–15.
73. Kawano H, Motoyama T, Hirashima O, Hirai N, Miyao Y, Sakamoto T, Kugiyama K, Ogawa H, Yasue H. Hyperglycemia rapidly suppresses flow-mediated endothelium- dependent vasodilation of brachial artery. J Am Coll Cardiol. 1999;34(1):146–54.
74. Shige H, Ishikawa T, Suzukawa M, Ito T, Nakajima K, Higashi K, Ayaori M, Tabata S, Ohsuzu F, Nakamura H. Endothelium-dependent flow-mediated vasodilation in the postprandial state in type 2 diabetes mellitus. Am J Cardiol. 1999;84(10):1272–4.
75. Haller H. Postprandial glucose and vascular disease. Diabet Med. 1997;14 Suppl 3:S50–6.
76. Lin KY, Ito AM, Asagami TM, Tsao PS, Adimoolam S, Kimoto M, Tsuji H, Reaven GMM, Cooke JPM. Impaired nitric oxide synthase pathway in diabetes mellitus: role of asymmetric dimethylarginine and dimethylarginine dimethylaminohydrolase. Circulation. 2002;106(8):987–92.

77. Davignon J. Beneficial cardiovascular pleiotropic effects of statins. Circulation. 2004;109 (23 Supplement1):III39–43.
78. Dandona P, Aljada A. Endothelial dysfunction in patients with type 2 diabetes and the effects of thiazolidinedione antidiabetic agents. J Diabetes Complications. 2004;18(2):91–102.
79. Hamdy O, Ledbury S, Mullooly C, Jarema C, Porter SM, Ovalle K, Moussa A, Caselli A, Caballero AE, Economides PA, Veves A, Horton ES. Lifestyle modification improves endothelial function in obese subjects with the insulin resistance syndrome. Diabetes Care. 2003;26(7):2119–25.
80. Maiorana A, O'Driscoll G, Cheetham C, Dembo L, Stanton K, Goodman C, Taylor R, Green D. The effect of combined aerobic and resistance exercise training on vascular function in type 2 diabetes. J Am Coll Cardiol. 2001;38:860–6.
81. Green DJ, Walsh JH, Maiorana A, Best MJ, Taylor RR, O'Driscoll JG. Exercise-induced improvement in endothelial dysfunction is not mediated by changes in CV risk factors: pooled analysis of diverse patient populations. Am J Physiol Heart Circ Physiol. 2003;285(6):H2679–87.
82. Green DJ, Maiorana A, O'Driscoll G, Taylor R. Effect of exercise training on endothelium-derived nitric oxide function in humans. J Physiol. 2004; 561(1):1–25.
83. Ambrose JA, Barua RS. The pathophysiology of cigarette smoking and cardiovascular disease: an update. J Am Coll Cardiol. 2004;43:1731–7.
84. Haire-Joshu D, Glasgow RE, Tibbs TL. Smoking and diabetes. Diabetes Care. 2004;27:S74–5.
85. Celermajer DS, Sorensen KE, Georgakopoulos D, Bull CM, Thomas O, Robinson J, Deanfield JE. Cigarette smoking is associated with dose-related and potentially reversible impairment of endothelium-dependent dilation in healthy young adults. Circulation. 1993;88:2149–55.
86. Celermajer DS, Adams MR, Clarkson P, Robinson J, McCredie R, Donald A, Deanfield JE. Passive smoking and impaired endothelium-dependent arterial dilatation in healthy young adults. N Engl J Med. 1996;334:150–4.
87. Poredos P, Orehek M, Tratnik E. Smoking is associated with dose-related increase of intima-media thickness and endothelial dysfunction. Angiology. 1999;50:201–8.
88. Johnson HM, Gossett LK, Piper ME, Aeschlimann SE, Korcarz CE, Baker TB, Fiore MC, Stein JH. Effects of smoking and smoking cessation on endothelial function: 1-year outcomes from a randomized clinical trial. J Am Coll Cardiol. 2010;55: 1988–95.
89. Guerci B, Bohme P, Kearney-Schwartz A, Zannad F, Drouin P. Endothelial dysfunction and type 2 diabetes. Part 2: altered endothelial function and the effects of treatments in type 2 diabetes mellitus. Diabetes Metab. 2001;27:436–47.
90. Schalkwijk CG, Stehouwer CDA. Vascular complications in diabetes mellitus: the role of endothelial dysfunction. Clin Sci. 2005;109:143–59.
91. Bagg W, Whalley GA, Gamble G, Drury PL, Sharpe N, Braatvedt GD. Effects of improved glycaemic control on endothelial function in patients with type 2 diabetes. Intern Med J. 2001;31:322–8.
92. Rask-Madsen C, King GL. Mechanisms of Disease: endothelial dysfunction in insulin resistance and diabetes. Nat Clin Pract Endocrinol Metab. 2007;3:46–56.
93. Evans M, Anderson RA, Smith JC, Khan N, Graham JM, Thomas AW, Morris K, Deely D, Frenneaux MP, Davies JS, Rees A. Effects of insulin lispro and chronic vitamin C therapy on postprandial lipaemia, oxidative stress and endothelial function in patients with type 2 diabetes mellitus. Euro J Clin Invest. 2003;33:231–8.
94. Gaenzer H, Neumayr G, Marschang P, Sturm W, Lechleitner M, Foger B, Kirchmair R, Patsch J. Effect of insulin therapy on endothelium-dependent dilation in type 2 diabetes mellitus. Am J Cardiol. 2002;89:431–4.
95. Vehkavaara S, Makimattila S, Schlenzka A, Vakkilainen J, Westerbacka J, Yki-Jarvinen H. Insulin Therapy Improves Endothelial Function in Type 2 Diabetes. Arterioscler Thromb Vasc Biol. 2000;20:545–50.
96. Vehkavaara S, Yki-Jarvinen H. 3.5 Years of insulin therapy with insulin glargine improves in vivo endothelial function in type 2 diabetes. Arterioscler Thromb Vasc Biol. 2004;24:325–30.
97. Rask-Madsen C, Ihlemann N, Krarup T, Christiansen E, Kober L, Kistorp CN, Torp-Pedersen C. Insulin therapy improves insulin-stimulated endothelial function in patients with type 2 diabetes and ischemic heart disease. Diabetes. 2001;50:2611–8.
98. Sundaresan P, Lykos D, Daher A, Diamond T, Morris R, Howes LG. Comparative effects of glibenclamide and metformin on ambulatory blood pressure and cardiovascular reactivity in NIDDM. Diabetes Care. 1997;20:692–7.
99. Williams S, Abbott D, Morfis L, Manwaring P, Diamond T, Howes LG. Effects of glibenclamide on blood pressure and cardiovascular responsiveness in non-insulin dependent diabetes mellitus. J Hypertens. 1998;16:705–11.
100. Spallarossa P, Schiavo M, Rossettin P, Cordone S, Olivotti L, Cordera R, Brunelli C. Sulfonylurea treatment of type 2 diabetic patients does Not reduce the vasodilator response to ischemia. Diabetes Care. 2001;24:738–42.
101. Wascher TC, Boes U. Forearm vascular reactivity is differentially influenced by gliclazide and glibenclamide in chronically treated type 2 diabetic patients. Clin Physiol Funct Imaging. 2005;25:40–6.
102. Abbink EJ, Pickkers P, Van Rosendaal AJ, Lutterman JA, Tack CJ, Russel FGM, Smits P. Vascular effects of glibenclamide vs. glimepiride and metformin in Type 2 diabetic patients. Diabet Med. 2002;19:136–43.

103. Manzella D, Grella R, Abbatecola AM, Paolisso G. Repaglinide administration improves brachial reactivity in type 2 diabetic patients. Diabetes Care. 2005;28:366–71.
104. Schmoelzer I, Wascher TC. Effect of repaglinide on endothelial dysfunction during a glucose tolerance test in subjects with impaired glucose tolerance. Cardiovasc Diabetol. 2006;5:9–12.
105. Mather KJ, Verma S, Anderson TJ. Improved endothelial function with metformin in type 2 diabetes mellitus. J Am Coll Cardiol. 2001;37:1344–50.
106. Natali A, Baldeweg S, Toschi E, Capaldo B, Barbaro D, Gastaldelli A, Yudkin JS, Ferrannini E. Vascular effects of improving metabolic control with metformin or rosiglitazone in type 2 diabetes. Diabetes Care. 2004;27:1349–57.
107. Gervois P, Fruchart JC, Staels B. Drug Insight: mechanisms of action and therapeutic applications for agonists of peroxisome proliferator-activated receptors. Nat Clin Pract Endocrinol Metab. 2007;3: 145–56.
108. Caballero AE, Saouaf R, Lim SC, Hamdy O, Abou-Elenin K, O'Connor C, LoGerfo FW, Horton ES, Veves A. The effects of troglitazone, an insulin-sensitizing agent, on the endothelial function in early and late type 2 diabetes: A placebo-controlled randomized clinical trial. Metabolism. 2003;52:173–80.
109. Suzuki M, Takamisawa I, Yoshimasa Y, Harano Y. Association between insulin resistance and endothelial dysfunction in type 2 diabetes and the effects of pioglitazone. Diabetes Res Clin Pract. 2007;76:12–7.
110. Martens FM, Visseren FL, de Koning EJ, Rabelink TJ. Short-term pioglitazone treatment improves vascular function irrespective of metabolic changes in patients with type 2 diabetes. J Cardiovasc Pharmacol. 2005;46:773–8.
111. Pistrosch F, Passauer J, Fischer S, Fuecker K, Hanefeld M, Gross P. In type 2 diabetes, rosiglitazone therapy for insulin resistance ameliorates endothelial dysfunction independent of glucose control. Diabetes Care. 2004;27:484–90.
112. Shimabukuro M, Higa N, Chinen I, Yamakawa K, Takasu N. Effects of a single administration of acarbose on postprandial glucose excursion and endothelial dysfunction in type 2 diabetic patients: a randomized crossover study. J Clin Endocrinol Metab. 2006;91:837–42.
113. Koska JM, Schwartz EP, Mullin MB, Schwenke DP, Reaven PM. Improvement of postprandial endothelial function after a single dose of exenatide in individuals with impaired glucose tolerance and recent-onset type 2 diabetes. Diabetes Care. 2010;33:1028–30.
114. Nystrom T, Gutniak MK, Zhang Q, Zhang F, Holst JJ, Ahren B, Sjoholm A. Effects of glucagon-like peptide-1 on endothelial function in type 2 diabetes patients with stable coronary artery disease. Am J Physiol Endocrinol Metab. 2004;287:E1209–15.
115. Ryan G, Briscoe TA, Jobe L. Review of pramlintide as adjunctive therapy in treatment of type 1 and type 2 diabetes. Drug Des Develop Ther. 2008;2:203–14.
116. Hoogwerf BJ, Doshi KB, Diab D. Pramlintide, the synthetic analogue of amylin: physiology, pathophysiology, and effects on glycemic control, body weight, and selected biomarkers of vascular risk. Vasc Health Risk Manag. 2008;4(2):355–62.
117. Wysham C, Lush C, Zhang B, Maier H, Wilhelm K. Effect of pramlintide as an adjunct to basal insulin on markers of cardiovascular risk in patients with type 2 diabetes. Curr Med Res Opin. 2007;24(1):79–85.
118. Hardman TC, Dubrey SW. Development and potential role of type-2 sodium-glucose transporter inhibitors for management of type 2 diabetes. Diabetes Ther. 2011;2(3):133–45.
119. Stocker R. Molecular mechanisms underlying the antiatherosclerotic and antidiabetic effects of probucol, succinobucol, and other probucol analogues. Curr Opin Lipidol. 2009;20(3):227–35.
120. Preik M, Kelm M, Rosen P, Tschhope D, Strauer BE. Additive effect of coexistent type 2 diabetes and arterial hypertension on endothelial dysfunction in resistance arteries of human forearm vasculature. Angiology. 2000;51(7):545–54.
121. Giacchetti G, Sechi LA, Rilli S, Carey RM. The renin-angiotensin-aldosterone system, glucose metabolism and diabetes. Trends Endocrinol Metab. 2005;16:120–6.
122. de Gasparo M. Angiotensin II and nitric oxide interaction. Heart Fail Rev. 2002;7:347–58.
123. Bijlstra PJ, Smits P, Lutterman JA, Thien T. Effect of long-term angiotensin-converting enzyme inhibition on endothelial function in patients with the insulin-resistance syndrome. J Cardiovasc Pharmacol. 1995;25:658–64.
124. Hermann TS, Li W, Dominguez H, Ihlemann N, Rask-Madsen C, Major-Pedersen A, Nielsen DB, Hansen KW, Hawkins M, Kober L, Torp-Pedersen C. Quinapril treatment increases insulin-stimulated endothelial function and adiponectin gene expression in patients with type 2 diabetes. J Clin Endocrinol Metab. 2006;91:1001–8.
125. Yilmaz MI, Axelsson J, Sonmez A, Carrero JJ, Saglam M, Eyileten T, Caglar K, Kirkpantur A, Celik T, Oguz Y, Vural A, Yenicesu M, Lindholm B, Stenvinkel P. Effect of renin angiotensin system blockade on pentraxin 3 levels in type-2 diabetic patients with proteinuria. Clin J Am Soc Nephrol. 2009;4:535–41.
126. O'Driscoll G, Green D, Maiorana A, Stanton K, Colreavy F, Taylor R. Improvement in endothelial function by angiotensin-converting enzyme inhibition in non-insulin-dependent diabetes mellitus. J Am Coll Cardiol. 1999;33:1506–11.
127. Ceriello A, Assaloni R, Da Ros R, Maier A, Piconi L, Quagliaro L, Esposito K, Giugliano D. Effect of atorvastatin and irbesartan, alone and in combination, on postprandial endothelial dysfunction, oxidative stress, and inflammation in type 2 diabetic patients. Circulation. 2005;111:2518–24.
128. Cheetham C, Collis J, O'Driscoll G, Stanton K, Taylor R, Green D. Losartan, an angiotensin type 1 receptor antagonist, improves endothelial function in

non-insulin-dependent diabetes. J Am Coll Cardiol. 2000;36:1461–6.
129. Cheetham C, O'Driscoll G, Stanton K, Taylor R, Green D. Losartan, an angiotensin type I receptor antagonist, improves conduit vessel endothelial function in Type II diabetes. Clin Sci. 2001;100: 13–7.
130. Flammer AJ, Hermann F, Wiesli P, Schwegler B, Chenevard R, Hurlimann D, Sudano I, Gay S, Neidhart M, Riesen W, Ruschitzka F, Luscher TF, Noll G, Lehmann R. Effect of losartan, compared with atenolol, on endothelial function and oxidative stress in patients with type 2 diabetes and hypertension. J Hypertens. 2007;25:785–91.
131. Davies JI, Band M, Morris A, Struthers AD. Spironolactone impairs endothelial function and heart rate variability in patients with type 2 diabetes. Diabetologia. 2004;47:1687–94.
132. Anderson TJ, Elstein E, Haber H, Charbonneau F. Comparative study of ace-inhibition, angiotensin ii antagonism, and calcium channel blockade on flow-mediated vasodilation in patients with coronary disease (BANFF Study). J Am Coll Cardiol. 2000;35:60–6.
133. Koh KK, Han SH, Ahn JY, Chung W-J, Lee Y, Shin EK. Amlodipine improves endothelial function and metabolic parameters in patients with hypertension. Int J Cardiol. 2009;133:23–31.
134. Oshima T, Ozono R, Yano Y, Higashi Y, Teragawa H, Miho N, Ishida T, Ishida M, Yoshizumi M, Kambe MM. Beneficial effect of t-type calcium channel blockers on endothelial function in patients with essential hypertension. Hypertens Res. 2005;28:889–94.
135. Kim KH, Jeong MH, Cho SH, Moon JY, Hong YJ, Park HW, Kim JH, Ahn Y, Cho JG, Park JC, Kang JC. Clinical effects of calcium channel blocker and angiotensin converting enzyme inhibitor on endothelial function and arterial stiffness in patients with angina pectoris. J Korean Med Sci. 2009;24:223–31.
136. Yilmaz MI, Carrero JJ, Martín-Ventura JL, Sonmez A, Saglam M, Celik T, Yaman H, Yenicesu M, Eyileten T, Moreno JA, Egido J, Blanco-Colio LM. Combined therapy with renin-angiotensin system and calcium channel blockers in type 2 diabetic hypertensive patients with proteinuria: Effects on soluble TWEAK, PTX3, and flow-mediated dilation. Clin J Am Soc Nephrol. 2010;5:1174–81.
137. Lim SC, Tan HH, Goh SK, Subramaniam T, Sum CF, Tan IK, Lee BL, Ong CN. Oxidative burden in prediabetic and diabetic individuals: evidence from plasma coenzyme $Q_{10}$. Diabet Med. 2006;23(12): 1344–9.
138. Villalba JM, Parrado C, Santos-Gonzalez M, Alcain FJ. Therapeutic use of coenzyme $Q_{10}$ and coenzyme $Q_{10}$-related compounds and formulations. Expert Opin Investig Drugs. 2010;19(4):535–54.
139. Watts GF, Playford DA, Croft KD, Ward NC, Mori TA, Burke V. Coenzyme $Q_{10}$ improves endothelial dysfunction of the brachial artery in Type II diabetes mellitus. Diabetologia. 2002;45(3):420–6.
140. Playford DA, Watts GF, Croft KD, Burke V. Combined effect of coenzyme Q10 and fenofibrate on forearm microcirculatory function in type 2 diabetes. Atherosclerosis. 2003;168(1):169–79.
141. Lim SC, Lekshminarayanan R, Goh SK, Ong YY, Subramaniam T, Sum CF, Ong CN, Lee BL. The effect of coenzyme $Q_{10}$ on microcirculatory endothelial function of subjects with type 2 diabetes mellitus. Atherosclerosis. 2008;196(2):966–9.
142. Ting H, Timimi F, Boles D, Creager SJ, Ganz P, Creager MA. Vitamin C improves endothelium-dependent vasodilation in patients with Non-insulin-dependent diabetes mellitus. J Clin Invest. 1996; 97(1):22–8.
143. Heitzer T, Finckh B, Albers S, Krohn K, Kohlschutter AM, Meinertz T. Beneficial effects of [alpha]-lipoic acid and ascorbic acid on endothelium-dependent, nitric oxide-mediated vasodilation in diabetic patients: relation to parameters of oxidative stress. Free Radic Biol Med. 2001;31(1):53–61.
144. Anderson RA, Evans LM, Ellis GR, Khan N, Morris K, Jackson SK, Rees A, Lewis MJ, Frenneaux MP. Prolonged deterioration of endothelial dysfunction in response to postprandial lipaemia is attenuated by vitamin C in Type 2 diabetes. Diabet Med. 2006;23(3):258–64.
145. Antoniades C, Tousoulis D, Tountas C, Tentolouris C, Toutouza M, Vasiliadou C, Tsioufis C, Toutouzas P, Stefanadis C. Vascular endothelium and inflammatory process, in patients with combined Type 2 diabetes mellitus and coronary atherosclerosis: the effects of vitamin C. Diabet Med. 2004;21(6):552–8.
146. Paolisso G, Tagliamonte MR, Barbieri M, Zito GA, Gambardella A, Varricchio G, Ragno E, Varricchio M. Chronic vitamin E administration improves brachial reactivity and increases intracellular magnesium concentration in type II diabetic patients. J Clin Endocrinol Metab. 2000;85(1):109–15.
147. Chowienczyk PJ, Brett SE, Gopaul NK, Meeking D, Mardhetti M, Russell-Jones DL, Anggard EE, Ritter JM. Oral treatment with an antioxidant (raxofelast) reduces oxidative stress and improves endothelial function in men with type II diabetes. Diabetologia. 2000;43(8):974–7.
148. Regensteiner JG, Popylisen S, Bauer TA, Lindenfeld J, Gill E, Smith S, Oliver-Pickett CK, Reusch JEB, Weil JV. Oral L-arginine and vitamins E and C improve endothelial function in women with type 2 diabetes. Vasc Med. 2003;8(3):169–75.
149. Tousoulis D, Antoniades C, Vasiliadou C, Kourtellaris P, Loniari K, Marinou K, Charakida M, Ntarladimas I, Siasos G, Stefanadis C. Effects of atorvastatin and vitamin C on forearm hyperaemic blood flow, asymmentrical dimethylarginine levels and the inflammatory process in patients with type 2 diabetes mellitus. Heart. 2007;93(2):244–6.
150. Darko D, Dornhorst A, Kelly FJ, Ritter JM, Chowienczyk PJ. Lack of effect of oral vitamin C on blood pressure, oxidative stress and endothelial function in Type II diabetes. Clin Sci. 2002;103(4): 339–44.

151. Chen H, Karne RJ, Hall G, Campia U, Panza JA, Cannon RO, Wang Y, Katz A, M L, Quon MJ. High-dose oral vitamin C partially replenishes vitamin C levels in patients with type 2 diabetes and low vitamin C levels but does not improve endothelial dysfunction or insulin resistance. Am J Physiol Heart Circ Physiol. 2006;290(1):H137–45.
152. Gazis A, White DJ, Page SR, Cockcroft JR. Effect of oral vitamin E (alpha-tocopherol) supplementation on vascular endothelial function in Type 2 diabetes mellitus. Diabet Med. 1999;16(4):304–11.
153. Beckman JA, Goldfine AB, Gordon MB, Garrett LA, Keaney JF, Creager MA. Oral antioxidant therapy improves endothelial function in type 1 but not type 2 diabetes mellitus. Am J Physiol Heart Circ Physiol. 2003;285(6):H2392–8.
154. Cordova AC, Jackson LS, Berke-Schlessel DW, Sumpio BE. The cardiovascular protective effect of red wine. J Am Coll Surg. 2005;200(3):428–39.
155. Dell'Agli M, Busciala A, Bosisio E. Vascular effects of wine polyphenols. Cardiovasc Res. 2004;63(4):593–602.
156. Napoli R, Cozzolino D, Guardasole V, Angelini V, Zarra E, Matarazzo M, Cittadini A, Sacca L, Torella R. Red wine consumption improves insulin resistance but not endothelial function in type 2 diabetic patients. Metabolism. 2005;54(3):306–13.
157. Heitzer T, Krohn K, Albers S, Meinertz T. Tetrahydrobiopterin improves endothelium-dependent vasodilation by increasing nitric oxide activity in patients with Type II diabetes mellitus. Diabetologia. 2000;43(11):1435–8.
158. Antoniades C, Shirodaria C, Warrick N, Cai S, de Bono J, Lee J, Leeson P, Neubauer S, Ratnatunga C, Pillai R, Refsum H, Channon KM. 5-Methyltetrahydrofolate rapidly improves endothelial function and decreases superoxide production in human vessels: effects on vascular tetrahydrobiopterin availability and endothelial nitric oxide synthase coupling. Circulation. 2006;114(11):1193–201.
159. van Etten RW, de Koning EJ, Verhaar M, Gaillard C, Rabelink T. Impaired NO-dependent vasodilation in patients with type II (non-insulin-dependent) diabetes mellitus is restored by acute administration of folate. Diabetologia. 2002;45(7):1004–10.
160. Mangoni AA, Sherwood RA, Asonganyi B, Swift CG, Thomas S, Jackson SHD. Short-Term oral folic acid supplementation enhances endothelial function in patients with type 2 diabetes. Am J Hypertens. 2005;18(2):220–6.
161. Title LM, Ur E, Giddens K, McQueen MJ, Nassar BA. Folic acid improves endothelial dysfunction in type 2 diabetes—an effect independent of homocysteine-lowering. Vasc Med. 2006;11(2):101–9.
162. Cyrus D, Akhil P, David L, Donald A, Fonseca VA. Acute and prolonged effects of sildenafil on brachial artery flow-mediated dilatation in type 2 diabetes. Diabetes Care. 2002;25:1336–9.
163. Hulley SM, Grady DM, Bush TP, Furberg CM, Herrington DM, Riggs BM, Vittinghoff EP. Randomized trial of estrogen plus progestin for secondary prevention of coronary heart disease in postmenopausal women. JAMA. 1998;280:605–13.
164. Manson JE, Hsia J, Johnson KC, Rossouw JE, et al. Estrogen plus progestin and the risk of coronary heart disease. N Engl J Med. 2003;349:523–34.
165. Rubanyi GM, Johns A, Kauser K. Effect of estrogen on endothelial function and angiogenesis. Vascul Pharmacol. 2002;38:89–98.
166. Lee SJ, Lee DW, Kim KS, Lee IK. Effect of estrogen on endothelial dysfunction in postmenopausal women with diabetes. Diabetes Res Clin Pract. 2001;54:S81–92.
167. Koh KK, Kang MH, Jin DK, Lee SK, Ahn JY, Hwang HY, Yang SH, Kim DS, Ahn TH, Shin EK. Vascular effects of estrogen in type II diabetic postmenopausal women. J Am Coll Cardiol. 2001;38:1409–15.
168. Silvestri A, Gambacciani M, Vitale C, Monteleone P, Ciaponi M, Fini M, Genazzani AR, Mercuro G, Rosano GMC. Different effect of hormone replacement therapy, DHEAS and tibolone on endothelial function in postmenopausal women with increased cardiovascular risk. Maturitas. 2005;50:305–11.
169. Howes JB, Tran D, Brillante D, Howes LG. Effects of dietary supplementation with isoflavones from red clover on ambulatory blood pressure and endothelial function in postmenopausal type 2 diabetes. Diabetes Obes Metab. 2003;5:325–32.
170. Herman SM, Robinson JTC, McCredie RJ, Adams MR, Boyer MJ, Celermajer DS. Androgen deprivation is associated with enhanced endothelium-dependent dilatation in adult men. Arterioscler Thromb Vasc Biol. 1997;17:2004–9.
171. Zitzmann M, Brune M, Nieschlag E. Vascular reactivity in hypogonadal men is reduced by androgen substitution. J Clin Endocrinol Metabol. 2002;87:5030–7.
172. Karakitsos D, Patrianakos AP, De Groot E, Boletis J, Karabinis A, Kyriazis J, Samonis G, Parthenakis FI, Vardas PE, Daphnis E. Androgen deficiency and endothelial dysfunction in men with end-stage kidney disease receiving maintenance hemodialysis. Am J Nephrol. 2006;26:536–43.
173. Akishita M, Hashimoto M, Ohike Y, Ogawa S, Iijima K, Eto M, Ouchi Y. Low testosterone level is an independent determinant of endothelial dysfunction in men. Hypertens Res. 2007;30:1029–34.
174. Mäkinen JI, Perheentupa A, Irjala K, Pöllänen P, Mäkinen J, Huhtaniemi I, Raitakari OT. Endogenous testosterone and brachial artery endothelial function in middle-aged men with symptoms of late-onset hypogonadism. Aging Male. 2011;14:237–42.
175. Mäkinen JI, Perheentupa A, Irjala K, Pöllänen P, Mäkinen J, Huhtaniemi I, Raitakari OT. Endogenous testosterone and serum lipids in middle-aged men. Atherosclerosis. 2008;197:688–93.

176. Sader MA, Griffiths KA, Skilton MR, Wishart SM, Handelsman DJ, Celermajer DS. Physiological testosterone replacement and arterial endothelial function in men. Clin Endocrinol. 2003;59: 62–7.
177. Kang S-M, Jang Y, Kim J-Y, Chung N, Cho S-Y, Chae JS, Lee J-H. Effect of oral administration of testosterone on brachial arterial vasoreactivity in men with coronary artery disease. Am J Cardiol. 2002;89:862–4.
178. Bilsborough W, O'Driscoll G, Stanton K, Weerasooriya R, Dembo L, Taylor R, Green D. Effect of lowering tumour necrosis factor-alpha on vascular endothelial function in Type II diabetes. Clin Sci. 2002;103:163–9.
179. Butler R, Morris AD, Belch JJF, Hill A, Struthers AD. Allopurinol normalizes endothelial dysfunction in type 2 diabetics with mild hypertension. Hypertension. 2000;35:746–51.
180. Fruchart JC, Sacks F, Hermans MP, Assmann G, for the Residual Risk Reduction initiative, et al. The residual risk reduction initiative: a call to action to reduce residual vascular risk in patients with dyslipidemia. Am J Cardiol. 2008;102(10, Supplement 1): 1K–34.
181. Taskinen R. Diabetic dyslipidaemia: from basic research to clinical practice. Diabetologia. 2003; 46(6):733–49.
182. Watts GF, Karpe F. Triglycerides and atherogenic dyslipidaemia: extending treatment beyond statins in the high-risk cardiovascular patient. Heart. 2011;97(5):350–6.
183. Nordestgaard BGM, Benn MM, Schnohr PM, Tybjaerg-Hansen AMD. Nonfasting triglycerides and risk of myocardial infarction, ischemic heart disease, and death in Men and women. JAMA. 2007;298(3):299–308.
184. Sarwar N, Danesh J, for the Triglyceride Coronary Disease Genetics Consortium and Emerging Risk Factors Collaboration. Triglyceride-mediated pathways and coronary disease: collaborative analysis of 101 studies. Lancet. 2010;375:1634–9.
185. Syvanne M, Taskinen MR. Lipids and lipoproteins as coronary risk factors in non-insulin-dependent diabetes mellitus. Lancet. 1997;350 Suppl 1: SI20–3.
186. Howard BV. Insulin resistance and lipid metabolism. Am J Cardiol. 1999;84(1, Supplement 1):28–32.
187. Adiels M, Boren J, Caslake MJ, Stewart P, Soro A, Westerbacka J, Wennberg B, Olofsson SO, Packard C, Taskinen MR. Overproduction of VLDL1 driven by hyperglycemia is a dominant feature of diabetic dyslipidemia. Arterioscler Thromb Vasc Biol. 2005;25(8):1697–703.
188. Adiels M, Taskinen MR, Packard C, Caslake MJ, Soro-Paavonen A, Westerbacka J, Vehkavaara S, Hakkinen A, Olofsson S, Yki-Jarvinen H, Boren J. Overproduction of large VLDL particles is driven by increased liver fat content in man. Diabetologia. 2006;49(4):755–65.
189. Cummings MH, Watts GF, Umpleby AM, Hennessy TR, Kelly JM, Jackson NC, Sonksen PH. Acute hyperinsulinemia decreases the hepatic secretion of very-low-density lipoprotein apolipoprotein B-100 in NIDDM. Diabetes. 1995;44(9):1059–65.
190. Malmstrom R, Packard CJ, Caslake M, Bedford D, Stewart P, Yki-Jarvinen H, Shepherd J, Taskinen MR. Defective regulation of triglyceride metabolism by insulin in the liver in NIDDM. Diabetologia. 1997;40(4):454–62.
191. Adiels M, Westerbacka J, Soro-Paavonen A, Hakkinen AM, Vehkavaara S, Caslake MJ, Packard C, Olofsson SO, Yki-Jarvinen H, Taskinen MR, Boren J. Acute suppression of VLDL1 secretion rate by insulin is associated with hepatic fat content and insulin resistance. Diabetologia. 2007;50(11):2356–65.
192. Chan DC, Watts GF. Dyslipidaemia in the metabolic syndrome and type 2 diabetes: pathogenesis, priorities, pharmacotherapies. Expert Opin Pharmacother. 2011;12(1):13–30.
193. De Man FHAF, Castro Cabezas M, Van Barlingen HHJJ, Erkelens DW, de Bruin TWA. Triglyceride-rich lipoproteins in non-insulin-dependent diabetes mellitus: post-prandial metabolism and relation to premature atherosclerosis. Eur J Clin Invest. 1996;26(2):89–108.
194. Watts GF, Mandalia S, Brunt JNH, Slavin BM, Coltart DJ, Lewis B. Independent associations between plasma lipoprotein subfraction levels and the course of coronary artery disease in the St. Thomas' Atherosclerosis Regression Study (STARS). Metabolism. 1993;42(11):1461–7.
195. Anber V, Griffin BA, McConnell M, Packard CJ, Shepherd J. Influence of plasma lipid and LDL-subfraction profile on the interaction between low density lipoprotein with human arterial wall proteoglycans. Atherosclerosis. 1996;124(2):261–71.
196. Syvanne M, Kahri J, Virtanen KS, Taskinen MR. Coronary heart disease/myocardial infarction/systemic vascular responses: HDLs containing apolipoproteins a-I and a-II (LpA-I: a-II) as markers of coronary artery disease in Men with Non-insulin-dependent diabetes mellitus. Circulation. 1995;92(3):364–70.
197. Syvanne M, Castro G, Dengremont C, De Geitere C, Jauhiaine M, Ehnholm C, Michelagnoli S, Franceschini G, Kahri J, Taskinen MR. Cholesterol efflux from Fu5AH hepatoma cells induced by plasma of subjects with or without coronary artery disease and non-insulin-dependent diabetes: importance of LpA-I:A-II particles and phospholipid transfer protein. Atherosclerosis. 1996;127(2):245–53.
198. Nofer JR, Kehrel B, Fobker M, Levkau B, Assmann G, von Eckardstein A. HDL and arteriosclerosis: beyond reverse cholesterol transport. Atherosclerosis. 2002;161(1):1–16.
199. Persegol L, Verges B, Foissac M, Gambert P, Duvillard L. Inability of HDL from type 2 diabetic patients to counteract the inhibitory effect of oxidised LDL on endothelium-dependent vasorelaxation. Diabetologia. 2006;49(6):1380–6.

200. Wilson DE, Hata A, Kwong LK, Lingam A, Shuhua J, Ridinger DN, Yeager C, Kaltenborn KC, Iverius PH, Lalouel JM. Mutations in exon 3 of the lipoprotein lipase gene segregating in a family with hypertriglyceridemia, pancreatitis, and Non-insulin-dependent diabetes. J Clin Invest. 1993;92(1):203–11.
201. Laakso M, Kesañniemi A, Kervinen K, Jauhiainen M, Pyorala K. Relation of coronary heart disease and apolipoprotein E phenotype in patients with non-insulin dependent diabetes. BMJ. 1991;303(6811):1159–62.
202. Li WW, Dammerman MM, Smith JD, Metzger S, Breslow JL, Leff T. Common genetic variation in the promoter of the human apo CIII gene abolishes regulation by insulin and May contribute to hypertriglyceridemia. J Clin Invest. 1995;96(6):2601–5.
203. Rigoli L, Raimondo G, Di Benedetto A, Romano G, Porcellini A, Campo S, Corica F, Riccardi G, Squadrito G, Cucinotta D. Apolipoprotein AI-CIII-AIV genetic polymorphisms and coronary heart disease in type 2 diabetes mellitus. Acta Diabetol. 1995;32(4):251–6.
204. Ukkola O, Savolainen MJ, Salmela PI, von Dickhoff K, Kesañniemi YA. DNA polymorphisms at the locus for human cholesteryl ester transfer protein (CETP) are associated with macro- and microangiopathy in non-insulin-dependent diabetes mellitus. Clin Genet. 1994;46(3):217–27.
205. American Diabetes Association. Standards of medical care in diabetes-2010. Diabetes Care. 2010;33:S11–61.
206. Third Report of the National Cholesterol Education Program (NCEP) Expert Panel on Detection. Evaluation, and treatment of high blood cholesterol in adults (adult treatment panel III) final report. Circulation. 2002;106(25):3143–421.
207. Fujioka K. Benefits of moderate weight loss in patients with type 2 diabetes. Diabetes Obes Metab. 2010;12(3):186–94.
208. Pi-Sunyer X, Blackburn G, Brancati F, Bray G, Bright R, Clarke J. Reduction in weight and cardiovascular disease risk factors in individuals with type 2 diabetes. Diabetes Care. 2007;30(6):1374–83.
209. Wing R, Bahnson JL, Bray GA, Clark JM, for The Look AHEAD Research Group, et al. Long-term effects of a lifestyle intervention on weight and cardiovascular risk factors in individuals with type 2 diabetes mellitus: four-year results of the look AHEAD trial. Arch Intern Med. 2010;170(17):1566–75.
210. Alam S, Stolinski M, Pentecost C, Boroujerdi MA, Jones RH, Sonksen PH, Umpleby M. The effect of a six-month exercise program on very Low-density lipoprotein apolipoprotein B secretion in type 2 diabetes. J Clin Endocrinol Metab. 2004;89(2):688–94.
211. Deedwania P, Barter P, Carmena R, Fruchart JC, Grundy SM, Haffner S, Lastelein JJP, La Rosa JC, Schachner H, Shepherd J, Waters DD. Reduction of low-density lipoprotein cholesterol in patients with coronary heart disease and metabolic syndrome: analysis of the treating to New targets study. Lancet. 2006;368:919–28.
212. The Diabetes Atorvastin Lipid Intervention (DALI) Study Group. The effect of aggressive versus standard lipid lowering by atovastatin on diabetic dyslipidemia: the DALI study: a double-blind, randomized, placebo-controlled trial in. Diabetes Care. 2001;24(8):1335–41.
213. Isley WL, Miles JM, Patterson BW, Harris WS. The effect of high-dose simvastatin on triglyceride-rich lipoprotein metabolism in patients with type 2 diabetes mellitus. J Lipid Res. 2006;47(1):193–200.
214. Pontrelli L, Parris W, Adeli K, Cheung RC. Atorvastatin treatment beneficially alters the lipoprotein profile and increases low-density lipoprotein particle diameter in patients with combined dyslipidemia and impaired fasting glucose/type 2 diabetes. Metabolism. 2002;51(3):334–42.
215. Stein EA, Lane M, Laskarzewski P. Comparison of statins in hypertriglyceridemia. Am J Cardiol. 1998;81(4, Supplement 1):66B–9.
216. Stein E, Plotkin D, Bays H, Davidson M, Dujovne C, Korenman S, Stepanavage M, Mercuri M. Effects of simvastatin (40 and 80 mg/day) in patients with mixed hyperlipidemia. Am J Cardiol. 2000;86(4): 406–11.
217. Miller M, Cannon CP, Murphy SA, Qin J, Ray KK, Braunwald E. Impact of triglyceride levels beyond Low-density lipoprotein cholesterol after acute coronary syndrome in the PROVE IT-TIMI 22 trial. J Am Coll Cardiol. 2008;7:724–30.
218. Verges B, Florentin E, Baillot-Rudoni S, Monier S, Petit JM, Rageot D, Gambert P, Duvillard L. Effects of 20 mg rosuvastatin on VLDL1-, VLDL2-, IDL- and LDL-ApoB kinetics in type 2 diabetes. Diabetologia. 2008;51(8):1382–90.
219. Jun M, Foote C, Lv J, Neal B, Patel AM, Nicholls SJ, Grobbee DE, Cass A, Chalmers J, Perkovic V. Effects of fibrates on cardiovascular outcomes: a systematic review and meta-analysis. Lancet. 2010;375:1875–84.
220. Koskinen P, Manttari M, Manninen V, Huttunen JK, Heinonen OP, Frick MH. Coronary heart disease incidence in NIDDM patients in the Helsinki heart study. Diabetes Care. 1992;15(7):820–5.
221. Scott R, O'Brien R, Fulcher G, Pardy C, D'Emden M, Tse D, Taskinen MR, Ehnholm C, Keech A, on behalf of the Fenofibrate Intervention and Event Lowering in Diabetes (FIELD) Study Investigators. Effects of fenofibrate treatment On cardiovascular disease risk in 9,795 individuals with type 2 diabetes and various components of the metabolic syndrome. Diabetes Care. 2009;32(3):493–8.
222. Ginsberg HN, Elam MB, Lovato LC, for the ACCORD Study Group, et al. Effects of combination lipid therapy in type 2 diabetes mellitus. N Engl J Med. 2010;362(17):1563–74.
223. Karpe F, Frayn KN. The nicotinic acid receptor-a new mechanism for an old drug. Lancet. 2004;363:1892–4.
224. Shepherd J, Betteridge J, Van Gaal L. Nicotinic acid in the management of dyslipidaemia associated with diabetes and metabolic syndrome: a position paper

developed by a European Consensus Panel. Curr Med Res Opin. 2005;21(5):665–82.
225. Helen V. Niacin: a re-emerging pharmaceutical for the treatment of dyslipidaemia. Brit J Pharmacol. 2009;158:429–41.
226. Tunaru S, Kero J, Schaub A, Wufka C, Blaukat A, Pfeffer K, Offermanns S. PUMA-G and HM74 are receptors for nicotinic acid and mediate its anti-lipolytic effect. Nat Med. 2003;9(3):352–5.
227. Wise A, Foord SM, Fraser NJ, Barnes-Ashley A, Elshourbagy N, Eilert M, Ignar DM, Murdock PR, Steplewski K, Green A, Brown AJ, Sowell SJ, Szekeres PG, Hassall DG, Marshall FH, Wilson S, Pike NB. Molecular identification of high and Low affinity receptors for nicotinic acid. J Biol Chem. 2003;278(11):9869–74.
228. Soga T, Kamohara M, Takasaki J, Matsumoto S, Saito T, Ohishi TM, Hiyama H, Matsuo AM, Matsushime H, Furuichi K. Molecular identification of nicotinic acid receptor. Biochem Biophys Res Commun. 2003;303(1):364–9.
229. Tunaru S, Lattig J, Kero J, Krause G, Offermanns S. Characterization of determinants of ligand binding to the nicotinic acid receptor GPR109A (HM74A/PUMA-G). Mol Pharmacol. 2005;68(5):1271–80.
230. van der Hoorn JWA, de Haan W, Berbee JFP, Havekes LM, Jukema JW, Rensen PCN, Princen HMG. Niacin increases HDL by reducing hepatic expression and plasma levels of cholesteryl ester transfer protein in APOE*3Leiden. CETP mice. Arterioscler Thromb Vasc Biol. 2008;28(11):2016–22.
231. Watts GF, Chan DC. Mechanisms for therapeutic correction of dyslipidaemia in insulin resistance and diabetes. Atheroscler Suppl. 2010;11(1):61–4.
232. Ganji SH, Tavintharan S, Zhu D, Xing Y, Kamanna VS, Kashyap ML. Niacin noncompetitively inhibits DGAT2 but not DGAT1 activity in HepG2 cells. J Lipid Res. 2004;45(10):1835–45.
233. Guyton JR. Extended-release niacin for modifying the lipoprotein profile. Expert Opin Pharmacother. 2004;5(6):1385–98.
234. Kamanna VS, Kashyap ML. Mechanism of action of niacin on lipoprotein metabolism. Curr Atheroscler Rep. 2000;2(1):36–46.
235. Berge KG, Canner PL. Coronary drug project: experience with niacin. Eur J Clin Pharmacol. 1991;40(1):S49–51.
236. Canner PL, Berge KG, Wenger NK, Stamler J, Friedman L, Prineas R, Friedewald W. Fifteen year mortality in coronary drug project patients: long-term benefit with niacin. J Am Coll Cardiol. 1986;8(6):1245–55.
237. Chapman MJ, Redfern JS, McGovern ME, Giral P. Niacin and fibrates in atherogenic dyslipidemia: pharmacotherapy to reduce cardiovascular risk. Pharmacol Ther. 2010;126(3):314–45.
238. Canner PL, Furberg CD, Terrin ML, McGovern ME. Benefits of niacin by glycemic status in patients with healed myocardial infarction (from the coronary drug project). Am J Cardiol. 2005;95(2):254–7.
239. Canner PL, Furberg CD, McGovern ME. Benefits of niacin in patients with versus without the metabolic syndrome and healed myocardial infarction (from the coronary drug project). Am J Cardiol. 2006;97(4):477–9.
240. Brown BG, Zhao XQ, Chait A, Fisher LD, Cheung MC, Morse JS, Dowdy AA, Marino MS, Bolson EL, Alaupovic P, Frohlich J, Albers JJ. Simvastatin and niacin, antioxidant vitamins, or the combination for the prevention of coronary disease. N Engl J Med. 2001;345(22):1583–92.
241. Taylor AJ, Sullenberger LE, Lee HJ, Lee JK, Grace KA. Arterial biology for the investigation of the treatment effects of reducing cholesterol (ARBITER) 2: a double-blind, placebo-controlled study of extended-release niacin on atherosclerosis progression in secondary prevention patients treated with statins. Circulation. 2004;110(23):3512–7.
242. Taylor A, Lee H, Sullenberger LE. The effect of 24 months of combination statin and extended-release niacin on carotid intima-media thickness: ARBITER 3. Curr Med Res Opin. 2006;22(11):2243–50.
243. Taylor AJ, Villines TC, Stanek EJ, Devine PJ, Griffen L, Miklller M, Weissman NJ, Turco M. Extended-release niacin or ezetimibe and carotid intima-media thickness. N Engl J Med. 2009; 361(22):2113–22.
244. Boden WE, Probstfield JK, Anderson T, Chaitman BR, Koprowicz K, Teo K, Weintraub W. Niacin in patients with low HDL cholesterol levels receiving intensive statin therapy. New Engl J Med. 2011;365: 2255–67.
245. Heart Protection Study-2 and the Treatment of HDL to reduce the incidence of vascular events (HPS2-THRIVE) (http://clinical trials.gov). Accessed 20 Jan 2010.
246. GISSI-Prevenzionne Investigators. Dietary supplementation with n-3 polyunsaturated fatty acids and vitamin E after myocardial infarction: results of the GISSI-prevenzione trial. Lancet. 1999;354(9177):447–55.
247. Yokoyama M, Origasa H, Matsuzaki M, Matsuzawa Y, Saito Y, Ishidawa Y, Oikawa S, Sasaki J, Hishida H, Itakura H, Kita T, Kitabatake A, Nakaya N, Sakata T, Shimada K, Shirato K, for the Janan EPA lipid interventi study (JELIS) Investigators. Effects of eicosapentaenoic acid on major coronary events in hypercholesterolaemic patients (JELIS): a randomised open-label, blinded endpoint analysis. Lancet. 2007;369:1090–8.
248. Saravanan P, Davidson NC, Schmidt EB, Calder PC. Cardiovascular effects of marine omega-3 fatty acids. Lancet. 2010;376:540–50.
249. Brousseau ME, Diffenderfer MR, Millar JS, Nartsupha C, Asztalos BF, Welty FK, Wolfe ML, Rudling M, Bjorkhem I, Angelin B, Mancuso JP, Digenio AG, Rader DJ, Schaefer EJ. Effects of cholesteryl ester transfer protein inhibition on high-density lipoprotein subspecies, apolipoprotein A-1 metabolism, and fecal sterol excretion. Arterioscler Thromb Vas Biol. 2005;25:1057–64.

250. Millar JS, Brousseau ME, Diffenderfer MR, Barrett PHR, Welty FK, Faruqi A, Wolfe ML, Nartsupha C, Digenio AG, Mancuso JP, Dolnikowski GG, Schaefer EJ, Rader DJ. Effects of the cholesteryl ester transfer protein inhibitor torcetrapib on apolipoprotein B100 metabolism in humans. Arterioscler Thromb Vas Biol. 2006;26:1350–6.
251. Stalenhoef AFH, Davidson MH, Robinson JG, Burgess T, Duttlinger-Maddux R, Kallend D, Goldberg AC, Bays H. Efficacy and safety of dalcetrapib in type 2 diabetes mellitus and/or metabolic syndrome patients, at high cardiovascular disease risk. Diabetes Obes Metab. 2012;14:30–9.
252. Fayad ZA, Mani V, Woodward M, Kallend D, Abt M, Burgess T, Fuster V, Ballantyne CM, Stein EA, Tardif J-C, Rudd JHF, Farkouh ME, Tawakol A. Safety and efficacy of dalcetrapib on atherosclerotic disease using novel non-invasive multimodality imaging (dal-PLAQUE): A randomised clinical trial. Lancet. 2011;378:1547–59.
253. Collins R, Armitage J, Parish S, Sleigh P, Peto R. MRC/BHF heart protection study of cholesterol-lowering with simvastatin in 5963 people with diabetes: a randomised placebo-controlled trial. Lancet. 2003;361:2005–16.
254. Stroes ESG, Koomans HA, de Bruin TWA, Rabelink TJ. Vascular function in the forearm of hypercholesterolaemic patients off and on lipid-lowering medication. Lancet. 1995;346(8973):467–71.
255. O'Driscoll GMBB, Green DP, Taylor RRM. Simvastatin, an HMG-coenzyme a reductase inhibitor, improves endothelial function within 1 month. Circulation. 1997;95(5):1126–31.
256. van de Ree MA, Huisman MV, de Man FH, van der Vijver JC, Meinders AE, Blauw GJ. Impaired endothelium-dependent vasodilation in type 2 diabetes mellitus and the lack of effect of simvastatin. Cardiovasc Res. 2001;52(2):299–305.
257. van Etten RW, de Koning EJ, Honing ML, Stroes ES, Gaillard CA, Rabelink TJ. Intensive lipid lowering by statin therapy does not improve vasoreactivity in patients with type 2 diabetes. Arterioscler Thromb Vasc Biol. 2002;22(5):799–804.
258. Sheu WH, Juang BL, Chen YT, Lee WJ. Endothelial dysfunction is not reversed by simvastatin treatment in type 2 diabetic patients with hypercholesterolemia. Diabetes Care. 1999;22(7):1224–5.
259. Sheu WH-H, Chen YT, Lee WJ. Improvement in endothelial dysfunction with LDL cholesterol level <80 mg/dl in type 2 diabetic patients. Diabetes Care. 2001;24(8):1499–501.
260. Tsunekawa T, Hayashi T, Kano H, Sumi D, Matsui-Hirai H, Thakur NK, Egashira K, Iguchi A. Cerivastatin, a hydroxymethylglutaryl coenzyme a reductase inhibitor, improves endothelial function in elderly diabetic patients within 3 days. Circulation. 2001;104(4):376–9.
261. Tan KCB, Chow WS, Tam SCF, Ai VHG, Lam CHL, Lam KSL. Atorvastatin lowers C-reactive protein and improves endothelium-dependent vasodilation in type 2 diabetes mellitus. J Clin Endocrinol Metab. 2002;87(2):563–8.
262. Ceriello AM, Taboga CM, Tonutti LM, Quagliaro L, Piconi L, Bais B, Da Ros R, Motz E. Evidence for an independent and cumulative effect of postprandial hypertriglyceridemia and hyperglycemia on endothelial dysfunction and oxidative stress generation: effects of short- and long-term simvastatin treatment. Circulation. 2002;106(10):1211–8.
263. Dalla N, Passaro A, Zamboni PF, Calzoni F, Fellin R, Solini A. Atorvastatin improves metabolic control and endothelial function in type 2 diabetic patients: a placebo-controlled study. J Endocrinol Invest. 2003;26(1):73–8.
264. Rawlings R, Nohria A, Liu PY, Donnelly J, Creager MA, Ganz P, Selwyn A, Lial JK. Comparison of effects of rosuvastatin (10 mg) versus atorvastatin (40 mg) on Rho kinase activity in Caucasian Men with a previous atherosclerotic event. Am J Cardiol. 2009;103(4):437–41.
265. Brunetti ND, Maulucci G, Casavecchia GP, Distaso C, De Gennaro L, Pellegrino PL, Di Biase M. Improvement in endothelium dysfunction in diabetics treated with statins: a randomized comparison of atorvastatin 20 mg versus rosuvastatin 10 mg. J Interv Cardiol. 2007;20(6):481–7.
266. Adel A, Abdel-Salam Z, Nammas W. Low-dose statin therapy improves endothelial function in type 2 diabetic patients with normal serum total cholesterol: a randomized placebo-controlled study. J Clin Hypertens. 2010;12(10):820–5.
267. Economides PA, Caselli A, Tiani E, Khaodhiar L, Horton ES, Veves A. The effects of atorvastatin on endothelial function in diabetic patients and subjects at risk for type 2 diabetes. J Clin Endocrinol Metab. 2004;89(2):740–7.
268. Beishuizen ED, Tamsma JT, Jukema JW, van de Ree MA, van der Vijver JCM, Meinders AE, Huisman MV. The effect of statin therapy on endothelial function in type 2 diabetes without manifest cardiovascular disease. Diabetes Care. 2005;28(7):1668–74.
269. van Venrooij FV, van de Ree MA, Bots ML, Stolk RP, Huisman MV, Banga JD, on behalf of the DALI Study Group. Aggressive lipid lowering does Not improve endothelial function in type 2 diabetes: the diabetes atorvastatin lipid intervention (DALI) study: a randomized, double-blind, placebo-controlled trial. Diabetes Care. 2002;25(7):1211–6.
270. Balletshofer BM, Goebbel S, Rittig K, Enderle M, Schmelzer I, Wascher TC, Ferenc PA, Westermeier T, Petzinna D, Matthaei S, Hering HU. Intense cholesterol lowering therapy with a HMG-CoA reductase inhibitor does not improve nitric oxide dependent endothelial function in type-2-diabetes. Exp Clin Endocrinol Diabetes. 2005;6:324–30.
271. Tantikosoom W, Thinkhamrop B, Kiatchusakul S, Jarernsiripornkul N, Srinakarin J, Ojaongpian S. Randomized trial of atorvastatin in improving

endothelial function in diabetics without prior coronary disease and having average cholesterol level. J Med Assoc Thai. 2005;88(3):399–406.
272. Tran D, Lowy A, Howes JB, Howes LG. Effects of cerivastatin on forearm vascular responses, blood pressure responsiveness and ambulatory blood pressure in type 2 diabetic men. Diabetes Obes Metab. 2005;7(3):273–81.
273. Chan D. Regulation of proprotein convertase subtilisin/kexin type 9: Therapeutical perspectives. Atherosclerosis. 2011;217(1):77–9.
274. Ronald G. Improving glycemic and cholesterol control through an integrated approach incorporating colesevelam—a clinical perspective. Diabetes Metab Syndr Obes. 2009;2:11–21.
275. Fonseca VA, Handelsman Y, Staels B. Colesevelam lowers glucose and lipid levels in type 2 diabetes: the clinical evidence. Diabetes Obes Metab. 2010;12(5):384–92.
276. Akdim F, Visser ME, Tribble DL, Baker BF, Stroes ES, Yu R, Flaim JD, Su J, Stein EA, Kastelein JJ. Effect of mipomersen, an apolipoprotein B synthesis inhibitor, on Low-density lipoprotein cholesterol in patients with familial hypercholesterolemia. Am J Cardiol. 2010;105(10):1413–9.
277. Raal FJ, Santos RD, Blom DJ, Marais AD, Charng M-J, Cromwell WC, Lachmann RH, Gaudet D, Tan JL, Chasan-Taber S, Tribble DL, Flaim JD, Crooke ST. Mipomersen, an apolipoprotein b synthesis inhibitor, for lowering of ldl cholesterol concentrations in patients with homozygous familial hypercholesterolaemia: a randomised, double-blind, placebo-controlled trial. Lancet. 2010;375:998–1006.
278. Bell DA, Hooper AJ, Burnett JR. Mipomersen, an antisense apolipoprotein B synthesis inhibitor. Expert Opin Investig Drugs. 2011;20(2):265–72.
279. Malik J, Melenovsky V, Wichterle D, Haas T, Simek J, Ceska R, Hradec J. Both fenofibrate and atorvastatin improve vascular reactivity in combined hyperlipidaemia (fenofibrate versus atorvastatin trial–FAT). Cardiovasc Res. 2001;52(2):290–8.
280. Koh KK, Han SH, Quon MJ, Yeal Ahn J, Shin EK. Beneficial effects of fenofibrate to improve endothelial dysfunction and raise adiponectin levels in patients with primary hypertriglyceridemia. Diabetes Care. 2005;28(6):1419–24.
281. Playford DA, Watts GF, Best JD, Burke V. Effect of fenofibrate on brachial artery flow-mediated dilatation in type 2 diabetes mellitus. Am J Cardiol. 2002;90(11):1254–7.
282. Chew GT, Watts GF, Davis TME, Stuckey BGA, Beilin LJ, Thompson PL, Burke V, Currie PJ. Hemodynamic effects of fenofibrate and coenzyme $Q_{10}$ in type 2 diabetic subjects with left ventricular diastolic dysfunction. Diabetes Care. 2008;31(8):1502–9.
283. Evans M, Anderson RA, Graham J, Ellis GR, Morris K, Davies S, Jackson SK, Lewis MJ, Frenneaux MP, Rees A. Ciprofibrate therapy improves endothelial function and reduces postprandial lipemia and oxidative stress in type 2 diabetes mellitus. Circulation. 2000;101(15):1773–9.
284. Avogaro A, Miola M, Favaro A, Gottardo L, Pacini G, Manzato M, Zambon S, Sacerdoti D, Sacerdoti D, de Kreutzenberg S, Pillego T, Tiengo A, Del Prato S. Gemfibrozil improves insulin sensitivity and flow-mediated vasodilatation in type 2 diabetic patients. Eur J Clin Invest. 2001;31(7):603–9.
285. Fegan PG, Shore AC, Mawson D, Tooke JE, MacLeod KM. Microvascular endothelial function in subjects with type 2 diabetes and the effect of lipid-lowering therapy. Diabet Med. 2005; 22(12):1670–6.
286. Hiukka A, Westerbacka J, Leinonen ES, Watanabe H, Wiklund O, Hulten LM, Salonen JT, Tuomainen TP, Yki-Jarvinen H, Keech AC, Taskinen MR. Long-term effects of fenofibrate on carotid intima-media thickness and augmentation index in subjects with type 2 diabetes mellitus. J Am Coll Cardiol. 2008;52(25):2190–7.
287. Keech AC, Mitchell P, Summanen PA, O'Day J, Davis TME, Moffitt MS, Taskinen MR, Simes RJ, Tse D, Williamson E, Merrifield A, Laatikainen LT, d'Emden MC, O'Connell RL, Colman PG, for the FIELD study investigators. Effect of fenofibrate on the need for laser treatment for diabetic retinopathy (FIELD study): a randomised controlled trial. Lancet. 2007;370(9600):1687–97.
288. Davis T, Ting R, Best J, Donoghoe MW, Drury PL, Sullivan DR, Jenkins AJ, O'Connell RL, Whiting MJ, Glaziou PP, Simes RJ, Kesaniemi YA, Gebski VJ, Scott RS, Keech AC, on behalf of the FIELD Investigators. Effects of fenofibrate on renal function in patients with type 2 diabetes mellitus: the Fenofibrate Intervention and Event Lowering in Diabetes (FIELD) Study. Diabetologia. 2011;54(2):280–90.
289. Ismail-Beigi F, Craven T, Banerji MA, Basile J, for the ACCORD Trial Group, et al. Effect of intensive treatment of hyperglycaemia on microvascular outcomes in type 2 diabetes: an analysis of the ACCORD randomised trial. Lancet. 2010;376(9739):419–30.
290. Chew E, Ambrosius W, Davis M, Danis RP, for the ACCORD Study Group and the ACCORD Eye Study Group, et al. Effects of medical therapies on retinopathy progression in type 2 diabetes. N Engl J Med. 2010;363(3):233–44.
291. Benjo AM, Maranhao RC, Coimbra SR, Andrade ACM, Favarato D, Molina MS, Brandizzi LIV, da Luz PL. Accumulation of chylomicron remnants and impaired vascular reactivity occur in subjects with isolated low HDL cholesterol: effects of niacin treatment. Atherosclerosis. 2006;187(1):116–22.
292. Thoenes M, Oguchi A, Nagamia S, Vaccari CS, Hammoud R, Umpierrex GE, Khan BV. The effects of extended-release niacin on carotid intimal media thickness, endothelial function and inflammatory markers in patients with the metabolic syndrome. Int J Clin Pract. 2007;61(11):1942–8.

293. Mori TA, Woodman RJ. The independent effects of eicosapentaenoic acid and docosahexaenoic acid on cardiovascular risk factors in humans. Curr Opin Clin Nutr Metab Care. 2006;9(2):95–104.
294. McVeigh GE, Brennan GM, Johnston GD, McDermott BJ, McGrath LT, Henry WR, Andrews JW, Hayes JR. Dietary fish oil augments nitric oxide production or release in patients with Type 2 (non-insulin-dependent) diabetes mellitus. Diabetologia. 1993;36(1):33–8.
295. Woodman RJ, Mori TA, Burke V, Puddey IB, Watts GF, Beilin LJ. Effects of purified eicosapentaenoic acid and docosahexaenoic acid on platelet, fibrinolytic and vascular function in hypertensive type 2 diabetic patients. Atherosclerosis. 2003;166(1):85–93.
296. West SG, Hecker KD, Mustad VA, Nicholson S, Schoemer SL, Wagner P, Hinderliter AL, Ulbrecht J, Ruey P, Kris-Etherton PM. Acute effects of monounsaturated fatty acids with and without omega-3 fatty acids on vascular reactivity in individuals with type 2 diabetes. Diabetologia. 2005;48(1):113–22.
297. Hilpert KF, West SG, Kris-Etherton PM, Hecker KD, Sompson NM, Alaupovic P. Postprandial effect of n-3 polyunsaturated fatty acids on apolipoprotein B-containing lipoproteins and vascular reactivity in type 2 diabetes. Am J Clin Nutr. 2007;85(2): 369–76.
298. Mori TA, Watts GF, Burke V, Hilme E, Puddey I, Beilin LJ. Differential effects of eicosapentaenoic acid and docosahexaenoic acid on vascular reactivity of the forearm microcirculation in hyperlipidemic, overweight men. Circulation. 2000;102(11):1264–9.
299. Parthasarathy S, Young SG, Witztum JL, Pittman RC, Steinberg D. Probucol inhibits oxidative modification of low density lipoprotein. J Clin Invest. 1986;77:641–4.
300. Yokoi H, Daida H, Kuwabara Y, Nishikawa H, Takatsu F, Tomihara H, Nakata Y, Kutsumi Y, Ohshima S, Nishiyama S, Seki A, Kato K, Nishimura S, Kanoh T, Yamaguchi H. Effectiveness of an antioxidant in preventing restenosis after percutaneous transluminal coronary angioplasty: The probucol angioplasty restenosis trial. J Am Coll Cardiol. 1997;30:855–62.
301. Sawayama Y, Shimizu C, Maeda N, Tatsukawa M, Kinukawa N, Koyanagi S, Kashiwagi S, Hayashi J. Effects of probucol and pravastatin on common carotid atherosclerosis in patients with asymptomatic hypercholesterolemia: Fukuoka atherosclerosis trial (FAST). J Am Coll Cardiol. 2002;39:610–6.
302. Endo K, Miyashita Y, Sasaki H, Ebisuno M, Ohira M, Saiki A, Koide N, Oyama T, Takeyoshi M, Shirai K. Probucol and atorvastatin decrease urinary 8-hydroxy-2′-deoxyguanosine in patients with diabetes and hypercholesterolemia. J Atheroscler Thromb. 2006;13:68–75.
303. Colhoun PH, Betteridge PDJ, Durrington PP, Hitman GA, Neil HAW, Livingstone SJ, Thason MJ, Mackness MI, Charlton-Menys V, Fuller JH, on behalf of the CARDS Investigators. Primary prevention of cardiovascular disease with atorvastatin in type 2 diabetes in the collaborative atorvastatin diabetes study (CARDS): multicentre randomised placebo-controlled trial. Lancet. 2004;364(9435):685–96.
304. Shepherd J, Barter P, Camena R, Deedwania P, Fruchart JC, Haffner S, Hsia J, Breazna A, LaRosa J, Grundy S, Waters D, for the Treating to New Targets Investigators. Effect of lowering LDL cholesterol substantially below currently recommended levels in patients with coronary heart disease and diabetes: the treating to New targets (TNT) study. Diabetes Care. 2006;29(6):1220–6.
305. Kearney PM, Blackwell L, Collins R, for the Cholesterol Treatment Trialists (CTT) Collaborators, et al. Efficacy of cholesterol-lowering therapy in 18,686 people with diabetes in 14 randomised trials of statins: a meta-analysis. Lancet. 2008;371(9607): 117–25.
306. Athyros VG, Papageorgiou AA, Athyrou VV, Demitriadis DS, Kontopoulos AG. Atorvastatin and micronized fenofibrate alone and in combination in type 2 diabetes with combined hyperlipidemia. Diabetes Care. 2002;25(7):1198–202.
307. Durrington PN, Tuomilehto J, Hamann A, Kallend D, Smith K. Rosuvastatin and fenofibrate alone and in combination in type 2 diabetes patients with combined hyperlipidaemia. Diabetes Res Clin Pract. 2004;64(2):137–51.
308. Gavish D, Leibovitz E, Shapira I, Rubinstein A. Bezafibrate and simvastatin combination therapy for diabetic dyslipidaemia: efficacy and safety. J Intern Med. 2000;247(5):563–9.
309. Derosa G, Cicero AEG, Bertone G, Piccinni MN, Ciccarelli L, Roggeri DE. Comparison of fluvastatin + fenofibrate combination therapy and fluvastatin monotherapy in the treatment of combined hyperlipidemia, type 2 diabetes mellitus, and coronary heart disease: a 12-month, randomized, double-blind, controlled trial. Clin Ther. 2004;26(10):1599–607.
310. Hamilton SJ, Chew GT, Davis TME, Watts GF. Fenofibrate improves endothelial function in the brachial artery and forearm resistance arterioles of statin-treated type 2 diabetic patients. Clin Sci. 2010;118(10):607–15.
311. Muhlestein JB, May HT, Jensen JR, Horne BD, Lanman RB, Lavasani F, Wolfert RL, Pearson RR, Yannicelli HD, Anderson JL. The reduction of inflammatory biomarkers by statin, fibrate, and combination therapy among diabetic patients with mixed dyslipidemia: the DIACOR (diabetes and combined lipid therapy regimen) study. J Am Coll Cardiol. 2006;48(2):396–401.
312. Van JT, Pan J, Wasty T, Chan E, Wu X, Charles MA. Comparison of extended-release niacin and atorvastatin monotherapies and combination treatment of the atherogenic lipid profile in diabetes mellitus. Am J Cardiol. 2002;89(11):1306–8.
313. Kuvin JT, Ramet ME, Patel AR, Pandian NG, Mendelsohn ME, Karas RH. A novel mechanism for the beneficial vascular effects of high-density

lipoprotein cholesterol: Enhanced vasorelaxation and increased endothelial nitric oxide synthase expression. Am Heart J. 2002;144(1):165–72.
314. Warnholtz A, Wild P, Ostad MA, Elsner V, Stieber F, Schinzel R, Walter U, Peetz D, Lackner K, Blankenberh S, Munzel T. Effects of oral niacin on endothelial dysfunction in patients with coronary artery disease: Results of the randomized, double-blind, placebo-controlled INEF study. Atherosclerosis. 2009;204(1):216–21.
315. Lee JMS, Robson MD, Yu L-M, Shirodaria CC, Cunnington C, Kylintireas I, Digby JE, Bannister T, Handa A, Wiesmann F, Durrington PN, Channon KM, Neubauer S, Choudhury RP. Effects of high-dose modified-release nicotinic acid on atherosclerosis and vascular function: A randomized, placebo-controlled, magnetic resonance imaging study. J Am Coll Cardiol. 2009;54:1787–94.
316. Hamilton SJ, Chew GT, Davis TM, Watts GF. Niacin improves small artery vasodilatory function and compliance in statin-treated type 2 diabetic patients. Diabetes Vasc Dis Res. 2010;7(4):296–9.
317. Tousoulis D, Antoniades C, Vassiliadou C, Toutouza M, Pitsavos C, Tentolouris C, Trikas A, Stefanadis C. Effects of combined administration of low dose atorvastatin and vitamin E on inflammatory markers and endothelial function in patients with heart failure. Eur J Heart Fail. 2005;7(7):1126–32.
318. Watts GF, Castelluccio C, Rice-Evans C, Taub NA, Baum H, Quinn PJ. Plasma coenzyme Q (ubiquinone) concentrations in patients treated with simvastatin. J Clin Pathol. 1993;46(11):1055–7.
319. Littarru GP, Langsjoen P. Coenzyme $Q_{10}$ and statins: biochemical and clinical implications. Mitochondrion. 2007;7(Supplement 1):S168–74.
320. Hamilton SP, Chew G, Watts G. Coenzyme $Q_{10}$ improves endothelial dysfunction in statin-treated type 2 diabetic patients. Diabetes Care. 2009;32(5): 810–2.
321. Tiano L, Belardinelli R, Carnevali P, Principi F, Seddaiu G, Littarru GP. Effect of coenzyme $Q_{10}$ administration on endothelial function and extracellular superoxide dismutase in patients with ischaemic heart disease: a double-blind, randomized controlled study. Eur Heart J. 2007;28(18):2249–55.
322. Koh KK, Quon MJ, Han SH, Ahn JY, Jin DK, Kim HS, Sik KDS, Shin EK. Vascular and metabolic effects of combined therapy with ramipril and simvastatin in patients with type 2 diabetes. Hypertension. 2005;45(6):1088–93.
323. Martin-Ventura JL, Tunon J, Duran MC, Blanco-Colio LM, Vivanco F, Egido J. Vascular protection of dual therapy (atorvastatin-amlodipine) in hypertensive patients. J Am Soc Nephrol. 2006;17(12 suppl 3):S189–93.
324. Koh KK, Quon MJ, Han SH, Ahn JY, Lee Y, Shin EK. Combined therapy with ramipril and simvastatin has beneficial additive effects on tissue factor activity and prothrombin fragment 1+2 in patients with type 2 diabetes. Atherosclerosis. 2007;194:230–7.
325. Jukema JW, Zwinderman AH, van Boven AJ, Reiber JHC, Van der Laarse A, Lie KI, Bruschke AVG. Evidence for a synergistic effect of calcium channel blockers with lipid-lowering therapy in retarding progression of coronary atherosclerosis in symptomatic patients with normal to moderately raised cholesterol levels. Arterioscler Thromb Vasc Biol. 1996;16(3):425–30.
326. Jukema JW, van Boven AJ, Zwinderman AH, Van der Laarse A, Bruschke AVG. Proposed synergistic effect of calcium channel blockers with lipid-lowering therapy in retarding progression of coronary atherosclerosis. Cardiovasc Drugs Ther. 1998;12:111–8.
327. Fogari R, Derosa G, Lazzari P, Zoppi A, Fogari E, Rinaldi A, Mugellini A. Effect of amlodipine-atorvastatin combination on fibrinolysis in hypertensive hypercholesterolemic patients with insulin resistance. Am J Hypertens. 2004;17(9):823–7.
328. Simons L, Tonkon M, Masana L, Maccubbin D, Shah A, Lee M, Gumbiner B. Effects of ezetimibe added to on-going statin therapy on the lipid profile of hypercholesterolemic patients with diabetes mellitus or metabolic syndrome. Curr Med Res Opin. 2004;20(9):1437–45.
329. Fleg JL, Mete M, Howard BV, Umans KG, Roman MJ, Ratner RE, Silverman A, Galloway JM, Henderson JA, Weir MR, Wilsn C, Stylianou M, Howard WM. Effect of statins alone versus statins plus ezetimibe on carotid atherosclerosis in type 2 diabetes: the SANDS (stop atherosclerosis in native diabetics study) trial. J Am Coll Cardiol. 2008;52(25):2198–205.
330. Kastelein JJP, Duivenvoorden R, Deanfield J, de Groot E, Jukema JW, Kaski J-C, Münzel T, Taddei S, Lehnert V, Burgess T, Kallend D, Lüscher TF. Rationale and design of dal-vessel: A study to assess the safety and efficacy of dalcetrapib on endothelial function using brachial artery flow-mediated vasodilatation. Curr Med Res Opin. 2011;27:141–50.
331. Luescher TF, Taddei S, Kaski J, Jukema JW, Kallend D, Munzel T, Kastelein JJ, Deanfield JE, on behalf of the dal-VESSEL investigators. Conference abstract. http://www.escardio.org/congresses/esc-2011/congress-reports/Pages/706-3-dal-VESSEL.aspx#presenter, Accessed 13/01/12.
332. Grundy SM, Cleeman JI, Merz NB, Brewer HB, Clark LT, Hunninghake DB, Pasternak RC, Smith SC, Stone NJ. Implications of recent clinical trials for the national cholesterol education program adult treatment panel III guidelines. Circulation. 2004;110:227–39.
333. Brunzell J, Davidson M, Furberg C, Goldberg R, Howard BV, Stein JH, Witztum JL. Lipoprotein management in patients with cardiometabolic risk: consensus statement from the American diabetes association and the American college of cardiology foundation. Diabetes Care. 2008;31(4):811–22.
334. National Heart Foundation of Australia. The cardiac society of Australia and New Zealand. Lipid management guidelines—2001. Med J Aust. 2001;175(Supplement):S55–88.

335. Graham I, Atar D, Borch-Johnsen K, et al. European guidelines on cardiovascular disease prevention in clinical practice: executive summary. Eur Heart J. 2007;28(19):2375–414.
336. Reiner Z, Catapano AL, De Backer G, Graham I, Taskinen MR, Wiklund O, Agewall S, Alegria E, Chapman MJ, Durrington P, Erdine S, Halcox J, Hobbs R, Kjekshus J, Filardi PP, Riccardi G, Storey RF, Wood D. ESC/EAS Guidelines for the management of dyslipidaemias. Eur Heart J. 2011;32(14):1769–818.
337. Chapman MJ, Ginsberg HN, Amarenco P, for the European Atherosclerosis Society Consensus Panel, et al. Triglyceride-rich lipoproteins and high-density lipoprotein cholesterol in patients at high risk of cardiovascular disease: evidence and guidance for management. Eur Heart J. 2011; 32(11): 1345–61.
338. Miller MMF, Stone NJM, Ballantyne C, Bittner V, Criqui MH, Ginsberg HN, Goldberg AC, Howard WJ, Jacobson MS, Kris-Etherrton P, Lennie T, Levi M, Mazzone T, Pennathur S. Triglycerides and cardiovascular disease: a scientific statement from the American heart association. Circulation. 2011; 123(20):2292–333.

# Lipoproteins and Diabetic Nephropathy

# 14

Ville-Petteri Mäkinen, Nina Tolonen, and Per-Henrik Groop

## Introduction

Diabetic nephropathy is the most common cause for end-stage renal disease worldwide and has a significant impact on the quality of life and longevity. It may affect up to a third of all patients with type 1 diabetes [2, 38, 102], and nephropathy is also a significant complication of type 2 diabetes [10, 11, 85]. The clinical course varies substantially, but in a typical case, the first indications of kidney injury appear within two decades of diabetes: urinary albumin excretion increases, blood pressure rises, and gradually the glomerular filtration rate (GFR) begins to decline with a concurrent increase in mortality [31, 38, 39, 96]. Glycemic control is the critical modifiable factor to delay and prevent diabetic nephropathy and other comorbidities [59]. The detrimental vascular effects of impaired glycemic control could be mediated by lipids and lipoproteins, and therefore the connection between serum lipoprotein lipids and diabetic nephropathy is clinically important.

Patients with chronic kidney disease have a greater risk of atherosclerosis and adverse vascular events, and diabetes adds to this risk even further [98]. As kidney function declines, secondary metabolic effects and adverse changes in lipoprotein metabolism follow [54, 81]. For instance, increased triglycerides and decreased HDL cholesterol concentrations as well as impaired clearance of VLDL particles are commonly seen [114]. Cardiovascular disease is the most common cause of death in patients with end-stage renal disease both in patients with and without diabetes. But in diabetes, the crucial changes seem to occur earlier: for instance, patients with type 1 diabetes and albuminuria have a dramatically increased risk of premature death even before their glomerular reserve is lost to the point of end-stage renal disease (Fig. 14.1). In particular, the lipoprotein lipid profile is correlated with albuminuria and predicts adverse outcomes [48, 110]. However, the good news is that patients with type 1 diabetes without any signs of renal disease show no excess mortality beyond that of the general population [38, 78].

V.-P. Mäkinen • N. Tolonen
Folkhälsan Research Center, Folkhälsan Institute of Genetics, Biomedicum Helsinki, Haartmaninkatu 8, 00290 Helsinki, Finland

Department of Medicine, Division of Nephrology, Helsinki University Central Hospital, Helsinki, Finland

P.-H. Groop, M.D., D.M.Sc. (✉)
Folkhälsan Research Center, Folkhälsan Institute of Genetics, Biomedicum Helsinki, Haartmaninkatu 8, 00290 Helsinki, Finland

Department of Medicine, Division of Nephrology, Helsinki University Central Hospital, Helsinki, Finland

Baker IDI Heart & Diabetes Institute, Melbourne, VIC, Australia
e-mail: per-henrik.groop@helsinki.fi

A.J. Jenkins et al. (eds.), *Lipoproteins in Diabetes Mellitus*, Contemporary Diabetes,
DOI 10.1007/978-1-4614-7554-5_14, © Springer Science+Business Media New York 2014

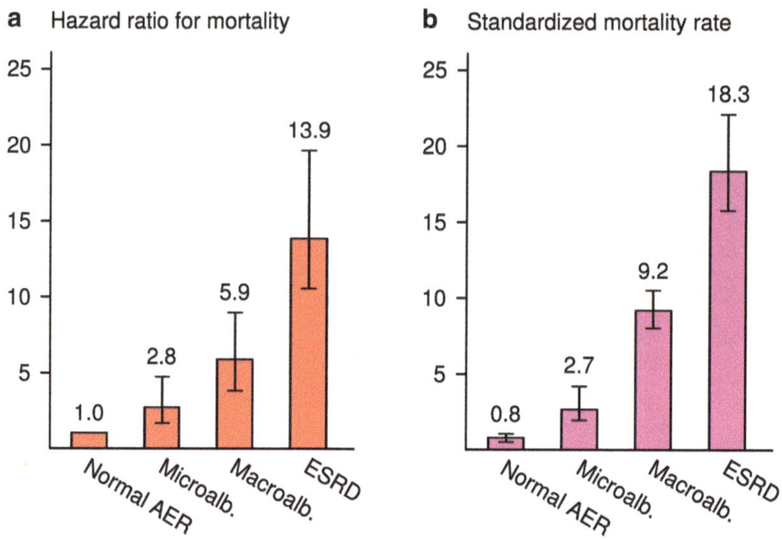


**Fig. 14.1** Prospective analysis of all-cause mortality in the FinnDiane cohort. Prospective analysis of all-cause mortality in the FinnDiane cohort of type 1 diabetes after an average of 7 years of follow-up. At baseline, 2,296 patients had normal AER, 504 had microalbuminuria, 579 had macroalbuminuria, and 293 had end-stage renal disease. Plot **a** depicts the adjusted hazard ratios with respect to normal AER. Plot **b** depicts the standardized mortality rate with respect to the age and sex groups in the Finnish background population (reference value was set to 1.0). The figure was adapted from [38]

The triad of poor glycemic control, obesity, and albuminuria indicates a high-risk vascular phenotype [68, 74]. All three risk factors overlap and are concurrently associated with dyslipidemia, particularly in the form of increased triglycerides and decreased HDL cholesterol. This also means that it is difficult to ascertain causal relationships between serum lipoproteins and diabetic kidney injury since both compartments may be parts of a larger complex of systemic atherogenic perturbations. Particularly in type 2 diabetes, lipid abnormalities such as high triglycerides, excessive postprandial lipidemia, small dense LDL cholesterol, and low levels of HDL cholesterol are frequently seen [106]. Hence, similar lipid abnormalities as in patients with end-stage renal disease are often observed in patients with type 2 diabetes even prior to the diagnosis of diabetes. The evidence regarding the kidney pathology is also unclear: it may be confounded by age-related phenomena and seems to be less related to urinary albumin excretion or GFR than in type 1 diabetes [32]. In this section, we primarily focus on the combined diagnostic and prognostic significance of kidney disease and lipoproteins in (type 1) diabetes and briefly discuss the biological implications to the lipoprotein composition and functionality.

## Conventional Lipoprotein Lipids, Albuminuria, and Kidney Function

Patients with type 1 diabetes but without complications show no adverse changes in their clinical lipid profile (total triglycerides, cholesterol, and HDL cholesterol), and patients with good glycemic control often have more favorable lipids than the background population [21, 76, 109]. On the other hand, plasma lipid abnormalities were reported in patients with nephropathy in a number of earlier studies [49, 50, 113], and the association between dyslipidemia and diabetic nephropathy has since been confirmed in several larger studies (Table 14.1).

**Table 14.1** Conventional lipid profile in patients with type 1 diabetes and diabetic nephropathy

| Study | Design | Albuminuria | Kidney dysfunction | Additional details |
|---|---|---|---|---|
| DCCT/EDIC [48] | Cross-sectional, N=968 | ↑TG, ↓HDL-C, ↑TotC, ↑LDL-C | n/a | HDL-C significant only in univariate analyses |
| DCCT/EDIC [24] | Progression from incident microalbuminuria to macroalbuminuria, N=325, 13-year follow-up | ↑TG, ↑TotC, ↑LDL-C | No findings | Lower baseline TG, TotC, and LDL-C associated with regression to normal AER |
| Estudio Diamante [25] | Cross-sectional, N=1,822 | ↑TG, ↑TotC | ↑TG, ↑TotC | LDL-C not reported |
| EURODIAB [65] | Cross-sectional, N=2,205 | ↑TG, ↓HDL-C, ↑TotC, ↑LDL-C | n/a | Sex-dependent findings on HDL-C |
| EURODIAB [12, 13] | Progression from normal AER, N=1,134, 7.3-year follow-up | ↑TG, ↓HDL-C, ↑TotC, ↑LDL-C | n/a | LDL-C and HDL-C significant when adjusted for diabetes duration, glycemic control, and baseline AER |
| EURODIAB [35] | Progression from microalbuminuria, N=352, 7.3-year follow-up | ↑TG | n/a | Lower baseline TG associated with regression to normal AER |
| FinnDiane [109] | Cross-sectional, N=2,927 | ↑TG, ↓HDL-C, ↑TotC, ↑LDL-C | ↑TG, ↓HDL-C, ↑TotC, ↑LDL-C | LDL-C and HDL-C significant in macroalbuminuria and ESRD |
| FinnDiane [110] | Progression to micro-, macroalbuminuria or ESRD, N=2,304, 5.4-year follow-up | ↑TG, ↑TotC | ↑TG, ↓HDL-C, ↑TotC, ↑LDL-C | |
| Pittsburgh [17] | Progression from normal AER, N=256, 2-year follow-up | ↑TG, ↑LDL-C | n/a | TotC not reported |
| Pittsburgh [77] | Progression to macroalbuminuria or ESRD, N=485, 10-year follow-up | ↑TG, ↑TotC, ↑LDL-C | ↑TG, ↑TotC, ↑LDL-C | Lipids significant only if progression within the first 5-year period |
| Nephropathy Family Study [64] | Progression from normal AER, N=895, 2.3-year follow-up | ↑TG, ↑TotC | n/a | Higher non-HDL cholesterol associated with progression |
| German Diabetes Documentation System [88] | Progression to micro-, macroalbuminuria or ESRD, N=27,805, 2.5-year follow-up | ↑TG, ↑TotC, ↑LDL-C | ↑TG, ↑TotC, ↑LDL-C | Dyslipidemia (TotC>200 mg/dL, LDL-C>160 mg/dL or TG>150 mg/dL) associated with progression |
| Angers cohort [41] | Progression to micro-, macroalbuminuria or ESRD, N=297, 7-year follow-up | ↑TG, ↓HDL-C | ↑TG, ↓HDL-C | Elevated plasma creatinine was used as an additional diagnostic category |
| Steno Diabetes Center [44] | Rate of GFR decline, N=301, 6.7-year follow-up | n/a | ↑TotC | Only TotC reported |
| Steno Diabetes Center [45] | Progression to micro- or macroalbuminuria, N=277, 18-year follow-up | See details | n/a | Lower baseline TotC associated with regression to normal AER<br>Only TotC reported |
| Joslin Study [83] | Regression from microalbuminuria, N=386, 6-year follow-up | See details | n/a | Lower baseline TG and TotC associated with AER reduction |

*Abbreviations*: *AER* urinary albumin excretion rate, *ESRD* end-stage renal disease, *TG* triglycerides, *TotC* total cholesterol, *HDL-C* HDL-cholesterol, *LDL-C* estimated LDL-cholesterol, *n/a* not available

## DCCT/EDIC

The Diabetes Control and Complications Trial (DCCT) was a multicenter clinical trial that compared intensive diabetes therapy with the current conventional treatment (between 1983 and 1993) in a cohort of 1,441 patients with type 1 diabetes. During the trial, the intensively treated patients had lower total triglycerides, total cholesterol, and calculated LDL cholesterol, but HDL cholesterol was unaffected [22]. At the same time, a significant reduction in the incidence of albuminuria was observed [23]. Specific analyses of urinary albumin excretion rate and serum lipoprotein lipids were made for the combined trial and follow-up period in the Epidemiology of Diabetes Interventions and Complications (EDIC) cohort of 968 patients [48]. Triglycerides, cholesterol, and calculated LDL cholesterol were increased in patients with microalbuminuria (40 < AER < 300 mg/24 h) and macroalbuminuria (AER > 300 mg/24 h) when tested for the overall trend and adjusted for age, diabetes duration, hypertension, hemoglobin A1c, body mass index (BMI), waist–hip ratio (WHR), and DCCT randomization group. A decreasing trend was observed for HDL cholesterol in women and in the full dataset, but these associations could be fully explained by the aforementioned risk factors and confounders.

The risk factors for long-term renal outcomes were examined in the 14th year of the EDIC Study in 325 patients [24] who developed persistent microalbuminuria (30 < AER < 300 mg/24 h) and were subsequently followed for regression to normal AER (36 %), progression of macroalbuminuria (30 %), and/or declining kidney function (18 %). Kidney function was determined by estimated glomerular filtration rate (eGFR). Total triglycerides, cholesterol, and calculated LDL cholesterol were associated with progression to macroalbuminuria (increased concentrations) and regression to normal AER (decreased concentration). No associations were detected for incident impaired eGFR, and HDL cholesterol failed to predict the renal outcomes altogether.

## EURODIAB

Cross-sectional associations between conventional lipoprotein measures and albuminuria were also seen in the EURODIAB IDDM Complications Study [65]. The set of 3,250 patients with type 1 diabetes were recruited from 16 European countries and represent age groups from 15 to 60 years. Increased concentrations of triglycerides, cholesterol, and calculated LDL cholesterol were observed for microalbuminuria (20 < AER < 200 μg/min) or macroalbuminuria (AER > 200 μg/min) for both sexes. Increased concentrations of triglycerides, cholesterol, and calculated LDL cholesterol were observed for microalbuminuria (20 < AER < 200 μg/min) or macroalbuminuria (AER > 200 μg/min) for both sexes. Furthermore, HDL cholesterol was decreased in patients with macroalbuminuria and, overall, the lipid abnormalities were more pronounced in the macroalbuminuric group. Of note, diabetes duration was highlighted as an important factor: associations between serum lipoprotein lipids and microalbuminuria were seen only in those patients with >5 years of duration.

A set of 1,134 patients with normal baseline AER were followed for a mean of 7.3 years in the EURODIAB Prospective Complication Study. The incidence of microalbuminuria was 12.6 %, which corresponds to 18 new cases per 1,000 person-years. In a multivariate model, baseline hemoglobin A1c, AER, triglycerides, and waist–hip ratio predicted the progression to microalbuminuria [12]. A sub-study of 352 patients with baseline microalbuminuria identified increased AER, suboptimal metabolic control, excess body fat, and peripheral neuropathy as significant risk factors for the progression to macroalbuminuria [35]. During an average of 7.3 years, 51 % regressed to normal AER, 36 % remained microalbuminuric, and 14 % progressed to macroalbuminuria. Overall, the lipoprotein lipids were not associated with the progressive kidney phenotype. However, fasting triglyceride concentration at baseline was a weak predictor of progression, and the lowest concentration was seen in the group that regressed.

## FinnDiane

The Finnish Diabetic Nephropathy Study (FinnDiane) represents a population-based sample of long-standing type 1 diabetes in Finland. In cross-sectional analyses of 2,927 patients, patients with normal urinary albumin excretion rate (AER < 30 mg/24 h) had the lowest, and those with macroalbuminuria (AER > 300 mg/24 h) had the highest triglyceride concentrations [109]. Glomerular filtration rate was also associated with lipid abnormalities: patients with impaired kidney function (eGFR < 60 mL/min/1.73 $m^2$) had higher triglycerides, total cholesterol, and lower HDL cholesterol than patients with normal kidney function (eGFR > 90 mL/min/1.73 $m^2$) or patients with mildly impaired kidney function (60 < eGFR < 90 mL/min/1.73 $m^2$).

In the prospective part of the FinnDiane Study, 2,304 patients with type 1 diabetes, followed for a mean of 5.4±2.0 years, were examined [110]. Baseline triglycerides predicted progression of kidney disease at all stages, including progression to micro- and macroalbuminuria and to end-stage renal disease. These associations could not be fully explained by conventional risk factors other than baseline AER. Several lipid variables predicted progression to end-stage renal disease, but when eGFR was included in the model, total cholesterol was the only significant lipid predictor.

The definition of the kidney disease phenotype may influence the results. In a model where normal AER and microalbuminuric groups were pooled, triglycerides predicted progression to macroalbuminuria, and the results could not be fully explained by either baseline AER or eGFR. When the patient set was divided into quartiles of triglycerides, the highest quartile had consistently higher hazard ratios for progression at all stages of nephropathy. From a practical point of view, however, no clear threshold could be observed for triglycerides and the progression of diabetic nephropathy.

## Pittsburgh EDC

A total of 658 patients with childhood onset of type 1 diabetes were included in the Pittsburgh Epidemiology of Diabetes Complications Study. A 2-year follow-up study of 256 patients indicated that poor glycemic control, increased LDL cholesterol, long duration of diabetes, and high systolic blood pressure at baseline were predictive of incident microalbuminuria, defined as AER>20 μg/min [17]. Glycemic control was a significant predictor in all subgroup analyses. In men, age and AER were also important predictors, whereas duration of diabetes and triglycerides were important in women. Calculated LDL cholesterol was significant in patients with type 1 diabetes duration <20 years, but triglycerides and systolic blood pressure predicted progression in the group with at least 20 years of duration. In a more recent study, 485 patients with or without overt nephropathy at baseline (AER < 200 μg/min) were followed for 10 years [77]. Estimated glucose disposal rate (a surrogate marker for insulin sensitivity) was predictive of overt nephropathy during the full follow-up. White blood cell count, triglycerides, calculated LDL cholesterol, non-HDL cholesterol, and systolic blood pressure predicted progression during the first 5 years of follow-up.

## German Diabetes Documentation System

The German Diabetes Documentation System cohort includes children, adolescents, and adults with a largely pediatric and adolescent onset of type 1 diabetes from Germany and Austria. A set of 27,805 patients were followed for an average of 2.5 years. The study revealed that triglycerides and LDL cholesterol were significant risk factors for the development of microalbuminuria [88]. Dyslipidemia, defined as at least one lipid variable over the cutoff level of >200 mg/dL for total cholesterol, >160 mg/dL for LDL cholesterol, and >150 mg/dL for triglycerides, was associated with the development of overt nephropathy.

## Nephropathy and Dyslipidemia in Type 2 Diabetes

Type 2 diabetes itself is strongly linked to similar lipoprotein abnormalities that are seen in patients with type 1 diabetes and microvascular complications, and it is therefore problematic to isolate the nephropathy-related changes from the background dyslipidemia. Nevertheless, more adverse lipid profiles are observed in patients with nephropathy, although the conventional lipids seem to hold limited prognostic utility. For instance, impaired kidney function was investigated in the Health Professionals Follow-Up Study (HPFS). In a cross-sectional sub-study of 732 men with type 2 diabetes [62], non-HDL cholesterol and triglycerides were increased from the highest (>90 mL/min/1.73 $m^2$) to the lowest eGFR category (<60 mL/min/1.73 $m^2$). On the other hand, a prospective analysis of 516 type 2 diabetic women from the Nurses' Health Study showed that an estimated eGFR decline of over 25 % during an 11-year follow-up was not associated with the conventional lipid profile [63].

A dyslipidemic pattern was observed in 275 Taiwanese patients [112]: increased total cholesterol and non-HDL cholesterol, especially when combined with hypertriglyceridemia, were significantly associated with albuminuria (defined as ACR > 30). In 1,557 Italian patients with type 2 diabetes, microalbuminuria was associated with diabetes duration, glycemic control, and blood pressure, but not with the lipid measures in univariate analyses [92].

The UK Prospective Diabetes Study examined patients with newly diagnosed type 2 diabetes and followed a subset of 4,031 patients with urinary albumin < 30 mg/L and a subset of 5,032 patients (criteria not mutually exclusive) with normal creatinine clearance (>60 mL/min/1.73 $m^2$) at baseline [90]. Increased plasma triglycerides were associated with incident micro- and macroalbuminuria, but not with declining creatinine clearance. The opposite was true for total and calculated LDL cholesterol: increased baseline concentrations predicted impaired creatinine clearance at follow-up. Decreased HDL cholesterol was also predictive of impaired creatinine clearance.

In a prospective study of 671 American Indians [28], high HDL cholesterol was inversely associated with incident increase in AER in women after 3.9 years of follow-up, and a suggestive positive association was found for triglycerides in men. Incident microalbuminuria (30 < AER < 300 mg/24 h) and macroalbuminuria (AER > 300 mg/24 h) were investigated in a set of 574 Israeli patients with a recent onset of type 2 diabetes [89]. The results were compatible with the previous reports: the combination of hypertension, increased total cholesterol, and poor glycemic control indicated the group at high risk for incident diabetic nephropathy.

A set of 3,667 type 2 diabetic patients with AER < 20 μg/min and eGFR > 60 mL/min/1.73 $m^2$ were examined in the Swedish National Diabetes Register for incident diabetic nephropathy [1]. Increased triglycerides and decreased HDL cholesterol at baseline predicted incident albuminuria (20 % of individuals) and both were also predictive of impaired eGFR. On the other hand, total or LDL cholesterol were not significant predictors. Of note, wider prescription of medications for lipidemia and hypertension were the most likely causes for overall decreases in LDL cholesterol and blood pressure at follow-up.

A study of the Hong Kong Diabetes Registry approached the issue from the opposite angle: the researchers reported that in a prospective cohort of 2,761 type 2 diabetic patients (2.8-year follow-up), macroalbuminuria predicted the incidence of abnormally high total cholesterol and calculated LDL cholesterol, while reduced eGFR predicted abnormally low HDL cholesterol [118].

## Interpretation of the Epidemiological Data

The cross-sectional analyses suggest that increased triglycerides, total cholesterol and LDL cholesterol, and a reduction in HDL cholesterol are typically seen in patients with diabetes and nephropathy. The dyslipidemia is more evident in advanced nephropathy, but this could be a conse-

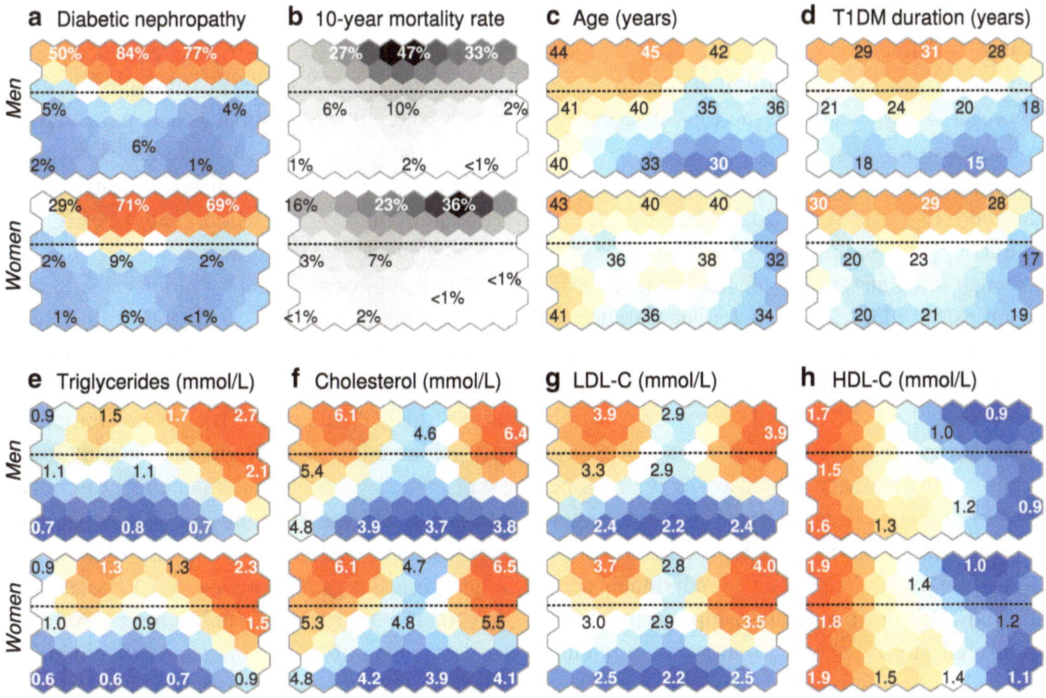


**Fig. 14.2** Self-organizing map analysis of 4,197 patients with type 1 diabetes from the FinnDiane Study. The figure can be interpreted the same way as a geographical map. Suppose the *rectangular* area is a map of a city, and the city is divided into *hexagonal* neighborhoods. In each neighborhood, the residents correspond to patients who are similar with respect to their serum and urine biochemical profiles. The locations of individuals were mathematically optimized by the self-organizing map algorithm (in a geographical map the locations would be physical coordinates). For the visualization, the *rectangular* map is colored based on the average characteristics in a neighborhood. For example, patients in the *top* part of the map show a high prevalence of diabetic nephropathy, which is indicated by the *red color* (Plot **a**). Diabetic nephropathy was defined as macroalbuminuria or end-stage renal disease. The figure was adapted from [68]

quence of poor glycemic control that, by itself, promotes the development of microvascular injuries. Furthermore, altered nutritional status and secondary effects of kidney failure may curb the increase in cholesterol but simultaneously cause an imbalance between triglycerides and HDL cholesterol when patients approach end-stage renal disease [14, 86].

Interestingly, when both hemoglobin A1c and BMI are high in type 1 diabetes, the lipid profile resembles that of the dyslipidemia typically observed in type 2 diabetes and the metabolic syndrome [68, 108]. The weight-adjusted insulin dose tends to be similar or even higher in these patients [70], which suggests that the dyslipidemia in today's type 1 diabetes could be at least partially related to increased insulin resistance rather than inadequate insulin administration. This fits to the concept of "double diabetes" and insulin resistance as major pathogenetic contributors to diabetic nephropathy [37, 58].

The classical linear analyses may hide the inherent complexity of the lipoprotein lipid profile. Figure 14.2 depicts the same dataset that was introduced in Fig. 14.1, but this time dissected by a multivariate nonlinear visualization method. Details of the self-organizing map (SOM) are available in supplements of previously published articles [68, 70]. Briefly, the method assigns a two-dimensional coordinate on the map for each patient based on the observed biochemical profiles. The map can then be colored according to a trait such as cholesterol concentration or prevalence of nephropathy in a given area. The idea is similar to coloring the world map based on average income or prevalence of diabetes—in that case the coordinates represent geographical locations. In Fig. 14.2, the map is always the same, so if a patient is located on the top-left corner in Plot a, he or she is also located in the top-left corner in every other plot.

The connection between diabetic nephropathy and mortality is obvious (Fig. 14.2a, b), as one would expect based on Fig. 14.1. The top part of the map contains most of the patients with nephropathy, older age, and longer duration of diabetes. The patterns of lipids are more complicated: low concentrations of triglycerides, total cholesterol, and LDL cholesterol consistently characterize the patients with no nephropathy, but greater diversity can be observed in the upper half. In linear analysis, triglycerides and cholesterol would emerge as positive regressors, but it is possible that only a subset of individuals actually show this positive relationship. Furthermore, HDL cholesterol appears to show a completely perpendicular pattern with respect to nephropathy, which could represent an additional independent modulating effect on vascular risk.

Figure 14.2 was created from a single cohort, the nonlinear method can lead to over-interpretation, and further work is needed to validate the observed patterns. Nevertheless, these results highlight the inherent biological complexity that may be missed by traditional approaches. For a practicing clinician, the heterogeneity is a challenge: those patients that have complications also show the greatest lipoprotein diversity. It is also possible that elevated cholesterol in one patient is more dangerous than in another, so additional information on the causal links is of great interest.

## Can Dyslipidemia Cause Nephropathy?

In prospective analyses, the picture is similar and conventional lipids are a part of the overall risk profile that is linked to poor glycemic control. In particular, total triglyceride concentration was a predictive marker at different stages of albuminuria in multiple studies: higher values were associated with progression and lower values with regression of albuminuria. Furthermore, dyslipidemia is associated with a faster progression of renal disease [65, 72, 77, 95, 97]. Although it is difficult to ascertain causal links based on the current clinical data, the practical message is clear: if lipids are abnormal, particularly in combination with smoking, hypertension, and obesity, the prognosis is considerably worse.

Atherosclerosis and glomerulosclerosis exhibit similar features [26] and it has been hypothesized that a compensatory increase in hepatic output of circulatory lipids follows the urinary loss of albumin. This in turn initiates a self-perpetuating cycle of glomerular and tubular events that aggravate and maintain progressive decline in kidney function [94]. There is some experimental evidence to support this theory. When guinea pigs and rats were fed cholesterol-rich food in a number of studies, they developed various forms of glomerular and other injuries, and the effects could be modulated by partial or unilateral nephrectomy and hypertension [41, 56, 84]. On the other hand, cholesterol alone may not be sufficient to initiate the disease processes since not all hyperlipidemic animals develop glomerular lesions. Moreover, nondiabetic human individuals with elevated cholesterol or triglycerides rarely develop kidney disease, so it is plausible that hyperglycemia (particularly in type 1 diabetes) and/or hypertension (particularly in type 2 diabetes) are necessary causative partners of hyperlipidemia on the path to diabetic kidney injury.

## Lipoprotein Subclasses and Albuminuria in Type 1 Diabetes

Chronic kidney disease per se is associated with multiple lipoprotein abnormalities, but before these direct effects of kidney insufficiency begin, dysfunctions in lipid transfer proteins, lipoprotein formation, and clearance may be present in albuminuric patients. There is also evidence of mechanistic links to lipotoxicity in the nephrons [94], and the epidemiological findings of increased triglycerides and cholesterol in the circulation suggest that lipoproteins provide the fuel for these lipotoxic processes. Lipoprotein particles comprise a heterogeneous group of lipid transport vehicles with diverse tasks and multiple characteristics such as size, density, and composition. In this respect, the conventional lipoprotein lipids are summary measures—more specific measurement techniques may reveal subtle lipoprotein defects that contribute to diabetic microvascular injury.

## VLDL Subclasses

In the DCCT/EDIC Study, lipoprotein subclasses were measured by a proton NMR spectroscopic method for 958 patients with type 1 diabetes [48, 79]. The strongest signals for albuminuria were obtained for the VLDL and HDL subclasses, whereas the LDL subclasses were weaker indicators of kidney disease. The total lipid contents in medium and small VLDL subclasses were significantly associated with AER, and the two were the only lipoprotein measures that were significant in women after adjusting for other risk factors. In men, all VLDL subclasses were increased in patients with increased AER, and differences were also observed in other lipoprotein measures. On the other hand, VLDL size was not associated with albuminuria.

Lipoprotein subclasses were measured by NMR in a subset of 325 type 1 diabetic patients from the FinnDiane cohort [69], although the methodology to extract subclass data from the NMR spectra was different from the one used in the DCCT/EDIC. The extra-large and large VLDL subclasses were significantly different between patients without (AER < 300 mg/24 h) or with macroalbuminuria (AER > 300 mg/24 h). The strongest positive correlations with continuous AER were observed for large VLDL cholesterol. Furthermore, the constituent lipids (such as triglycerides and phospholipids) in extra-large and medium VLDL subclasses were significant covariates of AER.

VLDL particles from ultracentrifugation and their relationships with the progression of diabetic nephropathy were investigated by Thomas et al. in a follow-up of 152 patients with type 1 diabetes [107]. No associations (when adjusted for other risk factors) were detected between VLDL measures and progression from normal AER (<20 mg/min at baseline), nor between VLDL and eGFR decline in the macroalbuminuric group (AER > 200 mg/min). On the other hand, VLDL triglycerides predicted progression from microalbuminuria (20 < AER < 200 μg/min at baseline).

## IDL and LDL Subclasses

The calculated Friedewald LDL cholesterol, which also includes cholesterol from IDL, was a significant covariate of AER in the DCCT/EDIC Study [48]. At subclass level, the lipid mass within IDL was increased in men with macroalbuminuria, but not in women. Only small LDL was significantly increased, and there was also evidence of gender interaction with AER. Men showed a decrease in LDL size, and both sexes showed an increase in LDL particle concentration in the macroalbuminuric group. Oxidation of LDL was investigated via fluorescence ratio and delta absorbance, but there were no differences between the AER categories. Of note, Lp(a) was also similar between the AER groups.

The Pittsburgh EDC Study Group employed the same NMR method as the DCCT/EDIC to examine 42 matched pairs of progressors and nonprogressors with respect to overt nephropathy (AER > 200 μg/min or serum creatinine > 153 μmol/L or renal failure). Decreased LDL particle size emerged as the most important lipoprotein measure [119], and the results also suggested that lipoprotein lipids are less important during the initial increase in AER, with larger effects in the later stages of albuminuria.

LDL subclass lipids were not significant indicators of albuminuria in the cross-sectional analysis of the subset from the FinnDiane Study [69]. In a prospective analysis, baseline IDL and LDL subclasses were associated with the progression of albuminuria, but not from macroalbuminuria (and impaired eGFR) to end-stage renal disease [70].

Thomas et al. reported that LDL cholesterol, LDL free cholesterol, and LDL mass, measured by ultracentrifugation, predicted the progression from normal AER [107]. Furthermore, IDL triglycerides predicted the progression from microalbuminuria, whereas only decreased LDL size was associated with declining eGFR in the macroalbuminuric group.

## Apolipoprotein B

Each lipoprotein particle in the VLDL–IDL–LDL cascade contains a single apolipoprotein B-100 molecule (apoB), and measuring apoB therefore works as a pooled measure of the circulating particle concentrations for these lipoproteins [19]. In the DCCT/EDIC Study, apoB was a significant covariate of AER and creatinine clearance for both sexes [48]. Furthermore, these associations could not be fully explained by confounders or traditional risk factors. Findings in the FinnDiane Study were similar: apoB was increased in microalbuminuric patients, even more in macroalbuminuric patients, and apoB was also associated with progression across the albuminuria categories [109, 110]. A nested case-control approach within the EURODIAB Prospective Complications Study found that in 224 patients with type 1 diabetes, apoB was significantly increased both in the micro- and macroalbuminuric groups [12, 13].

## HDL Subclasses

HDL cholesterol is decreased in patients with macroalbuminuria, and the size, function, and composition of HDL particles is altered during the course of diabetic kidney disease. In the DCCT/EDIC, the HDL subfraction was split into large HDL and small. Total lipid content of large HDL particles was decreased in patients with macroalbuminuria, but small HDL was increased in both men and women, which fits to the assumed roles [48]. Furthermore, HDL particle size was inversely correlated with AER.

The HDL subfraction was divided into four subclasses in the FinnDiane sub-study with serum NMR data [69]. Patients with macroalbuminuria had decreased cholesterol and other constituent lipids in large HDL (the second largest subclass), and weaker inverse associations were also detected for medium HDL lipids, esterified cholesterol in the largest HDL, and total lipids in small HDL. In the prospective analysis, depletion of large HDL cholesterol was observed in patients who progressed at shorter duration [70]. Surprisingly, the largest HDL subclass was positively correlated with LDL lipids and elevated in patients at risk for progression from normal AER or microalbuminuria.

The HDL subfraction can also be divided according to buoyancy: the $HDL_2$ subclass represents large buoyant particles, whereas the $HDL_3$ denotes smaller and denser particles. $HDL_3$ cholesterol was investigated by an enzymatic method in the main FinnDiane cohort. In cross-sectional analysis, both $HDL_2$ (estimated as non-$HDL_3$) and $HDL_3$ cholesterol were decreased in patients with macroalbuminuria and in patients with impaired eGFR [109]. In prospective analysis, the pattern was similar when progressors were compared with nonprogressors for each baseline nephropathy category [110]. However, the progressor groups were different with respect to gender and diabetes duration. When traditional risk factors were taken into account, $HDL_3$ cholesterol was positively associated with progression from normal AER to microalbuminuria.

## Apolipoproteins A-I and A-II

ApoA-I and apoA-II are major structural components of HDL particles, and their concentrations are correlated with HDL lipids [87]. Kahri et al. compared HDL particles between 52 patients with normal AER, 37 with microalbuminuria ($20 < AER < 200$ μg/min), and 64 with macroalbuminuria ($AER > 200$ μg/min). $HDL_2$ cholesterol was higher in patients with normal AER, but no differences were detected with respect to apoA-I or apoA-II, or HDL particles with or without apoA-II [52].

Surprisingly, apoA-I was a borderline positive covariate of albuminuria in men in the DCCT/EDIC, and there was also a positive association with creatinine clearance [48]. Results from the FinnDiane Study were also somewhat unexpected: neither A-I nor A-II showed a clear trend for AER or eGFR in cross-sectional analysis, but increased apoA-II and decreased apoA-I/A-II ratio predicted progression from normal AER in prospective analysis [109, 110]. In the subset of 325 patients from the main FinnDiane cohort, apoA-II was correlated with total cholesterol and serum phosphatidylcholine in a network model and increased in patients with a high risk of incident albuminuria [70].

## Lipoprotein Abnormalities in Chronic Kidney Disease and Their Relevance to Diabetic Nephropathy

Loss of kidney function results in multiple systemic effects on metabolism, and lipoproteins are also affected [7, 114]. The most marked changes can be summarized as (1) reduced clearance of apoB-containing lipoproteins and their remnants, (2) accumulation of small and dense and oxidized LDL particles, and (3) impaired maturation of HDL particles. Some of these effects may depend on the renal replacement therapies. For instance, peritoneal dialysis causes plasma albumin loss and is linked to increased LDL and total cholesterol due to increased cholesterol biosynthesis, whereas hemodialysis seems not to have similar adverse effects [6, 18]. Of note, excess apoB-containing lipoproteins have been observed in nephrotic proteinuria, where depletion of plasma albumin is also common [60].

Chylomicrons are large triglyceride-rich lipoprotein particles with a single apolipoprotein B-48, and they deliver dietary fatty acids from the intestine to the rest of the body. The VLDL particles are the hepatic counterparts with a single apolipoprotein B-100, and the triglyceride-poor remnants of both classes are taken up by the liver [73]. The release of the triglyceride content from VLDL particles requires apolipoproteins E and C-II from mature cholesterol-rich HDL particles [114]. In chronic kidney disease, however, HDL fails to mature properly [71], which then disrupts the normal release of triglycerides from the VLDL and their subsequent conversion to IDL and ultimately to triglyceride-free LDL that can be cleared by the liver.

The lipoprotein subclass data on diabetic nephropathy supports the concept of impaired clearance of VLDL, as elevated VLDL subclass lipids were observed in multiple studies and in different disease stages. However, patients with type 1 diabetes and albuminuria show signs of "double diabetes," and both impaired clearance and increased VLDL synthesis are likely to be responsible for the dyslipidemia [106, 115]. It is possible that the balance between VLDL synthesis and clearance changes as kidney injuries advance. Therefore, although increases in VLDL subclasses can be observed during the entire course of diabetic nephropathy, the causes may be different for low-grade albuminuria, proteinuria with a sufficient glomerular reserve, and end-stage renal disease.

Small and dense LDL particles are considered highly atherogenic and have been linked with increased risk of cardiovascular disease [80]. In addition, oxidation of LDL makes the particles more prone to infiltrate vascular walls and promote the inflammatory cascade that leads to intima-media thickening and accumulation of atherosclerotic plaque [116]. Decreased LDL size was a significant predictor for the progression of diabetic nephropathy in several studies, and increased concentration of small LDL lipids was also observed. This modification of LDL subclass distributions is probably connected to the clearance of the entire VLDL–IDL–LDL pool [47, 53]. In the DCCT, oxidation of LDL was not found to be different between AER categories [48], but more studies are needed to ascertain if LDL oxidation is important in the pathogenesis of diabetic nephropathy.

The HDL fraction contains a complex set of multifunctional particles at different stages of maturation [36]. In general, HDL particles are protective against vascular diseases: they are able to remove excess cholesterol from peripheral tissues, attenuate oxidative stress, and may have anti-inflammatory properties [3, 67, 93]. When kidney function declines, HDL fails to mature properly to its cholesterol-rich form and remains as a small lipid-poor particle, and this may explain the inverse association with the conventional HDL cholesterol [54]. Decreased HDL subclasses were detected in a number of studies on diabetic nephropathy, but results on apolipoproteins A-I and A-II (the major structural proteins) were conflicting, and it is difficult to say if the number of particles is affected. Nevertheless, an inverse correlation between HDL size and AER was observed, and increased small HDL (a correlate of insulin resistance and elevated triglycerides) may predict nephropathy, which fits to the concept of impaired HDL maturation as a significant defect also in diabetic nephropathy.

## Lipid Medications and Diabetic Nephropathy

In the previous sections we have discussed the various lipoprotein defects that are associated with kidney injury. Several pharmacological agents are available to correct atherogenic changes in lipoprotein metabolism, and their beneficial effects in the general population have been established in numerous studies. Statins are effective cholesterol-lowering drugs due to their direct inhibitory effect on the HMG-CoA reductase, which is a central enzyme in hepatic cholesterol synthesis [61]. Fenofibrates are synthetic ligands to the peroxisome proliferator-activated receptor alpha (PPARα), and the lipid-lowering mechanisms include the activation of lipoprotein lipase, reduced production of apolipoprotein C-III, and the subsequent clearance of VLDL and IDL particles [8]. A summary of clinical trials where renal outcomes were investigated is listed in Table 14.2. The discussion here is centered on the potential renoprotective effects of the drugs, and therefore explicit results on cardioprotection are omitted. It is, however, important to stress that in many of the studies a significant reduction in cardiovascular events was seen, especially in patients with early stages of nephropathy.

### Effect of Statins on Kidney Function or Urinary Albumin Excretion

Pravastatin or simvastatin treatments produced a modest reduction in the rate of eGFR decline, and atorvastatin was associated with eGFR improvement in people with (or at risk of) coronary heart disease [5, 46, 100, 111]. In a meta-analysis of 39,704 patients with and without diabetes, eGFR decline was 1.22 mL/min per year slower with statin treatment [99]. However, the majority of participants already had cardiovascular disease, the between-study heterogeneity in the effect of statins was substantial, and subgroup analyses showed no statistical significant differences in patients with diabetic kidney disease. Albuminuria or proteinuria (1,323 patients) was modestly reduced (0.6 units of SD) in statin recipients, but again the between-study heterogeneity in the effect of statins was large. In another meta-analysis regarding the effects of statins on albuminuria in 1,384 patients with and without diabetes, a proportional reduction in albuminuria and proteinuria was seen in 13 of 15 studies [27].

In a study with 197,551 veterans, statin treatment was associated with a 13 % decrease in the development of renal dysfunction, possibly by other than lipid-dependent mechanisms [104]. The Heart Protection Study (HPS), including patients with diabetes or occlusive arterial disease, found that simvastatin treatment was associated with a smaller decrease in eGFR, and the effect was slightly larger among patients with diabetes [15]. The Collaborative Atorvastatin Diabetes Study (CARDS), including patients with type 2 diabetes without prior cardiovascular disease, found that atorvastatin treatment was associated with a modest improvement in the annual change in estimated GFR, and this was most apparent in patients with albuminuria, but no significant influence on the incidence of albuminuria was seen [16]. In a sub-study of the Treating to New Targets (TNT) trial in patients with coronary artery disease, both 10 and 80 mg of atorvastatin increased eGFR in patients with diabetes, with or without moderate chronic kidney disease, and with a higher increase in eGFR in patients treated with the 80 mg atorvastatin dose [101].

**Table 14.2** Lipid-lowering treatment and progression of diabetic nephropathy

| Study | Design | Intervention | Renal outcome | Details |
|---|---|---|---|---|
| DAIS [4] | T2DM without nephropathy, *N*=314, 3.3-year follow-up | Fenofibrate 200 mg or placebo | Reduced progression to microalbuminuria | Higher AER at trial end for 8 % on fenofibrate and 18 % on placebo |
| FIELD [57] | T2DM, majority without overt nephropathy, *N*=9,795, 5-year follow-up | Fenofibrate 200 mg or placebo | Small reduction in progression of albuminuria | Statistically significant if pooled with regression of albuminuria |
| FIELD washout sub-study [20] | T2DM, *N*=661 | Fenofibrate 200 mg or placebo | Slower decline in eGFR, reduction in ACR | Initial but reversible increase in plasma creatinine |
| ACCORD [34] | T2DM, high vascular risk, *N*=5,518, 4.7-year follow-up | Fenofibrate 160 mg and Simvastatin 20–40 mg or placebo and Simvastatin 20–40 mg | Small reduction in progression to micro- or macroalbuminuria | Reduced dose of fenofibrate if eGFR < 50 mL/min per 1.73 $m^2$ |
| Heart protection study [15] | T1DM (3 %), T2DM (26 %), and arterial disease without diabetes (71 %), *N*=20,270, 4.6-year follow-up | Simvastatin 40 mg or placebo | Slightly slower decline in eGFR | Effect on eGFR larger in patients with diabetes |
| CARDS [16] | T2DM, no prior CVD, 34 % impaired eGFR, *N*=2,838, 3.9-year follow-up | Atorvastatin 10 mg or placebo | Minor improvement in eGFR | No effect on albuminuria incidence |
| TNT [101] | T2DM, coronary heart disease, *N*=1,431, 4.8-year follow-up | Atorvastatin 10 mg or Atorvastatin 80 mg | Improvement in eGFR in both treatment groups | |
| ALERT [29] | Renal transplant recipients, 13 % diabetes, *N*=2,102, 6-year follow-up | Fluvastatin 40 mg or Fluvastatin 80 mg or placebo | No effect | GFR was measured directly in a subset of 439 patients |
| SHARP [9] | Dialysis or pre-dialysis patients, 20 % diabetes, *N*=9,270, 4.9-year follow-up | Simvastatin 20 mg and Ezetimibe 10 mg or placebo | No effect on renal disease progression | Simvastatin 20 mg alone in 1,054 patients for 1 year |

*Abbreviations*: *T1DM* and *T2DM* type 1 and type 2 diabetes, *AER* urinary albumin excretion rate, *ACR* urinary albumin-to-creatinine ratio, *eGFR* estimated glomerular filtration rate, *CVD* cardiovascular disease

## Statins and Chronic Kidney Disease

Statins modestly reduced proteinuria (311 patients, –0.73 g/24 h), but did not improve eGFR (548 patients) in a meta-analysis of patients with chronic kidney disease [103]. Fatal and nonfatal cardiovascular events were reduced, but no significant effect on all-cause mortality was seen. In another meta-analysis of only pre-dialysis patients [75], statins reduced all-cause mortality (18,781 patients, relative risk 0.81), and in a third meta-analysis including nine trials with atorvastatin treatment for 4,194 patients with pre-dialysis chronic kidney disease, a significant effect on eGFR was reported [105].

Atorvastatin showed a suggestive preventive effect on cardiovascular events but failed to reduce cerebrovascular events or mortality in Die Deutsche Diabetes Dialyse (4D) trial of 1,225 patients with type 2 diabetes on hemodialysis [117]. Another statin drug, rosuvastatin, was not effective in the prevention of cardiovascular events in A Study to Evaluate the Use of Rosuvastatin in Subjects on Regular Hemodialysis: Assessment of Survival and Cardiovascular Events (AURORA) of 2,779 hemodialysis patients [30]. Rosuvastatin did reduce the number of first cardiovascular events and all-cause mortality by more than 40 % during an average of 2 years of follow-up in patients with only modest kidney disease [91] in the Justification for the Use of Statins in Prevention—an Intervention Trial Evaluating Rosuvastatin (JUPITER). However, no effect on eGFR was seen at 12 months of follow-up.

A combination therapy of simvastatin and ezemitibe (an inhibitor of cholesterol absorption in the gut) reduced the number of major atherosclerotic events by 17 % in 9,270 patients in the Study of Heart and Renal Protection (SHARP) trial [9]. The study set included both pre-dialysis and dialysis patients, but the study was underpowered to analyze the endpoints in these groups separately. Measures of kidney disease in predialysis patients were not significantly affected by the combination therapy.

Fluvastatin treatment had no significant effect on the incidence of renal graft loss, doubling of serum creatinine, decline in GFR, or major adverse cardiac events during a 5-year follow-up of 2,102 renal transplant recipients in the Assessment of Lescol in Renal Transplantation (ALERT) study [29, 42]. Of note, fewer nonfatal myocardial infarctions and cardiac deaths were observed in the fluvastatin group. In a subsequent analysis of the study population after a 7-year follow-up, open-label fluvastatin treatment reduced the risk of the first major cardiac event by 21 %, but no significant difference in graft loss or total mortality was seen [43].

## Fenofibrates

Fenofibrate treatment of patients with type 2 diabetes reduced the progression of microalbuminuria in the Diabetes Atherosclerosis Intervention (DAIS) and in the Fenofibrate Intervention and Event Lowering in Diabetes (FIELD) studies [4, 33, 57]. However, the effect sizes were modest. In an additional study of the FIELD cohort with a washout period, an initial and reversible increase was seen in plasma creatinine, but during a follow-up of 5 years, fenofibrate slowed eGFR loss, and a greater benefit of eGFR preservation with fenofibrate treatment was seen in those with baseline dyslipidemia [20]. A combination of fenofibrate and simvastatin modestly reduced progression to micro- or macroalbuminuria compared to simvastatin treatment alone in the Action to Control Cardiovascular Risk in Diabetes (ACCORD) trial [34]. In a meta-analysis of fibrate studies including albuminuria data from the studies above (15,731 patients), fenofibrate reduced the risk of albuminuria progression by 14 % [52].

## Clinical Utility of Lipid Treatment in Diabetic Nephropathy

Overall, lipid-modifying treatments seem to have a modest effect on the development of albuminuria and the decline of eGFR. As discussed in the previous sections, the causal links between lipoprotein lipids and kidney injury are tentative, which may explain the lack of strong effects. Of note, improving glycemic control and aggressive treatment of hypertension are effective in protecting the kidneys [23, 82], and life style interventions have beneficial effects on the total systemic metabolism, including lipids. Most of the evidence on lipid drugs comes from patients with detectable vascular problems; it is not known if lipid-based interventions in an earlier phase could provide benefits that are lost at later stages of diabetic nephropathy. Furthermore, trials with hard renal endpoints and direct GFR measurements (not only estimated GFR which is dependent on creatinine production and excretion) are needed to clarify the situation.

Should the dyslipidemia in patients with diabetic nephropathy be medicated? There is a consistent body of evidence that reducing the atherogenicity of lipoproteins is beneficial in most population groups. Accordingly, diabetic patients with albuminuria but without kidney failure should be medicated, perhaps even more aggressively than the general population. Unfortunately, end-stage renal disease with or without diabetes seems to be a tough problem to solve. Several trials reported reduced rates of cardiovascular deaths, which is enough to warrant the prescription of these drugs, but the net effects on mortality have been less spectacular. It is possible that the atherosclerotic processes that are related to dyslipidemia become less important as declining kidney function causes secondary physiological and metabolic disturbances. Heart failure, arrhythmias, and hypertensive cardiomyopathy, for instance, contribute to the increased cardiovascular risk in end-stage renal disease, and therefore the usefulness of lipid medication should be carefully assessed for these patients.

## Concluding Remarks

Clinical and other research has established a strong link with lipoprotein metabolism and cardiovascular disease during the past century. At the same time, the sequence of events from the first signs of albuminuria, followed by persistent proteinuria and culminating in cardiovascular deaths and/or end-stage renal disease, has been

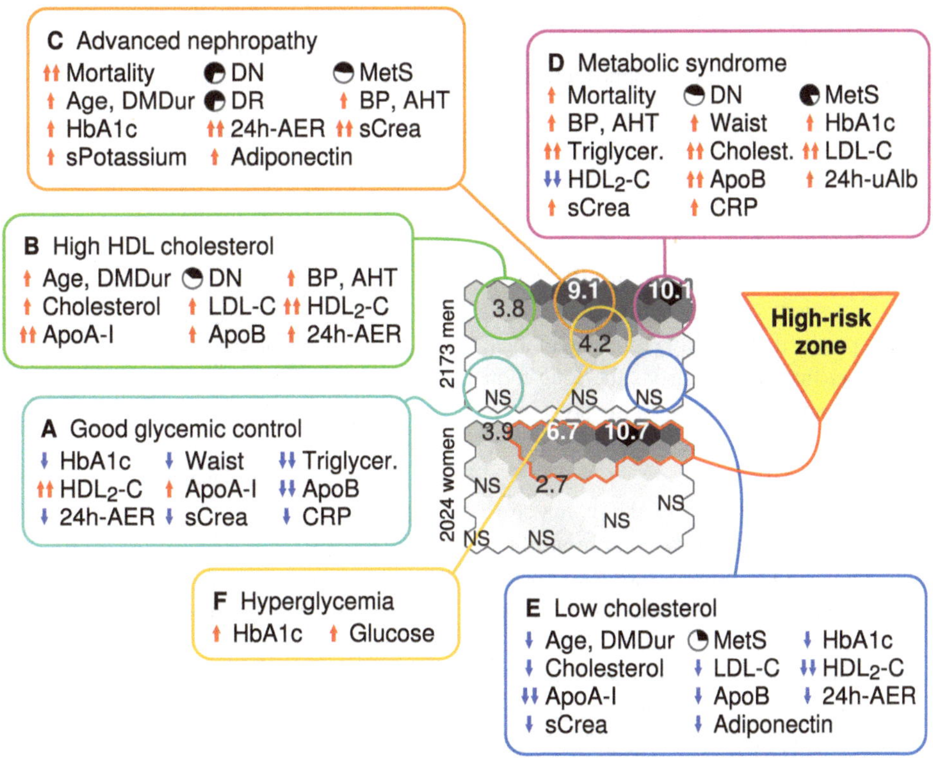


**Fig. 14.3** Exploratory analysis of 4,197 patients with type 1 diabetes by a self-organizing map (SOM) of biochemical measures [68]. The SOM algorithm produces a two-dimensional layout of the individuals based on their biochemical profiles: the distance on the map is proportional to the similarity of the biochemical profiles, which means that a specific region on the map contains patients with mutually similar metabolic features, whereas the patients on opposite sides are metabolically different. The map itself is just the layout, but this layout can be colored with respect to different clinical traits, or subgroups of patients. Here, men and women were visualized separately (although both were analyzed with the same map). The *grayscale* on the two colorings was determined based on the vitality status of the patients during an average of 8-year follow-up. The numbers on the map depict the relative mortality rate compared with the background population of similar age. The results show that patients with the characteristics of the metabolic syndrome (Phenotype D) and patients with advanced nephropathy (Phenotype C) are at high risk of premature death. Patients with favorable lipids show lower mortality compared to the metabolic syndrome phenotype despite a higher age and similar prevalence of diabetic nephropathy (Phenotype B vs. D). *Abbreviations*: *AER* urinary albumin extretion rate, *AHT* anti-hypertensive treatment, *BP* blood pressure, *CRP* C-reactive protein, *DMDur* type 1 diabetes duration, *DN* diabetic nephropathy, *DR* diabetic retinopathy, *MetS* metabolic syndrome, *sCrea* serum creatinine

described in patients with diabetes. It is therefore plausible that the interplay between dyslipidemia and diabetic kidney disease may form the basis for the excess mortality in diabetes.

Figure 14.3 depicts a multivariate summary of the FinnDiane Cohort. This data-driven visualization is essentially the clinical picture of Finnish patients with a long-standing type 1 diabetes, and the six model phenotypes from A to F could be real patients walking into the clinic for a checkup. Advanced kidney disease is associated with the highest absolute mortality (Phenotype C), but age-adjusted risk for premature death is, in fact, equally high in younger patients with the dyslipidemic, metabolic syndrome characteristics (Phenotypes D). In contrast, patients with the opposite pattern have an overall favorable metabolic profile without any excess mortality (Phenotype A). How much of the differences between A and D are due to a patient's life choices and the quality of care and how much of it comes from genetic heterogeneity? At this point, our knowledge is insufficient to answer this question. Nevertheless, Phenotype A and the lipid profile therein may represent an ideal treatment target that protects from the long-term complications, and any means from life style interventions to new pharmacological agents should be employed to achieve it.

Observational data supports the connection between micro- and macrovascular complications, and lipids are the prime candidates for the connecting agents. However, specific trials on dyslipidemia as a predictor or causative factor to the onset of diabetic kidney disease are sparse. In particular, most lipid drug trials have focused on late vascular events such as myocardial infarctions, and at that point it may be too late to investigate diabetic nephropathy. Primary prevention is most effective before significant atherosclerotic lesions develop, and in this respect the potential links between serum lipid profile and early stages of diabetic nephropathy—as a proxy for a vulnerable vascular phenotype—should be investigated more thoroughly.

Finally, patients with diabetic kidney disease may be more vulnerable to the effects of dyslipidemia than the general population. For instance, the commonly used threshold for triglycerides may be too high for patients with type 1 diabetes, since the majority of patients are below the limit while still having a high incidence of cardiovascular disease and microvascular complications. It is also important to remember that cholesterol in the modern world is typically twice as high as in hunter-gatherer communities, regardless of diabetes status. Tighter lipid control is therefore warranted in situations of impaired glycemic control to avoid a double hit on vascular health.

## References


1. Afghahi H, Cederholm J, Eliasson B, Zethelius B, Gudbjörnsdottir S, Hadimeri H, Svensson MK. Risk factors for the development of albuminuria and renal impairment in type 2 diabetes—the Swedish National Diabetes Register. Nephrol Dial Transplant. 2011;26:1236–43.
2. Allen KV, Walker JD. Microalbuminuria and mortality in long-duration type 1 diabetes. Diabetes Care. 2003;26:2389–91.
3. Andrews KL, Moore XL, Chin-Dusting JP. Anti-atherogenic effects of high-density lipoprotein on nitric oxide synthesis in the endothelium. Clin Exp Pharmacol Physiol. 2010;37:736–42.
4. Ansquer JC, Foucher C, Rattier S, Taskinen MR, Steiner G, DAIS Investigators. Fenofibrate reduces progression to microalbuminuria over 3 years in a placebo-controlled study in type 2 diabetes: results from the Diabetes Atherosclerosis Intervention Study (DIAS). Am J Kidney Dis. 2005;45:485–93.
5. Athyros VG, Mikhailidis DP, Papageorgiou AA, Symeonidis AN, Pehlivanidis AN, Bouloukos VI, Elisaf M. The effect of statins versus untreated dyslipidaemia on renal function in patients with coronary heart disease. A subgroup analysis of the Greek atorvastatin and coronary heart disease evaluation (GREACE) study. J Clin Pathol. 2004;57:728–34.
6. Attman PO, Samuelsson O, Johansson AC, Moberly JB, Alaupovic P. Dialysis modalities and dyslipidemia. Kidney Int. 2003;84:S110–2.
7. Attman PO, Samuelsson O, Alaupovic P. The effect of decreasing renal function on lipoprotein profiles. Nephrol Dial Transplant. 2011;26:2572–5.
8. Auwerx J, Schoonjans K, Fruchart JC, Staels B. Regulation of triglyceride metabolism by PPARs: fibrates and thiazolidinediones have distinct effects. J Atheroscler Thromb. 1996;3:81–9.
9. Baigent C, Landray MJ, Reith C, Emberson J, Wheeler DC, Tomson C, Wanner C, Krane V, Cass A, Craig J, Neal B, Jiang L, Hooi LS, Levin A, Agodoa L, Gaziano M, Kasiske B, Walker R, Massy ZA, Feldt-Rasmussen B, Krairittichai U, Ophascharoensuk V, Fellström B, Holdaas H, Tesar

V, Wiecek A, Grobbee D, de Zeeuw D, Grönhagen-Riska C, Dasgupta T, Lewis D, Herrington W, Mafham M, Majoni W, Wallendszus K, Grimm R, Pedersen T, Tobert J, Armitage J, Baxter A, Bray C, Chen Y, Chen Z, Hill M, Knott C, Parish S, Simpson D, Sleight P, Young A, Collins R, SHARP Investigators. The effects of lowering LDL cholesterol with simvastatin plus ezetimibe in patients with chronic kidney disease (Study of Heart and Renal Protection): a randomised placebo-controlled trial. Lancet. 2011;377:2181–92.
10. Bakris G, Vassalotti J, Ritz E, Wanner C, Stergiou G, Molitch M, Nesto R, Kaysen GA, Sowers JR, CKD Consensus Working Group. National Kidney Foundation consensus conference on cardiovascular and kidney diseases and diabetes risk: an integrated therapeutic approach to reduce events. Kidney Int. 2010;78(8):726–36.
11. Brown WV. Microvascular complications of diabetes mellitus: renal protection accompanies cardiovascular protection. Am J Cardiol. 2008;102(12A):10L–3.
12. Chaturvedi N, Bandinelli S, Mangili R, Penno G, Rottiers RE, Fuller JH. Microalbuminuria in type 1 diabetes: rates, risk factors and glycemic threshold. Kidney Int. 2001;60:219–27.
13. Chaturvedi N, Fuller JF, Taskinen MR. Differing associations of lipid and lipoprotein disturbances with the macrovascular and microvascular complications of type 1 diabetes. Diabetes Care. 2001;24: 2071–7.
14. Choudhury D, Luna-Salazar C. Preventive health care in chronic kidney disease and end-stage renal disease. Nat Clin Pract Nephrol. 2008;4:194–206.
15. Collins R, Armitage J, Parish S, Sleigh P, Peto R, Heart Protection Study Collaborative G. MRC/BHF heart protection study of cholesterol-lowering with simvastatin in 5963 people with diabetes: a randomised placebo-controlled trial. Lancet. 2003; 361:2005–16.
16. Colhoun HM, Betteridge DJ, Durrington PN, Hitman GA, Neil HAW, Livingstone SJ, Charlton-Menys V, DeMicco DA, Fuller JH. Effects of atorvastatin on kidney outcomes and cardiovascular disease in patients with diabetes: an analysis from the collaborative atorvastatin diabetes study (CARDS). Am J Kidney Dis. 2009;54:810–9.
17. Coonrod BA, Ellis D, Becker DJ, Bunker CH, Kelsey SF, Lloyd CE, Drash AL, Kuller LH, Orchard TJ. Predictors of microalbuminuria in individuals with IDDM. Pittsburgh Epidemiology of Diabetes Complications Study. Diabetes Care. 1993;16:1376–83.
18. Dautin G, Soltani Z, Ducloux D, Gautier T, Pais de Barros JP, Gambert P, Lagrost L, Masson D. Hemodialysis reduces plasma apolipoprotein C-I concentration making VLDL a better substrate for lipoprotein lipase. Kidney Int. 2007;72:871–8.
19. Davidson MH. Apolipoprotein measurements: is more widespread use clinically indicated? Clin Cardiol. 2009;32:482–6.
20. Davis TM, Ting R, Best JD, Donoghoe MW, Drury PL, Sullivan DR, Jenkins AJ, O'Connell RL, Whiting MJ, Glasziou PP, Simes RJ, Kesäniemi YA, Gebski VJ, Scott RS, Keech AC, Fenofibrate Intervention and Event Lowering in Diabetes Study investigators. Effects of fenofibrate on renal function in patients with type 2 diabetes mellitus: the Fenofibrate Intervention and Event Lowering in Diabetes (FIELD) Study. Diabetologia. 2011;54: 280–90.
21. DCCT. Lipid and lipoprotein levels in patients with IDDM diabetes control and complication. Trial experience. The DCCT research group. Diabetes Care. 1992;15:886–94.
22. DCCT. Effect of intensive diabetes management on macrovascular events and risk factors in the Diabetes Control and Complications Trial. Am J Cardiol. 1995;75:894–903.
23. DCCT. Effect of intensive therapy on the development and progression of diabetic nephropathy in the Diabetes Control and Complications Trial. Kidney Int. 1995;47:1703–20.
24. de Boer IH, Rue TC, Cleary PA, Lachin JM, Molitch ME, Steffes MW, Sun W, Zinman B, Brunzell JD, Diabetes Control and Complications Trial/ Epidemiology of Diabetes Interventions and Complications Study Research Group, White NH, Danis RP, Davis MD, Hainsworth D, Hubbard LD, Nathan DM. Long-term renal outcomes of patients with type 1 diabetes mellitus and microalbuminuria: an analysis of the Diabetes Control and Complications Trial/Epidemiology of Diabetes Interventions and Complications cohort. Arch Intern Med. 2011;171: 412–20.
25. Diamante. Estudio Diamante: Renal involvement in type 1 diabetes in Spain. Diabetes Res Clin Pract. 1997;38:129–37.
26. Diamond JR, Karnovsky MJ. Focal and segmental glomerulosclerosis: analogies to atherosclerosis. Kidney Int. 1988;33:917–24.
27. Douglas K, O'Malley PG, Jackson JL. Meta-analysis: the effect of statins on albuminuria. Ann Intern Med. 2006;145:117–24.
28. Fagot-Campagna A, Nelson RG, Knowler WC, Pettitt DJ, Robbins DC, Go O, Welty TK, Lee ET, Howard BV. Plasma lipoproteins and the incidence of abnormal excretion of albumin in diabetic American Indians: the Strong Heart Study. Diabetologia. 1998;41:1002–9.
29. Fellström B, Holdaas H, Jardine AG, Holme I, Nyberg G, Fauchald P, Grönhagen-Riska C, Madsen S, Neumayer HH, Cole E. Effect of fluvastatin on renal end points in the assessment of Lescol in renal transplant (ALERT) trial. Kidney Int. 2004;66:1549–55.
30. Fellström BC, Jardine AG, Schmieder RE, Holdaas H, Bannister K, Beutler J, Chae DW, Chevaile A, Cobbe SM, Grönhagen-Riska C, the AURORA Study Group. Rosuvastatin and cardiovascular events in patients undergoing hemodialysis. N Engl J Med. 2009;360:1395.

31. Finne P, Reunanen A, Stenman S, Groop PH, Grönhagen-Riska C. Incidence of end-stage renal disease in patients with type 1 diabetes. JAMA. 2005;294(14):1782–7.
32. Fioretto P, Mauer M. Diabetic nephropathy: diabetic nephropathy—challenges in pathologic classification. Nat Rev Nephrol. 2010;6:508–10.
33. Forsblom C, Hiukka A, Leinonen ES, Sundvall J, Groop PH, Taskinen MR. Effects of long-term fenofibrate treatment on markers of renal function in type 2 diabetes: the FIELD Helsinki substudy. Diabetes Care. 2010;33:215–20.
34. Ginsberg HN, Elam MB, Lovato LC, for The ACCORD Study Group, et al. Effects of combination lipid therapy in type 2 diabetes mellitus. N Engl J Med. 2010;362:1563–74.
35. Giorgino F, Laviola L, Cavallo Perin P, Solnica B, Fuller J, Chaturvedi N. Factors associated with progression to macroalbuminuria in microalbuminuric Type 1 diabetic patients: the EURODIAB Prospective Complications Study. Diabetologia. 2004;47: 1020–8.
36. Gordon SM, Hofmann S, Askew DS, Davidson WS. High density lipoprotein: it's not just about lipid transport anymore. Trends Endocrinol Metab. 2011;22:9–15.
37. Groop PH, Forsblom C, Thomas MC. Mechanisms of disease: pathway-selective insulin resistance and microvascular complications of diabetes. Nat Clin Pract Endocrinol Metab. 2005;1(2):100–10.
38. Groop PH, Thomas MC, Moran JL, Wadèn J, Thorn LM, Mäkinen VP, Rosengård-Bärlund M, Saraheimo M, Hietala K, Heikkilä O, Forsblom C, FinnDiane Study Group. The presence and severity of chronic kidney disease predicts all-cause mortality in type 1 diabetes. Diabetes. 2009;58(7):1651–8.
39. Gross JL, de Azevedo MJ, Silveiro SP, Canani LH, Caramori ML, Zelmanovitz T. Diabetic nephropathy: diagnosis, prevention, and treatment. Diabetes Care. 2005;28:164–76.
40. Gröne HJ, Walli AK, Gröne EF. Arterial hypertension and hyperlipidemia as determinants of glomerulosclerosis. Clin Investig. 1993;71:834–9.
41. Hadjadj S. Duly-Bouhanick B, Bekherraz A, BrIdoux F, Gallois Y, Mauco G, Ebran J, Marre M. Serum triglycerides are a predictive factor for the development and the progression of renal and retinal complications in patients with type 1 diabetes. Diabetes Metab. 2004;30:43–51.
42. Holdaas H, Fellström B, Jardine AG, Holme I, Nyberg G, Fauchald P, Grönhagen-Riska C, Madsen S, Neumayer HH, Cole E. Effect of fluvastatin on cardiac outcomes in renal transplant recipients: a multicentre, randomised, placebo-controlled trial. Lancet. 2003;361:2024–31.
43. Holdaas H, Fellström B, Cole E, Nyberg G, Olsson A, Pedersen T, Madsen S, Grönhagen-Riska C, Neumayer HH, Maes B. Long-term cardiac outcomes in renal transplant recipients receiving fluvastatin: the ALERT extension study. Am J Transplant. 2005;5:2929–36.
44. Hovind P, Rossing P, Tarnow L, Smidt UM, Parving HH. Progression of diabetic nephropathy. Kidney Int. 2001;59:702–9.
45. Hovind P, Tarnow L, Rossing P, Jensen BR, Graae M, Torp I, Binder C, Parcing HH. Predictors for the development of microalbuminuria and macroalbuminuria in patients with type 1 diabetes: inception cohort study. BMJ. 2004;328:1105.
46. Huskey J, Lindenfeld J, Cook T, Targher G, Kendrick J, Kjekshus J, Pedersen T, Chonchol M. Effect of simvastatin on kidney function loss in patients with coronary heart disease: findings from the Scandinavian simvastatin survival study (4S). Atherosclerosis. 2009;205:202–6.
47. Ikewaki K, Schaefer JR, Frischmann ME. Delayed in vivo catabolism of intermediate-density lipoprotein and low-density lipoprotein in hemodialysis patients as potential cause of premature atherosclerosis. Arterioscler Thromb Vasc Biol. 2005;25: 2615–22.
48. Jenkins AJ, Lyons TJ, Zheng D, Otvos JD, Lackland DT, McGee D, Garvey WT, Klein RL. Lipoproteins in the DCCT/EDIC cohort: associations with diabetic nephropathy. Kidney Int. 2003;64:817–28.
49. Jensen T, Stender S, Deckert T. Abnormalities in plasma concentrations of lipoproteins and fibrinogen in type 1 (insulin dependent) diabetic patients with increased urinary albumin excretion. Diabetologia. 1988;31:142–5.
50. Jones SL, Close CF, Mattock MB, Jarret RJ, Keen H, Viberti GC. Plasma lipid and coagulation factor concentrations in insulin dependent diabetics with microalbuminuria. BMJ. 1989;298:487–90.
51. Jun M, Foote C, Lv J, Neal B, Patel A, Nicholls SJ, Grobbee DE, Cass A, Chalmers J, Perkovic V. Effects of fibrates on cardiovascular outcomes: a systematic review and meta-analysis. Lancet. 2010;375:1875–84.
52. Kahri J, Groop PH, Elliott T, Viberti G, Taskinen MR. Plasma cholesteryl ester transfer protein and its relationship to plasma lipoproteins and apolipoprotein A-I containing lipoproteins in IDDM patients with microalbuminuria and clinical nephropathy. Diabetes Care.1994;17:412–419.
53. Kastarinen H, Hörkkö S, Kauma H, Karjalainen A, Savolainen MJ, Kesäniemi YA. Low-density lipoprotein clearance in patients with chronic renal failure. Nephrol Dial Transplant. 2009;24:2131–5.
54. Kaysen GA. Lipid and lipoprotein metabolism in chronic kidney disease. J Ren Nutr. 2009;19:73–7.
55. Kaysen GA. New insights into lipid metabolism in chronic kidney disease. J Ren Nutr. 2011; 2011(21):120–3.
56. Keane WF, Kasiske BL, O'Donnell MP, Kim Y. The role of altered lipid metabolism in the progression of renal disease: experimental evidence. Am J Kidney Dis. 1991;17:38–42.
57. Keech A, Simes RJ, Barter P, Best J, Scott R, Taskinen MR, Forder P, Pillai A, Davis T, Glasziou P, Drury P, Kesäniemi YA, Sullivan D, Hunt D, Colman P, d'Emden M, Whiting M, Ehnholm C,

Laakso M, FIELD study investigators. Effect of long-term fenofibrate therapy on cardiovascular events in 9795 people with type 2 diabetes mellitus (the FIELD study): randomised controlled trial. Lancet. 2005;366:1849–61.
58. Kilpatrick ES, Rigby AS, Atkin SL. Insulin resistance, the metabolic syndrome, and complication risk in type 1 diabetes: "double diabetes" in the Diabetes Control and Complications Trial. Diabetes Care. 2007;30(3):707–12.
59. Kilpatrick ES, Rigby AS, Atkin SL. The diabetes control and complications trial: the gift that keeps giving. Nat Rev Endocrinol. 2009;5(10):537–45.
60. Kronenberg F. Dyslipidemia and nephrotic syndrome: recent advances. J Ren Nutr. 2005;15: 195–203.
61. Lennernäs H, Fager G. Pharmacodynamics and pharmacokinetics of the HMG-CoA reductase inhibitors. Similarities and differences. Clin Pharmacokinet. 1997;32:403–25.
62. Lin J, Hu FB, Rimm EB, Rifai N, Curhan GC. The association of serum lipids and inflammatory biomarkers with renal function in men with type 2 diabetes mellitus. Kidney Int. 2006;69(2):336–42.
63. Lin J, Hu FB, Mantzoros C, Curhan GC. Lipid and inflammatory biomarkers and kidney function decline in type 2 diabetes. Diabetologia. 2010;53(2): 263–7.
64. Marcovecchio ML, Dalton RN, Prevost AT, Acerini CL, Barrett TG, Cooper JD, Edge J, Neil A, Shield J, Widmer B, Todd JA, Dunger DB. Prevalence of abnormal lipid profiles and the relationship with the development of microalbuminuria in adolescents with type 1 diabetes. Diabetes Care. 2009;32:658–63.
65. Mattock MB, Cronin N, Cavallo-Perin P, Idzior-Walus B, Penno G, Bandinelli S, Standl E, Kofinis A, Fuller JH. Plasma lipids and urinary albumin excretion rate in Type 1 diabetes mellitus: the EURODIAB IDDM Complications Study. Diabetic Med. 2001;18:59–67.
66. Mulec H, Johnsen SA, Wiklund O, Björck S. Cholesterol: a renal risk factor in diabetic nephropathy? Am J Kidney Dis. 1993;22:196–201.
67. Murphy AJ, Chin-Dusting JP, Sviridov D, Woollard KJ. The anti-inflammatory effects of high density lipoproteins. Curr Med Chem. 2009;16:667–75.
68. Mäkinen V, Forsblom C, Thorn LM, Wadén J, Gordin D, Heikkilä O, Hietala K, Kyllönen L, Kytö J, Rosengård-Bärlund M, Saraheimo M, Tolonen N, Parkkonen M, Kaski K, Ala-Korpela M, Groop P. Metabolic phenotypes, vascular complications, and premature deaths in a population of 4,197 patients with type 1 diabetes. Diabetes. 2008;57:2480–7.
69. Mäkinen V-P, Tynkkynen T, Soininen P, Forsblom C, Peltola T, Kangas AJ, Groop P-H, Ala-Korpela M. Sphingomyelin is associated with kidney disease in type 1 diabetes (The FinnDiane Study). Metabolomics. 2011;8(3):369–75.
70. Mäkinen VP, et al. Metabolic diversity of progressive kidney disease in 325 patients with type 1 diabetes. J Proteome Res. 2012;11(3):1782–90.
71. Moradi H, Yuan J, Ni Z, Norris K, Vaziri ND. Reverse cholesterol transport pathway in experimental chronic renal failure. Am J Nephrol. 2009;30: 147–54.
72. Mänttäri M, Tiula E, Alikoski T, Manninen V. Effects of hypertension and dyslipidemia on the decline in renal function. Hypertension. 1995;26: 670–5.
73. Nakajima K, Nakano T, Tokita Y, Nagamine T, Inazu A, Kobayashi J, Mabuchi H, Stanhope KL, Havel PJ, Okazaki M, Ai M, Tanaka A. Postprandial lipoprotein metabolism: VLDL vs. chylomicrons. Clin Chim Acta. 2011;412:1306–18.
74. Natali A, Pucci G, Boldrini B, Schillaci G. Metabolic syndrome: at the crossroads of cardiorenal risk. J Nephrol. 2009;22(1):29–38.
75. Navaneethan SD, Pansini F, Perkovic V, Manno C, Pellegrini F, Johnson DW, Craig JC, Strippoli GF. HMG CoA reductase inhibitors (statins) for people with chronic kidney disease not requiring dialysis. Cochrane Database Syst Rev. 2009;2, CD007784.
76. Nikkilä EA, Hormila P. Serum lipids and lipoproteins in insulin-treated diabetes: demonstrations of increased high-density lipoprotein concentrations. Diabetes. 1978;27:1078–86.
77. Orchard TJ, Chang Y-F, Ferrel RE, Petro N, Ellis DE. Nephropathy in type 1 diabetes: a manifestation of insulin resistance and multiple genetic susceptibilities? Kidney Int. 2002;62:963–70.
78. Orchard TJ, Secrest AM, Miller RG, Costacou T. In the absence of renal disease, 20 year mortality in type 2 diabetes is comparable to that of the general population: a report from the Pittsburgh Epidemiology of Diabetes Complications Study. Diabetologia. 2010;53:2312–9.
79. Otvos JD. Measurement of lipoprotein subclass profiles by nuclear magnetic resonance spectroscopy. Clin Lab. 2002;48(3–4):171–80.
80. Packard CJ. Small dense low-density lipoprotein and its role as an independent predictor of cardiovascular disease. Curr Opin Lipidol. 2006;17:412–7.
81. Palmer SC, Hayen A, Macaskill P, Pellegrini F, Craig JC, Elder GJ, Strippoli GF. Serum levels of phosphorus, parathyroid hormone, and calcium and risks of death and cardiovascular disease in individuals with chronic kidney disease: a systematic review and meta-analysis. JAMA. 2011;305(11):1119–27.
82. Parving HH. The impact of hypertension and antihypertensive treatment on the course and prognosis of diabetic nephropathy. J Hypertens. 1990;8: S187–91.
83. Perkins BA, Ficociello LH, Silva KH, Finkelstein DM, Warram JH, Krolewski AS. Regression of microalbuminuria in type 1 diabetes. N Engl J Med. 2003;348:2285–93.
84. Peric-Golia L, Peric-Golia M. Aortic and renal lesions in hypercholesterolemic adult, male, virgin Sprague-Dawley rats. Atherosclerosis. 1983;46: 57–65.
85. Postma MJ, de Zeeuw D. The economic benefits of preventing end-stage renal disease in patients with

type 2 diabetes mellitus. Nephrol Dial Transplant. 2009;24(10):2975–83.
86. Prichard SS. Impact of dyslipidemia in end-stage renal disease. J Am Soc Nephrol. 2003;14: S315–20.
87. Rader DJ. Molecular regulation of HDL metabolism and function: implications for novel therapies. J Clin Invest. 2006;116:3090–100.
88. Raile K, Galler A, Hofer S, Herbst A, Dunstheimer D, Busch P, Holl RW. Diabetic nephropathy in 27,805 children, adolescents, and adults with type 1 diabetes: effect of diabetes duration, A1C, hypertension, dyslipidemia, diabetes onset, and sex. Diabetes Care. 2007;30:2523–8.
89. Ravid M, Brosh D, Ravid-Safran D, Levy Z, Rachmani R. Main risk factors for nephropathy in type 2 diabetes mellitus are plasma cholesterol levels, mean blood pressure, and hyperglycemia. Arch Intern Med. 1998;158:998–1004.
90. Retnakaran R, Cull CA, Thorne KI, Adler AI, Holman RR, the UKPDS Study Group. Risk factors for renal dysfunction in type 2 diabetes. Diabetes. 2006;55:1832–9.
91. Ridker PM, Macfadyen J, Cressman M, Glynn RJ. Efficacy of rosuvastatin among men and women with moderate chronic kidney disease and elevated high-sensitivity C-reactive protein: a secondary analysis from the JUPITER (Justification for the Use of Statins in Prevention—an Intervention Trial Evaluating Rosuvastatin) trial. J Am Coll Cardiol. 2010;55(12):1266–73.
92. Rossi MCE, Nicolucci A, Pellegrini F, Comaschi M, Ceriello A, Cucinotta D, Giorda C, Valentini U, Vespasiani G, De Cosmo S. Identifying patients with type 2 diabetes at high risk of microalbuminuria: results of the DEMAND (Developing Education on Microalbuminuria for Awareness of reNal and cardiovascular risk in Diabetes) study. Nephrol Dial Transplant. 2008;23:1278–84.
93. Rothblat GH, Phillips MC. High-density lipoprotein heterogeneity and function in reverse cholesterol transport. Curr Opin Lipidol. 2010;21:229–38.
94. Ruan XZ, Varghese Z, Moorhead JF. An update on the lipid nephrotoxicity hypothesis. Nat Rev Nephrol. 2009;5:713–21.
95. Samuelsson O, Mulec H, Knight-Gibson C, Attman PO, Kron B, Larsson R, Weiss L, Wedel H, Alaupovic P. Lipoprotein abnormalities are associated with increased rate of progression of human chronic renal insufficiency. Nephrol Dial Transplant. 1997;12:1908–15.
96. Secrest AM, Becker DJ, Kelsey SF, Laporte RE, Orchard TJ. Cause-specific mortality trends in a large population-based cohort with long-standing childhood-onset type 1 diabetes. Diabetes. 2010; 59:3216–22.
97. Schaeffner ES, Kurth T, Curhan GC, Glynn RJ, Rexrode KM, Baigent C, Buring JE, Gaziano JM. Cholesterol and the risk of renal dysfunction in apparently healthy men. J Am Soc Nephrol. 2003; 14:2084–91.
98. Shamseddin MK, Parfrey PS. Sudden cardiac death in chronic kidney disease: epidemiology and prevention. Nat Rev Nephrol. 2011;7(3):145–54.
99. Sandhu S, Wiebe N, Fried LF, Tonelli M. Statins for improving renal outcomes: a meta-analysis. J Am Soc Nephrol. 2006;17:2006–16.
100. Shepherd J, Kastelein JJ, Bittner V, Deedwania P, Breazna A, Dobson S, Wilson DJ, Zuckerman A, Wenger NK, Treating to New Targets I. Effect of intensive lipid lowering with atorvastatin on renal function in patients with coronary heart disease: the treating to new targets (TNT) study. Clin J Am Soc Nephrol. 2007;2:1131–9.
101. Shepherd J, Kastelein JP, Bittner VA, Carmena R, Deedwania PC, Breazna A, Dobson S, Wilson DJ, Zuckerman AL, Wenger NK, Treating to New Targets Steering Committee and Investigators. Intensive lipid lowering with atorvastatin in patients with coronary artery disease, diabetes, and chronic kidney disease. Mayo Clin Proc. 2008;83:870–9.
102. Stadler M, Auinger M, Anderwald C, Kästenbauer T, Kramar R, Feinböck C, Irsigler K, Kronenberg F, Prager R. Long-term mortality and incidence of renal dialysis and transplantation in type 1 diabetes mellitus. J Clin Endocrinol Metab. 2006;91:3814–20.
103. Strippoli GF, Navaneethan SD, Johnson DW, Perkovic V, Pellegrini F, Nicolucci A, Craig JC. Effects of statins in patients with chronic kidney disease: meta-analysis and meta-regression of randomised controlled trials. BMJ. 2008;336:645–51.
104. Sukhija R, Bursac Z, Kakar P, Fink L, Fort C, Satwani S, Aronow WS, Bansal D, Mehta JL. Effect of statins on the development of renal dysfunction. Am J Cardiol. 2008;101:975–9.
105. Takagi H, Umemoto T. A meta-analysis of randomized trials for effects of atorvastatin on renal function in chronic kidney disease. Int J Cardiol. 2011;152: 242–4.
106. Taskinen MR. Diabetic dyslipidaemia: from basic research to clinical practice. Diabetologia. 2003;46: 733–49.
107. Thomas MC, Rosengård-Bärlund M, Mills V, Rönnback M, Thomas S, Forsblom C, Cooper ME, Taskinen MR, Viberti G, Groop PH. Serum lipids and the progression of nephropathy in type 1 diabetes. Diabetes Care. 2006;29(2):317–22.
108. Thorn LM, Forsblom C, Wadén J, Saraheimo M, Tolonen N, Hietala K, Groop PH, Finnish Diabetic Nephropathy Study Group. Metabolic syndrome as a risk factor for cardiovascular disease, mortality, and progression of diabetic nephropathy in type 1 diabetes. Diabetes Care. 2009;32(5):950–2. Epub 2009 Feb 5.
109. Tolonen N, Forsblom C, Thorn L, Wadén J, Rosengård-Bärlund M, Saraheimo M, Heikkilä O, Pettersson-Fernholm K, Taskinen MR, Groop PH, FinnDiane Study Group. Relationship between lipid profiles and kidney function in patients with type 1 diabetes. Diabetologia. 2008;51(1):12–20.
110. Tolonen N, Forsblom C, Thorn L, Wadén J, Rosengård-Bärlund M, Saraheimo M, Feodoroff M,

Mäkinen VP, Gordin D, Taskinen MR, Groop PH, FinnDiane Study Group. Lipid abnormalities predict progression of renal disease in patients with type 1 diabetes. Diabetologia. 2009;52(12):2522–30.
111. Tonelli M, Isles C, Craven T, Tonkin A, Pfeffer MA, Shepherd J, Sacks FM, Furberg C, Cobbe SM, Simes J, West M, Packard C, Curhan GC. Effect of pravastatin on rate of kidney function loss in people with or at risk for coronary disease. Circulation. 2005;112:171–8.
112. Tseng CH. Lipid abnormalities associated with urinary albumin excretion rate in Taiwanese type 2 diabetic patients. Kidney Int. 2005;67:1547–53.
113. Vannini P, Ciavarella A, Flammini M, Bargossi AM, Forlani G, Borgnino LC, Orsoni G. Lipid abnormalities in insulin-dependent diabetic patients with albuminuria. Diabetes Care. 1984;7:151–4.
114. Vaziri ND. Causes of dysregulation of lipid metabolism in chronic renal failure. Semin Dial. 2009; 22:644–51.
115. Vergès B. Abnormal hepatic apolipoprotein B metabolism in type 2 diabetes. Atherosclerosis. 2010;211:353–60.
116. Verhoye E, Langlois MR, Asklepios Investigators. Circulating oxidized low-density lipoprotein: a biomarker of atherosclerosis and cardiovascular risk? Clin Chem Lab Med. 2009;47:128–37.
117. Wanner C, Krane V, März W, Olschewski M, Mann JF, Ruf G, Ritz E, German Diabetes and Dialysis Study Investigators. Atorvastatin in patients with type 2 diabetes mellitus undergoing hemodialysis. N Engl J Med. 2005;353:238–49.
118. Yang X, So WY, Ma R, Ko G, Kong A, Lam C, Ho CS, Cockram C, Chow C-C, Tong P, Chan J. Effects of albuminuria and renal dysfunction on development of dyslipidaemia in type 2 diabetes — the Hong Kong Diabetes Registry. Nephrol Dial Transplant. 2008;23:2834–40.
119. Yishak A, Costacou T, Virella G, Zgibor J, Fried L, Walsh M, Evans RW, Lopes-Virella M, Kagan VE, Otvos J, Orchard TJ. Novel predictors of overt nephropathy in subjects with type 1 diabetes. A nested case control study from the Pittsburgh Epidemiology of Diabetes Complications cohort. Nephrol Dial Transplant. 2006;21:93–100.

# Roles of Extravasated and Modified Plasma Lipoproteins in Diabetic Retinopathy

# 15

Mingyuan Wu and Timothy J. Lyons

## Core Messages

- Diabetic retinopathy (DR) is generally viewed as a consequence of hyperglycemia, but to a large extent, it may be driven by effects of plasma lipoproteins.
- The effects of plasma lipoproteins in DR have been underestimated because of their indirect nature, i.e., they are predominantly consequences of lipoprotein leakage (extravasation) through damaged inner and outer blood-retinal barriers, rather than a direct initiation of vascular damage. After extravasation, lipoproteins become severely modified by glycation and oxidation and, as a result, toxic towards numerous types of retinal cells. They then promote not only further vascular damage and leakage but also a generalized retinal injury.
- The extent of capillary leakage is a more critical determinant of lipoprotein-mediated retinal injury in diabetes than the extent of dyslipidemia. In contrast to the arterial intima, the unique structure of retinal capillaries means that no lipoprotein extravasation occurs under normal conditions (i.e., with intact blood-retinal barriers in the absence of diabetes), making dyslipidemia largely irrelevant to retinal health. In diabetes, blood-retinal barrier breakdown develops only slowly, explaining why the associations between plasma lipoproteins and severity of DR are relatively weak (although statistically significant) and disguising the subsequent importance of lipoproteins in propagating retinal injury.

## Introduction: Diabetic Retinopathy

With sufficiently long survival, almost everyone with diabetes mellitus eventually develops some degree of retinal damage (diabetic retinopathy (DR)), but the rate of progression and its severity vary greatly among individuals. This is true even when conventional risk factors such as duration of diabetes and severity of long-term hyperglycemia are taken into account. DR is one of the most feared complications of diabetes [1] and is a leading cause of blindness in the working-age population [2]. According to a report from the (US) National Eye Institute, about 50 % of people with diabetes have at least some degree of retinopathy, and in the USA, approximately 1 person in 400 has sight-threatening retinal disease caused by diabetes [3]. In type 1 diabetes, in which the duration of diabetes is clear-cut (there is no prolonged asymptomatic phase as in type 2 diabetes), clinical disease typically does not develop within the first 5 years, yet even during this phase, it is evident that subclinical retinal injury is taking place. This was elegantly demonstrated in a dog model

M. Wu • T.J. Lyons, M.D., F.R.C.P. (✉)
Section of Endocrinology & Diabetes, Harold Hamm Oklahoma Diabetes Center, University of Oklahoma Health Sciences Center, 1000 N. Lincoln Blvd., HHODC 2900, Oklahoma City, OK 73104-5020, USA
e-mail: timothy-lyons@ouhsc.edu

A.J. Jenkins et al. (eds.), *Lipoproteins in Diabetes Mellitus*, Contemporary Diabetes, DOI 10.1007/978-1-4614-7554-5_15, © Springer Science+Business Media New York 2014

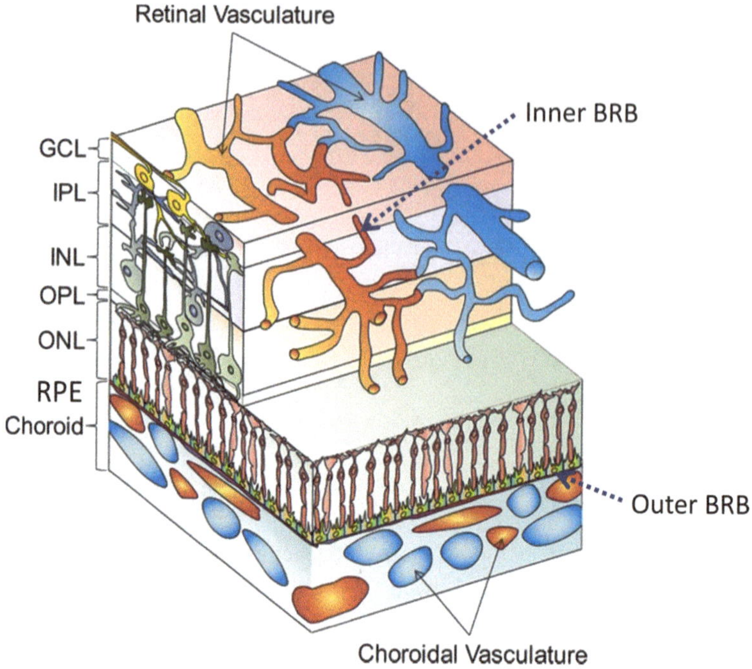


**Fig. 15.1** Retinal cells and blood supply: (Modified from: Fulton, A.B. et al., Retinal degenerative and hypoxic ischemic disease. Doc Ophthalmol. 2009;118:55–61; and reproduced with permission). *Abbreviations*: *GCL* ganglion cell layer, *IPL* inner plexiform layer, *INL* inner nuclear layer, *OPL* outer plexiform layer, *ONL* outer nuclear layer, *RPE* retinal pigment epithelium, *BRB* blood-retinal barrier

of DR by Engerman and Kern [4]. Once present, DR may broadly be classified into three stages: background disease, non-proliferative diabetic retinopathy (NPDR), and an advanced, sight-threatening-phase, proliferative diabetic retinopathy (PDR). Fortunately, the latter develops in only a minority of patients [5]. PDR is characterized by the growth, in response to retinal ischemia, of abnormal new, fragile blood vessels. These vessels invade the vitreous humor and are leaky and prone to hemorrhage.

The normal retina is a highly specialized tissue bounded on the inside by the inner limiting membrane and on the outside by the basement membrane of the retinal pigment epithelium (RPE) (Bruch's membrane) (Fig. 15.1). Counterintuitively, the light-sensing rods and cones are located in the outer retina, immediately inside the RPE, so that light must pass through the overlying retinal "circuitry" (ganglion cell nuclei and plexiform layers) and blood vessels to reach them. Signals to the brain pass inward from the rods and cones, through the ganglion cell layers, to axons which travel across the innermost layer of the retina to reach the optic disc and optic nerve. "Müller cells" are glial cells which span all the layers of the retina vertically: they are essential to retinal health and perform a macrophage-like function. Sooner or later, all types of retinal cell may be injured in diabetes. Most, but not all, investigators believe that the initial lesion is in the microvasculature.

The retina has a dual blood supply. The central retinal artery, a branch of the ophthalmic artery, enters the eye at the optic nerve head and branches across the inner retina. It is readily visualized with an ophthalmoscope, and in diabetes, perhaps because of this easy visual access, abnormalities of its vascular tree serve to define the severity of DR. The capillaries of this inner retinal circulation are highly specialized: endothelial cells have tight junctions which form the inner blood-retinal barrier (IBRB), while pericytes are more numerous than in any other capillary bed, equaling the number of endothelial cells. The pericytes are contractile and regulate retinal blood flow (the highest in the body per gram of tissue); they also regulate the growth and maintain the function of the endothelial cells and IBRB. On the outside of the retina, the ophthalmic artery also supplies the choroidal circulation, which lies between Bruch's membrane and the underlying sclera. This vascular bed is separated from the neural retina by the outer blood-retinal barrier (OBRB), which is formed by tight junctions between the RPE monolayer. The choroidal circulation provides a majority (65–70 %) of the oxygen and nutrients consumed by the retina [6], but it is not visible with the ophthalmoscope, and so in this location, the effects of diabetes are less well-defined.

As mentioned, early DR is defined by damage to the inner retinal capillaries, specifically pericyte loss and leakage of the IBRB. Ophthalmoscopically, "microaneurysms" appear and are thought to be the result of proliferation of endothelial cells following loss of pericytes. Other features include "hard exudates," which are accretions of lipid-rich material following vascular leakage, and "soft exudates," areas of retinal edema resulting from ischemia. Later in the disease process, macular edema and neovascularization may be evident, and both are major causes of vision loss as a result of retinal detachment and/or hemorrhage [1, 2, 7–9].

For decades, two assumptions dominated DR research. First, DR was viewed as a "microvascular complication of diabetes": one in which the retinal insult is primarily or entirely vascular in both its origin and its progression, specifically involving damage to the highly specialized inner retinal capillaries. Second, hyperglycemia has been viewed as the primary cause of both early and advanced disease. While both of these contentions still hold strong elements of truth, it has also become clear that they are oversimplifications. The injury in DR is not confined to the capillaries (and consequent ischemia) but rather affects many (perhaps all) varieties of retinal cell. Hyperglycemia is now regarded as necessary, but not sufficient, for DR to develop: other factors modulate disease severity, and understanding these will bring new opportunities for prevention and therapeutic intervention. In this chapter, we describe the development of a new lipoprotein-related concept for the propagation of DR which is consistent with a generalized retinal injury and which adds a new mechanism, in addition to effects of elevated glucose levels.

## The Initiation of DR

The earliest preclinical event in the evolution of DR is unclear. It is likely to vary from one person to another, to involve several simultaneous insults, and to be scattered in space and time across the retina. Breakdown of the IBRB is an early feature: it may result from metabolic or osmotic injury from high (and fluctuating) plasma glucose levels or intermittent exposure of the capillary endothelium to the severe metabolic stresses that accompany uncontrolled diabetes ("diabetic ketoacidosis"). Such stresses include acidosis, osmotic stress, and elevation of plasma ketone bodies and free fatty acids. Supporting this, it is thought that recurrent diabetic ketoacidosis may be a risk factor for retinopathy [10]. Another early feature of DR, pericyte loss, may occur independently of, or as a result of, injury to endothelial cells and/or the IBRB but, regardless, will itself lead to endothelial injury and IBRB leakage [9]. Such leakage can be detected by fluorescein angiography and occurs at the preclinical phase [11]. Furthermore, studies using microspheres show that particles as large as 100 nm diameter can leak from retinal capillaries in the early, preclinical stages of DR in vivo in animal studies [12]. This is of relevance to our present subject, since all major classes of plasma lipoproteins are smaller than these microspheres (HDL: ~9 nm; LDL: ~20 nm; VLDL: 50–70 nm) and therefore can become extravasated early in the course of DR.

In summary, metabolic stresses of diabetes, including exposure to elevated glucose, free fatty acids, osmotic stress, and other factors, may initiate inner retinal capillary leakage, allowing the retina to be flooded with plasma constituents that normally are rigorously excluded. It is also possible that the earliest stages of diabetes, prior to IBRB leakage, may lead directly to dysfunction of other cell types (Müller cells, neurons, RPE, the choroidal circulation), but these effects are not yet well-defined. We contend that, while hyperglycemia and inner retinal capillary damage may indeed be dominant initial causal factors and features of retinal injury in DR, they are soon followed by a cascade of events in which extravasated, glycated, and oxidized lipoproteins are important promoters of endothelial, IBRB, and pericyte injury. As vicious cycles of vascular injury ensue, these modified lipoproteins may promote a generalized retinal injury. As detailed in this chapter, there is evidence that these processes are well advanced by the time clinical retinopathy becomes detectable.

## Treatment Considerations for DR

The ideal treatment for DR would arrest its development in the pre-clinical phase. Efforts in this regard currently focus on control of modifiable risk factors, most notably hyperglycemia, and indeed, it appears that complete control of glycemia would completely prevent DR. Unfortunately, in the foreseeable future, it is very unlikely that normalization of glucose levels will be achieved for more than a small proportion of people affected by the diabetes epidemic worldwide. Fortunately, new knowledge of disease mechanisms means that specific measures may be developed to block progression even in the presence of hyperglycemia. For example, treatments that would enhance the integrity of the IBRB would hold promise. Existing treatments for DR address only advanced disease. Laser treatment entirely ablates areas of the retina that are ischemic, removing the angiogenic stimulus that drives PDR in neighboring regions, but in effect it sacrifices peripheral vision to save central vision. More recently, specific anti-angiogenic therapies given by intermittent intravitreal injection also aim to inhibit PDR but, by definition, are effective only when an ischemia-induced angiogenic stimulus has already developed, i.e., at a late stage in disease development.

## Evidence Supporting a Role for Plasma Lipoproteins in DR

Numerous studies have sought to define associations between lipoprotein levels and severity of DR, either cross-sectionally or prospectively. There are many challenges to this work: large numbers of subjects must be studied, the plasma lipoprotein system is highly complex (there are many potential metrics), DR severity and progression over time must be assessed objectively (even the fact that a person has two eyes creates challenges), disease progression takes years, and there are numerous confounding clinical variables to be considered (age, sex, diabetes duration, long-term glycemia, renal function, medications over time, and many others). Despite these challenges, a consistent message has emerged from studies over the past 50 years [13–41] (including some recent large cohort studies reviewed below [39–41]), revealing significant associations between adverse lipoprotein levels and DR. Despite this, interest has been muted because the strength of these associations has been weak compared with (a) that between DR and hyperglycemia [42, 43] and (b) those between plasma lipoproteins and risk for atherosclerosis [44, 45].

The term "dyslipidemia" requires definition: it will be used to describe both quantitative and qualitative alterations of lipoproteins found in plasma. The former usage is the standard one and refers to altered levels of simple measures of plasma lipids, e.g., total or LDL cholesterol, HDL cholesterol, and triglycerides. The latter usage includes modification of lipoprotein particles (e.g., by glycation of apolipoproteins and phospholipids, and/or oxidation of any component, but especially unsaturated fatty acids), structural changes, altered distribution of subclasses defined in various ways, and compositional changes in the ratios of component lipids and individual apolipoproteins. Many of these qualitative changes result from or are enhanced by the presence of diabetes, most obviously glycation and oxidation. While enhanced glycation of lipoproteins occurs in plasma in diabetes [46], oxidation predominantly occurs outside the circulation, after extravasation and sequestration in vessel walls, as is established in atherogenesis. Strictly speaking, these extravascular modifications and effects of lipoproteins are distinct from properties found in plasma, i.e., they are not "dyslipidemia."

In the past, many cross-sectional studies in type 1 and type 2 diabetes have described correlations between retinopathy and standard measures of plasma cholesterol, including total and LDL-cholesterol and LDL:HDL cholesterol ratio [14–24, 38] while some found correlations with plasma triglycerides [17, 18, 25, 28]. A series of studies from the 1960s suggested that lipid-lowering interventions, specifically clofibrate, may reduce retinal hard exudates [29–38]. Recently, two large and important prospective studies of patients with type 2 diabetes, Action to Control Cardiovascular Risk in Diabetes (ACCORD) [47] and the Fenofibrate Intervention and Event Lowering in Diabetes (FIELD) Study [48], demonstrated very significant benefits of another fibrate drug, fenofibrate, in preventing the need for laser treatment for DR. The mechanisms for this beneficial effect are currently unknown but under investigation.

More recently, associations of plasma lipoproteins with DR have been addressed in more detail. We studied 988 type 1 diabetic patients (440 women and 548 men) from the Diabetes Control and Complications Trial (DCCT) [41]. We measured detailed lipoprotein characteristics, including conventional lipid profiles, nuclear magnetic resonance lipoprotein subclass profile (NMR-LSP), apoA1, apoB, lipoprotein(a), and susceptibility of LDL to oxidation [41], to DR as assessed by the rigorous DCCT protocol (serial seven-field stereo retinal photographs read centrally [43, 49]). In brief, the lipid parameters that were positively associated with DR included serum triglycerides, serum concentrations of low-density lipoprotein (LDL), LDL particle concentration, and ApoB. The severity of retinopathy was negatively associated with HDL-cholesterol. In men, but not in women, higher levels of small-dense LDL and lower levels of large buoyant LDL were associated with severe DR, and for HDL, similar size-based associations were observed. In general, an atherogenic plasma lipoprotein profile was associated with more severe retinal disease (and of note, DR is a known risk factor for atherosclerosis in people with diabetes [50]). The Hoorn study [39], which included 2,484 50- to 74-year-old Caucasians, yielded similar findings in type 1 and type 2 diabetes (including newly diagnosed and known diabetes) in a population-based cross-sectional study. The prevalence of retinopathy was positively associated with serum cholesterol and triglyceride levels, and elevated plasma total and LDL-cholesterol levels showed associations with retinal hard exudates. Furthermore, the Pittsburgh Epidemiology of Diabetes Complications (EDC) Study [40] of a large type 1 diabetes cohort demonstrated that serum triglycerides and, to a lesser extent, higher levels of LDL-cholesterol were associated with the progression of retinopathy. Progression to proliferative retinopathy was related to higher LDL-cholesterol, serum triglycerides, as well as albumin excretion rate, and glycated hemoglobin. Furthermore, a recent report demonstrated that apoAI, apoB, and the apoB:apoAI ratio were significantly and independently associated with DR in a cross-sectional study of 224 diabetic patients (85 type 1; 139 type 2) [51].

Overall, several points are notable. The associations between the plasma lipoprotein characteristics and DR are, in general, statistically highly significant, but only moderate in magnitude. Also, in people who do not have diabetes, dyslipidemia does not cause retinal disease. Finally, dyslipidemia is very clearly associated with atherosclerosis not only in the presence [52–56] but also in the absence of diabetes. Taken together, the evidence suggests an indirect effect of plasma lipoproteins in the retina, one which is contingent upon unique properties of that tissue and upon unique effects of diabetes. We posit that this relates to the presence of the IBRB and its breakdown in diabetes.

## Extravasated, Modified LDL in the Pathogenesis of DR

In atherosclerosis, elevated plasma levels of LDL and/or modified LDL (oxidized LDL: ox-LDL) are associated with cardiovascular disease [52–56], but both the modification of LDL and its harmful effects occur primarily in the arterial intima, not in plasma. We have developed a new concept: that LDL (and by extension, other plasma lipoproteins) mediate a significant proportion of retinal injury in diabetes, but do so indirectly, not by initiating vascular damage, but rather by becoming extravasated through leaking inner (and perhaps) outer blood-retinal barriers, subsequently being modified by glycation and oxidation, thereby becoming toxic towards any cells in the vicinity. Initially, such damage is patchy and the nearby cells are vascular, but later with more severe leakage, extravasated lipoproteins could permeate throughout all layers of the retina, which is only ~249 μm in total thickness [57].

## Effects of Modified LDL on Retinal Capillary Vascular Cells

We have accrued considerable evidence of injurious effects of modified LDL towards a variety of retinal cell species in culture. Generally we employed two control conditions: not only native (N-)LDL (i.e., unmodified LDL), comparing its effects to modified forms, but also serum-free medium, recognizing that in the healthy retina, no extravasation of plasma lipoproteins occurs. We utilized degrees of in vitro modification and LDL concentrations designed to simulate conservatively the stresses present in diabetes in vivo. Initially, we investigated the effects of normal and mildly modified human LDL (from healthy donors) on bovine retinal capillary endothelial cell and pericytes. These modified LDLs, prepared in vitro, were intended to simulate characteristics of circulating, plasma lipoproteins, not those that had undergone more severe oxidation after extravasation. This work was intended to address the question of whether mild glycation and/or oxidation of plasma LDL might contribute to the initiation of retinal capillary injury. We found that indeed, survival of both endothelial cells and pericytes decreased with exposure to low levels of modified LDL and that toxicity increased in the following order: glycation < mild oxidation < combined glycation/mild oxidation [58].

In our more recent cell culture work, we have employed more severe degrees of LDL modification, again imposed in vitro on LDL from healthy donors, to simulate lipoproteins that have become extravasated. To prepare "highly-oxidized glycated LDL" (HOG-LDL), N-LDL was first glycated (as would happen in plasma in diabetes), then copper oxidized to simulate its fate after extravasation [59–61]. In all of this work, it is essential to maintain conditions that are pathophysiologically relevant. It is of interest that antibodies raised against copper-oxidized LDL (that had been prepared by a similar protocol to our own) recognized in vivo oxidized LDL in atheromatous plaque and, in our hands, in human diabetic retinae (see below). The concentration of LDL employed is also critical. In our work, cells are typically exposed to a range of concentrations, of which the highest is about half of typical plasma levels. Tissue levels in the diabetic retina are unknown, but estimates of ApoB levels in atheromatous plaque suggest they may be 2–79 times *higher* than in plasma [62, 63]. This surprising finding may be explained by extensive sequestration of LDL in vessel walls as a result of covalent cross-linking, and it is reasonable to expect a similar effect in the diabetic retina.

## Modified LDL Mediates Apoptosis of Retinal Capillary Endothelial Cells and Pericytes

As detailed above, our early studies demonstrated that mild modification of LDL resulting from separate or combined processes of glycation and oxidation is implicated in chronic retinal capillary injury and thus perhaps to the initiation of DR [58], acting in concert with hyperglycemia. Using more severely modified HOG-LDL, we showed that oxidative stress and inflammation are associated with LDL-induced retinal cell death. HOG-LDL enhanced intracellular reactive oxygen species (ROS), 3-nitrotyrosine (3-NT), tyrosine nitration of prostacyclin synthase, peroxynitrite ($ONOO^-$) formation, inducible nitric oxide synthase (iNOS) expression, and nitric oxide (NO) production, in parallel with induction of monocyte chemoattractant protein-1 (MCP-1) secretion and nuclear factor-kappaB (NF-kappaB) activation in human retinal capillary pericytes [64, 65]. Thus, HOG-LDL has pro-inflammatory and pro-oxidant effects on retinal pericytes. HOG-LDL also induced DNA fragmentation, activated the caspase cascade, and inhibited cell proliferation in pericytes, consistent with a possible contributory role in the apoptotic pericyte loss that occurs in vivo in DR [61, 66]. Exposure to HOG-LDL versus N-LDL induced similar phosphorylation of mitogen-activated protein kinase (MAPK) signaling pathways including extracellular signal-regulated kinase (ERK), p38, and Jun N-terminal kinase (JNK), and blockade of the ERK, p38, and JNK pathways did not inhibit apoptosis of pericyte induced by HOG-LDL, suggesting that apoptosis induced by HOG-LDL is independent of the activation of MAPK signaling pathways [60]. Recently, we implicated Wnt signaling pathways in DR [67, 68]. Wnt signaling pathways regulate cell proliferation and differentiation, apoptosis, stem cell maintenance, angiogenesis, inflammation, fibrosis, and carcinogenesis [69]. In our studies, modified LDL resulted in Wnt pathway activation via oxidative stress [68], and further studies are in progress. In conclusion, this body of cell culture work indicates that modified LDL, if it comes in contact with specialized retinal cells, can activate multiple intracellular pathways consistent with known characteristics of DR.

## Modified LDL Influences Gene Expression in Human Retinal Capillary Pericytes

Complementing the studies described above, we used gene array studies to investigate the effects of 24 h exposure to HOG-LDL versus N-LDL in human retinal pericytes [61]. These revealed 60 genes that were altered, including members of functional pathways involving fatty acid, eicosanoid, and cholesterol metabolism; fibrinolytic regulation; cell growth and proliferation; cell stress responses; the kinin system; and angiogenesis, indicating that HOG-LDL elicits gene expression in retinal pericytes that may contribute to pericyte loss and other retinal abnormalities in DR. Pro-apoptotic and pro-angiogenic responses to HOG-LDL may be of particular importance in this regard [70]. Microarray analysis also showed that matrix metalloproteinase 1 (MMP1), MMP2, MMP11, MMP14, and MMP25 and tissue inhibitor of metalloproteinase1 (TIMP1), TIMP2, TIMP3, and TIMP4 were expressed in pericytes. Of these, only TIMP3 mRNA showed altered regulation, being expressed at significantly lower levels in response to HOG-LDL versus N-LDL [56]. Quantitative PCR and immunoblotting of cell/matrix proteins confirmed the reduction in TIMP3 mRNA and protein in response to HOG-LDL. In contrast to cellular TIMP3 protein, analysis of secreted TIMP1, TIMP2, and MMP1 and collagenase activity indicated no changes in their production in response to modified LDL. Thus, HOG-LDL selectively influences tissue inhibitor of metalloproteinase-3 gene expression and protein production among in pericytes and might contribute to microvascular abnormalities in DR [59].

## Aminoguanidine Mitigates Toxicity in Human Retinal Capillary Pericytes Exposed to HOG-LDL

Much evidence suggests beneficial effects of aminoguanidine in experimental DR, including prevention of abnormal endothelial cell proliferation [71], reduction of pericyte dropout [71, 72], inhibition of the development of retinal microaneurysms [72] and acellular capillaries [72], prevention of arteriolar thrombosis [73], and reduction of retinal capillary-associated basement membrane thickening [74]. These benefits have been found in various animal models including diabetic dogs [72], streptozotocin-induced diabetic rats [71, 74], and diabetic and hypertensive rats [73]. Typically, aminoguanidine was administered by intraperitoneal (i.p.) injection (~25–50 mg/kg) or adding into diet (~3.0 g/kg) or drinking water (~50 mg/100 ml). In vitro, we found that remarkably low concentrations of aminoguanidine (in the nanomolar range) blocked cytotoxic modification of LDL exposed to stresses including oxidation and glycation that simulate the diabetic environment [75], thus protecting retinal capillary cells from previously modified LDL. This action may contribute to the beneficial effects of aminoguanidine observed in experimental DR. The efficacy of aminoguanidine at nanomolar concentrations suggests an action through scavenging reactive carbonyls (whether generated by oxidative or metabolic processes) rather than by NOS inhibition that occurs at higher concentrations [75, 76]. Unfortunately, in a clinical trial of oral aminoguanidine (300 mg/day), three patients developed glomerulonephritis [77], and further human studies have not taken place. However, local administration of this drug to the eye could still represent a potential intervention, potentially bringing its beneficial effects while avoiding systemic side effects.

## Effects of Pigment Epithelium Derived Factor

PEDF is a glycoprotein with neurotrophic, anti-oxidative, and anti-angiogenic properties. Previous studies have shown that decreased ocular levels of PEDF are associated with DR [78–80]. Intravitreal injection of PEDF reduced vascular leakage in rat models of diabetes and oxygen-induced retinopathy (OIR), likely resulting from the decreased levels of retinal inflammatory factors including VEGF, VEGF receptor-2, MCP-1, tumor necrosis factor alpha (TNF-α), and intercellular adhesion molecular-1 (ICAM-1) [81]. In cultured retinal capillary endothelial cells, PEDF treatment decreased TNF alpha and ICAM-1 expression under hypoxia. Downregulation of PEDF expression by siRNA leads to increased levels of VEGF and TNF alpha secretion in retinal Müller cells. Taken together, PEDF is a novel endogenous anti-inflammatory factor in the eye. As stated above, HOG-LDL, but not N-LDL, significantly increased ONOO(−) formation, NO production, and iNOS expression in human retinal capillary pericytes [65]. These changes were alleviated by PEDF. Moreover, PEDF significantly ameliorated HOG-LDL-induced ROS generation through upregulation of superoxide dismutase 1 expression [65]. Overall, PEDF is a potential candidate for the prevention or inhibition of DR, operating at least in part by inhibiting the effects of oxidized LDL [65, 81].

## Immunologic Consequences

An intriguing possibility is that extravasated and modified LDL may trigger an immune response and the resulting modified LDL immunocomplexes might mediate retinal injury (Fig. 15.2). Such effects have been implicated in atherogenesis. Increased levels of oxidized LDL immunocomplexes are associated with the development of coronary calcification [82, 83]. In addition, oxidized LDL and advanced glycation end product-modified LDL (AGE-LDL) in circulating immunocomplexes are associated with progression and increased levels of carotid intima-media thickness (IMT), demonstrating that ox-LDL immune complexes have pro-inflammatory and proatherogenesis properties in type 1 diabetes [82, 83]. However, the potential roles and mechanisms of modified LDL immunocomplexes in DR have not been addressed.

## Evidence for the Presence of Modified Lipoproteins in the Diabetic Retina

Clearly, our hypothesis requires demonstration of the actual presence of modified lipoproteins in the diabetic retina and their absence in the healthy retina. Recently, we obtained characterized human retinae postmortem from nondiabetic and type 2 diabetic individuals with varying degrees of DR [61] (Fig. 15.3) and performed immunohistochemistry to detect oxidized LDL and ApoB (ApoB100, a marker of LDL and VLDL). Staining was absent in non-diabetic subjects but present in those with diabetes, correlating with severity of retinopathy across three categories (no clinical retinopathy, non-proliferative DR, and PDR). Thus, lipoprotein extravasation in diabetic retinae

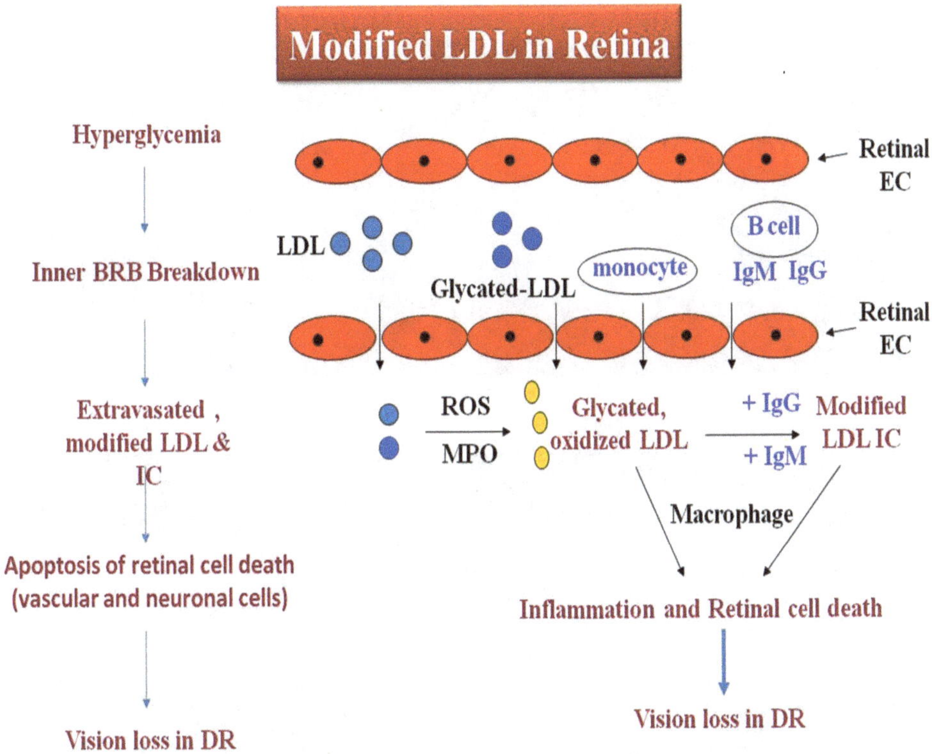


**Fig. 15.2** Potential consequences of extravasated LDL in the progression of retinal injury in diabetic retinopathy: After extravasation, LDL becomes severely modified by glycation and oxidation and, as a result, toxic towards numerous types of retinal cells. In addition, extravasated and modified LDL may trigger an immune response, and the resulting modified LDL immunocomplexes may mediate retinal injury

was clear-cut and was present even in subjects with no clinical DR (consistent with a causative role for future DR), but was entirely absent in healthy retinae from non-diabetic individuals. Ox-LDL was prominent in inner retina (ganglion cell layer (GCL)) where most blood flow is from the central retinal artery. In PDR, ox-LDL was also present in the outer retina, near the RPE, which is supplied by the choroidal circulation. This could represent permeation of extravasated LDL from the inner to all retinal layers, or it could suggest leakage of the OBRB as an additional mechanism for DR. Besides ox-LDL, intra-retinal immunofluorescence of ApoB was also present in diabetic human retinae, paralleling the findings with ox-LDL and correlating with the severity of DR [61]. In addition, in retinal sections from subjects with PDR, macrophage infiltration was prominent—suggesting significant inflammation and another parallel with atherogenesis.

In summary, the data suggest that lipoproteins from plasma may play a central, and heretofore unrecognized, role in propagating retinal injury, even though the associations of plasma lipoproteins with the severity of retinopathy are relatively weak. Ox-LDL is known to be toxic to many cell types, including vascular and neural cells, and may therefore perpetuate retinal injury. These observations support the concept that plasma lipoproteins (which we can study relatively easily) may modulate disease risk, but extravasated lipoproteins (much less accessible and likely to be significantly modified) are the direct mediators of DR. From this it follows that effective treatments must correct not only adverse quantitative plasma lipoprotein levels but also a spectrum of qualitative abnormalities in both plasma and tissues and, perhaps most important, the processes that lead to IBRB leakage and those by which lipoproteins and cells interact in tissues, at the sites of disease.

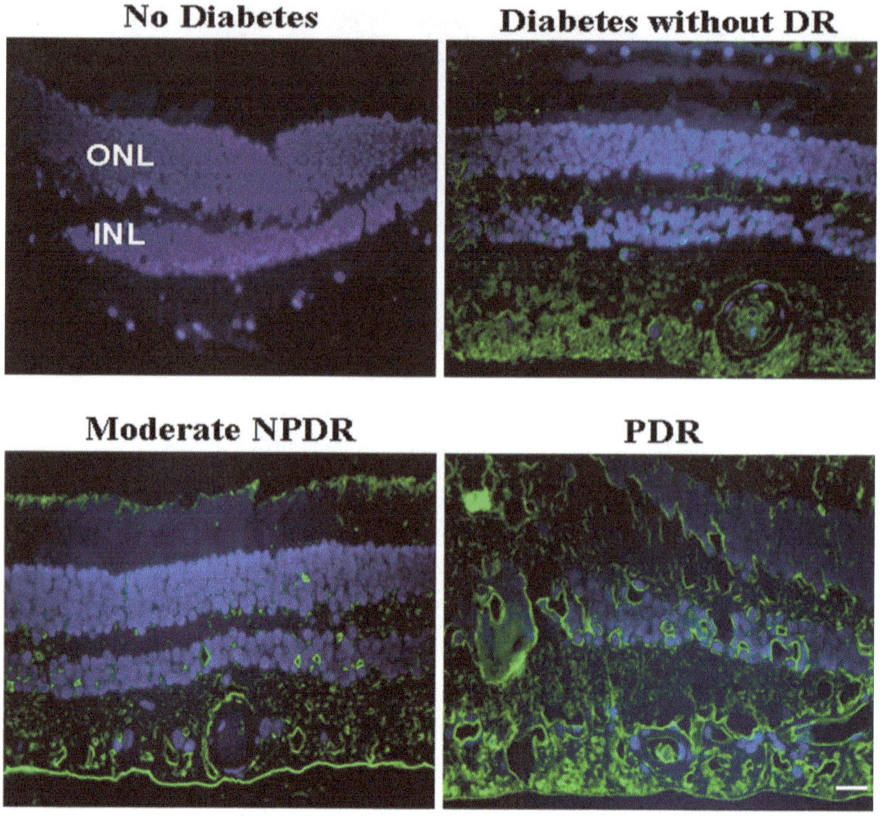


**Fig. 15.3** Immunostaining for ox-LDL in retinae from type 2 diabetic patients: Staining was observed in all diabetic groups, even before the onset of clinically detectable DR. The fluorescent signal intensity increased with DR severity, but was absent in non-diabetic retinae. Image reproduced with permission from Wu, M., et al., Intraretinal leakage and oxidation of LDL in diabetic retinopathy. Invest Ophthalmol Vis Sci, 2008; 49: 2679–85. *Abbreviations*: *ONL* outer nuclear layer, *INL* inner nuclear layer

## Conclusion

Diabetes and its vascular complications including DR is epidemic worldwide. In many settings, the disease process proceeds unchecked for years or decades before detection. Better identification of risk factors, better understanding of disease mechanisms, and the development of effective screening, prevention, and treatment strategies are critical in meeting these challenges. Residual risk (plasma lipoprotein abnormalities that persist after conventional treatment) is a new concept in the role of dyslipidemia in the pathogenesis of vascular disease. The described effects of modified LDL (and by extension, other lipoproteins) in the retina are analogous to effects in atherogenesis in cardiovascular diseases, but represent an entirely new area in ocular and DR research. As stated above, extravasated LDL and subsequently modified LDL (ox-LDL) are present in diabetic human retinae, correlating with severity of DR. Modified LDL has toxic effects on retinal cells, most thoroughly defined in pericytes, contributing to retinal dysfunction and vision loss. Further studies are necessary to elucidate more details regarding these mechanisms, such as involvement of the Wnt pathway [67, 68, 84] and endoplasmic reticulum (ER) stress [85–87], and to explore new interventions that may prevent IBRB leakage or the effects of modified lipoproteins in the retina after extravasation. These new treatments will address the earliest, pre-clinical stages of DR and could obviate the need for today's late-stage interventions. They have potential for a major impact on the health of the nation and the world and on health-care costs.

## References


1. Grassi G. Diabetic retinopathy. Minerva Med. 2003; 94(6):419–35.
2. Gardner TW, Antonetti DA. A prize catch for diabetic retinopathy. Nat Med. 2007;13(2):131–2.
3. Kowluru RA, Chan PS. Oxidative stress and diabetic retinopathy. Exp Diabetes Res. 2007;2007:43603.
4. Engerman RL, Kern TS. Progression of incipient diabetic retinopathy during good glycemic control. Diabetes. 1987;36(7):808–12.
5. Engerman RL. Pathogenesis of diabetic retinopathy. Diabetes. 1989;38(10):1203–6.
6. Alm A. Ocular circulation. In: Hart WM, editor. Adler's physiology of the eye. St. Louis, MO: Mosby-year book; 1992. p. 198–227.
7. Garner A. Histopathology of diabetic retinopathy in man. Eye (Lond). 1993;7(Pt 2):250–3.
8. Hammes HP. Pericytes and the pathogenesis of diabetic retinopathy. Horm Metab Res. 2005;37 Suppl 1:39–43.
9. Hammes HP, et al. Pericytes and the pathogenesis of diabetic retinopathy. Diabetes. 2002;51(10):3107–12.
10. Kingsley LA, et al. An epidemiologic approach to the study of retinopathy: the Pittsburgh diabetic morbidity and retinopathy studies. Diabetes Res Clin Pract. 1988;4(2):99–109.
11. Lobo CL, Bernardes RC, Cunha-Vaz JG. Alterations of the blood-retinal barrier and retinal thickness in preclinical retinopathy in subjects with type 2 diabetes. Arch Ophthalmol. 2000;118(10):1364–9.
12. Qaum T, et al. VEGF-initiated blood-retinal barrier breakdown in early diabetes. Invest Ophthalmol Vis Sci. 2001;42(10):2408–13.
13. Dornan TL, et al. Low density lipoprotein cholesterol: an association with the severity of diabetic retinopathy. Diabetologia. 1982;22(3):167–70.
14. Keiding NR, et al. Serum lipoproteins and cholesterol levels in normal subjects and in young patients with diabetes in relation to vascular complications. Diabetes. 1952;1(6):434–40.
15. Lowy Jr AD, Barach JH. A study of serum lipoprotein and cholesterol determinations in 901 diabetics. Diabetes. 1957;6(4):342–53.
16. Bhan CK, Kumar V, Ahuja MM. Studies on neutral fat, lipoproteins and lipoprotein lipase in relation to vascular disease in young Indian diabetics. Acta Diabetol Lat. 1971;8(4):638–48.
17. Kissebah AH, et al. Plasma-lipids and glucose/insulin relationship in non-insulin-requiring diabetics with and without retinopathy. Lancet. 1975;1(7916): 1104–8.
18. Eckel RH, et al. Plasma lipids and microangiopathy in insulin-dependent diabetes mellitus. Diabetes Care. 1981;4(4):447–53.
19. Dornan TL, et al. Genetic susceptibility to the development of retinopathy in insulin-dependent diabetics. Diabetes. 1982;31(3):226–31.
20. Mohan R, et al. Increased LDL cholesterol in non-insulin-dependent diabetics with maculopathy. Acta Diabetol Lat. 1984;21(1):85–9.
21. Chakraborty A, et al. Serum lipids and lipoproteins in diabetic retinopathy. J Assoc Physicians India. 1986;34(9):631–2.
22. Miccoli R, et al. Circulating lipid levels and severity of diabetic retinopathy in type I diabetes mellitus. Ophthalmic Res. 1987;19(1):52–6.
23. Kostraba JN, et al. The epidemiology of diabetes complications study. IV. Correlates of diabetic background and proliferative retinopathy. Am J Epidemiol. 1991;133(4):381–91.
24. Sinav S, et al. Plasma lipids and lipoproteins in retinopathy of type I (insulin-dependent) diabetic patients. Ann Ophthalmol. 1993;25(2):64–6.
25. West KM, Erdreich LJ, Stober JA. A detailed study of risk factors for retinopathy and nephropathy in diabetes. Diabetes. 1980;29(7):501–8.
26. Nathan DM, et al. Retinopathy in older type II diabetics. Association with glucose control. Diabetes. 1986;35(7):797–801.
27. Agardh CD, et al. Plasma lipids and plasma lipoproteins in diabetics with and without proliferative retinopathy. Acta Med Scand. 1988;223(2):165–9.
28. Dhir SP, et al. Serum lipoprotein cholesterol profile in diabetic retinopathy. Indian J Ophthalmol. 1984; 32(2):89–91.
29. Van Eck WF. The effect of a low fat diet on the serum lipids in diabetes and its significance in diabetic retinopathy. Am J Med. 1959;27:196–211.
30. King RC, Dobree JH. Corn oil in the treatment of exudative diabetic retinopathy. Proc R Soc Med. 1963; 56:759–60.
31. Ernest I, Linner E, Svanborg A. Carbohydrate-rich, fat-poor diet in diabetes. Am J Med. 1965;39(4):594–600.
32. Cullen JF, Ireland JT, Oliver MF. A controlled trial of atromid therapy in exudative diabetic retinopathy. Trans Ophthalmol Soc U K. 1964;84:281–95.
33. Duncan LJ, et al. A three-year trial of atromid therapy in exudative diabetic retinopathy. Diabetes. 1968; 17(7):458–67.
34. Houtsmuller AJ. Treatment of exudative diabetic retinopathy with atromid-S. Ophthalmologica. 1968; 156(1):2–5.
35. Vannas S, Esila R, Tuovinen E. Observations on the effect of ethyl a-p chlorophenoxyisobutyrate (CPIB) therapy on serum lipid levels and on diabetic and some other retinopathies. Acta Ophthalmol (Copenh). 1968;46(2):162–70.
36. Harrold BP, Marmion VJ, Gough KR. A double-blind controlled trial of clofibrate in the treatment of diabetic retinopathy. Diabetes. 1969;18(5):285–91.

37. Gordon B, et al. The effects of lipid lowering on diabetic retinopathy. Am J Ophthalmol. 1991;112(4): 385–91.
38. Janknecht P, Schumann M, Hansen LL. Reduction of retinal exudates in diabetic retinopathy after heparin-induced extracorporeal LDL-precipitation (HELP). A case report. Eur J Ophthalmol. 1996;6(3):340–2.
39. van Leiden HA, et al. Blood pressure, lipids, and obesity are associated with retinopathy: the hoorn study. Diabetes Care. 2002;25(8):1320–5.
40. Lloyd CE, et al. The progression of retinopathy over 2 years: the Pittsburgh Epidemiology of Diabetes Complications (EDC) Study. J Diabetes Complications. 1995;9(3):140–8.
41. Lyons TJ, et al. Diabetic retinopathy and serum lipoprotein subclasses in the DCCT/EDIC cohort. Invest Ophthalmol Vis Sci. 2004;45(3):910–8.
42. Fong DS, et al. Retinopathy in diabetes. Diabetes Care. 2004;27 Suppl 1:S84–7.
43. The effect of intensive treatment of diabetes on the development and progression of long-term complications in insulin-dependent diabetes mellitus. The Diabetes Control and Complications Trial Research Group. N Engl J Med. 1993;329(14):977–86.
44. Jialal I, Devaraj S. Low-density lipoprotein oxidation, antioxidants, and atherosclerosis: a clinical biochemistry perspective. Clin Chem. 1996;42(4):498–506.
45. Mora S, et al. LDL particle subclasses, LDL particle size, and carotid atherosclerosis in the multi-ethnic study of atherosclerosis (MESA). Atherosclerosis. 2007;192(1):211–7.
46. Lyons TJ, et al. Glycosylation of low density lipoprotein in patients with type 1 (insulin-dependent) diabetes: correlations with other parameters of glycaemic control. Diabetologia. 1986;29(10):685–9.
47. Chew EY, et al. Effects of medical therapies on retinopathy progression in type 2 diabetes. N Engl J Med. 2010;363(3):233–44.
48. Keech AC, et al. Effect of fenofibrate on the need for laser treatment for diabetic retinopathy (FIELD study): a randomised controlled trial. Lancet. 2007;370(9600):1687–97.
49. Fundus photographic risk factors for progression of diabetic retinopathy. ETDRS report number 12. Early Treatment Diabetic Retinopathy Study Research Group. Ophthalmology. 1991;98 5 Suppl:823–33.
50. Cheung N, et al. Diabetic retinopathy and the risk of coronary heart disease: the Atherosclerosis Risk in Communities Study. Diabetes Care. 2007;30(7): 1742–6.
51. Sasongko MB, et al. Serum apolipoprotein AI and B are stronger biomarkers of diabetic retinopathy than traditional lipids. Diabetes Care. 2011;34(2):474–9.
52. Stephens JW, Khanolkar MP, Bain SC. The biological relevance and measurement of plasma markers of oxidative stress in diabetes and cardiovascular disease. Atherosclerosis. 2009;202(2):321–9.
53. Forrest KY, et al. Are predictors of coronary heart disease and lower-extremity arterial disease in type 1 diabetes the same? A prospective study. Atherosclerosis. 2000;148(1):159–69.
54. Luc G, et al. Lipoprotein (a) as a predictor of coronary heart disease: the PRIME Study. Atherosclerosis. 2002;163(2):377–84.
55. Meisinger C, et al. Plasma oxidized low-density lipoprotein, a strong predictor for acute coronary heart disease events in apparently healthy, middle-aged men from the general population. Circulation. 2005;112(5):651–7.
56. Stephens JW, et al. Increased plasma markers of oxidative stress are associated with coronary heart disease in males with diabetes mellitus and with 10-year risk in a prospective sample of males. Clin Chem. 2006;52(3):446–52.
57. Alamouti B, Funk J. Retinal thickness decreases with age: an OCT study. Br J Ophthalmol. 2003;87(7): 899–901.
58. Lyons TJ, et al. Toxicity of mildly modified low-density lipoproteins to cultured retinal capillary endothelial cells and pericytes. Diabetes. 1994;43(9):1090–5.
59. Barth JL, et al. Oxidised, glycated LDL selectively influences tissue inhibitor of metalloproteinase-3 gene expression and protein production in human retinal capillary pericytes. Diabetologia. 2007;50(10):2200–8.
60. Diffley M, Wu M, Sohn M, Song W, Hammad SM, Lyons TJ. Apoptosis induction by oxidized glycated LDL in human retinal capillary pericytes is independent of activation of MAPK signaling pathways. Mol Vis. 2009;15:135–45.
61. Wu M, et al. Intraretinal leakage and oxidation of LDL in diabetic retinopathy. Invest Ophthalmol Vis Sci. 2008;49(6):2679–85.
62. Nishi K, et al. Oxidized LDL in carotid plaques and plasma associates with plaque instability. Arterioscler Thromb Vasc Biol. 2002;22(10):1649–54.
63. Smith EB, Staples EM. Plasma protein concentrations in interstitial fluid from human aortas. Proc R Soc Lond B Biol Sci. 1982;217(1206):59–75.
64. Zou MH, et al. Tyrosine nitration of prostacyclin synthase is associated with enhanced retinal cell apoptosis in diabetes. Am J Pathol. 2011;179(6):2835–44.
65. Zhang SX, et al. Pigment epithelium-derived factor mitigates inflammation and oxidative stress in retinal pericytes exposed to oxidized low-density lipoprotein. J Mol Endocrinol. 2008;41(3):135–43.
66. Wu M, Lyons TJ. Treatment approaches for diabetes and dyslipidemia. Horm Res Paediatr. 2011;76 Suppl 1:76–80.
67. Chen Y, et al. Activation of the Wnt pathway plays a pathogenic role in diabetic retinopathy in humans and animal models. Am J Pathol. 2009;175(6):2676–85.
68. Zhou T, et al. The role of lipid peroxidation products and oxidative stress in activation of the canonical wingless-type MMTV integration site (WNT) pathway in a rat model of diabetic retinopathy. Diabetologia. 2011;54(2):459–68.

69. Mattson MP. Roles of the lipid peroxidation product 4-hydroxynonenal in obesity, the metabolic syndrome, and associated vascular and neurodegenerative disorders. Exp Gerontol. 2009;44(10):625–33.
70. Song W, et al. Effects of oxidized and glycated LDL on gene expression in human retinal capillary pericytes. Invest Ophthalmol Vis Sci. 2005;46(8): 2974–82.
71. Hammes HP, et al. Aminoguanidine treatment inhibits the development of experimental diabetic retinopathy. Proc Natl Acad Sci USA. 1991;88(24):11555–8.
72. Kern TS, Engerman RL. Pharmacological inhibition of diabetic retinopathy: aminoguanidine and aspirin. Diabetes. 2001;50(7):1636–42.
73. Hammes HP, et al. Aminoguanidine inhibits the development of accelerated diabetic retinopathy in the spontaneous hypertensive rat. Diabetologia. 1994; 37(1):32–5.
74. Gardiner TA, Anderson HR, Stitt AW. Inhibition of advanced glycation end-products protects against retinal capillary basement membrane expansion during long-term diabetes. J Pathol. 2003;201(2):328–33.
75. Lyons TJ, et al. Aminoguanidine and the effects of modified LDL on cultured retinal capillary cells. Invest Ophthalmol Vis Sci. 2000;41(5):1176–80.
76. Yu Y, et al. Effects of D- and L-glucose and mannitol on retinal capillary cells: inhibition by nanomolar aminoguanidine. Am J Pharmacol Toxicol. 2007;2(4): 148–58.
77. Bolton WK, et al. Randomized trial of an inhibitor of formation of advanced glycation end products in diabetic nephropathy. Am J Nephrol. 2004;24(1):32–40.
78. Boehm BO, et al. Low content of the natural ocular anti-angiogenic agent pigment epithelium-derived factor (PEDF) in aqueous humor predicts progression of diabetic retinopathy. Diabetologia. 2003;46(3): 394–400.
79. Ogata N, et al. Unbalanced vitreous levels of pigment epithelium-derived factor and vascular endothelial growth factor in diabetic retinopathy. Am J Ophthalmol. 2002;134(3):348–53.
80. Ogata N, et al. Pigment epithelium-derived factor in the vitreous is low in diabetic retinopathy and high in rhegmatogenous retinal detachment. Am J Ophthalmol. 2001;132(3):378–82.
81. Zhang SX, et al. Pigment epithelium-derived factor downregulates vascular endothelial growth factor (VEGF) expression and inhibits VEGF-VEGF receptor 2 binding in diabetic retinopathy. J Mol Endocrinol. 2006;37(1):1–12.
82. Lopes-Virella MF, et al. Oxidized LDL immune complexes and coronary artery calcification in type 1 diabetes. Atherosclerosis. 2011;214(2):462–7.
83. Lopes-Virella MF, et al. Levels of oxidized LDL and advanced glycation end products-modified LDL in circulating immune complexes are strongly associated with increased levels of carotid intima-media thickness and its progression in type 1 diabetes. Diabetes. 2011;60(2):582–9.
84. Chen Y, et al. Very low density lipoprotein receptor, a negative regulator of the wnt signaling pathway and choroidal neovascularization. J Biol Chem. 2007; 282(47):34420–8.
85. Li J, et al. Endoplasmic reticulum stress is implicated in retinal inflammation and diabetic retinopathy. FEBS Lett. 2009;583(9):1521–7.
86. Li J, Wang JJ, Zhang SX. Preconditioning with endoplasmic reticulum stress mitigates retinal endothelial inflammation via activation of X-box binding protein 1. J Biol Chem. 2011;286(6):4912–21.
87. Zhong Y, Wang JJ, Zhang SX. Intermittent but not constant high glucose induces ER stress and inflammation in human retinal pericytes. Adv Exp Med Biol. 2012;723:285–92.

# Effects of Lifestyle (Diet, Plant Sterols, Exercise) and Glycemic Control on Lipoproteins in Diabetes

16

Peter Clifton

## Abbreviations

| | |
|---|---|
| ADA | American Diabetes Association |
| Apo | Apolipoprotein |
| HDL | High-density lipoprotein |
| LDL | Low-density lipoprotein |
| P:S | Polyunsaturated to saturated fat ratio |
| TG | Triglycerides |
| VLDL | Very low density lipoprotein |

## General Considerations

Lipid changes occur quickly in response to diet, and in two weeks 80 % of the maximal effect is seen, with no further change beyond four weeks. If diet is maintained, then the effect on circulating lipid levels is persistent. Regardless of the background diet, or if the study is parallel or crossover, then contrasting the effect of two diets on lipids at the end of four weeks is more than adequate to see a clear effect. Washout periods are not required. BMI, diabetes control, nor type of diabetes does not appear to interact with responses to fat or fiber, but they do appear to be related to response to cholesterol and plant sterols.

**Lipid Conversion Units**: To convert mmol/L of cholesterol to mg/dL, multiply by 38.8, and to convert mmol/L of triglyceride to mg/dL, multiply by 88.5.

P. Clifton, M.B.B.S., B.Med.Sci., F.R.A.C.P., Ph.D. (✉)
Sansom Institute University of South Australia, Adelaide, SA, Australia
e-mail: Peter.Clifton@unisa.edu.au

## Dietary Fat and Lipoproteins

### Saturated, n6 Polyunsaturated, and Monounsaturated Fat

In non-diabetic subjects the effects of dietary saturated, polyunsaturated, and monounsaturated fat are well described in a meta-analysis of 60 clinical trials published in 2003 by Mensink et al. [1]. In this paper 1 % of energy from saturated fat elevated LDL-cholesterol by 0.03 mmol/L when it replaced carbohydrate, while n6 polyunsaturated fat lowered LDL-cholesterol levels by 0.02 mmol/L when it replaced carbohydrate. The concentration of HDL-cholesterol was elevated by about 0.01 mmol/L by saturated and unsaturated fat in comparison with carbohydrate. Thus an absolute 10 % energy reduction in saturated fat (a very large change) and replacement of this fat entirely with n6 polyunsaturated fat would lower LDL-cholesterol levels by 0.5 mmol/L (or about 14–15 %). If the 10 % saturated fat were replaced entirely by carbohydrate, then LDL-cholesterol would fall by 0.3 mmol/L, HDL-cholesterol would fall by 0.1 mmol/L, and triglyceride levels would rise by 0.24 mmol/L. Is there any evidence that people with diabetes behave in a different way to changes in dietary fat composition? Somewhat surprisingly, it is difficult to answer this question as there have been a very limited number of studies in people with diabetes—either type 1 or type 2 diabetes—and much of the focus has been on glycemic rather

A.J. Jenkins et al. (eds.), *Lipoproteins in Diabetes Mellitus*, Contemporary Diabetes,
DOI 10.1007/978-1-4614-7554-5_16, © Springer Science+Business Media New York 2014

than lipid control. All studies contained very small numbers of volunteers, except for the Oxford study.

The Oxford study was begun at a time (1973) when the standard dietary advice was a high fat (40 % of energy), low-carbohydrate diet (maximum of 40 % of energy) and little attention was paid to the type of fat in the diet, which was mostly saturated. The study contrasted the standard diet with a modified fat diet of 30 % of energy with a polyunsaturated/saturated (P/S) fat ratio of 0.9 or above. Two hundred and fifty people with newly diagnosed type 2 diabetes were enrolled between 1973 and 1976 [2]. Total cholesterol levels were 0.7 mmol/L lower on the modified fat diet averaged over 1, 3, and 5 years, which is consistent with an estimated reduction in saturated fat of about 15 % and an increase in polyunsaturated fat of 10 % [3]. Dietary records were not collected.

In a controlled study by Storm et al. [4], a palmitic acid-rich diet (16 % of energy) increased total cholesterol compared with a carbohydrate-rich diet or a stearic acid-rich diet (13 % of energy) for 3 weeks each, but surprisingly LDL- and HDL-cholesterol were not different. However, only 15 volunteers with type 2 diabetes were included in this relatively short study, and the difference in LDL-Cholesterol levels (based on total cholesterol changes) may have been about 0.2–0.3 mmol/L, which is about half of that expected. A 6-week study in 16 patients with type 2 diabetes compared 20 % of energy as saturated fat with 20 % as monounsaturated fat and a 20 % trans monounsaturated fat diet [5]. Lipids, lipoprotein, and apoB levels were the same on the three diets, which would not have been expected. A very small study in Pima Indians ($n=7$) by Abbott et al. [6] showed a fall in LDL-cholesterol levels by 17 % with a change in saturated fat of 14 % of energy, and the changes were very similar to those seen in the nondiabetic subjects in the same study. Kinetic studies showed that these changes were due to slower conversion of VLDL to LDL. HDL-cholesterol and fasting TG concentrations were not significantly altered. Heine et al. [7] performed a 30-week study of two diets, one with a low polyunsaturated to saturated fat ratio (P:S 0.3) and one with a P:S of 1.0, in 14 patients with type 2 diabetes in a crossover study. Total dietary fat was 37–38 % with linoleic acid increasing from 4.2 to 10.9 %. LDL-cholesterol levels declined by 9.8 % ($p<0.01$) during the high P:S diet. The change in LDL-cholesterol levels of 0.4 mmol/L is what would be expected based on the Mensink meta-analysis. A combination of weight loss and reduced dietary saturated fat lowered LDL-cholesterol levels by 10–17 % with a high-carbohydrate or high-monounsaturated fat diet respectively [8].

Overall, despite the small number of studies, the data suggest that people with type 2 diabetes respond to dietary lipid changes in the same way as non-diabetic subjects. However, a Cochrane review in 2007 [9] of dietary advice for adults with type 2 diabetes, which examined 18 trials of more than six months duration with 1,467 participants and a wide variety of dietary interventions, concluded that there was insufficient data to conclude anything other than that exercise lowered HbA1c.

## Dietary Fat vs. Carbohydrate

Much of the major disagreements in nutrition over the last 20 years for people with type 2 diabetes have related to replacing saturated fat with carbohydrate as opposed to unsaturated fat. For many years (1970s–1990s), a very high-carbohydrate (and high-fiber) diet was strongly advocated, although some researchers suggested high-carbohydrate diets were theoretically not optimal because of the lowering of HDL-cholesterol and elevation of fasting triglyceride levels (which is also seen to the same degree in non-diabetic subjects). The meta-analysis ($n=133$ subjects, nine studies) of Garg in 1998 [10] focused on comparing high-carbohydrate diets (49–60 % of energy) with high-monounsaturated fat diets (24–33 % monounsaturated fat, 37–50 % total fat). A high-monounsaturated fat diet was associated with a reduction in fasting triglyceride levels of 0.36 mmol/L (19 %) and a reduction in VLDL-cholesterol levels of 22.5 %. HDL-cholesterol levels increased by 0.05 mmol/L or 4 %. The remainder of the fat in both diets was 7–21 %, presumably about 5 % polyunsaturated fat with the remainder being saturated fat, but surprisingly in the meta-analysis, neither of these two fats was mentioned. LDL-cholesterol levels were not different between the two diets, but the data are uninterpretable in relation to the effect of saturated fat, and one can only assume that saturated fat was not different between diets. The lack of difference between carbohydrate and monounsaturated fat on LDL-cholesterol levels is consistent with the Mensink data [1] in non-diabetic subjects.

A later meta-analysis by Kodama et al. [11] examined 19 studies with 306 patients and again showed no effect of a high-carbohydrate diet on LDL-cholesterol levels with a rise in triglycerides of 13 % and a lowering of HDL-cholesterol levels of 8 %. These changes are similar to that expected in non-diabetic subjects [12]. Whether these changes with a high-carbohydrate diet promote an increased risk of cardiovascular disease (CVD) is not clear, but there are no data available to refute this suggestion. Secondary intervention studies in non-diabetic subjects suggest that replacing saturated fat with carbohydrate is not beneficial, whereas replacing it with n6 polyunsaturated fat is beneficial [13]. A (pro-atherogenic) smaller LDL particle size in those following a high-carbohydrate diet may contribute to the adverse effect [12].

Replacing carbohydrate with protein and/or polyunsaturated fat would be expected to have similar effects to replacing it with monounsaturated fat. This was demonstrated by Thompson et al. [14] and a small ($n = 11$ participants) study of a high protein, lower carbohydrate Paleolithic diet that showed a reduction in triglycerides levels of 0.4 mmol/L and an increase in HDL-cholesterol levels of 0.08 mmol/L [15]. Although the Paleolithic diet had a lower glycemic load than the standard American Diabetes Association (ADA) diet, it was also reduced in energy and the 3 kg weight loss may account for some or all of these effects.

## Relationship Between Diet and Coronary Events in People with Type 2 Diabetes

Although there is now considerable controversy about the role of dietary saturated fat and cholesterol in promoting CVD, the data in people with type 2 diabetes are relatively clear in the US Nurses' Health Study [16]. Between 1980 and 1998, 619 new cases of CVD (nonfatal myocardial infarction, fatal coronary heart disease, and stroke) occurred in 5,672 women with type 2 diabetes. The relative risk (RR) of CVD for an increase of 200 mg cholesterol/1,000 kcal was 1.37 ($p = 0.003$). Each 5 % of energy intake from saturated fat, as compared with equivalent energy from carbohydrates, was associated with a 29 % greater risk of CVD (RR: 1.29 $p = 0.04$). Keys score (1.26 × (2 x% saturated fat − % polyunsaturated fat) + 1.5 × square root dietary cholesterol in mg/1000 kcal) was the most powerful predictor after multivariate adjustment ($p = 0.001$). The ratio of polyunsaturated to saturated fat was inversely associated with the risk of *fatal* CVD ($p = 0.007$). Replacement of 5 % of energy from saturated fat with equivalent energy from monounsaturated fat was associated with a 37 % lower risk of CVD.

## Fish Oil

A Cochrane meta-analysis in 2008 examined 23 randomized controlled trials (1,075 participants with type 2 diabetes), with a mean treatment duration of 8.9 weeks [17]. The mean dose of omega-3 PUFA used in the trials was 3.5 g/day. Among those taking omega-3 PUFA circulating triglyceride levels were significantly lowered by 0.45 mmol/L ($p < 0.00001$) and levels of VLDL-cholesterol lowered by 0.07 mmol/L ($p = 0.04$). LDL-cholesterol levels were raised by 0.11 mmol/L ($p = 0.05$). No significant changes in levels of total or HDL-cholesterol, HbA1c, fasting glucose, fasting insulin, or in body weight were observed. The decrease in VLDL-cholesterol levels was significant only in trials of longer duration and in hypertriglyceridemic patients.

## Dietary Cholesterol

A meta-analysis of 17 studies of dietary cholesterol in non-diabetic subjects showed that the addition of 100 mg dietary cholesterol/day increased the ratio of total to HDL-cholesterol by 0.020 U, total cholesterol concentrations by

0.056 mmol, LDL-cholesterol by 0.05 mmol/L, and HDL-cholesterol concentrations by 0.008 mmol/L [18].

Dietary cholesterol had little effect either on total- or LDL-cholesterol-in 31 overweight, insulin-resistant postmenopausal women over four weeks, and the effect was no different to the 34 women who were insulin sensitive [19]. A further 4-week study in insulin-sensitive individuals consuming four eggs/day showed a significant increase in non-HDL-cholesterol levels and in inflammatory markers in insulin-sensitive individuals, which was not observed in lean or obese insulin-resistant individuals, but the difference between the groups was not statistically different [20].

## Cholesterol Synthesis and Absorption

Cholesterol synthesis can be assessed by the circulating level of lathosterol, an intermediate in the cholesterol synthetic pathway, while absorption can be assessed by measuring the level of plant sterols sitosterol and campesterol or the level of an endogenous bacterial cholesterol metabolite, cholestanol. All of these are transported in lipoproteins and the higher the lipoprotein level, the higher the sterol level, so adjustment needs to be made for the level of the carrier.

Insulin-sensitive individuals had higher plant sterol levels and lower lathosterol levels, indicative of higher cholesterol absorption and lower cholesterol synthesis. In 761 men of varying degrees of glucose tolerance, including 76 with type 2 diabetes, cholesterol synthesis markers were lowest and absorption markers highest in normoglycemia. Sitosterol was lower in subjects with impaired fasting glucose, impaired glucose tolerance, and type 2 diabetes compared with normoglycemic subjects (111–115 ± 7 vs. 136 ± 3 μmol × 100/mmol of cholesterol, $p<0.05$). Campesterol levels were also significantly lower in these groups relative to the normoglycemic control subjects. Peripheral insulin sensitivity evaluated by the Matsuda index was associated with the lathosterol/sitosterol ratio in the entire population ($r=-0.457$, $p<0.001$) and with that of lathosterol/cholestanol independently of obesity [21].

Clinical research on dietary cholesterol and diabetes management is very limited, and there are no clinical intervention trials that have investigated the role of egg consumption in people with type 2 diabetes.

A small study in ten male volunteers with type 1 diabetes showed that 800 mg/day of cholesterol for three weeks increased LDL-cholesterol levels by 12 % with a 7 % increase in control subjects. HDL-cholesterol levels remained the same but tended to increase in control subjects [22]. High-cholesterol absorption markers, e.g., sitosterol or campesterol, and low-cholesterol synthesis markers, e.g., lathosterol, appear to characterize type 1 diabetes [23], and these differ from people with type 2 diabetes [24].

Obesity is inversely related to fractional cholesterol absorption both in diabetic and non-diabetic subjects [25], but absorption is lower in subjects with type 2 diabetes [26]. Cholesterol absorption efficiency was 29 ± 1 % in obese subjects with diabetes vs. 42 ± 2 % in the obese control subjects ($p<0.01$). Cholesterol synthesis was higher (17 ± 1 vs. 14 ± 1 mg/kg/day; $p<0.05$) and neutral sterol and bile acid excretion and cholesterol turnover tended to be higher in the group with diabetes than in the control group. Blood glucose (measured twice one week apart) was positively related to cholesterol synthesis in the diabetic group ($r=0.663$, $p<0.01$) and in the control group ($r=0.590$, $p<0.05$), suggesting that the higher blood glucose level, the higher the cholesterol synthesis. In 16 obese patients with type 2 diabetes, baseline cholesterol absorption and synthesis were related to respective serum sex hormone-binding globulin, glucose, and insulin values. Weight reduction of 6 kg increased cholesterol absorption efficiency and the ratio of serum plant sterols to cholesterol—indicators of cholesterol absorption—increased by 28 % ($p<0.01$) and 20–31 % ($p<0.05$ for both) and reduced blood glucose by 14 %. Serum cholesterol levels did not change but serum triglyceride levels fell by 13 % [26].

## Plant Sterols

Plant sterols are the plant equivalent of cholesterol and are found in cell walls and membranes. They differ from cholesterol by small changes to the side chain. They can be found naturally in oil seeds and cooking oils and are a normal part of the diet—up to 400–800 mg/day. Stanols are the same except for the removal of a double bond in the cholesterol nucleus. Some foods such as milk, margarine, orange juice, cheese, and chocolate are sometimes supplemented with sterols or stanols and deliver 2–2.5 g/day when consumed as directed.

*Type 2 diabetes*. The data above would suggest that obese subjects with type 2 diabetes would be less sensitive to dietary cholesterol and in turn less sensitive to the effects of dietary plant sterols. However, plant sterols appear to be just as efficacious in people with type 2 diabetes as in nondiabetic subjects. Plant sterols (1.8 g/day) for 21 days significantly reduced ($p<0.05$) LDL-cholesterol concentrations from baseline levels in 15 nondiabetic and 14 type 2 diabetic subjects by 15.1 and 26.8 %, respectively, and these were not statistically different from each [27]. A meta-analysis of five clinical trials, involving seven groups ($n=148$ subjects with type 2 diabetes, with follow-up range of 3–12 weeks) found the use of sterols/stanols significantly reduced LDL-cholesterol levels by 0.30 mmol/L (9 %, $p<0.01$), with no apparent effect on triglycerides and a trend towards raising HDL-cholesterol levels. These results are exactly the same as those seen in a meta-analysis of nondiabetic subjects [28].

*Type 1 diabetes*. Excellent efficacy of plant sterols is also seen in patients with type 1 diabetes with [29] or without [30] the concomitant use of statins.

## Epidemiology of Cholesterol Intake and CVD

Despite the limited effect of dietary cholesterol on fasting lipids, egg consumption of one per day doubles the risk of coronary heart disease in women and all-cause mortality in men with type 2 diabetes compared with an intake of one egg per week [31, 32]. The incidence of type 2 diabetes is also increased with higher egg intake [33, 34].

## Fiber

Very high fiber diets were actively promoted and studied in the 1980s both for glycemic and lipid control [35–38], but interest faded as patients found the diets too difficult or they were found in some studies to be ineffective [39–41].

A more recent small intervention study, published in the *New England Journal of Medicine* [42], in 13 patients with type 2 diabetes compared a high-fiber diet which provided 50 g of total fiber per day (as soluble and insoluble fiber 25 g each), with the standard ADA diet containing 24 g of total fiber per day, with 8 g as soluble fiber and 16 g as insoluble fiber. No fiber supplements were used. As compared with the ADA diet, the high-fiber diet resulted in a lower fasting plasma total cholesterol concentration (by 6.7 %, $p=0.02$), a lower plasma triglyceride concentration (by 10.2 %, $p=0.02$), and a lower plasma VLDL-cholesterol concentration (by 12.5 %, $p=0.01$). The fasting plasma LDL-cholesterol concentration was 6.3 % lower with the high-fiber diet, but this was not statistically significant ($p=0.11$), almost certainly due to the small size of the study. There were no significant differences between the two diets in fasting plasma HDL-cholesterol concentrations.

A 6-month Canadian study [43] compared a low-glycemic-index (GI) diet with a high-fiber diet in 210 participants with type 2 diabetes. The high-cereal fiber diet included 35 g of fiber, GI of 86, and glycemic load of 201. The low-GI diet included 42 g of fiber, GI of 62, and glycemic load of 141. There was an increase of HDL-cholesterol levels in the low-GI diet by 1.7 mg/dL compared with a decrease of HDL-cholesterol by −0.2 mg/dL in the high-cereal fiber diet ($p=0.005$), but this occurred only after about 16 weeks and was not associated with a change in triglyceride levels, so it is hard to conceive of a mechanism and may just be noise, although HbA1c improved modestly in the low-GI diet. LDL-cholesterol levels did not change.

The effects of specific types of dietary fibre are now summarized.

*Wheat bran* has no effect on lipid levels in type 2 diabetes [44] nor does adherence to a high-fiber, high-vegetable Mediterranean diet [45], admittedly in a small study.

*Psyllium* in a low dose (3.5 g three times/day) in 40 participants for 2 months does not appear to significantly lower LDL-cholesterol or triglyceride levels compared to a control group [46]. However, higher doses of psyllium (15 g/day) can significantly lower triglyceride levels compared with control when enough participants are studied ($n=125$) [47]. Psyllium has also been demonstrated to lower LDL-cholesterol levels in some studies [48, 49].

*Oat bran* can lower LDL-cholesterol—an extra 15 g of fiber from oat bran lowered LDL-cholesterol levels by 0.77 mol/L, but this study [50] was very small ($n=8$).

*Stabilized rice bran* (20 g/day for 12 weeks) lowered LDL-cholesterol levels by 13.7 % compared with the control group in a parallel study in 28 subjects with type 2 diabetes [51]. Triglyceride levels were also lowered by 0.5 mmol/L.

*Guar gum* is well established as being able lower LDL-cholesterol levels [52–54], but is not widely used. It would appear from the limited number of studies (except for guar) that soluble fiber can reduce LDL-cholesterol and triglyceride levels to the same degree as in nondiabetic subjects [55].

## Low-Glycemic-Index Carbohydrate

As noted above, replacing fat with carbohydrate lowers HDL-cholesterol and increases triglyceride levels. In most of these studies, the GI of the carbohydrate was not assessed. Low-GI carbohydrate may have lesser effects on these lipid levels compared with high-GI carbohydrates. A meta-analysis was performed by Opperman et al. [56] in 2004 who examined lipid changes in 13 studies (eight in people with type 2 diabetes). Seven of the ten studies found an improvement in mean LDL-cholesterol concentrations on a low-GI diet. Overall, low-GI diets tended to decrease LDL-cholesterol concentrations; however, it was not statistically significant (change 0.15 (95 % CI 0.31, 0.00) mmol/L; $p=0.06$). The GI of the diets was decreased by 21 (SD 10) units. In type 2 diabetes subjects, it appeared that LDL-cholesterol concentrations were decreased to a greater extent (0.18 mmol/L, $p=0.06$) than in healthy subjects. Only six of the 13 studies showed an improvement in triglyceride concentrations with a low-GI diet, and the overall change was not statistically significant (change 0.03 mmol/L, $p=0.73$). When divided into subgroups, no significant difference was found within type 2 diabetes, coronary heart disease, or healthy subjects. No effect was observed when only subjects with elevated triglyceride concentrations were included. Lowering the GI of food did not cause an overall significant change in mean HDL-cholesterol levels.

In a 1-year Canadian study [57], subjects with type 2 diabetes managed by diet alone ($n=162$) were randomly assigned to receive high-carbohydrate, high-glycemic-index (high-GI), high-carbohydrate, low-glycemic-index (low-GI), or low-carbohydrate, high-monounsaturated fat (low-CHO) diets. With the low-GI diet, overall mean triglyceride levels were 12 % higher and HDL-cholesterol levels were 4 % lower than with the low-CHO diet ($p<0.05$), despite a 26 % lower glycemic load. The lack of benefit of a low-GI/low-GL diet on triglyceride and HDL-cholesterol levels confirms the short-term meta-analytic results, but it is not clear why there were adverse changes. LDL-cholesterol responses were not different between the diets.

Epidemiological studies, such as the Zutphen Elderly Study [58] and the EURODIAB Complications Study [59], failed to show a relationship between LDL-cholesterol concentrations and low-GI diets, while other cross-sectional studies, such as the Survey of British Adults (1986–1987) [60] and the Third National Health and Nutrition Examination Survey (1988–1994) [61], found an increase in HDL-cholesterol concentrations with long-term low-GI diets. No relationship was found between low-GI diets and triglyceride concentrations [58, 59].

## Fructose

Fructose for many years was promoted as very suitable for people with diabetes because it lowered plasma glucose and insulin levels and improved HbA1c levels when it replaced starch, glucose, or sucrose. Gannon [62] showed a high-fruit and high-vegetable diet with little starch lowered 24 hour blood glucose levels without adverse effects on triglyceride levels compared with a high-starch diet or a usual American diet. 30–60 g/day of pure fructose supplementation (6–12 % of energy) for 3–12 months had no adverse effects on lipids [63–67] or lipid metabolism [68]. A very high intake of fructose (>20 % of energy) has been found to elevate lipids in some studies [69–72], but not in others [73, 74].

## Weight Loss

### Non-diabetic Subjects

Aucott [75] conducted a systematic review of studies that included lifestyle interventions for adults (18–65 years), with a mean baseline BMI <35 kg/m$^2$, with weight and lipid differences over 2 years. Between 1990 and 2010, 14 studies were identified. From meta-regression they found that a 1 kg maintained weight loss in the long term (2–3 years) could be expected to result in reductions of 1.3 % in total cholesterol, 1.6 % for triglycerides, and 0.34 % for LDL-cholesterol levels with a 4 % increase of HDL-cholesterol levels.

An earlier meta-analysis by Poobalan [76] of 13 long-term studies (both cohort and surgical and non-surgical and drug-based weight loss interventions) with a follow-up of more than two years found that total cholesterol concentrations had a significant positive linear relationship with weight change ($r=0.89$), where change in weight explained about 80 % of the cholesterol difference variation. For every 10 kg weight loss, a drop of 0.23 mmol/L in total cholesterol levels may be expected (about 5 %). Triglycerides and LDL-cholesterol concentrations were similarly related to weight loss, with a 10 kg change producing a 0.25 mmol/L and a 0.20 mmol/L change respectively. HDL-cholesterol changes were not related to weight loss. Participants in the two long-term meta-analyses could be on lipid-lowering medication.

In a meta-analysis of 70 short-term dietary weight loss studies in nondiabetic subjects, Dattilo and Kris Etherton [77] found that for every kilogram decrease in body weight, there was a 0.05 mmol/L decrease in total cholesterol levels (about 8–10 %, $p<0.0$ 1), a 0.02 mmol/L decrease in LDL-cholesterol levels ($p<0.001$), a 0.007 mmol/L decrease in HDL-cholesterol for active weight loss ($p<0.05$), a 0.009 mmol/L increase in HDL-cholesterol for stabilized weight loss ($p<0.01$), and a 0.015 mmol/L decrease in triglyceride levels ($p<0.05$). Correlations between weight loss and lipid changes were of the order of 0.3–0.4 and were much lower than in the long-term studies.

In the LIFE study [78] of 212 participants without diabetes, BMI fell in women from 35 to 33.7 kg/m$^2$ over 30 months and from 35 to 33 kg/m$^2$ in men, with a nadir at 12 months in both. In women, multivariate-adjusted HDL-cholesterol concentrations at 6-month follow-up was significantly lower than at baseline, and at subsequent time points HDL-cholesterol concentration was significantly higher than at 6-month follow-up, with no significant differences between the later time points, which however were not significantly different from baseline. In men the small decrease at six months was not statistically significant but later rises in HDL-cholesterol levels were, with a maximum change at 18 months of about 10 %. Triglyceride levels were significantly lower than baseline at six months but rose back to and beyond baseline in women, but remained low in men.

### Diabetic Subjects

For participants with diabetes, there are much fewer studies available. The Look Ahead study was a very large randomized study ($n=5{,}145$)

of intensive lifestyle interventions (ILI) or standard treatment (DSE) in overweight or obese individuals with type 2 diabetes [79]. After four years, ILI participants had a greater percentage of weight loss than DSE participants (−6.15 vs. −0.88 %; $p<0.001$) and superior improvements in HDL-cholesterol levels (3.7 vs. 2.0 mg/dL; $p<0.001$) and triglyceride levels (−25.6 vs. −19.75 mg/dL; $p<0.001$) averaged across all 4 years. Reductions in LDL-cholesterol levels were greater in DSE than ILI participants (−11.3 vs. 12.8 mg/dL; $p=0$ 0.009) owing to greater use of medications to lower lipid levels in the DSE group. The effects on triglyceride levels were not statistically significant at four years but the HDL-cholesterol level difference was consistent across all four years. These effects on lipid levels were lower than those in the long-term meta-analyses quoted above, but not different from those of the 2-year studies in nondiabetic subjects from Shai and Sacks [80, 81]. However, HDL-cholesterol changes were very similar to the meta-analysis of short-term studies by Dattilo and Kris Etherton [77].

A weight loss of 4.5 kg in 2,906 patients in the UKPDS reduced triglyceride levels by 0.41 mmol/L in men and 0.23 mmol/L in women with an HDL-cholesterol increase of 0.02 and 0.01 mmol/L, respectively. LDL-cholesterol levels did not change [82].

## Glycemic Control

In 2,220 type 2 diabetic patients (aged 35–91 years; male/female ratio, 1.07), HbA1c levels showed direct and significant correlations with total cholesterol, triglyceride, and LDL-cholesterol levels and inverse correlation with levels of HDL-cholesterol [83]. In Italian diabetes outpatient clinics, abnormal lipids were associated with markedly higher HbA1c levels [84] in 12,222 patients. On multiple regression, triglyceride levels were associated with HbA1c after adjustment for age, BMI and diabetes treatment, and a variety of other factors, while HDL-cholesterol levels were related to HbA1c levels in men only.

## Interventions to Improve Glycemic Control

A Dutch study [85] which targeted a strict fasting capillary glucose of <6.5 mmol/L vs. a less strict regimen of <8.5 mmol/L in 214 patients over two years looked at individual changes in HbA1c vs. lipid changes. Individuals in whom HbA1c levels decreased had significant favorable concurrent changes in triglycerides $r=0.26$ with HbA1c changes ($p=0.001$) with an absolute difference of 0.25 mmol/L between those whose HbA1c fell (−0.17 mmol/L) vs. those whose HbA1c rose (0.08 mmol/L). Changes in LDL- and HDL-cholesterol levels were not statistically significant. The difference in HbA1c between the two groups was 1.09 %.

In the Veterans Affairs Cooperative study in 513 male type 2 diabetes patients over two years, triglyceride levels decreased in the intensive-treatment arm from 2.25±0.27 to 1.54±0.14 mmol/L at 1 year ($p=0.004$) and to 1.74±0.18 mmol/L at 2 years ($p=0.03$); there was no change in the standard-treatment arm. Total cholesterol levels decreased in the intensive-treatment arm at 1 year from 5.4±0.21 to 4.99±0.13 mmol/L ($p=0.02$); there was no change in the standard-treatment arm. Levels of LDL- and HDL-cholesterol decreased in the standard-treatment arm only after two years, from 3.44±0.13 to 3.16±0.10 mmol/L ($p=0.02$) and from 1.10±0.03 to 1.00±0.03 mmol/L ($p<0.001$), respectively. Levels of apolipoprotein B decreased in both treatment arms ($p<0.001$), and apolipoprotein A1 levels decreased in the standard-treatment arm ($p<0.01$). A 2.1 % difference in HbA1c levels was achieved over the 2-year period [86].

The DCCT study [87] and the study by Cusp et al. [88] have shown falls in LDL-cholesterol with intensive diabetes treatment. The latter study was very small ($n=12$) and the fall in HbA1c achieved with 80 IU of insulin was 3.7 % over 16 weeks. In the DCCT with 1,441 patients with type 1 diabetes, changes in LDL-cholesterol levels were small, 0.1–0.2 mmol/L, but the risk of developing an LDL-cholesterol level of >4 mmol/L was reduced by 40 % in the intensive diabetes treatment group, although rates were about 1 per 100 patient years or less. Mean HbA1c level in the intensive- and conventional-treatment groups differed by about 2% throughout the follow-up period (7.2 vs. 9.1 %, respectively, $p<0.001$).

## Alcohol Intake

A moderate alcohol intake is associated with about a 30 % lower incidence of type 2 diabetes but high alcohol intake and binge drinking increases the risk of type 2 diabetes [89, 90]. Alcohol intake in people with type 2 diabetes in the EPIC study [91] did not reduce mortality, although a prospective cohort study in older people showed an 80 % reduction in death due to coronary heart disease with 14 g or more of alcohol/day [92] before and after adjustment for levels of HDL-cholesterol and total cholesterol. In Japanese men with type 2 diabetes, alcohol intake was directly related to HDL-cholesterol levels and hypertension, but the lowest triglyceride level was in the 1–22 g alcohol/day intake group compared with the nondrinker group [93]. There appear to be no alcohol intervention studies in people with diabetes.

## Exercise

In a Cochrane meta-analysis [94], 14 randomized controlled trials comparing supervised or well-documented (aerobic, resistance, or mixed) exercise against "no exercise" in type 2 diabetes were identified involving 377 participants. Most studies had three 30–60 min exercise sessions per week. Trials ranged from eight weeks to 12 months duration. No specific exercise program was given to the control group, but there were no reports on their incidental activity. The exercise intervention significantly decreased plasma triglyceride levels (−0.25 mmol/L, 95 % CI −0.48 to −0.02). No significant difference was found between groups in plasma cholesterol levels or LDL-cholesterol or HDL-cholesterol levels.

## Smoking

A recent meta-analysis [95] of observational studies in 130,000 people with diabetes showed the relative risk comparing smokers with non-smokers was 1.48 for total mortality (27 studies), 1.36 for cardiovascular mortality (nine studies), 1.54 for CHD (13 studies), 1.44 for stroke (nine studies), and 1.52 for MI (seven studies). The increased risk of smoking is similar to people without diabetes. Smoking lowers HDL-cholesterol levels. The major lipid-related effect of smoking cessation is an increase (of about 0.1 mmol/L or 3.9 mg/dl) [96].

## New Research Areas

Given the association between cholesterol intake and CVD events in people with diabetes, a cholesterol-feeding trial in people with both type 1 and type 2 diabetes needs to be done, focused not just on LDL- and HDL-cholesterol levels, but adhesion molecules and other inflammatory markers.

Long-term dietary intervention studies examining low salt, low saturated fat, high polyunsaturated fat, and high fruit, vegetables, and fiber over a 3-year period need to be done with surrogate cardiovascular measures such as carotid intima-medial thickness as an endpoint.

## Conclusions

There is a very limited amount of data related to the lifestyle effects on lipoproteins specifically involving people with diabetes. What data are available suggest they respond in a similar way to people without diabetes to lifestyle measures. The expected responses of LDL-cholesterol levels to dietary changes are summarized in Table 16.1. The effect of dietary cholesterol needs further exploration.

**Table 16.1** Effects of dietary changes on circulating LDL-cholesterol levels

| Dietary component | LDL-cholesterol lowering (%) |
|---|---|
| Saturated fat reduction 15–10 % | 5 |
| Polyunsaturated fat increase 5–10 % | 3 |
| Plant sterols 2 g/day | 10 |
| Oat bran 15 g/day | 5 |
| Low-GI carbohydrate in place of high-GI | 5 |
| Total possible change | 28 |

## References


1. Mensink RP, Zock PL, Kester AD, Katan MB. Effects of dietary fatty acids and carbohydrates on the ratio of serum total to HDL cholesterol and on serum lipids and apolipoproteins: a meta-analysis of 60 controlled trials. Am J Clin Nutr. 2003;77(5):1146–55.
2. Simpson RW, Mann JI, Eaton J, Moore RA, Carter R, Hockaday TDR. Improved glucose control in maturity-onset diabetes treated with high-carbohydrate-modified fat diet. BMJ. 1979;1:1753–6.
3. Howard-Williams J, Patel P, Jelfs R, et al. Polyunsaturated fatty acids and diabetic retinopathy. Br J Ophthalmol. 1985;69:15–8.
4. Storm H, Thomsen C, Pedersen E, Rasmussen O, Christiansen C, Hermansen K. Comparison of a carbohydrate-rich diet and diets rich in stearic or palmitic acid in NIDDM patients. Effects on lipids, glycemic control, and diurnal blood pressure. Diabetes Care. 1997;20(12):1807–13.
5. Christiansen E, Schneider S, Palmvig B, Tauber-Lassen E, Pedersen O. Intake of a diet high in trans monounsaturated fatty acids or saturated fatty acids. Effects on postprandial insulinemia and glycemia in obese patients with NIDDM. Diabetes Care. 1997;20(5):881–7.
6. Abbott WG, Swinburn B, Ruotolo G, Hara H, Patti L, Harper I, Grundy SM, Howard BV. Effect of a high-carbohydrate, low-saturated-fat diet on apolipoprotein B and triglyceride metabolism in Pima Indians. J Clin Invest. 1990;86(2):642–50.
7. Heine RJ, Mulder C, Popp-Snijders C, van der Meer J, van der Veen EA. Linoleic-acid-enriched diet: long-term effects on serum lipoprotein and apolipoprotein concentrations and insulin sensitivity in noninsulin-dependent diabetic patients. Am J Clin Nutr. 1989;49(3):448–56.
8. Heilbronn LK, Noakes M, Clifton PM. Effect of energy restriction, weight loss, and diet composition on plasma lipids and glucose in patients with type 2 diabetes. Diabetes Care. 1999;22(6):889–95.
9. Nield L, Moore HJ, Hooper L, Cruickshank JK, Vyas A, Whittaker V, Summerbell CD. Dietary advice for treatment of type 2 diabetes mellitus in adults. Cochrane Database Syst Rev. 2007;3, CD004097.
10. Garg A. High-monounsaturated-fat diets for patients with diabetes mellitus: a meta-analysis. Am J Clin Nutr. 1998;67(3 Suppl):577S–82.
11. Kodama S, Saito K, Tanaka S, Maki M, Yachi Y, Sato M, Sugawara A, Totsuka K, Shimano H, Ohashi Y, Yamada N, Sone H. Influence of fat and carbohydrate proportions on the metabolic profile in patients with type 2 diabetes: a meta-analysis. Diabetes Care. 2009;32(5):959–65.
12. Krauss RM, Blanche PJ, Rawlings RS, Fernstrom HS, Williams PT. Separate effects of reduced carbohydrate intake and weight loss on atherogenic dyslipidemia. Am J Clin Nutr. 2006;83(5):1025–31.
13. Mozaffarian D, Micha R, Wallace S. Effects on coronary heart disease of increasing polyunsaturated fat in place of saturated fat: a systematic review and meta-analysis of randomized controlled trials. PLoS Med. 2010;7(3):e1000252. Review.
14. Thomsen C, Rasmussen OW, Hansen KW, Vesterlund M, Hermansen K. Comparison of the effects on the diurnal blood pressure, glucose, and lipid levels of a diet rich in monounsaturated fatty acids with a diet rich in polyunsaturated fatty acids in type 2 diabetic subjects. Diabet Med. 1995;12(7):600–6.
15. Jönsson T, Granfeldt Y, Ahrén B, Branell UC, Pålsson G, Hansson A, Söderström M, Lindeberg S. Beneficial effects of a Paleolithic diet on cardiovascular risk factors in type 2 diabetes: a randomized cross-over pilot study. Cardiovasc Diabetol. 2009;8:35.
16. Tanasescu M, Cho E, Manson JE, Hu FB. Dietary fat and cholesterol and the risk of cardiovascular disease among women with type 2 diabetes. Am J Clin Nutr. 2004;79:999–1005.
17. Hartweg J, Perera R, Montori V, Dinneen S, Neil HA, Farmer A. Omega-3 polyunsaturated fatty acids (PUFA) for type 2 diabetes mellitus. Cochrane Database Syst Rev. 2008;1, CD003205.
18. Weggemans RM, Zock PL, Katan MB. Dietary cholesterol from eggs increases the ratio of total cholesterol to high-density lipoprotein cholesterol in humans: a meta-analysis. Am J Clin Nutr. 2001; 73(5):885–91.
19. Reaven GM. Insulin resistance, dietary cholesterol, and cholesterol concentration in postmenopausal women. Metabolism. 2001;50:594–7.
20. Tannock LR, O'Brien KD, Knopp RH, et al. Cholesterol feeding increases C-reactive protein and serum amyloid A levels in lean insulin-sensitive subjects. Circulation. 2005;111:3058–62.
21. Gylling H, Hallikainen M, Pihlajamäki J, Simonen P, Kuusisto J, Laakso M, Miettinen TA. Insulin sensitivity regulates cholesterol metabolism to a greater extent than obesity: lessons from the METSIM Study. J Lipid Res. 2010;51(8):2422–7. Epub 2010 May 1.
22. Romano G, Tilly-Kiesi MK, Patti L, et al. Effects of dietary cholesterol on plasma lipoproteins and their subclasses in IDDM patients. Diabetologia. 1998;41: 193–200.

23. Gylling H, Tuominen JA, Koivisto VA, Miettinen TA. Cholesterol metabolism in type 1 diabetes. Diabetes. 2004;53(9):2217–22.
24. Miettinen TA, Gylling H, Tuominen J, Simonen P, Koivisto V. Low synthesis and high absorption of cholesterol characterize type 1 diabetes. Diabetes Care. 2004;27(1):53–8.
25. Simonen PP, Gylling HK, Miettinen TA. Diabetes contributes to cholesterol metabolism regardless of obesity. Diabetes Care. 2002;25(9):1511–5.
26. Simonen P, Gylling H, Howard AN, Miettinen TA. Introducing a new component of the metabolic syndrome: low cholesterol absorption. Am J Clin Nutr. 2000;72:82–8.
27. Lau VW, Journo M, Jones PJ. Plant sterols are efficacious in lowering plasma LDL and non-HDL cholesterol in hypercholesterolemic type 2 diabetic and nondiabetic persons. Am J Clin Nutr. 2005;81(6): 1351–8.
28. Abumweis SS, Barake R, Jones PJ. Plant sterols/stanols as cholesterol lowering agents: a meta-analysis of randomized controlled trials. Food Nutr Res. 2008;52. doi: 10.3402/fnr.v52i0.1811.
29. Hallikainen M, Kurl S, Laakso M, Miettinen TA, Gylling H. Plant stanol esters lower LDL cholesterol level in statin-treated subjects with type 1 diabetes by interfering the absorption and synthesis of cholesterol. Atherosclerosis. 2011;217(2):473–8. Epub 2011 Apr 5.
30. Hallikainen M, Lyyra-Laitinen T, Laitinen T, Moilanen L, Miettinen TA, Gylling H. Effects of plant stanol esters on serum cholesterol concentrations, relative markers of cholesterol metabolism and endothelial function in type 1 diabetes. Atherosclerosis. 2008;199(2):432–9. Epub 2007 Dec 11.
31. Hu FB, Stampfer MJ, Rimm EB, et al. A prospective study of egg consumption and risk of cardiovascular disease in men and women. JAMA. 1999;281: 1387–94.
32. Djousse L, Gaziano JM. Egg consumption in relation to cardiovascular disease and mortality: the physicians' health study. Am J Clin Nutr. 2008;87:964–9.
33. Liese AD, Weis KE, Schulz M, Tooze JA. Food intake patterns associated with incident type 2 diabetes: the insulin resistance atherosclerosis study. Diabetes Care. 2009;32:263–8.
34. Djousse L, Gaziano JM, Buring JE, Lee IM. Egg consumption and risk of type 2 diabetes in men and women. Diabetes Care. 2009;32:295–300.
35. Rivellese A, Riccardi G, Giacco A, Pacioni D, Genovese S, Mattioli PL, Mancini M. Effect of dietary fibre on glucose control and serum lipoproteins in diabetic patients. Lancet. 1980;2(8192):447–50.
36. Karlström B, Vessby B, Asp NG, Boberg M, Gustafsson IB, Lithell H, Werner I. Effects of an increased content of cereal fibre in the diet of type 2 (non-insulin-dependent) diabetic patients. Diabetologia. 1984;26(4):272–7.
37. Riccardi G, Rivellese A, Pacioni D, Genovese S, Mastranzo P, Mancini M. Separate influence of dietary carbohydrate and fibre on the metabolic control in diabetes. Diabetologia. 1984;26(2):116–21.
38. Lousley SE, Jones DB, Slaughter P, Carter RD, Jelfs R, Mann JI. High carbohydrate-high fibre diets in poorly controlled diabetes. Diabet Med. 1984;1(1): 21–5.
39. Scott AR, Attenborough Y, Peacock I, Fletcher E, Jeffcoate WJ, Tattersall RB. Comparison of high fibre diets, basal insulin supplements, and flexible insulin treatment for non-insulin dependent (type II) diabetics poorly controlled with sulphonylureas. BMJ. 1988;297:707–10.
40. Hollenbeck CB, Coulston AM, Reaven M. To what extent does increased dietary fiber improve glucose and lipid metabolism in patients with noninsulin-dependent diabetes mellitus (NIDDM). Am J Clin Nutr. 1986;43:16–24.
41. Beattie VA, Edwards CA, Hosker JP, Cullen DR, Ward JD, Read NW. Does adding fibre to a low energy, high carbohydrate, low fat diet confer any benefit to the management of newly diagnosed overweight type II diabetics? Br Med J (Clin Res Ed). 1988;296(6630):1147–9.
42. Chandelier M, Garg A, Lutjohann D, von Bergmann K, Grundy SM, Brinkley LJ. Beneficial effects of high dietary fiber intake in patients with type 2 diabetes mellitus. N Engl J Med. 2000;342(19):1392–8.
43. Jenkins DJ, Kendall CW, McKeown-Eyssen G, Josse RG, Silverberg J, Booth GL, Vidgen E, Josse AR, Nguyen TH, Corrigan S, Banach MS, Ares S, Mitchell S, Emam A, Augustin LS, Parker TL, Leiter LA. Effect of a low-glycemic index or a high-cereal fiber diet on type 2 diabetes: a randomized trial. JAMA. 2008;300(23):2742–53.
44. Jenkins DJ, Kendall CW, Augustin LS, Martini MC, Axelsen M, Faulkner D, Vidgen E, Parker T, Lau H, Connelly PW, Teitel J, Singer W, Vandenbroucke AC, Leiter LA, Josse RG. Effect of wheat bran on glycemic control and risk factors for cardiovascular disease in type 2 diabetes. Diabetes Care. 2002;25(9):1522–8.
45. Itsiopoulos C, Brazionis L, Kaimakamis M, Cameron M, Best JD, O'Dea K, Rowley K. Can the Mediterranean diet lower HbA1c in type 2 diabetes? Results from a randomized cross-over study. Nutr Metab Cardiovasc Dis. 2011;21(9):740–7. Epub 2010 Jul 31.
46. Sartore G, Reitano R, Barison A, Magnanini P, Cosma C, Burlina S, Manzato E, Fedele D, Lapolla A. The effects of psyllium on lipoproteins in type II diabetic patients. Eur J Clin Nutr. 2009;63(10):1269–71. Epub 2009 Jul 22.
47. Rodriguez-Moran M, Guerrero-Romero F, Lazcano-Burciaga GJ. Lipid- and glucose-lowering efficacy of Plantago Psyllium in type II diabetes. J Diabetes Complications. 1998;12:273–8.
48. Anderson JW, Allgood LD, Turner J, Oeltgen PR, Daggy BP. Effects of psyllium on glucose and serum lipid responses in men with type 2 diabetes and hypercholesterolemia. Am J Clin Nutr. 1999;70(4): 466–73.

49. Sierra M, García JJ, Fernández N, Diez MJ, Calle AP. Therapeutic effects of psyllium in type 2 diabetic patients. Eur J Clin Nutr. 2002;56(9):830–42.
50. Pick ME, Hawrysh ZJ, Gee MI, Toth E, Garg ML, Hardin RT. Oat bran concentrate bread products improve long-term control of diabetes: a pilot study. J Am Diet Assoc. 1996;96(12):1254–61.
51. Cheng HH, Huang HY, Chen YY, Huang CL, Chang CJ, Chen HL, Lai MH. Ameliorative effects of stabilized rice bran on type 2 diabetes patients. Ann Nutr Metab. 2010;56(1):45–51. Epub 2009 Dec 15.
52. Uusitupa M, Siitonen O, Savolainen K, Silvasti M, Penttilä I, Parviainen M. Metabolic and nutritional effects of long-term use of guar gum in the treatment of noninsulin-dependent diabetes of poor metabolic control. Am J Clin Nutr. 1989;49(2):345–51.
53. Lalor BC, Bhatnagar D, Winocour PH, Ishola M, Arrol S, Brading M, Durrington PN. Placebo-controlled trial of the effects of guar gum and metformin on fasting blood glucose and serum lipids in obese, type 2 diabetic patients. Diabet Med. 1990; 7(3):242–5.
54. Vuorinen-Markkola H, Sinisalo M, Koivisto VA. Guar gum in insulin-dependent diabetes: effects on glycemic control and serum lipoproteins. Am J Clin Nutr. 1992;56(6):1056–60.
55. Anderson JW, Allgood LD, Lawrence A, Altringer LA, Jerdack GR, Hengehold DA, et al. Cholesterol-lowering effects of psyllium intake adjunctive to diet therapy in men and women with hypercholesterolemia: meta-analysis of 8 controlled trials. Am J Clin Nutr. 2000;71:472–9.
56. Opperman AM, Venter CS, Oosthuizen W, Thompson RL, Vorster HH. Meta-analysis of the health effects of using the glycaemic index in meal-planning. Br J Nutr. 2004;92(3):367–81.
57. Wolever TM, Gibbs AL, Mehling C, Chiasson JL, Connelly PW, Josse RG, Leiter LA, Maheux P, Rabasa-Lhoret R, Rodger NW, Ryan EA. The Canadian Trial of Carbohydrates in Diabetes (CCD), a 1-y controlled trial of low-glycemic-index dietary carbohydrate in type 2 diabetes: no effect on glycated hemoglobin but reduction in C-reactive protein. Am J Clin Nutr. 2008;87(1):114–25.
58. Van Dam RM, Visscher AWJ, Feskens EJM, Verhoef P, Kromhout D. Dietary glycemic index in relation to metabolic risk factors and incidence of coronary heart disease: the Zutphen Elderly Study. Eur J Clin Nutr. 2000;54:729–31.
59. Buyken AE, Toeller M, Heitkamp G, Karamaros B, Rottiers R, Muggeo M, Fuller J, The EURODIAB IDDM Complications Study Group. Glycemic index in the diet of European outpatients with type 1 diabetes: relations to glycated hemoglobin and serum lipids. Am J Clin Nutr. 2001;73:574–81.
60. Frost G, Leeds AA, Doré CJ, Madeiros S, Brading S, Dornhorst A. Glycaemic index as a determinant of serum HDL-cholesterol concentration. Lancet. 1999;353(9158):1045–8.
61. Ford ES, Liu S. Glycemic index and serum high-density lipoprotein cholesterol concentration among us adults. Arch Intern Med. 2001;161(4):572–6.
62. Gannon MC, Nuttall FQ, Westphal SA, Fang S, Ercan-Fang N. Acute metabolic response to high-carbohydrate, high-starch meals compared with moderate-carbohydrate, low-starch meals in subjects with type 2 diabetes. Diabetes Care. 1998;21(10): 1619–26.
63. Osei K, Bossetti B. Dietary fructose as a natural sweetener in poorly controlled type 2 diabetes: a 12 month crossover study of effects on glucose, lipoprotein, and apolipoprotein metabolism. Diabet Med. 1989;6:506–11.
64. Osei K, Falko J, Bossetti BM, Holland GC. Metabolic effects of fructose as a natural sweetener in the physiologic meals of ambulatory obese patients with type II diabetes. Am J Med. 1987;83(2):249–55.
65. Grigoresco C, Rizkalla SW, Halfon P, Bornet F, Fontvielle AM, Bros M, Dauchy F, Tchobroutsky G, Slama G. Lack of detectable deleterious effects on metabolic control of daily fructose ingestion for 2 mo in NIDDM patients. Diabetes Care. 1988;11:546–50.
66. Anderson JW, Story LJ, Zettwoch NC, Gustafson NJ, Jefferson BS. Metabolic effects of fructose supplementation in diabetic individuals. Diabetes Care. 1989;12:337–44.
67. McAteer EJ, O'Reilly G, Hadden DR. The effects of one month high fructose intake on plasma glucose and lipid levels in non-insulin-dependent diabetes. Diabet Med. 1987;4(1):62–4.
68. Thorburn AW, Crapo PA, Beltz WF, Wallace P, Witztum JL, Henry RR. Lipid metabolism in non-insulin-dependent diabetes: effects of long-term treatment with fructose-supplemented mixed meals. Am J Clin Nutr. 1989;50:1015–22.
69. Crapo PA, Kolterman OG, Henry RR. Metabolic consequence of two-week fructose feeding in diabetic subjects. Diabetes Care. 1986;9:111–9.
70. Bantle JP, Swanson JE, Thomas W, Laine DC. Metabolic effects of dietary fructose in diabetic subjects. Diabetes Care. 1992;15:1468–76.
71. Bantle JP. Dietary fructose and metabolic syndrome and diabetes. J Nutr. 2009;139(6):1263S–8.
72. Abraha A, Humphreys SM, Clark ML, Matthews DR, Frayn KN. Acute effects of fructose on postprandial lipaemia in diabetic and non-diabetic subjects. Br J Nutr. 1998;80:169–75.
73. Koivisto VA, Yki-Järvinen H. Fructose and insulin sensitivity in patients with type 2 diabetes. J Intern Med. 1993;233:145–53.
74. Malerbi DA, Paiva ES, Duarte AL, Wajchenberg BL. Metabolic effects of dietary sucrose and fructose in type II diabetic subjects. Diabetes Care. 1996;19:1249–56.
75. Aucott L, Gray D, Rothnie H, Thapa M, Waweru C. Effects of lifestyle interventions and long-term weight loss on lipid outcomes – a systematic review. Obes Rev. 2011;12(5):e412–25.

76. Poobalan A, Aucott L, Smith WCS, Avenel A, Jung R, Broom J, Grant AM. Effects of weight loss in overweight/obese individuals and long-term lipid outcomes – a systematic review. Obes Rev. 2004;5(1):43–50.
77. Dattilo AM, Kris-Etherton PM. Effects of weight reduction on blood lipids and lipoproteins: a meta-analysis. Am J Clin Nutr. 1992;56:320–8.
78. Yatsuya H, Jeffery RW, Erickson DJ, Welsh EM, Flood AP, Jaeb MA, Laqua PS, Mitchell NR, Langer SL, Levy RL. Sex-specific HDL cholesterol changes with weight loss and their association with anthropometric variables: the LIFE study. Obesity (Silver Spring). 2011;19(2):429–35.
79. Look AHEAD Research Group, Wing RR. Long-term effects of a lifestyle intervention on weight and cardiovascular risk factors in individuals with type 2 diabetes mellitus: four-year results of the Look AHEAD trial. Arch Intern Med. 2010;170(17):1566–75.
80. Shai I, Schwarzfuchs D, Henkin Y, Shahar DR, Witkow S, Greenberg I, Golan R, Fraser D, Bolotin A, Vardi H, Tangi-Rozental O, Zuk-Ramot R, Sarusi B, Brickner D, Schwartz Z, Sheiner E, Marko R, Katorza E, Thiery J, Fiedler GM, Blüher M, Stumvoll M, Stampfer MJ. Dietary intervention randomized controlled trial (DIRECT) group. Weight loss with a low-carbohydrate, Mediterranean, or low-fat diet. N Engl J Med. 2008;359(3):229–41.
81. Sacks FM, Bray GA, Carey VJ, Smith SR, Ryan DH, Anton SD, McManus K, Champagne CM, Bishop LM, Laranjo N, Leboff MS, Rood JC, de Jonge L, Greenway FL, Loria CM, Obarzanek E, Williamson DA. Comparison of weight-loss diets with different compositions of fat, protein, and carbohydrates. N Engl J Med. 2009;360(9):859–73.
82. Manley SE, Stratton IM, Cull CA, Frighi V, Eeley EA, Matthews DR, Holman RR, Turner RC, Neil HA, United Kingdom Prospective Diabetes Study Group. Effects of three months' diet after diagnosis of type 2 diabetes on plasma lipids and lipoproteins (UKPDS 45). Diabet Med. 2000;17(7):518–23.
83. Ahmad Khan H. Clinical significance of HbA1c as a marker of circulating lipids in male and female type 2 diabetic patients. Acta Diabetol. 2007;44(4):193–200. Epub 2007 Sep 1.
84. Comaschi M, Coscelli C, Cucinotta D, Malini P, Manzato E, Nicolucci A, SFIDA Study Group-Italian Association of Diabetologists (AMD). Cardiovascular risk factors and metabolic control in type 2 diabetic subjects attending outpatient clinics in Italy: the SFIDA (survey of risk factors in Italian diabetic subjects by AMD) study. Nutr Metab Cardiovasc Dis. 2005;15(3):204–11.
85. Becker A, van der Does FE, van Hinsbergh VW, Heine RJ, Bouter LM, Stehouwer CD. Improvement of glycaemic control in type 2 diabetes: favourable changes in blood pressure, total cholesterol and triglycerides, but not in HDL cholesterol, fibrinogen, Von Willebrand factor and (pro)insulin. Neth J Med. 2003;61(4):129–36.
86. Emanuele N, Azad N, Abraira C, et al. Effect of intensive glycemic control on fibrinogen, lipids, and lipoproteins: veterans affairs cooperative study in type II diabetes mellitus. Arch Intern Med. 1998;158: 2485–90.
87. The Diabetes Control and Complications Trial (DCCT) Research Group. Effect of intensive diabetes management on macrovascular events and risk factors in the diabetes control and complications trial. Am J Cardiol. 1995;75:894–903.
88. Cusi K, Cunningham GR, Comstock JP. Safety and efficacy of normalizing fasting glucose with bedtime NPH insulin alone in NIDDM. Diabetes Care. 1995;18:843–5.
89. Carlsson S, Hammar N, Grill V, Kaprio J. Alcohol consumption and the incidence of type 2 diabetes: a 20-year follow-up of the Finnish twin cohort study. Diabetes Care. 1998;21(10):1619–26.
90. Koppes LL, Dekker JM, Hendriks HF, Bouter LM, Heine RJ. Moderate alcohol consumption lowers the risk of type 2 diabetes: a meta-analysis of prospective observational studies. Diabetes Care. 2005;28(3):719–25.
91. Sluik D, Boeing H, Bergmann MM, Schütze M, Teucher B, Kaaks R, Tjønneland A, Overvad K, Arriola L, Ardanaz E, Bendinelli B, Agnoli C, Tumino R, Ricceri F, Mattiello A, Spijkerman AM, Beulens JW, Grobbee DE, Nilsson PM, Melander O, Franks PW, Rolandsson O, Riboli E, Gallo V, Romaguera D, Nöthlings U. Alcohol consumption and mortality in individuals with diabetes mellitus. Br J Nutr. 2011; 15:1–9.
92. Valmadrid CT, Klein R, Moss SE, Klein BE, Cruickshanks KJ. Alcohol intake and the risk of coronary heart disease mortality in persons with older-onset diabetes mellitus. JAMA. 1999;282(3):239–46.
93. Wakabayashi I. Association between alcohol drinking and metabolic syndrome in Japanese male workers with diabetes mellitus. J Atheroscler Thromb. 2011;18(8):684–92.
94. Thomas DE, Elliott EJ, Naughton GA. Exercise for type 2 diabetes mellitus. Cochrane Database Syst Rev. 2006;3, CD002968.
95. Qin R, Chen T, Lou Q, Yu D. Excess risk of mortality and cardiovascular events associated with smoking among patients with diabetes: meta-analysis of observational prospective studies. Int J Cardiol. 2013;167(2):342–50.
96. Maeda K, Noguchi Y, Fukui T. The effects of cessation from cigarette smoking on the lipid and lipoprotein profiles: a meta-analysis. Prev Med. 2003;37:283–290.

# About Randomised Clinical Trials Related to Lipoproteins in Diabetes Mellitus

17

Anthony Keech, Alicia J. Jenkins, and Val Gebski

## Introduction

Many wise people have made statements relevant to the practice of medicine, including Hippocrates (c. 460 BC–370 BC) who commented that "Life is short, the art of medicine long; the opportunity is fleeting, experience perilous, and decisions difficult". More recently, in 1982 Richard Doll stated that "Every time a doctor treats a patient…he is performing an experiment". Fortunately in this era of evidence-based medicine, we have many studies and, specifically, randomized controlled trials (RCTs) to guide clinical practice, including individual patient care, the development of treatment algorithms and guidelines, and to inform public health policy.

As diabetes mellitus, dyslipidemia and their vascular complications are increasingly common and costly, both in personal and economic terms, many research studies related to the management of lipoproteins in people with diabetes have been conducted, are in progress and are in development. The most directly relevant to clinical practice is the randomised controlled trial (RCT). Most RCTs in the field of lipoproteins in diabetes relate to adults with type 2 diabetes mellitus or to an admixture of people with type 1 diabetes and type 2 diabetes. Lipid drug studies are sometimes conducted specifically in youth with type 1 diabetes, such as part of the Adolescent type 1 Diabetes cardio-renal Intervention Trial (AdDIT) study which is evaluating the effects of a statin and an ACE inhibitor (or their combination) on surrogate vascular end points [1]. The conduct of such studies and their translation from the research setting to clinical practice has undoubtedly contributed to the improving outcomes of diabetes and its risk of cardiovascular disease. In this chapter we describe the elements of a good RCT, the challenges to its conduct, aspects to consider when reporting or reading and assessing a clinical trial, including its generalizability to clinical practice and the future of RCTs.

## Definition

An RCT is a prospective scientific experiment comparing the effects of a specific treatment strategy in an experimental group with an alternate strategy in a similar (control) group, in which chance (randomization) determines to which group each subject is allocated, so as to reduce bias [2].

A. Keech
NHMRC Clinical Trials Centre, University of Sydney, Sydney, NSW, Australia
e-mail: tony@ctc.usyd.edu.au

A.J. Jenkins, M.D., F.R.A.C.P. (✉)
Section of Endocrinology and Diabetes, University of Oklahoma Health Sciences Center, 941 Stanton L. Young Blvd., BSEB 302F, Oklahoma City, OK 73104, USA

NHMRC Clinical Trials Centre, University of Sydney, Sydney, NSW, Australia
e-mail: alicia-jenkins@ouhsc.edu; alicia.jenkins@ctc.usyd.edu.au

V. Gebski
NHMRC Clinical Trials Centre, University of Sydney, Sydney, NSW, Australia

A.J. Jenkins et al. (eds.), *Lipoproteins in Diabetes Mellitus*, Contemporary Diabetes, DOI 10.1007/978-1-4614-7554-5_17, 

Most RCTs related to lipoproteins in diabetes evaluate the clinical effects of a single lipid drug vs. a placebo, as in the Scandinavian Simvastatin Survival Study (4S) Study [3], Collaborative Atorvastatin Diabetes Study (CARDS) [4] and Fenofibrate Intervention and Event Lowering in Diabetes (FIELD) [5] Study, or test a combination vs. a single treatment, such as in the Action to Control Cardiovascular Risk in Diabetes (ACCORD)-LIPID [6] study, which tested fenofibrate and simvastatin vs. placebo and simvastatin in adults with type 2 diabetes. In the Heart Protection Study (HPS) [7], simvastatin vs. placebo and combination antioxidant vitamins E, C and beta-carotene vs. placebo were evaluated in a 2×2 factorial designed trial.

Common RCT end points are usually hard clinical events such as mortality, myocardial infarction, leg amputation, nephropathy or retinopathy or a combination thereof. Some alternate RCT end points are intermediate measures of vascular damage such as carotid intima medial thickness, the results of pulse-wave analysis or lipoprotein-related measures such as LDL-cholesterol levels. Rather than testing a drug, some RCTs related to lipoproteins in diabetes will test the effects of a diet or lifestyle, as discussed in another chapter in this book.

## Precursors to and Phases of an RCT

*Preclinical Research.* An RCT usually stems from many years of costly biochemical, cell-based, animal and human preclinical research. Prior to and after the conduct of an RCT testing a pharmaceutical agent, there are several general "phases" of trials. A drug may be tested in more than one phase simultaneously, in different trials, and some trials may overlap two phases. Many regulatory and ethics committee approvals are also required, ideally including trial registration.

There are five phases of trials, as described below [8].

*Phase 0.* A phase 0 trial is an exploratory study usually conducted in a small number of subjects (often less than 20) using subtherapeutic doses.

*Phase 1.* Phase 1 studies are early stage testing in human subjects, predominantly to evaluate the safety and pharmacologic aspects such as drug absorption, distribution, excretion and half-life. Subjects are usually healthy volunteers and often young adults. Usually small numbers of subjects (10–20) are tested, often in specialised facilities.

*Phase 2.* Phase 2 studies are usually conducted in larger groups (often 100–300) of people with the condition of interest, in this case diabetes, so as to demonstrate safety and efficacy. A phase 2 study of a lipid drug in people with diabetes may report side effects, effects on renal and liver function and on glycemia and lipid levels.

*Phase 3.* Phase 3 studies aim to provide conclusive evidence with regard to the safety and effectiveness of a test drug. A phase 3 RCT usually involves hundreds to thousands, even tens of thousands of subjects, with the condition of interest (e.g. diabetes) in multiple centers in multiple countries.

*Phase 4.* After regulatory body approval (e.g. by the USA's Federal and Drug Administration (FDA)), phase 4 studies monitor long-term safety and efficacy, and are essential, as often people given the drug differ clinically from those subjects in whom the earlier phase studies were conducted. If there are sufficient concerns, drugs may be removed from clinical use at this stage.

## Elements of a Good RCT

The quality of RCTs and the evidence resulting from them can vary; hence it is important not only that the clinicians, scientists and statisticians involved in their planning and conduct have a good understanding of optimal RCT design and conduct, and also that people who may utilize RCT results in their clinical practice or in their own research can assess study quality [2].

Important elements of an RCT include subject selection, randomization and masking, study end point choice and measurement, statistical power and data analysis, the reporting and interpretation of study outcomes, recognition of potential confounders and relevance to clinical practice.

*General Study Considerations.* An RCT must be of sufficient scientific quality to be able to satisfactorily answer the questions of interest; to account for the potential confounders, such as arising from different responses to treatment between men and women or between younger and older subjects; and to control for statistical uncertainty (Type 1 and Type 2 errors, discussed below). Scientific quality would include ensuring sufficient numbers of participants are recruited, accuracy in the measurement of the study outcomes, appropriate number of repeated measurements (where required), well-implemented methods of randomization and allocation concealment and minimal attrition and low rates of missing/incomplete observations on patients. Study outcomes refer to measurements pertaining to an individual patient, such as success/failure, time to an event or levels/scores in the case of continuous measurements. Study end points on the other hand generally refer to the summary measures of the benefit of the intervention over the control and are usually differences in mean levels (for continuous outcomes), odds ratios or differences in proportions (binary outcomes) and hazard or risk ratios (time to event).

Sample size calculations in an RCT are usually based on the minimum clinical difference that is deemed worthwhile between the control and intervention groups in the primary study outcome. This chosen difference to seek is usually based on results of previous studies, if they exist, on clinical judgement, from epidemiologic studies and from likely cost of treatment, and reflects the potential importance and value of the benefit which could be provided by the intervention in clinical practice. If the study outcome is a clinical vascular event, larger studies for several years are usually required. Further, the phenomenon of metabolic memory may delay the clinical manifestations of modifying lipoprotein levels. Study size impacts on the statistical power of a study (and vice versa). The statistical power of a study is the likelihood that the study will correctly identify a true advantage of a tested intervention compared with control, i.e. it is the probability that a true effect of a certain (usually clinically useful) size will be detected, and a statistically significant result will be obtained from an RCT of a given size. In general this likelihood is fixed in the study design and generally set at 80 or 90 %, based on numerous assumptions. Thus if a study on many thousands of patients (not likely to be repeated) is planned, the investigators would want the chance of the study "missing the targeted effect" (if it really is beneficial) to be small, usually 1 in 10 chance—i.e. 90 % power, or a 9 in 10 chance of the study correctly declaring a significant difference. For other studies (e.g. cancer trials), a 4 in 5 chance is often deemed sufficient. The chance of missing the targeted effect is referred to as the Type 2 error (a statistical term) and is the complement of the power, i.e. power + Type 2 error = 1. Fixing the power is required to determine the sample size of the study, and so the calculations underpinning the planned sample size (including assumed control group event rates, expected compliance losses, designed power, chosen level of significance [*p* value] and size of treatment effect being sought) are usually performed in the design stage before the RCT begins and need to be included in applications for RCT funding and also in the study reports.

The inclusion and exclusion criteria are important parts of an RCT and subsequently impact on the translation of the trial results to clinical practice. Both should be carefully considered in study design and described in detail in all RCT reports. Ideally the subjects included will represent those who are expected to benefit from the treatment being tested in the RCT and are representative of the majority with the condition of interest. The exclusion criteria are usually designed to avoid participation of those perceived to be at high risk of potential harm by either treatment or who may confound the study outcomes, such as those with limited life expectancy from other causes or with, for example, severe renal or liver disease.

*Randomization* is the process used to allocate willing and eligible participants to one or other study treatment, hence into either the intervention or the control arm of an RCT, and aims to ensure similarity between the two groups at baseline, such that any observed differences emerging from the trial are related to the intervention (or to the play of chance (*p* values and confidence intervals quantify the likelihood of chance differences of the magnitude observed)). The randomization process intends to preferential assignment to any of the RCT arms. When the randomization is not equal (e.g. 2:1), the treatment assignment is still randomly allocated but weighted to the group receiving the higher number of patients. Subjects should generally only be randomized after written informed consent has been provided, and they (and usually also the investigators) should remain masked to which treatment group they have been allocated (discussed below). In most RCTs, randomization is done "centrally", away from the investigators and trial participants, and often involves telephone, the Internet or interactive voice-activated programmes, which must be available around the clock, particularly for international multicenter RCTs. If the randomization procedure has worked well, the major demographic groups of the treatment arms at baseline should not differ significantly regarding such variables as age, sex, diabetes duration, baseline lipids, blood pressure, smoking status and glycemic control (e.g. HbA1c levels), except occasionally by chance alone.

There are several types of randomization in common use [9]. In a *simple randomization* process, each trial subject has an equal chance of being assigned to the intervention arm or the control group. This type of randomization can be achieved using random numbers from a statistical textbook or more commonly using a computer-generated algorithm.

*Stratified randomization* is sometimes used to achieve better balance between groups on factors which are known to influence study outcomes. For example, separate random allocation sequences may be used for men and for women or for people with diabetes with, vs. without, prior diabetic renal damage or cardiovascular disease to ensure better balance between groups on these factors.

*Permuted block randomization* is commonly used for small RCTs (of less than 1,000 subjects), as simple randomization can sometimes result in large chance differences in factors (e.g. such as gender) between treatment groups. In block randomization, blocks having equal numbers of control and intervention allocations (e.g. two controls (C) and two intervention (I) subjects in a block of four) are used, with the order of treatments in the block being randomly permuted. For example, a block of four subjects has six possible treatment arrangements: CCII, CICI, CIIC, IICC, ICIC and ICCI. A random number sequence is used to choose the particular block, which then sets the allocation order. A minor drawback of block randomization however is that, if at the end of the study there are numerous incompleted blocks in use across many centers, there may still be a substantial overall imbalance in the number of participants allocated to each of the treatment(s). A further limitation is that, unless the block sizes are allowed to vary randomly in length (e.g. 4, 6, 4, 8, 6), the overall sequence can sometimes be identified, resulting in the potential ability to predict the next treatment allocation to be issued should you choose to randomize a particular patient.

*Dynamic random allocation* methods, also known as adaptive allocation, are an alternate randomization procedure. This process allocates trial participants to the RCT treatment arms by first checking the allocation tallies of similar participants who have already been randomised, so as to achieve the best balance between treatment groups across all nominated stratification variables. Stratified minimisation and dynamic balanced randomization are two examples. Computer-based algorithms are able to facilitate this process.

*Unsuitable randomization methods* include alternate allocation to control or intervention groups, or allocation based on the day of clinic attendance or birth date, or sealed envelopes held at the site. With these methods, it cannot be guaranteed that the process has not been breached (e.g. by transilluminating envelopes or by re-scheduling a patient's randomization day) and that each patient was truly randomly allocated to their originally assigned treatment.

The allocation status should of course be concealed from the site staff and the participant. This process is called allocation concealment.

*Blinding or Masking*. RCTs in the field of lipoproteins in diabetes usually involve subjects being randomized to one of two groups, one of which will receive a single active drug and the other of which will receive a matching placebo, as in CARDS [4]. In some RCTs, one active drug that is usually the best currently available treatment is given to all subjects, and one test drug or matching placebo is added (such as in the ACCORD–LIPID study). Masking refers to the process by which the treatment allocation is hidden from the people involved in the study [10].

*Double blind* refers to both the participant and the investigators being unaware of the treatment allocation. This process serves to minimize potential for observer bias to occur and also for participants dropping out because of knowledge of treatment arm or, if possible, through other means of acquiring one of the treatments, for example, if they were determined to receive a specific treatment. The masking of whether a treatment is active or placebo is more feasible in RCTs with tablet therapies, unlike surgical trials or device-related trials; however when there are very common and specific drug effects, such as flushing with nicotinic acid, this can be difficult. For example, in the recent AIM-HIGH trial, [11] low-dose nicotinic acid was added to the "placebo" to induce some flushing, but the dose used was sufficient to elevate HDL-C levels. With lipoprotein-related studies, a potential confounder is that some trial participants and their general practitioners, either inadvertently or in a desire to try to work out if the person is receiving the active drug, will order and discuss a lipid profile. In our experience this has resulted in some trial participants choosing to cease participation in the trial as they determined (rightly or wrongly) that they were not allocated to the active treatment arm.

*Outcomes*. There are usually multiple outcomes in RCTs, and what the primary, secondary and sometimes even tertiary outcomes are should be prestated and the trial planned with appropriate study duration to be able to detect realistic changes, to provide adequate statistical power to avoid Type 1 or Type 2 errors, and to enable appropriate subgroup analyses. Outcomes, which are usually measured for each study participant, may range from hard clinical events, e.g. death, to intermediate measures such as carotid IMT, to lipid levels.

*Statistical Power and Data Analysis*. Statistical analysis of RCT data provides an estimate of the magnitude of difference in outcome rates between the groups, and the probability that the trial results could have occurred by chance alone. A commonly used cut-off at which statistical significance is taken is at $p<0.05$, meaning that the probability of the trial result (e.g. drug benefit over placebo) occurring by chance alone is less than 5 %. This value is referred to as the significance level of the trial, and the complement (95 %) the confidence level. It may be thought of as the level we are prepared to accept of a false-positive result. If there are multiple RCT end points, statistical significance may be taken at lower $p$ values. There are two types of statistical errors that can occur in an RCT: Type 1 error (chance of a false-positive result) and Type 2 error (chance of missing a true benefit).

*Type 1 error* refers to concluding that there is a real difference between treatments (or groups) when none exists, i.e. rejecting the null hypothesis when it is correct.

*Type 2 error* refers to concluding that there is no effect of treatment when one does truly exist, i.e. accepting the null hypothesis when it is incorrect.

Clinical significance is a judgement that an effect is large enough to change the way a patient should be treated. Clinicians and those devising treatment algorithms and health policy can be assisted in these judgements by calculations of the number of patients needed to treat (NNT) to derive benefit (discussed below) and the hazard or odds ratios. The hazard ratio is the proportion of subjects in the intervention arm of the RCT (as the numerator) compared with the proportion of subjects in the control arm (as the denominator) having a (predefined) event during the RCT time period.

*The number needed to treat* is the number of patients who must be treated to prevent one specified event. It is the reciprocal of the absolute risk reduction. The NNT with a particular drug may vary according to the subject characteristics. For example, in the FIELD study the NNT with fenofibrate for approximately 5 years to prevent one amputation in all FIELD subjects was 197, but the NNT to prevent one amputation in patients with a previous foot ulcer or amputation was only 25 [12].

## Challenges of Conducting an RCT Related to Lipoproteins in Diabetes Mellitus

There are many challenges to conducting and interpreting the results of an RCT related to lipoproteins in diabetes. Some can be at least partially, if not fully, controlled by study design, but others cannot, but still should be addressed. Challenges include aspects related to diabetes and its complications and to lipoproteins, study outcome definitions and their measurement and study reporting and generalizability. It is also important to recognise that people who participate in an RCT can enjoy lower adverse clinical outcome rates, even if allocated to a placebo arm, than those who do not. This phenomenon of people tending to perform better when in a study is called the Hawthorne effect and was first described in a Harvard-based study evaluating the relationship between productivity and the work environment in an industrial setting, the Hawthorne Works Plant [13]. The day-to-day efforts of a person with diabetes, including attention to their diet, exercise, non-smoking status, foot care and adherence to recommended treatments, can all substantially impact their weight, vascular risk factors and development of diabetes complications and potentially the magnitude of observed response, or lack thereof, to a lipoprotein-targeted intervention.

### Different Types and Stages of Diabetes

The type of diabetes, be it type 1 or type 2 diabetes, the stage and duration of diabetes and the level of glucose control can impact lipoprotein levels and potentially the response to treatment being tested in an RCT. The amount of endogenous insulin production and degree of insulin resistance can differ substantially in both types of diabetes, and this and the level of glycemic control, usually reflected by HbA1c levels, can impact lipoproteins. Hypertriglyceridemia and low HDL-cholesterol levels are more common in type 2 diabetes than in type 1 diabetes, and this dyslipidemic profile is accentuated by poor glycemic control, obesity or renal dysfunction [14, 15]. The number of people with type 1 or type 2 diabetes, their glucose control modality and level and complication status, should be considered and reported and subgroup analyses performed if there are enough subjects available to provide adequate statistical power.

### Multiple Risk Factors for Complications Including Genetic and Epigenetic Effects

As mentioned above, lipoprotein levels are impacted by many variables, some of which are fixed, for example, genotypes affecting lipoprotein levels [16] and treatment response [17], and others may vary over time, such as diet, smoking, exercise and medication adherence. All these things tend to balance out between treatment arms in larger studies but may still confound trial results in smaller trials of just a few hundred people. Epigenetic effects may enable environmental factors and even the lipoprotein-targeting drug to modulate the effects of the inherited genotype [18].

Whilst abnormal lipid levels are major risk factors for both the macrovascular and microvascular complications of diabetes [14, 15], other factors such as age, diabetes duration, family history, poor glycaemic control, hypertension, smoking, obesity and periodontal disease [19] contribute to the development and progression of vascular disease in diabetes and hence may impact rates of complication development.

### Slow Vascular Disease Development

Atherosclerosis and its related clinical events of myocardial infarction (which is often silent in people with diabetes), stroke, claudication, gangrene and amputation, retinopathy, nephropathy and neuropathy develop over years to decades. Atherosclerosis can begin in youth, even in the absence of diabetes, and the process of this inflammatory process is accelerated in diabetes [20]. Because of this, if vascular events or even some intermediate measures of vascular damage such as carotid intima media thickness (IMT) are RCT outcomes, then the lipid-related study will need to last for years to modify these. Many lipid drug trials in diabetes with vascular event end points have a 5-year intervention period, and to increase the number of events that will accrue and statistical power, large numbers (thousands) of subjects are included. The use of intermediate end points, such as vascular function (e.g. flow-mediated dilation, pulse-wave analysis) and structural changes (such as assessed by coronary artery intravascular ultrasound (IVUS), carotid IMT), which may change over shorter time frames are sometimes used in RCTs. These studies usually still take several years to complete and may have lesser impact on clinical practice. An additional factor to consider is that of metabolic memory (also known as the legacy effect) of glucose control, which has been demonstrated in both type 1 and type 2 diabetes [21, 22].

## Metabolic Memory or the Legacy Effect

These comparable terms were coined in relationship to the DCCT/EDIC (type 1 diabetes) and the 10-year follow-up of the United Kingdom Progression of Diabetes Study (UKPDS) type 2 diabetes studies. The legacy effect refers to the phenomenon by which the body's tissues, including arteries, retinae, kidneys and nerves, continue to respond to poor or good glycemic control for years after the glucose control has improved or worsened. This memory can last for years. The UKPDS data demonstrates a legacy effect of glycemia for 10 years after 10 years with an HbA1c≈7.0 % [21]. This is in keeping with the time frame of metabolic memory in type 1 diabetes evidenced by the DCCT/EDIC study, in which≈5.9 years of intensive vs. conventional diabetes management (HbA1c 9 vs. 7 %) lowered vascular complication rates for 8–12 or more years [22]. It is not yet clear if there is a threshold level for metabolic memory and how long this effect is maintained for a given time at each HbA1c level across the full HbA1c spectrum.

This legacy effect may also apply to other non-glucose vascular risk factors. The UKPDS also examined if there was a legacy effect for tight vs. less-tight blood pressure control. Whilst the UKPDS showed clear vascular complication benefit for lower blood pressure levels, the UKPDS follow-up study did not find evidence for persistence of benefit beyond the randomised period [23]. Potential mitigating circumstances are the relatively high blood pressure targets during the UKPDS.

*What about lipid memory?* Some early lipid diet or drug trials with post-trial follow-up found persistent cardiovascular and mortality benefit in those with lower on-trial lipid levels, even though lipid level differences ceased soon after study end [24, 25–28]. As yet, there are no specific lipid-related studies exclusively in diabetes for which the legacy effect has been published, and given the major benefit of lipid-lowering drugs in type 2 diabetes, it could be ethically difficult to conduct such a study in the future.

Such metabolic memory for glucose, and potentially for lipid levels, means that the full impact of a lipoprotein-targeted intervention in diabetes may not be fully evident until many years after its commencement. The extremely high human and economic costs of running large and long-duration RCTs related to lipoproteins in people with diabetes usually require major pharmaceutical industry support and/or support from multiple funding agencies.

## Variability in Some RCT End Points

When considering RCTs related to vascular damage in diabetes, one should consider the variability of the vascular end point measure. Microaneurysms, a commonly used indicator of diabetic retinopathy, can regress [29].

Albuminuria, a commonly used measure of diabetic nephropathy, is highly variable within an individual, being affected by such factors as exercise, blood pressure and glycemia. Even without a specific intervention, such as angiotensin-converting enzyme (ACE) inhibitor drugs, increased albuminuria levels can spontaneously regress in people with type 1 diabetes [30]. It is now recognised that in people with diabetes, renal function, reflected by glomerular filtration rate or creatinine clearance, may still decline even in the absence of increased urinary albumin loss [31]. Other renal function measures commonly used to characterise trial subjects and which may be an RCT end point include serum creatinine levels, time till doubling of serum creatinine levels, circulating cystatin C levels, end-stage renal disease and commencement of renal dialysis or renal transplantation [32]. Renal function effects in RCTs may differ according to which renal function end point is chosen.

Measurement issues can also impact RCT results. Factors such as subject preparation (e.g. prandial status will greatly alter triglyceride levels), biological variation (e.g. circadian and seasonal effects), issues related to sample collection, storage and processing, the quality of the assays chosen, operator-dependent factors and any human or undetected instrument error may impact RCT biomarker levels.

In RCTs traditional lipid levels (and other detailed lipoprotein-related characteristics such as lipoprotein composition, size, apolipoprotein content, related enzyme activities, lipoprotein modifications (discussed in other book chapters) such as non-enzymatic glycation and oxidation and lipoprotein function) can vary greatly over time. Whilst circulating lipoproteins exist only for hours to days, in most RCTs related to lipoproteins in diabetes, measures of lipoprotein quantity or quality are usually only evaluated at several time points, which may be months, sometimes years apart. Whilst HbA1c levels reflect mean blood glucose levels over the previous 2–3 months, as yet there are no equivalents for lipid levels. Furthermore for lipoprotein and vascular disease-related RCTs, it must be remembered that lipoprotein levels in blood are measured, yet this is not the site of disease. It is the amount of lipoprotein that has accumulated within the vasculature that is of major importance to clinical events. As an example, oxidized LDL is more atherogenic than unmodified (normal) LDL, and oxidized LDL levels are 70-fold higher in the arterial wall than in blood [33], yet intravascular oxidized levels cannot be measured in an RCT. Similarly, inflammatory markers, such as serum C-reactive protein (CRP) and soluble forms of the vascular cell adhesion molecules (CAMs), are often measured in serum samples from RCTs [34, 35], yet it is likely the level of inflammation within the arteries, retinae and renal tissue that matters most. Indeed many blood- and urine-based biomarkers that are measured in RCTs are not at the site of disease, though still often correlate with the risk of event and/or treatment benefit. In some studies the study outcome is the circulating level or quality of a lipoprotein.

## Pleiotropic Effects

Drug treatments used in RCTs related to lipoproteins in diabetes may also have pleiotropic effects which can favorably or unfavorably affect study end-points. Many pleiotropic effects of some lipid drugs, such as statins and fibrates, are relevant to vascular health and include anti-inflammatory, antioxidant, antiplatelet and anticlotting effects, vasodilation, angiogenesis-related effects and alterations in cell signalling and genetic effects [36, 37]. Not all pleiotropic effects are potentially vasoprotective, for example, fenofibrate increases levels of the vascular risk marker homocysteine [38].

It is important to consider the potential contribution of pleiotropic drug effects in RCT reporting and assessment, though it cannot be readily quantified. Whilst lipid levels, including elevated triglycerides and low HDL-cholesterol levels, are commonly associated with and predictive of the vascular complications of diabetes and of regression of increased albuminuria [14, 15], fenofibrate, which substantially lowers triglyceride levels and increases apoA1 and HDL levels, was associated with significant improvements in diabetic retinopathy [39], nephropathy [40] and amputations [12] in the FIELD study. In the FIELD study most of these major microvascular benefits were reported not to clearly relate to changes in traditional lipid levels. Preliminary data analyses of combined microvascular and combined macrovascular end points in the FIELD study support independent associations with factors related to oxidative stress, inflammation and adipokines and effects of fenofibrate on circulating levels of many of these biomarkers.

## Reporting and Interpreting RCT Results

In reporting or assessing and interpreting the results of an RCT, the underlying hypothesis, aims, methods and results should be clearly presented, along with a balanced discussion of the study outcomes, strengths and weaknesses of the study design, similarities and differences with previous studies, remaining or new questions and clinical implications. The appropriateness and limitations of the study design (e.g. length of intervention), subject inclusion and exclusion criteria, clinical and laboratory tools used and statistical power should be considered, and the authors, prompted if need be by their manuscript reviewers and editors, should provide sufficient detail to enable a thorough assessment [41].

## Adverse Events

There must be sufficient detail collected and reported in an RCT to judge the severity and relationship of possible adverse events to the treatment(s) allocated. A definition of adverse events has been adopted by the International Conference on Harmonization [42], which is a collaboration between drug marketing regulatory bodies in the USA, the European Union and Japan. "An adverse event is any untoward medical occurrence in a patient or clinical investigation subject administered a pharmaceutical product and which does not necessarily have a causal relationship with this treatment. An adverse event therefore can be any unfavorable and unintended sign (including an abnormal laboratory finding), symptom or disease temporarily associated with the use of a medicinal (investigational) product, whether or not related to the medicinal (investigational) product." A subset of adverse events is that of adverse drug reactions, which are those unfavorable conditions that may reasonably be related to the drug, provided it was used in the approved dose range in the target population for the treatment of the appropriate disease.

Adverse events or drug reactions can be classified as serious or non-serious. A serious adverse event is one that (a) causes death, (b) is life-threatening, (c) necessitates or prolongs an inpatient hospital stay, (d) causes persistent or significant disability or (e) causes a birth defect. An example of a serious adverse event in a lipid drug RCT is that of rhabdomyolysis possibly due to statin treatment (sometimes aggravated by another concomitant medication) and non-serious adverse events may include headache, rash or lethargy. Non-serious adverse events are usually divided into those that can confidently be regarded as not being drug related, whilst others are classified as those that are either definitely or possibly drug related.

So as to enable comparison between different RCTs, adverse events are usually listed by body system, e.g. cardiovascular, gastrointestinal and renal. Commonly used schemes are those of the International Classification of Diseases (ICD) [43] and the Medical dictionary for regulatory activities (MedRA) [44].

As stated by the Declaration of Helsinki World Medical Association, "it is the duty of the physician in medical research to protect the life, health, privacy and dignity of the human subject" [45]. To facilitate this in RCTs, the research subjects should be advised to report any changes in their well-being, and the trial nurses and doctors should document and report the details. A data safety and monitoring committee (DSMC) or board of independent, preappointed and appropriately experienced people can review the events whilst unmasked to treatment allocation. They play a vital role in ensuring RCT subject safety and can mandate the early cessation of an RCT as soon as it is evident that the treatment being tested is harmful or beneficial overall. For example, the ILLUMINATE trial of a CETP inhibitor, torcetrapib, was ceased early due to an excess of harm (including death and severe hypertension) [46]. CARDS [4] was intended to be a 4-year primary prevention double-blind trial of atorvastatin 10 mg/day vs. matching placebo in patients with type 2 diabetes with an LDL-cholesterol level ≤160 mg/dL, fasting triglycerides ≤600 mg/dL and at least one additional cardiovascular risk factor. The study end was to take place after 304 primary end points, but there was substantial benefit of atorvastatin seen on the planned interim analysis, after 149 primary end points, and the independent steering committee recommended that the study should be stopped early. This (CARDS) result and similar findings among people with diabetes from the Heart Protection Study [7] were some of the major RCT findings in this area to influence clinical practice, such that many people with type 2 diabetes are now offered statin treatment to reduce CVD risk.

## Generalizability of RCT Results to Clinical Practice

In 1980, Bernard Fisher said "I consider the prospective randomized trial mechanism one of the most important advances of this century and the most effective method available for transferring medical practice from an art to a science".

One of the main purposes for conducting RCTs is to guide clinical practice. In making clinical decisions for individual patients, preparing guidelines or deciding public policy, major factors to be considered include the relevance of the RCT to the clinical question, the similarity of the RCT participants to those in question, the quality of the RCT and whether other evidence, including the outcomes of other RCTs, agree.

RCTs often focus on one or two interventions which are given to specially selected well-motivated and usually treatment-adherent subjects who will be monitored relatively closely compared to usual clinical practice. In the "real world", patients may differ from subjects in the RCT, and because of this need to compare applicability to the clinical care setting, subject inclusion and exclusion criteria and demographics should be described in detail. Potential differences relate to age—clinical care subjects may be older or younger or of different ethnic background to the RCT participants. They may have multiple co-morbidities, which may include renal or liver dysfunction, which may impact drug handling. They may be taking many other medications, excess alcohol or recreational drugs which may increase the risk of drug interactions. As another example, two major RCTs of fenofibrate in people with type 2 diabetes demonstrated protective effects against diabetic retinopathy [39, 47], but this evidence may not apply directly to people with type 1 diabetes. Such a trial has been planned (see FAME 1 Eye study at trials.gov), but not yet conducted. Whilst RCTs of statins have shown vascular benefit in tens of thousands of subjects, those with advanced renal or liver disease, or moderate degrees or both, which are not uncommon in clinical practice, have usually been excluded. (The SHARP trial has now demonstrated benefits of simvastatin and ezetimibe in combination to reduce. cardiovascular events in people with advanced renal disease [48].) It is because of such factors that the (Phase 4) marketing surveillance and reporting of major adverse events and drug interactions are very important. Regulatory bodies can add safety warnings or even withdraw a therapy after its approval for use in clinical practice. For example, the FDA has issued safety warnings against the use of full-dose (80 mg) simvastatin, due to higher rates of myositis [49]. Post-marketing surveillance also led to warnings against the combination of a statin with a fibrate other than fenofibrate, due to the higher risk of myositis [50].

Apart from the efficacy of a therapy in treating lipoprotein disorders in people with diabetes, other aspects should be considered. This includes the rates and types of adverse effects of the treatment and the acceptability of the treatment regimen and any required monitoring. As dyslipidemia per se is not associated with symptoms (unless there is severe hypertriglyceridemia, which can cause acute pancreatitis and eruptive xanthomata [51]) and long-term treatment is needed, the ease of adherence should be high and side effects minimal to achieve good long-term compliance in practice. Another important aspect to consider in the translation of RCT results to clinical practice is the economic costs to the individual and others who cover the treatment costs. Health economics analyses and quality of life data related to an RCT can be helpful in this regard.

## Landmark Trials of Lipoprotein Treatments in Diabetes

In recent decades several RCTs related to lipoprotein treatments in diabetes have resulted in changes to clinical practice. Effects on clinical practice are usually greater after two or more large RCTs are supportive. As summarised in Table 17.1, the major statin trials addressing the value of lowering LDL-cholesterol in diabetes have been the HPS, ALLHAT-LLT, ASCOT-LLA, CARDS, 4D, ASPEN and MEGA trials and A-Z, TNT, IDEAL and SEARCH trials, all of which have included more than 1,000 individuals with diabetes in their trials, though of these, only the CARDS, 4D and ASPEN trials were conducted solely among people with diabetes [52]. Furthermore, only the HPS and ALERT trials have included more than 200 individuals each with type 1 diabetes (Table 17.2) [53].

Collectively, however, they provide in meta-analysis (see below) strong evidence of the value of statin therapy in reducing vascular risk among people with both type 1 and type 2 diabetes (Fig. 17.1) [53].

The trials of fibrate therapy have also been of great interest for the treatment of people with diabetes. Both the FIELD study and then the ACCORD-LIPID study were conducted exclusively among people with type 2 diabetes, and both demonstrated large benefits to lower CVD risk among those individuals with dyslipidemia (low HDL-c and high TG), despite negative overall primary end points among all subjects [5, 6, 54]. This has been a highly consistent finding in all of the large fibrate trials. Further, both studies demonstrated highly significant and large reductions in measures of retinopathy [39, 47], in both cases a prespecified other end point. FIELD in addition demonstrated reduced amputations with fenofibrate [12], and in both trials, new or progression of albuminuria was reduced with treatment [6, 40].

Major results in individuals with diabetes are keenly awaited from the currently underway large scale trials of Proprotein Convertase Subtilisin/Kexin type 9 (PCSK9) inhibitors, which demonstrate a profound lowering of LDL-cholesterol levels, even when added to high dose statin therapy [55, 56].

## Combining Results from RCTs

*Systematic Reviews*: A systematic review is a synthesis of published results and conclusions of previous relevant investigations. There are explicit methods for the literature search, study appraisals and data analysis to answer a clearly stated a priori research question. The related term "meta-analysis" refers to the statistical techniques used in a systematic review, which pool the results of several RCTs. Both RCTs and systematic reviews of RCTs can provide valuable health-care decision support. RCTs are often helpful to address a specific question such as whether low- or high-dose statin therapy is more effective at reducing cardiovascular events, and sometimes a single RCT will provide clear-cut evidence, such as in the CARDS. However when the effect sizes in the RCT results are contrasting or modest, a systematic review can be helpful. An example of a helpful systematic review relates to the use of statins in people with diabetes (discussed above). The Cholesterol Trialists Treatment Collaboration was able to demonstrate benefit of statin therapy for people with type 1 diabetes [53], among other findings.

*The Art of Medicine*: There are not always clear-cut results of RCTs available to answer all clinical questions related to the treatment of lipoproteins in people with diabetes. This may relate to lack of resources to conduct the required stud-

**Table 17.1** Baseline characteristics and eligibility criteria of participating trials

| | Number of patients | Treatment comparison (mg/day) | Median follow-up in survivors (years)[a] | Mean age (years) | Baseline LDL-C (mmol/L) | Prior CHD[b] | Other vascular disease[c] | No prior vascular disease | Women | LDL-C difference at 1 year (mmol/L) |
|---|---|---|---|---|---|---|---|---|---|---|
| *Statin vs. control* | | | | | | | | | | |
| SSSS | 4,444 | S20-40 vs. placebo | 5.4 | 59 | 4.88 | 4,444 (100 %) | 126 (3 %) | 0 (0 %) | 827 (19 %) | −1.77 |
| WOSCOPS | 6,595 | P40 vs. placebo | 4.8 | 55 | 4.96 | 338 (5 %) | 193 (3 %) | 6,096 (92 %) | 0 (0 %) | −1.07 |
| CARE | 4,159 | P40 vs. placebo | 5.0 | 59 | 3.58 | 4,159 (100 %) | 0 (0 %) | 0 (0 %) | 576 (14 %) | −1.03 |
| Post CABG | 1,351 | L40-80 vs. L2.5-5 | 4.3 | 61 | 4.02 | 1,351 (100 %) | 37 (3 %) | 0 (0 %) | 102 (8 %) | −1.07 |
| AFCAPS/TexCaps | 6,605 | L20-40 vs. placebo | 5.2 | 58 | 3.89 | 10 (1 %) | 9 (0 %) | 6,586(0.99 %) | 997 (15 %) | −0.94 |
| LIPID | 9,014 | P40 vs. placebo | 6.0 | 61 | 3.88 | 9,014 (100 %) | 905 (10 %) | 0 (0 %) | 1,516 (17 %) | −1.03 |
| GISSI-P | 4,271 | P20 vs. no treatment | 2.0 | 59 | 3.92 | 4,271 (100 %) | 179 (4 %) | 0 (0 %) | 587 (14 %) | −0.35 |
| LIPS | 1,677 | F80 vs. placebo | 3.9 | 60 | 3.42 | 1,677 (100 %) | 142 (8 %) | 0 (0 %) | 271 (16 %) | −0.92 |
| HPS | 20,536 | S40 vs. placebo | 5.4 | 63 | 3.38 | 13,386 (65 %) | 8,865 (43 %) | 3,161 (15 %) | 5,082 (25 %) | −1.29 |
| PROSPER | 5,804 | P40 vs. placebo | 3.3 | 75 | 3.79 | 1,881 (32 %) | 1,026 (18 %) | 3,254 (56 %) | 3,000 (52 %) | −1.04 |
| ALLHAT-LLT | 10,355 | P40 vs. usual care | 4.9 | 67 | 3.76 | 1,188 (11 %) | 1,788 (17 %) | 8,037 (78 %) | 5,051 (49 %) | −0.54 |
| ASCOT-LLA | 10,305 | A10 vs. placebo | 3.3 | 63 | 3.44 | 15 (1 %) | 1,435 (14 %) | 8,860 (86 %) | 1,942 (19 %) | −1.07 |
| ALERT | 2,102 | F40 vs. placebo | 5.5 | 50 | 4.14 | 400 (19 %) | 241 (11 %) | 1,702 (81 %) | 715 (34 %) | −0.84 |
| CARDS | 2,838 | A10 vs. placebo | 4.1 | 62 | 3.03 | 9 (1 %) | 97 (3 %) | 2,738 (96 %) | 909 (32 %) | −1.14 |
| ALLIANCE | 2,442 | A10-80 vs. usual care | 4.7 | 61 | 3.80 | 2,442 (100 %) | 162 (7 %) | 0 (0 %) | 434 (18 %) | −1.16 |
| 4D | 1,255 | A20 vs. placebo | 4.0 | 66 | 3.25 | 630 (50 %) | 666 (53 %) | 344 (27 %) | 578 (46 %) | −0.89 |
| ASPEN | 2,410 | A10 vs. placebo | 4.0 | 61 | 2.93 | 578 (24 %) | 302 (13 %) | 1,663 (69 %) | 811 (34 %) | −0.99 |
| MEGA[d] | 8,214 | P10-20 vs. usual care | 5.0 | 58 | 4.05 | 42 (1 %) | 53 (1 %) | 8,119 (99 %) | 5,547 (68 %) | −0.67 |
| JUPITER | 17,802 | R20 vs. placebo | 2.0 | 66 | 2.70 | 0 (0 %) | 0 (0 %) | 17,802 (100 %) | 6,801 (38 %) | −1.09 |
| GISSI-HF | 4,574 | R10 vs. placebo | 4.2 | 67 | 3.06 | 1,797 (39 %) | 4,574 (100 %) | 0 (0 %) | 1,032 (23 %) | −0.92 |
| AURORA | 2,773 | R10 vs. placebo | 4.6 | 64 | 2.58 | 659 (24 %) | 743 (27 %) | 1,663 (60 %) | 1,050 (38 %) | −0.99 |
| CORONA | 5,011 | R10 vs. placebo | 3.0 | 73 | 3.55 | 4,377 (87 %) | 5,011 (100 %) | 0 (0 %) | 1,180 (24 %) | −1.19 |
| *Subtotal (22 trials)* | 134,537 | – | 4.8[e] | 63[e] | 3.70[e] | 52,668 (39 %) | 26,554 (20 %) | 70,025 (52 %) | 39,008 (29 %) | −1.08‖ |

| | | | | | | | | | | |
|---|---|---|---|---|---|---|---|---|---|---|
| *More vs. less statin* | | | | | | | | | | |
| PROVE-IT | 4,162 | A80 vs. P40 | 2.1 | 58 | 2.62[f] | 4,162 (100 %) | 328 (8 %) | 0 (0 %) | 911 (22 %) | −0.65 |
| A to Z | 4,497 | S40 then S80 vs. placebo then S20 | 2.0 | 60 | 2.09[f] | 4,497 (100 %) | 479 (11 %) | 0 (0 %) | 1,100 (24 %) | −0.30 |
| TNT | 10,001 | A80 vs. A10 | 5.0 | 61 | 2.52 | 10,001 (100 %) | 1,537 (15 %) | 0 (0 %) | 1,902 (19 %) | −0.62 |
| IDEAL | 8,888 | A40-80 vs. S20-40 | 4.8 | 62 | 2.64[f] | 8,888 (100 %) | 971 (11 %) | 0 (0 %) | 1,702 (19 %) | −0.55 |
| SEARCH | 12,064 | S80 vs. S20 | 7.0 | 64 | 2.50 | 12,064 (100 %) | 1,062 (9 %) | 0 (0 %) | 2,052 (17 %) | −0.39 |
| *Subtotal (5 trials)* | 39,612 | – | 5.1[e] | 62[e] | 2.53[e] | 39,612 (100 %) | 4,377 (11 %) | 0 (0 %) | 7,667 (19 %) | −0.51‖ |
| *Total (27 trials)* | 174,149 | – | 4.9[e] | 63[e] | – | 92,280 (53 %) | 30,931 (18 %) | 70,025 (40 %) | 46,675 (27 %) | – |

Trials are ordered by their date of publication

*A* atorvastatin, *F* fluvastatin, *L* lovastatin, *P* pravastatin, *R* rosuvastatin, *S* simvastatin, *LDL-C* LDL cholesterol, *CHD* coronary heart disease, *4D* Die Deutsche Diabetes Dialyse Studie, *A to Z* Aggrastat to Zocor, *AFCAPS/TexCAPS* Air Force/Texas Coronary Atherosclerosis Prevention Study, *ALERT* Assessment of Lescol in Renal Transplantation, *ALLHAT-LLT* Antihypertensive and Lipid-Lowering Treatment to Prevent Heart Attack Trial, *ALLIANCE* Aggressive Lipid-Lowering Initiation Abates New Cardiac Events, *ASCOT-LLA* Anglo-Scandinavian Cardiac Outcomes Trial–Lipid Lowering Arm, *ASPEN* Atorvastatin Study for Prevention of Coronary Heart Disease Endpoints in Non-Insulin-Dependent Diabetes Mellitus, *AURORA* A Study to Evaluate the Use of Rosuvastatin in Subjects on Regular Hemodialysis: An Assessment of Survival and Cardiovascular Events, *CARDS* Collaborative Atorvastatin Diabetes Study, *CARE* Cholesterol And Recurrent Events, *GISSI-HF* Gruppo Italiano per lo Studio della Sopravvivenza nell'Insufficienza cardiac, *GISSI–P* Gruppo Italiano per lo Studio della Sopravvivenza nell'Infarto Miocardico, *HPS* Heart Protection Study, *IDEAL* Incremental Decrease in End Points Through Aggressive Lipid Lowering Study Group, *JUPITER* Justification for the Use of Statins in Prevention: an Intervention Trial Evaluating Rosuvastatin study group, *LIPID* Long–term Intervention with Pravastatin in Ischaemic Disease, *LIPS* Lescol Intervention Prevention Study, *MEGA* Management of Elevated Cholesterol in the Primary Prevention Group of Adult Japanese Study Group, *Post-CABG* Post-Coronary Artery Bypass Graft, *PROSPER* PROspective Study of Pravastatin in the Elderly at Risk, *PROVE-IT* Pravastatin or Atorvastatin Evaluation and Infection Therapy, *SEARCH* Study of the Effectiveness of Additional Reductions in Cholesterol and Homocysteine, *SSSS* Scandinavian Simvastatin Survival Study, *TNT* Treating to New Targets, *WOSCOPS* West of Scotland Coronary Prevention Study

[a] Estimated with standard Kaplan–Meier methods, with patients censored at their date of death

[b] History of MI or other symptomatic CHD

[c] History of intracerebral bleed, transient ischaemic attack, ischaemic stroke, unknown stroke, peripheral artery disease or heart failure (if known)

dIncludes 382 randomised patients who were excluded from the trialists' primary publication

[e] Median follow-up, and mean age, baseline LDL-C and LDL-C difference at 1 year are weighted by the trial-specific variances of the observed logrank (o-e) statistic for major vascular events

[f] These three trials did not have active run-in periods; the values shown are the estimated on-treatment LDL cholesterol levels in the standard statin group

**Table 17.2** Number of participants with diabetes by trial

| | Diabetes mellitus | | | No diabetes |
|---|---|---|---|---|
| | Type 1 | Type 2[a] | Any type | |
| 4S | 24 (0.5 %) | 178 (4.0 %) | 202 (4.5 %) | 4,242 (95.5 %) |
| WOSCOPS | 8 (0.1 %) | 68 (1.0 %) | 76 (1.2 %) | 6,519 (98.8 %) |
| CARE | 193 (4.6 %) | 393 (9.4 %) | 586 (14.1 %) | 3,573 (85.9 %) |
| Post CABG | 27 (2.0 %) | 89 (6.6 %) | 116 (8.6 %) | 1,235 (91.4 %) |
| AFCAPS/TexCAPS | 0 | 155 (2.3 %) | 155 (2.3 %) | 6,450 (97.7 %) |
| LIPID | 106 (1.2 %) | 676 (7.5 %) | 782 (8.7 %) | 8,232 (91.3 %) |
| GISSI-P | 120 (2.8 %) | 462 (10.8 %) | 582 (13.6 %) | 3,689 (86.4 %) |
| LIPS | 39 (2.3 %) | 163 (9.7 %) | 202 (12.0 %) | 1,475 (88.0 %) |
| HPS | 615 (3.0 %) | 5,348 (26.0 %) | 5,963 (29.0 %) | 14,573 (71.0 %) |
| PROSPER | 51 (0.9 %) | 572 (9.9 %) | 623 (10.7 %) | 5,181 (89.3 %) |
| ALLHAT-LLT | 0 | 3,638 (35.1 %) | 3,638 (35.1 %) | 6,717 (64.9 %) |
| ASCOT-LLA | 0 | 2,527 (24.5 %) | 2,527 (24.5 %) | 7,778 (75.5 %) |
| ALERT | 280 (13.3 %) | 116 (5.5 %) | 396 (18.8 %) | 1,706 (81.2 %) |
| CARDS | 3 (0.1 %) | 2,835 (99.9 %) | 2,838 (100 %) | 0 |
| Total | 1,466 (1.6 %) | 17,220 (19.1 %) | 18,686 (20.7 %) | 71,370 (79.3 %) |

Data are number (%)
[a]Includes 13 participants with diabetes of unknown type
(Reprinted from The Lancet, 371(9607), Cholesterol Treatment Trialists' (CTT) Collaborators, Kearney PM, Blackwell L, Collins R, Keech A, Simes J, Peto R, Armitage J, Baigent C. Efficacy of cholesterol-lowering therapy in 18,686 people with diabetes in 14 randomised trials of statins: a meta-analysis., pp:117–25. Copyright (2008), with permission from Elsevier.)

ies, contrasting results of similar RCTs, or be due to a suitable RCT still being in progress. For example, there are no RCTs of statins in only people with type 1 diabetes for the primary prevention of cardiovascular disease, nor are there RCTs related to the use of fibrates or a fibrate and a statin to reduce microvascular events in type 1 diabetes. In these situations, expert opinion groups or the individual clinician must decide. Factors they may take into consideration are the results of RCTs in related groups (e.g. they may use the results of RCTs in type 2 diabetes patients or in nondiabetic subjects to decide treatment recommendations for people with type 1 diabetes). Results of case series, pilot studies and judgement based on knowledge of the disease process and effects of treatment may also be influential. The physician should discuss the reasons and risks behind their treatment recommendations, which may include not using a drug treatment, with the patient and regularly review the medical evidence and adjust their treatment recommendations accordingly. Such is the art of medicine.

## Other Resources

The purpose of this chapter has been to provide an overview of relevant issues to the conduct and interpretation of RCTs related to lipoproteins in diabetes. This proper design, conduct and reporting of an RCT is a large enough topic for several textbooks [57, 58] and courses. For readers who wish to learn more about RCTs, there are many courses, papers, websites and textbooks that may be of assistance. Discussions with trialists and studying or working as part of a multidisciplinary team experienced in RCTs are also valuable tools.

## The Future of RCTs of Treatments Related to Lipoproteins in Diabetes

Diabetes mellitus and lipid problems are common and costly health conditions. Existent nonpharmacologic and drug therapies for the treatment of lipid disorders have already improved clinical outcomes for people with diabetes, but residual

| Groups | Events (%) Treatment | Events (%) Control | RR (CI) | Test for heterogenity or trend |
|---|---|---|---|---|
| **Type of diabetes:** | | | | |
| Type 1 diabetes | 147 (20·5%) | 196 (26·2%) | 0·79 (0·62–1·01) | $\chi^2_1$=0·0; p=1·0 |
| Type 2 diabetes | 1318 (15·2%) | 1586 (18·5%) | 0·79 (0·72–0·87) | |
| **Sex:** | | | | |
| Men | 1082 (17·2%) | 1332 (21·4%) | 0·78 (0·71–0·86) | $\chi^2_1$=0·1; p=0·7 |
| Women | 383 (12·4%) | 450 (14·6%) | 0·81 (0·67–0·97) | |
| **Age (years):** | | | | |
| ≤65 | 701 (13·1%) | 898 (17·1%) | 0·77 (0·68–0·87) | $\chi^2_1$=0·5; p=0·5 |
| >65 | 764 (18·9%) | 884 (21·8%) | 0·81 (0·71–0·92) | |
| **Currently treated hypertension:** | | | | |
| Yes | 1030 (16·3%) | 1196 (19·1%) | 0·82 (0·74–0·91) | $\chi^2_1$=2·7; p=0·1 |
| No | 435 (14·2%) | 586 (19·3%) | 0·73 (0·63–0·85) | |
| **Body-mass index:** | | | | |
| <25·0 | 276 (15·7%) | 362 (20·4%) | 0·78 (0·64–0·95) | |
| ≥25·0–<30·0 | 639 (15·9%) | 774 (19·8%) | 0·77 (0·68–0·88) | $\chi^2_1$=0·5; p=0·5 |
| ≥30·0 | 532 (15·1%) | 628 (17·6%) | 0·82 (0·71–0·95) | |
| **Systolic blood pressure (mm Hg):** | | | | |
| <160 | 993 (15·0%) | 1276 (19·1%) | 0·76 (0·69–0·85) | $\chi^2_1$=1·3; p=0·3 |
| ≥160 | 472 (17·1%) | 505 (19·2%) | 0·83 (0·71–0·96) | |
| **Diastolic blood pressure (mm Hg):** | | | | |
| ≤90 | 1176 (16·5%) | 1417 (19·8%) | 0·81 (0·73–0·89) | $\chi^2_1$=1·7; p=0·2 |
| >90 | 288 (12·9%) | 364 (17·1%) | 0·73 (0·61–0·87) | |
| **Smoking status:** | | | | |
| Current smokers | 266 (17·5%) | 347 (22·5%) | 0·78 (0·64–0·96) | $\chi^2_1$=0·0; p=0·9 |
| Non-smokers | 1199 (15·2%) | 1435 (18·5%) | 0·79 (0·72–0·87) | |
| **Estimated GFR (mL/min/1·73m²):** | | | | |
| <60 | 415 (20·6%) | 477 (24·0%) | 0·83 (0·71–0·97) | |
| ≥60–<90 | 816 (15·5%) | 961 (18·4%) | 0·81 (0·72–0·91) | $\chi^2_1$=2·9; p=0·09 |
| ≥90 | 194 (12·5%) | 286 (18·7%) | 0·65 (0·50–0·84) | |
| **Predicted risk of major vascular event (per year):** | | | | |
| <4·5% | 474 (8·4%) | 631 (11·2%) | 0·74 (0·64–0·85) | |
| ≥4·5–<8·0% | 472 (23·2%) | 540 (27·3%) | 0·80 (0·66–0·96) | $\chi^2_1$=1·8; p=0·2 |
| ≥8·0% | 519 (30·5%) | 611 (35·8%) | 0·82 (0·70–0·95) | |
| **All diabetes** | **1465 (15·6%)** | **1782 (19·2%)** | **0·79 (0·74–0·84)** | |

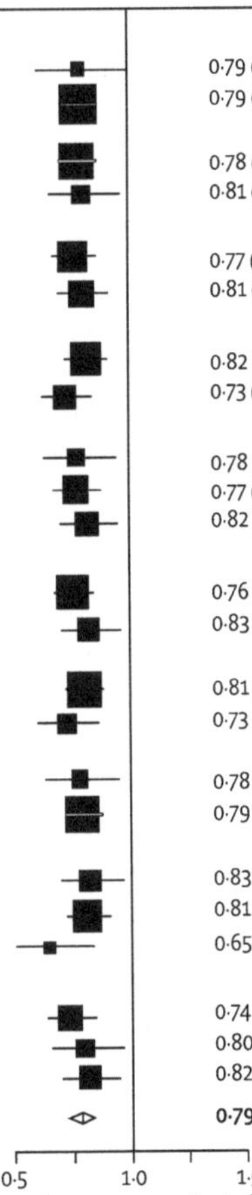


Global test for heterogeneity within subtotals: $\chi^2_{13}$=13·9: p=0·4

■ RR (99% CI)

◇ RR (95% CI)

**Fig. 17.1** Proportional effects on major vascular events per mmol/L reduction in LDL cholesterol by baseline prognostic factors in participants with diabetes
Rate ratios (RRs) are plotted comparing outcome in participants who were allocated statin treatment to that in those allocated control, along with their CIs. The area of each square is proportional to the amount of statistical information in that particular category. Diamonds or squares to the left of the solid line indicate benefi t with treatment, but this is significant (i.e., p<0·05 and p<0·01, respectively) only if the diamond or horizontal line does not overlap the solid line. The RRs are weighted to represent the reduction in the rate per 1 mmol/L LDL cholesterol reduction achieved by treatment at 1 year after randomisation. Tests for trend are shown for subgroups involving three categories, heterogeneity tests for those involving two. GFR glomerular filtration rate.
(Reprinted from The Lancet, 371(9607), Cholesterol Treatment Trialists' (CTT) Collaborators, Kearney PM, Blackwell L, Collins R, Keech A, Simes J, Peto R, Armitage J, Baigent C. Efficacy of cholesterol-lowering therapy in 18,686 people with diabetes in 14 randomised trials of statins: a meta-analysis., pp:117-25. Copyright (2008), with permission from Elsevier.)

risk remains high, including some related to quantitative and qualitative changes in lipoproteins. As discussed in another chapter, additional treatments, including more efficient drugs from existent drug classes, new classes of drugs and gene-based therapies agents, are emerging. After rigorous preclinical testing and testing in phases 0, 1 and 2 clinical trials, some therapies will reach the (phase 3) RCT stage and, if successful, clinical practice and post-marketing (phase 4) surveillance. The size, workload and cost of such RCTs are usually extremely high. To maximise the knowledge gained from RCTs and the cost-effectiveness of relevant research, it is desirable, and usual practice, to obtain consent for and store blood, including DNA, and urine for future analyses. Sometimes the biomarkers subsequently quantified were not known of at the time, or the earlier available assays lacked sensitivity or specificity. With the evolution of medical science, increasingly sophisticated biomarkers are available. Such tools as MRIs, IVUS, PET scans, microRNAs, microparticles, circulating stem cells, epigenetics, proteomics and metabolomics can help evaluate the disease process in living subjects and assay results can provide mechanistic insights. Often these studies require separate research funding, but existent data and a biorepository from a well-conducted RCT make this type of research extremely cost-effective and also usually time-effective. Most importantly, RCTs related to lipoproteins in diabetes have made substantial contributions to the well-being of people with diabetes, and further RCTs in this area should continue to do so in the future.

**Acknowledgements** The Clinical Trials Centre is partly supported by funding from the Australian National Health and Medical Research Council.

## References

1. The Adolescent type 1 Diabetes cardio-renal Intervention Trial Research Group. Adolescent type 1 diabetes cardio-renal intervention trial (AdDIT). BMC Pediatr. 2009;9:79.
2. Gebski V, Beller E, Keech A, Ven Der Weyden M. In: Keech A, Gebski V, Pike R. Interpreting and reporting clinical trials: a guide to the CONSORT statement and the principles of randomised controlled trials. Sydney: Australasian Medical Publishing Company; 2007. Chapter 1.
3. The Scandinavian Simvastatin Survival Study (4S) group. Randomised trial of cholesterol lowering in 4444 patients with coronary heart disease: the Scandinavian Simvastatin Survival Study (4S). Lancet. 1994;344(8934):1383–9.
4. Colhoun HM, Betteridge DJ, Durrington PN, Hitman GA, Neil HA, Livingstone SJ, Thomason MJ, Mackness MI, Charlton-Menys V, Fuller JH, CARDS investigators. Primary prevention of cardiovascular disease with atorvastatin in type 2 diabetes in the Collaborative Atorvastatin Diabetes Study (CARDS): multicentre randomised placebo-controlled trial. Lancet. 2004;364(9435):685–96.
5. Keech A, Simes RJ, Barter P, Best J, Scott R, Taskinen MR, Forder P, Pillai A, Davis T, Glasziou P, Drury P, Kesaniemi YA, Sullivan D, Hunt D, Colman P, d'Emden M, Whiting M, Ehnholm C, Laakso M. FIELD study investigators. Effects of long-term fenofibrate therapy on cardiovascular events in 9795 people with type 2 diabetes mellitus (the FIELD study): randomised controlled trial. Lancet. 2005; 366(9500):1849–61. Erratum in: Lancet. 2006 Oct 21; 368(9545):1415. Lancet. 2006 Oct 21;368(9545):1420. PubMed PMID: 16310551.
6. ACCORD Study Group, Ginsberg HN, Elam MB, Lovato LC, Crouse 3rd JR, Leiter LA, Linz P, Friedewald WT, Buse JB, Gerstein HC, Probstfield J, Grimm RH, Ismail-Beigi F, Bigger JT, Goff Jr DC, Cushman WC, Simons-Morton DG, Byington RP. Effects of combination lipid therapy in type 2 diabetes mellitus. N Engl J Med. 2010;362(17):1563–74.
7. Heart Protection Study Collaborative Group. MRC/BHF Heart Protection Study of cholesterol-lowering with simvastatin in 20,536 high-risk individuals: randomised placebo-controlled trial. Lancet. 2002;360:7–22.
8. Keech A, Gebski V. Interpreting and reporting clinical trials: a guide to the CONSORT statement and the principles of randomised controlled trials. Sydney: Australasian Medical Publishing Company; 2007. Chapter 3, pg 12.
9. Beller E, Gebski V, Keech A. Interpreting and reporting clinical trials: A guide to the CONSORT statement and the principles of randomised controlled trials. Sydney: Australasian Medical Publishing Company; 2007. Chapter 8.
10. Forder P, Gebski V, Keech A. Interpreting and reporting clinical trials: a guide to the CONSORT statement and the principles of randomised controlled trials. Sydney: Australasian Medical Publishing Company; 2007. Chapter 9.
11. AIM-HIGH Investigators. The role of niacin in raising high-density lipoprotein cholesterol to reduce cardiovascular events in patients with atherosclerotic cardiovascular disease and optimally treated low-density lipoprotein cholesterol rationale and study design. The atherothrombosis intervention in metabolic syndrome with low HDL/high triglycerides: impact on global health outcomes (AIM-HIGH). Am Heart J. 2011;161(3):471–7.
12. Rajamani K, Colman PG, Li LP, Best JD, Voysey M, D'Emden MC, Laakso M, Baker JR, Keech AC, on behalf of the FIELD study investigators. Effect of fenofibrate on amputation events in people with type 2 diabetes mellitus (FIELD study): a prespecified analysis of a randomised controlled trial. Lancet. 2009;373(9677):1780–8.
13. French JRP. Field experiments: changing group productivity. In: Miller JM, editor. Experiments in social process: a symposium on social psychology. New York, NY: McGraw-Hill; 1950. p. 82.
14. Jenkins AJ, Best JD, Klein RL, Lyons TJ. 'Lipoproteins, glycoxidation and diabetic angiopathy'. Diabetes Metab Res Rev. 2004;20(5):349–68.
15. Jenkins AJ, Rowley KG, Lyons TJ, Best JD, Hill MA, Klein RL. Lipoproteins and diabetic microvascular complications. Curr Pharm Des. 2004;10(27):3395–418.
16. Sóter MO, Gomes KB, Fernandes AP, Md C, Pinheiro PS, Bosco AA, Silva DD, Sousa MO. -1131T>C and SW19 polymorphisms in APOA5 gene and lipid lev-

els in type 2 diabetic patients. Mol Biol Rep. 2012;39(7):7541–8.
17. Deshmukh HA, Colhoun HM, Johnson T, McKeigue PM, Betteridge DJ, Durrington PN, Fuller JH, Livingstone S, Charlton-Menys V, Neil A, Poulter N, Sever P, Shields DC, Stanton AV, Chatterjee A, Hyde C, Calle RA, Demicco DA, Trompet S, Postmus I, Ford I, Jukema JW, Caulfield M, Hitman GA, CARDS, ASCOT, and PROSPER Investigators. Genome-wide association study of genetic determinants of LDL-c response to atorvastatin therapy: importance of Lp(a). J Lipid Res. 2012;53(5):1000–11.
18. Villeneuve LM, Reddy MA, Natarajan R. Epigenetics: deciphering its role in diabetes and its chronic complications. Clin Exp Pharmacol Physiol. 2011;38(7): 451–9.
19. Saremi A, Nelson RG, Tulloch-Reid M, Hanson RL, Sievers ML, Taylor GW, Shlossman M, Bennett PH, Genco R, Knowler WC. Periodontal disease and mortality in type 2 diabetes. Diabetes Care. 2005; 28(1):27–32.
20. Strong JP, Malcom GT, Newman 3rd WP, Oalmann MC. Early lesions of atherosclerosis in childhood and youth: natural history and risk factors. J Am Coll Nutr. 1992;11:51S–4.
21. Holman RR, Paul SK, Bethel MA, Matthews DR, Neil HA. 10-Year follow-up of intensive glucose control in type 2 diabetes. N Engl J Med. 2008;359(15): 1577–89.
22. White NH, Sun W, Cleary PA, Danis RP, Davis MD, Hainsworth DP, Hubbard LD, Lachin JM, Nathan DM. Prolonged effect of intensive therapy on the risk of retinopathy complications in patients with type 1 diabetes mellitus: 10 years after the diabetes control and complications trial. Arch Ophthalmol. 2008; 126(12):1707–15.
23. Holman RR, Paul SK, Bethel MA, Neil HA, Matthews DR. Long-term follow-up after tight control of blood pressure in type 2 diabetes. N Engl J Med. 2008;359(15):1565–76.
24. Jermendy G. Vascular memory: can we broaden the concept of the metabolic memory? Cardiovasc Diabetol. 2012;11(1):44.
25. Pedersen TR, Wilhelmsen L, Faergeman O, Strandberg TE, Thorgeirsson G, Troedsson L, Kristianson J, Berg K, Cook TJ, Haghfelt T, Kjekshus J, Miettinen T, Olsson AG, Pyörälä K, Wedel H. Follow-up study of patients randomized in the Scandinavian simvastatin survival study (4S) of cholesterol lowering. Am J Cardiol 2000;86:257–62.
26. Bulbulia R, Bowman L, Wallendszus K, Parish S, Armitage J, Peto R, Collins R for the Heart Protection Study. Effects of 11-year mortality and morbidity of lowering LDL cholesterol with simvastatin for about 5 years in 20536 high-risk individuals: a randomised controlled trial. Lancet 2011;378;2013–2020.
27. Ford I, Murray H, Packard CJ, Shepherd J, MacFarlane PW, Cobbe SM, for the West of Scotland Coronary Prevention Study Group. Long-term follow-up of the West of Scotland Coronary Prevention Study. N Eng J Med 2007;357;1477–1486.
28. Sever PS, Chang CL, Gupta AK, Whitehouse A, Poulter NR. ASCOT Investigators. The Anglo-Scandinavian Cardiac Outcomes Trial: 11-year mortality follow-up of the lipid-lowering arm in the UK. Eur Heart J 2011;32:2525–32.
29. Sjølie AK, Klein R, Porta M, Orchard T, Fuller J, Parving HH, Bilous R, Aldington S, Chaturvedi N. Retinal microaneurysm count predicts progression andregression of diabetic retinopathy. Post-hoc results from the DIRECT Programme. Diabet Med. 2011;28(3):345–51.
30. Perkins BA, Ficociello LH, Silva KH, Finkelstein DM, Warram JH, Krolewski AS. Regression of microalbuminuria in type 1 diabetes. N Engl J Med. 2003;348(23):2285–93.
31. Halimi JM. The emerging concept of chronic kidney disease without clinical proteinuria in diabetic patients. Diabetes Metab. 2012;38(4):291–7. doi: 10.1016/j.diabet.2012.04.001. Epub 2012 May 22. Review. PubMed PMID: 22622176.
32. Rigalleau V, Beauvieux MC, Gonzalez C, Raffaitin C, Lasseur C, Combe C, Chauveau P, De la Faille R, Rigothier C, Barthe N, Gin H. Estimation of renal-function in patients with diabetes. Diabetes Metab. 2011;37(5):359–66.
33. Tsmikas S, Shortal BP, Witztum JL, Palinski W. In vivo uptake of radiolabeled MDA2, an oxidation specific monoclonal antibody, provides an accurate measure of atherosclerotic lesions rich in oxidized LDL and is highly sensitive to their regression. Arterioscler Thromb Vasc Biol. 2000;20:689–97.
34. Jenkins AJ, Rothen M, Klein RL, Moller K, Eldridge L, Zheng D, Durazo-Arvizu R, McGee D, Lackland D, Thorpe SR, Garvey WT, Lyons TJ, DCCT/EDIC Research Group. Cross-sectional associations of C-reactive protein with vascular risk factors and vascular complications in the DCCT/EDIC cohort. J Diabetes Complications. 2008;22(3):153–63.
35. Lopes-Virella MF, Carter RE, Gilbert GE, Klein RL, Jaffa M, Jenkins AJ, Lyons TJ, Garvey WT, Virella G, Diabetes Control and Complications Trial/ Epidemiology of Diabetes Intervention and Complications Cohort Study Group. Risk factors related to inflammation and endothelial dysfunction in the DCCT/EDIC cohort and their relationship with nephropathy and macrovascular complications. Diabetes Care. 2008;31(10):2006–12.
36. Florentin M, Liberopoulos EN, Kei A, Mikhailidis DP, Elisaf MS. Pleiotropic effects of nicotinic acid: beyond high density lipoprotein cholesterol elevation. Curr Vasc Pharmacol. 2011;9(4):385–400.
37. Mihos CG, Salas MJ, Santana O. The pleiotropic effects of the hydroxy-methyl-glutaryl-CoA reductase inhibitors in cardiovascular disease: a comprehensive review. Cardiol Rev. 2010;18(6):298–304.
38. Foucher C, Brugère L, Ansquer JC. Fenofibrate, homocysteine and renal function. Curr Vasc Pharmacol. 2010;8(5):589–603.

39. Keech AC, Mitchell P, Summanen PA, O'Day J, Davis TM, Moffitt MS, Taskinen MR, Simes RJ, Tse D, Williamson E, Merrifield A, Laatikainen LT, d'Emden MC, Crimet DC, O'Connell RL, Colman PG, FIELD study investigators. Effect of fenofibrate on the need for laser treatment for diabetic retinopathy (FIELD study): a randomised controlled trial. Lancet. 2007;370(9600):1687–97.
40. Davis TM, Ting R, Best JD, Donoghoe MW, Drury PL, Sullivan DR, Jenkins AJ, O'Connell RL, Whiting MJ, Glasziou PP, Simes RJ, Kesäniemi YA, Gebski VJ, Scott RS, Keech AC, on behalf of the FIELD Study investigators. Effects of fenofibrate on renal function in patients with type 2 diabetes mellitus: the fenofibrate intervention and event lowering in diabetes (FIELD) study. Diabetologia. 2011;54(20):280–90.
41. Keech AC, Pike R, Granger R, Gebski V. Interpreting the results of a clinical trial (Chapter 20). In: Keech AC, Gebski VJ, Pike R, editors. Interpreting and reporting clinical trials: a guide to the CONSORT statement and the principles of randomised controlled trials. Sydney: AMPCo. 2007;143–148
42. Note for guidance on good clinical practice (CPMP/ICH/135/95). ICH topic E6. European Agency for the Evaluation of Medicinal Products, 2002.
43. World Health Organization. International statistical classification of diseases and related health problems, 10th revision. Geneva: World Health Organization; 1992.
44. International Conference on Harmonization. Medical dictionary for regulatory activities (MedDRA); 2003.
45. World Medical Association. Declaration of Helsinki: ethical principles for medical research involving human subjects. Helsinki: World Medical Association; 2000.
46. Barter PJ, Caulfield M, Eriksson M, Grundy SM, Kastelein JJ, Komajda M, Lopez-Sendon J, Mosca L, Tardif JC, Waters DD, Shear CL, Revkin JH, Buhr KA, Fisher MR, Tall AR, Brewer B, ILLUMINATE Investigators. Effects of torcetrapib in patients at high risk for coronary events. N Engl J Med. 2007; 357(21):2109–22.
47. ACCORD Study Group, ACCORD Eye Study Group, Chew EY, Ambrosius WT, Davis MD, Danis RP, Gangaputra S, Greven CM, Hubbard L, Esser BA, Lovato JF, Perdue LH, Goff Jr DC, Cushman WC, Ginsberg HN, Elam MB, Genuth S, Gerstein HC, Schubart U, Fine LJ. Effects of medical therapies on retinopathy progression in type 2diabetes. N Engl J Med. 2010;363(3):233–44.
48. Baigent C, Landray MJ, Reith C, Emberson J, Wheeler DC, Tomson C, Wanner C, Krane V, Cass A, Craig J, Neal B, Jiang L, Hooi LS, Levin A, Agodoa L, Gaziano M, Kasiske B, Walker R, Massy ZA, Feldt-Rasmussen B, Krairittichai U, Ophascharoensuk V, Fellström B, Holdaas H, Tesar V, Wiecek A, Grobbee D, de Zeeuw D, Grönhagen-Riska C, Dasgupta T, Lewis D, Herrington W, Mafham M, Majoni W, Wallendszus K, Grimm R, Pedersen T, Tobert J, Armitage J, Baxter A, Bray C, Chen Y, Chen Z, Hill M, Knott C, Parish S, Simpson D, Sleight P, Young A, Collins R, SHARP Investigators. The effects of lowering LDL cholesterol with simvastatin plus ezetimibe in patients with chronic kidney disease (study of heart and renal protection): a randomised placebo-controlled trial. Lancet. 2011;377(9784): 2181–92.
49. www.fda.gov/Drugs/DrugSafety/PostmarketDrugSafetyInformationforPatientsandProviders/ucm204882.htm. FDA alert 28 Feb 2011.
50. Jones PH, Davidson MH. Reporting rate of rhabdomyolysis with fenofibrate + statin versus gemfibrozil + any statin. Am J Cardiol. 2005;95(1):120–2.
51. Sandhu S, Al-Sarraf A, Taraboanta C, Frohlich J, Francis GA. Incidence of pancreatitis, secondary causes, and treatment of patients referred to a specialty lipid clinic with severe hypertriglyceridemia: a retrospective cohort study. Lipids Health Dis. 2011;10:157.
52. Cholesterol Treatment Trialists' (CTT) Collaboration, Baigent C, Blackwell L, Emberson J, Holland LE, Reith C, Bhala N, Peto R, Barnes EH, Keech A, Simes J, Collins R. Efficacy and safety of more intensive lowering of LDL cholesterol: a meta-analysis of data from 170 000 participants in 26 randomised trials. Lancet. 2010;376(9753):1670–81.
53. Cholesterol Treatment Trialists' Collaborators, Kearney PM, Blackwell L, Collins R, Keech A, Simes J, Peto R, Armitage J, Baigent C. Efficacy of cholesterol-lowering therapy in 18,686 people with diabetes in 14 randomised trials of statins: a meta-analysis. Lancet. 2008;371:117–25.
54. Scott R, O'Brien R, Fulcher G, Pardy C, d'Emden M, Tse D, Taskinen MR, Ehnholm C, Keech A, on behalf of the FIELD Study Investigators. The effects of fenofibrate treatment on cardiovascular disease risk in 9795 people with type 2 diabetes and various components of the metabolic syndrome: the FIELD study. Diabetes Care. 2009;32(3):493–8.
55. Robert PG, Nihar RD, Payal K, William JR, Ransi S, Fannie H, Thomas L, Satishkumar M, Elaine BH, Shannon TM, Timothy EA, Scott MW, Robert S, Marc SS. For the LAPLACE-TIMI 57 Investigators, Efficacy, safety, and tolerability of a monoclonal antibody to proprotein convertase subtilisin/kexin type 9 in combination with a statin in patients with hypercholesterolemia (LAPLACE-TIMI 57): a randomized, placebo-controlled, dose-ranging, phase 2 study. The Lancet 2012;380(9858, 8–14):2007–2017.
56. Stein EA, Gipe D, Bergeron J, Gaudet D, Weiss R, Dufour R, Wu R, Pordy R. Effect of a monoclonal antibody to PCSK9, REGN727/SAR236553, to reduce low-density lipoprotein cholesterol in patients with heterozygous familial hypercholesterolaemia on stable statin dose with or without ezetimibe therapy: a phase 2 randomised controlled trial. Lancet 2012;380:29–36.
57. Keech A, Gebski V, Pike R. Interpreting and reporting clinical trials: a guide to the CONSORT statement and the principles of randomised controlled trials. Sydney: Australasian Medical Publishing Company; 2007.
58. Liu MB, Davis K. A clinical trials manual from the Duek Clinical Research Institute. Lessons from a horse named Jim. 2nd ed. Oxford. UK: Wiley-Blackwell; 2010.

# Statin Therapy: Impact on Dyslipidemia and Cardiovascular Events in Diabetic Patients

# 18

Seth S. Martin, Parag H. Joshi, and Steven R. Jones

## Introduction

This chapter begins by briefly discussing the basic biologic impact of HMG-CoA reductase inhibitor or "statin" therapy on dyslipidemia in diabetic patients, emphasizing the important distinction between cholesterol and lipoprotein particles. Next, section II focuses on randomized clinical trials that have investigated the impact of statin therapy on cardiovascular events in diabetic patients. This section selectively discusses the details of four large trials, which account for the majority of data supporting the use of statins in patients with diabetes mellitus. We then place the evidence in perspective and describe an example of implementing the evidence in practice. Finally, section III addresses the observation that despite the notable impact of statin therapy, there remain a significant number of patients in the treatment arms of clinical trials who continue to sustain cardiovascular events. This "residual risk," along with the biology of dyslipidemia, invokes the potential role of lipoprotein targets that may serve as more accurate measurements of atherosclerotic risk than current cholesterol parameters and, therefore, better guide statin treatment in diabetic patients.

S.S. Martin • P.H. Joshi
Johns Hopkins University, Baltimore, MD, USA

S.R. Jones, M.D. (✉)
Department of Medicine, Cardiology Division,
The Johns Hopkins Hospital, Zayed 7125U,
1800 Orleans Street, Baltimore, MD 21287, USA
e-mail: sjones64@jhmi.edu

## Section I: Impact of Statin Therapy on Dyslipidemia

Understanding the central impact of statin therapy on dyslipidemia requires attention to the key role of atherogenic lipoprotein particles in the basic biology of atherosclerosis itself. Atherosclerosis begins with lipoprotein deposition in the arterial wall, which propagates through further lipoprotein deposition and subsequent inflammatory responses [1, 2]. The lipoprotein is made up of a core of lipid elements including cholesteryl esters and triglycerides surrounded by surface phospholipids and apolipoproteins. Atherogenic lipoproteins include low-density lipoprotein (LDL), intermediate-density lipoprotein (IDL), very low-density lipoproteins (VLDL) and their remnants, and lipoprotein (a) (Lp(a)). Each of these atherogenic lipoproteins contains one copy of apolipoprotein B (apoB) on their surface. Proteoglycans in the arterial wall contain binding sites that recognize apoB, leading to retention of the particles, and therefore the presence of more circulating atherogenic particles translates into an increased risk of initiation and propagation of atherosclerosis. Lipoprotein matrix interactions are discussed in detail in Chaps. 9 and 11.

A.J. Jenkins et al. (eds.), *Lipoproteins in Diabetes Mellitus*, Contemporary Diabetes,
DOI 10.1007/978-1-4614-7554-5_18, © Springer Science+Business Media New York 2014

Notably, in the presence of diabetic dyslipidemia, the atherogenic particle concentration in plasma is frequently underestimated by lipoprotein cholesterol measurements. Along with higher levels of triglycerides and smaller high-density lipoprotein (HDL) particles, there is a trend towards small dense LDL (sdLDL) [3], particularly in those with type 2 diabetes. Because of the predominance of sdLDL in diabetic subjects, atherogenic potential is better reflected by measurements of apoB than LDL-C, which frequently underestimates the concentration of LDL particles in this setting. Diabetic patients commonly have normal LDL-C, but elevated apoB, which may be substantially contributory to the particularly high diabetic vascular risk despite largely normal LDL-C.

While statin therapy exerts some effect on all lipid parameters, the most important effect is on apoB-containing lipoproteins. Statin therapy lowers LDL-C and non-HDL-C levels to a larger degree than LDL particle concentration (LDL-P) and overall atherogenic particle concentration as measured by apoB [4]. For example, in the combined analysis of the Treating to New Targets (TNT) and the Incremental Decrease in End Points through Aggressive Lipid-Lowering (IDEAL) trials, LDL-C, non-HDL-C, and apoB levels were measured in nearly 19,000 patients with established coronary heart disease who were assigned to usual-dose or high-dose statin treatment [5]. In the patients on moderate statin doses (either atorvastatin 10 mg, simvastatin 20 mg, or 40 mg), LDL-C (101–102 mg/dL) and non-HDL-C (129–132 mg/dL) were reduced to the 30–35th percentile for the American population; however, the corresponding apoB levels (107–113 mg/dL) were still markedly high relative to the American population at the 56–64th percentile. In the high statin dose arms (atorvastatin 80 mg), LDL-C (75–80 mg/dL) and non-HDL-C (101–102 mg/dL) levels were reduced to the 10–14th percentile for the American population. The corresponding apoB levels (84–91 mg/dL) were at the 20–31st percentile for the American population. The discrepancy between cholesterol reduction and particle reduction was also evident in the type 2 diabetic patients treated with statin therapy in the Collaborative Atorvastatin Diabetes Study (CARDS); LDL-C and non-HDL-C were lowered by 40.9 and 38.1 %, while apoB levels were reduced by only 24.3 % [6]. While numerous studies have undoubtedly shown the effect of statin therapy in reducing cardiovascular events in diabetic patients, the discordance between cholesterol and particle reduction may in part explain the high residual risk remaining after statin therapy.

## Section II: Impact of Statin Therapy on Cardiovascular Events in Diabetic Patients

### Evidence from Key Randomized Clinical Trials

#### Heart Protection Study

The TIMRC/BHF Heart Protection Study (HPS) opened a new clinical era by providing the first clear justification for routine use of statin therapy in diabetic patients at sufficiently high risk for major cardiovascular events [7, 8]. Prior to HPS, only ~1,500 secondary prevention and ~200 primary prevention diabetic patients had participated in randomized statin trials. The HPS enrolled 5,963 diabetic patients (2,912 were free of occlusive arterial disease) and an additional 14,573 nondiabetic patients in the United Kingdom between 1994 and 1997. HPS included 615 type 1 diabetic and 5,348 type 2 diabetic subjects. Patients aged 40–80 years with non-fasting total cholesterol concentrations ≥3.5 mmol/L (135 mg/dL) were randomized to 40 mg of simvastatin daily versus matching placebo. Average statin use was 85 % in the statin-allocated group compared with 17 % in the placebo-allocated group, yielding an average LDL-C difference of ~1 mmol/L (39 mg/dL).

In line with results from the total study population, statin-treated diabetic patients had a 22 % (95 % CI 13–30) relative risk reduction (RRR, event rate 20.2 % versus 25.1 %, $p<0.0001$) in the first occurrence of major coronary events, stroke, or revascularization compared with their placebo-allocated counterparts [8]. Similar reductions were seen in those without baseline occlusive arterial disease (RRR 33 % [95 % CI

17–46], $p=0.0003$) and those with baseline LDL-C levels <3.0 mmol/L (116 mg/dL) (RRR 27 % [95 % CI 13–40], $p=0.0007$). The risk reduction due to statin therapy did not depend on diabetes type, duration, or intensity of glycemic control; age; or hypertension. In sum, HPS showed that statin therapy improves outcomes across a broad range of patients with diabetes.

### Anglo-Scandinavian Cardiac Outcomes Trial

The Anglo-Scandinavian Cardiac Outcomes Trial Lipid-Lowering Arm (ASCOT-LLA) addressed lipoprotein lowering in hypertensive patients in a 2×2 factorial investigation [9, 10]. Recruitment occurred between 1998 and 2000 at family practices in the United Kingdom, Ireland, and Nordic countries. Patients aged 40–79 years without a history of coronary heart disease, with untreated blood pressure ≥160/100 mmHg or treated blood pressure ≥140/90 mmHg, and additional risk factors, including type 2 diabetes mellitus, were randomized to antihypertensive treatment. Of the 19,342 randomized patients, the 10,305 patients with non-fasting total cholesterol concentrations ≤6.5 mmol/L entered the lipid-lowering arm and were randomized to 10 mg of atorvastatin daily versus placebo. A baseline diagnosis of diabetes was present in 2,532 of participants. After a median follow-up of 3.3 years, total and LDL-C concentrations among diabetic patients treated with atorvastatin were ~1 mmol/L (39 mg/dL) lower than those allocated to placebo, and the study was stopped early for efficacy. Like HPS, the proportional risk reduction in diabetic participants was similar to patients without diabetes [10]. There were 116 (9.2 %) major cardiovascular events or procedures in atorvastatin allocated diabetic patients and 151 (11.9 %) events in the placebo group (hazard ratio 0.77 [95 % CI 0.61–0.98], $p=0.04$). For the individual components of the composite end point, analyses were underpowered.

### Collaborative Atorvastatin Diabetes Study

Concentrating on diabetic patients in a primary prevention context, the Collaborative Atorvastatin Diabetes Study (CARDS) enrolled subjects from the United Kingdom and Ireland from 1997 to 2001 [11]. Participating patients were 40–75 years in age with type 2 diabetes plus at least one additional risk factor, including hypertension, retinopathy, proteinuria, or smoking. The CARDS trial randomized 2,838 patients to atorvastatin 10 mg daily versus placebo. CARDS met its pre-specified early stopping rule for efficacy two years early after accumulating an average follow-up of 3.9 years. An acute coronary event, coronary revascularization, or stroke occurred in 127 patients allocated placebo and 83 allocated atorvastatin (RRR 37 % [95 % CI 17–52], $p=0.001$). Relative risk reductions by individual outcomes were 36 % for acute coronary events, 31 % for coronary revascularizations, and 48 % for stroke. A non-significant 27 % reduction in mortality was also noted in favor of atorvastatin.

### Antihypertensive and Lipid-Lowering Treatment to Prevent Heart Attack Trial

The lipid-lowering trial (LLT) component of the Antihypertensive and Lipid-Lowering Treatment to Prevent Heart Attack Trial (ALLHAT) [12] was conducted from 1994 to 1998 primarily in community-based North American centers, included 3,638 diabetic participants aged ≥55 years, and similar in design to ASCOT-LLT. The ALLHAT investigators demonstrated a neutral effect of pravastatin 20–40 mg daily versus usual care on cardiovascular events over a mean follow-up of 4.8 years. The findings of this trial do not contradict the aforementioned trials because there was a statin drop-in effect in the usual care arm. Nearly a third of usual care patients started lipid-lowering therapy during the trial. As a result, there was only a modest differential in total cholesterol (9.6 %) between groups. This difference between treatment groups would not be expected to yield meaningful differences in risk for cardiovascular events. Combined with other major limitations of the trial, including its non-blinded design, the trial's neutrality is not unanticipated.

### Meta-Analysis

The strength of evidence supporting statin therapy for diabetic patients is summarized in a prospective meta-analysis from the Cholesterol

**Table 18.1** Randomized clinical trials of statin therapy in diabetic patients

| Randomized clinical trial | Original publication year | Diabetic subjects (*n*) | Study focus group | Statin type (mg/day) | Average follow-up (years) | Primary enrollment locations |
|---|---|---|---|---|---|---|
| 4S | 1994 | 202 | CHD | Simva 20–40 | 5.4 | Scandinavia |
| WOSCOPS | 1995 | 76 | PP (men) | Prava 40 | 4.9 | Scotland |
| CARE | 1996 | 586 | Post-MI | Prava 40 | 5 | USA and Canada |
| Post-CABG | 1997 | 116 | CABG | Lova 2.5–80 | 4.3 | USA |
| AFCAPS | 1998 | 155 | PP | Lova 20–40 | 5.2 | USA |
| LIPID | 1998 | 782 | CHD | Prava 40 | 6.1 | Australia and New Zealand |
| GISSI | 2000 | 582 | Post-MI | Prava 20 | 2 | Italy |
| HPS | 2002 | 5,963 | High-risk | Simva 40 | 5.3 | UK |
| PROSPER | 2002 | 623 | Elderly | Prava 40 | 3.2 | Scotland, Ireland, Netherlands |
| ALLHAT | 2002 | 3,638 | HTN | Prava 20–40 | 4.8 | USA and Canada |
| LIPS | 2002 | 202 | Post-PCI | Fluva 80 | 3.9 | Europe, Canada, Brazil |
| ASCOT | 2003 | 2,527 | HTN | Atorva 10 | 3.3 | UK, Ireland, Nordic countries |
| ALERT | 2003 | 396 | Renal Txp | Fluva 40 | 5.1 | Europe, Canada |
| CARDS | 2004 | 2,838 | DM | Atorva 10 | 4 | UK and Ireland |

*CHD* coronary heart disease, *PP* primary prevention, *HTN* hypertension, *PCI* percutaneous coronary intervention, *Txp* transplant, *DM* diabetes mellitus

Treatment Trialists' (CTT) Collaborators [13]. The four trials discussed above, HPS, ASCOT-LLA, CARDS, and ALLHAT-LLT, account for 14,996 of the 18,686 patients (83 %) included in the CTT meta-analysis. Of the 10,355 diabetic patients enrolled in the trial, 35 % had type 2 diabetes. The 14 trials included in the analysis (see Table 18.1 for details) were agreed upon before the results of trials were known and analyses were pre-specified. The pooled dataset provided greater power to assess the impact of statin therapy on individual outcomes in diabetic patients and perform subgroup analyses.

During an average follow-up of 4.3 years, 3,247 major vascular events occurred in diabetic patients. All-cause mortality was reduced by 9 % per 1 mmol/L reduction in LDL-C in diabetic patients (RR 0.91 [99 % CI 0.82–1.01], $p=0.02$), which was similar to patients without diabetes. As expected, the mortality reduction was attributable to lower vascular mortality (RR 0.87 [99 % CI 0.76–1.00], $p=0.008$) with no effect on non-vascular mortality. Major vascular events were reduced by 21 % per 1 mmol/L reduction in LDL-C (RR 0.79 [99 % CI 0.72–0.86], $p<0.0001$). Individually, each component endpoint was reduced: myocardial infarction or coronary death (RR 0.78 [99 % CI 0.69–0.87], $p<0.0001$), coronary revascularization (RR 0.75 [99 % CI 0.64–0.88], $p<0.0001$), and stroke (RR 0.79 [99 % CI 0.67–0.93], $p=0.0002$). Findings were not dependent on pre-treatment lipoprotein parameters and there was no threshold below which benefit was absent. The proportional therapeutic benefits of statins in diabetic patients were also similar irrespective of type of diabetes, sex, age, hypertension, body mass index, smoking, kidney disease, or overall risk category (Fig. 18.1).

## Putting the Evidence in Perspective

Based on the CTT meta-analysis [13], in adults who have diabetes, it was estimated that a low-potency statin would prevent approximately 45 patients per 1,000 from having a major vascular event over five years. Given that high-potency statins are roughly two and one-half times as effective as low potency ones, a high-potency statin prevents approximately 113 patients per 1,000 from having a major vascular event over 5 years with a number needed to treat (NNT) of 9. This is approximately half the 5-year number needed to treat of 20 for a major vascular event found in the Justification for the Use of statins in Prevention: An Intervention Trial Evaluating Rosuvastatin (JUPITER) trial [14], a primary prevention trial of a potent statin, rosuvastatin 20 mg daily, that excluded diabetic patients. Economic analyses of randomized trials,

| Groups | Events (%) Treatment | Events (%) Control | RR (CI) | Test for heterogenity or trend |
|---|---|---|---|---|
| **Type of diabetes:** | | | | |
| Type 1 diabetes | 147 (20·5%) | 196 (26·2%) | 0·79 (0·62–1·01) | $\chi^2_1$=0·0; p=1·0 |
| Type 2 diabetes | 1318 (15·2%) | 1586 (18·5%) | 0·79 (0·72–0·87) | |
| **Sex:** | | | | |
| Men | 1082 (17·2%) | 1332 (21·4%) | 0·78 (0·71–0·86) | |
| Women | 383 (12·4%) | 450 (14·6%) | 0·81 (0·67–0·97) | $\chi^2_1$=0·1; p=0·7 |
| **Age (years):** | | | | |
| ≤65 | 701 (13·1%) | 898 (17·1%) | 0·77 (0·68–0·87) | $\chi^2_1$=0·5; p=0·5 |
| >65 | 764 (18·9%) | 884 (21·8%) | 0·81 (0·71–0·92) | |
| **Currently treated hypertension:** | | | | |
| Yes | 1030 (16·3%) | 1196 (19·1%) | 0·82 (0·74–0·91) | $\chi^2_1$=2·7; p=0·1 |
| No | 435 (14·2%) | 586 (19·3%) | 0·73 (0·63–0·85) | |
| **Body-mass index:** | | | | |
| <25·0 | 276 (15·7%) | 362 (20·4%) | 0·78 (0·64–0·95) | |
| ≥25·0–<30·0 | 639 (15·9%) | 774 (19·8%) | 0·77 (0·68–0·88) | $\chi^2_1$=0·5; p=0·5 |
| ≥30·0 | 532 (15·1%) | 628 (17·6%) | 0·82 (0·71–0·95) | |
| **Systolic blood pressure (mm Hg):** | | | | |
| <160 | 993 (15·0%) | 1276 (19·1%) | 0·76 (0·69–0·85) | $\chi^2_1$=1·3; p=0·3 |
| ≥160 | 472 (17·1%) | 505 (19·2%) | 0·83 (0·71–0·96) | |
| **Diastolic blood pressure (mm Hg):** | | | | |
| ≤90 | 1176 (16·5%) | 1417 (19·8%) | 0·81 (0·73–0·89) | $\chi^2_1$=1·7; p=0·2 |
| >90 | 288 (12·9%) | 364 (17·1%) | 0·73 (0·61–0·87) | |
| **Smoking status:** | | | | |
| Current smokers | 266 (17·5%) | 347 (22·5%) | 0·78 (0·64–0·96) | $\chi^2_1$=0·0; p=0·9 |
| Non-smokers | 1199 (15·2%) | 1435 (18·5%) | 0·79 (0·72–0·87) | |
| **Estimated GFR (mL/min/1·73m²):** | | | | |
| <60 | 415 (20·6%) | 477 (24·0%) | 0·83 (0·71–0·97) | |
| ≥60–<90 | 816 (15·5%) | 961 (18·4%) | 0·81 (0·72–0·91) | $\chi^2_1$=2·9; p=0·09 |
| ≥90 | 194 (12·5%) | 286 (18·7%) | 0·65 (0·50–0·84) | |
| **Predicted risk of major vascular event (per year):** | | | | |
| <4·5% | 474 (8·4%) | 631 (11·2%) | 0·74 (0·64–0·85) | |
| ≥4·5–<8·0% | 472 (23·2%) | 540 (27·3%) | 0·80 (0·66–0·96) | $\chi^2_1$=1·8; p=0·2 |
| ≥8·0% | 519 (30·5%) | 611 (35·8%) | 0·82 (0·70–0·95) | |
| **All diabetes** | **1465 (15·6%)** | **1782 (19·2%)** | **0·79 (0·74–0·84)** | |

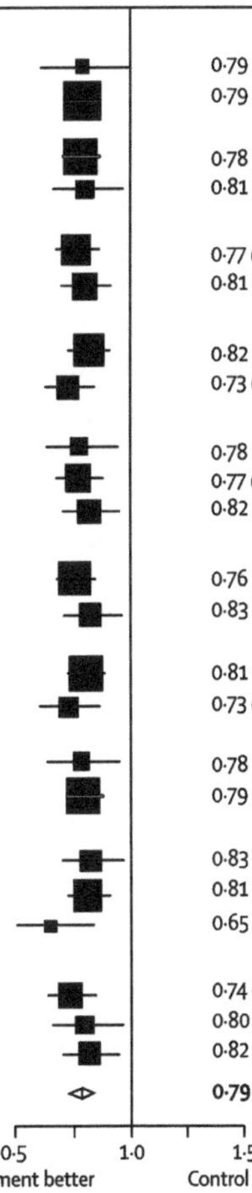


Global test for heterogeneity within subtotals: $\chi^2_{13}$=13·9: p=0·4
■ RR (99% CI)
◇ RR (95% CI)

**Fig. 18.1** Proportional effects on major vascular events per mmol/L reduction in LDL cholesterol by baseline subgroups in diabetic patients. Rate ratios (RRs) are plotted comparing outcome in participants who were allocated statin treatment to control, along with their CIs. The area of each *square* is proportional to the amount of statistical information in that particular category. *Diamonds* or *squares* to the *left* of the *solid line* indicate benefit with treatment, which is significant (i.e., $p<0.05$ and $p<0.01$, respectively) if the *diamond* or *horizontal line* does not overlap the *solid line*. The RRs are weighted to represent the reduction in the rate per 1 mmol/L LDL cholesterol reduction achieved by treatment at 1 year after randomization. GFR = glomerular filtration rate. Figure reproduced with permission from Elsevier [13]

including the HPS [15], have shown statin therapy is cost-effective, if not cost saving, for a wide range of diabetic patients.

## Implementing the Evidence in Practice

In the Steno-2 study, investigators from Denmark randomly assigned 160 patients with type 2 diabetes and microalbuminuria to a multifactorial intervention (lipid-lowering therapy, aspirin, renin-angiotensin inhibition, and tight glucose control) versus conventional therapy [16]. The study completed follow-up in 2006 after a mean duration of treatment of 7.8 years and additional mean observation period of 5.5 years. During the intervention phase, 85 % of the treatment group took statins (mean attained LDL-C 83 mg/dL from 133 mg/dL at baseline) compared with 22 % of the conventional therapy group (mean attained LDL-C 126 mg/dL from 137 mg/dL at baseline). More than eight in ten patients in both groups went on to take statins in the observation phase with mean LDL-C concentrations converging near 70 mg/dL; however, survival curves continued to diverge.

Upon completion of follow-up, compared with 40 deaths in the conventional therapy group, only 24 patients who received multifactorial intervention died (hazard ratio 0.54 [95 % CI 0.32–0.89], $p=0.02$). Multifactorial intervention reduced cardiovascular mortality (hazard ratio 0.43 [95 % CI 0.19–0.94], $p=0.04$) and cardiovascular events (hazard ratio 0.41 [95 % CI 0.25–0.67], $p<0.001$). Even with imperfect implementation (proportion of patients achieving ideal treatment targets was modest), the NNTs over the full study period (7.8 years of intervention and an additional 5.5 years of follow-up) were impressively low: three patients to prevent one cardiovascular event, five patients to prevent death from any cause, and eight patients to prevent a cardiovascular death. It was concluded that statins and antihypertensive therapies were the two most influential therapies in reducing risk. In sum, Steno-2 demonstrates that early implementation of statin therapy as part of a multifaceted approach to risk reduction achieves dramatic reductions in absolute risk, and thus low numbers needed to treat, making primary prevention strategies incorporating statin therapy in diabetic patients second to few if any other medical therapies in modern medicine.

## Section III: Residual Risk of Cardiovascular Events in Diabetic Patients on Statin Therapy

### Residual Risk Data

In the HPS there was a 22 % relative risk reduction in major coronary events, stroke, or revascularization compared with placebo [7]. However, there remained a residual risk where 78 % of events in diabetics treated with simvastatin therapy were not prevented. In ASCOT-LLA there was a similar 23 % relative risk reduction in events, leaving a residual risk of 77 % [9]. Both HPS and ASCOT-LLA showed a reduction in LDL-C of approximately 40 mg/dL from baseline. Similarly, in the summary meta-analysis from the CTT Collaborators, for every approximate 40 mg/dL decrease in LDL-C, there was a relative risk reduction of major vascular events of 21 % [13].

The residual risk in these treated diabetic subjects can be attributed to a number of factors, some of which may be related to lipoproteins. Accordingly, with regard to reducing residual risk with statin therapy, there are two potential areas of focus: (1) the target lipoprotein parameter measured (i.e., LDL-C, non-HDL-C, apoB, LDL-P) and (2) the target level of lipoprotein reduction.

### Lipoprotein Epidemiology and the Ideal Therapeutic Target

Prospective observational studies have confirmed that vascular event risk is more accurately predicted by measurements of atherogenic particle concentration than total cholesterol or LDL-C [17]. Non-HDL-C is the currently recommended method of estimating risk and treatment in patients with hypertriglyceridemia, as there is considerable variation in the distribution of cholesterol content across particle classes [18]. In such instances, non-HDL-C is a better estimator of the cholesterol content of all apoB-containing particles and has high correlations with apoB; however, on an individual patient basis, there is a significant degree of discordance between non-HDL-C and apoB [4].

Nevertheless, it has been substantially demonstrated that apoB and LDL particle measurements consistently outperform cholesterol measurements epidemiologically [17]. For example, in the Multi-Ethnic Study of Atherosclerosis (MESA), 6,814 patients without cardiovascular disease were enrolled and followed for cardiovascular events. LDL particle concentration was measured and compared to LDL-C levels (Fig. 18.2). Discordance between the two measurements was defined as LDL-C and particle values differing by 12 percentile points (an arbi-

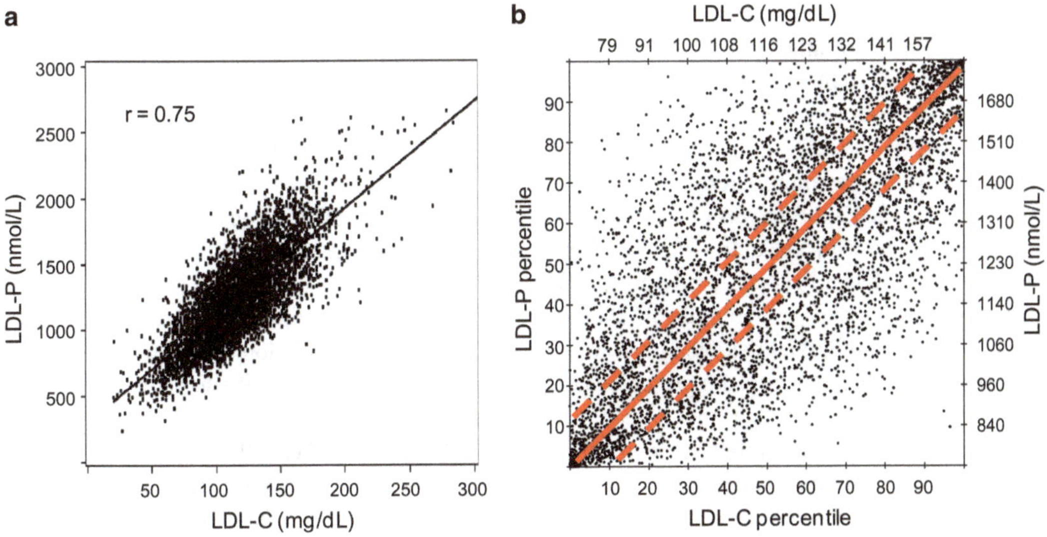


**Fig. 18.2** Relations between LDL-C and LDL-P among 5,598 MESA participants. (**a**) Relation of LDL-C and LDL-P concentrations. (**b**) Relation of LDL-C and LDL-P levels given in percentile units. The *dashed lines bracket* concordant LDL-C and LDL-P values defined as those within ±12 percentile units. Reprinted with permission from Elsevier [19]

trary value so that 50 % of the population was discordant). In patients with concordance, both LDL-C and particle concentration were associated with incident events. However, in those patients with discordance, only LDL particle concentration was associated with incident events [19]. This suggests that risk in those patients with elevated levels of circulating LDL particles may be underestimated by solely measuring cholesterol levels. In a comprehensive meta-analysis including 12 independent reports involving more than 230,000 subjects with nearly 23,000 events, as markers of cardiovascular risk, apoB (RRR 1.43; 95 % CI 1.35–1.51) outperformed non-HDL-C (RRR 1.34; 95 % CI 1.24–1.44) which outperformed LDL-C (RRR 1.25; 95 % CI 1.18–1.33) [20].

## Guidelines

In measuring the lipoprotein-based risk for sustaining acute cardiovascular events, the marker of choice has progressed from total cholesterol followed by LDL-C to the evolving recommendation of non-HDL-C levels. These cholesterol-based levels have served as an imperfect proxy for the concentration of circulating apoB-containing particles, and due to its wide implementation in clinical medicine with a simple measurement platform, it has been argued that these measurements should not be abandoned. However, heterogeneity in particle sizes, cholesterol content, and lipoprotein phenotypes among and within individuals suggests that cholesterol-based measurements are not a sufficiently accurate measurement of atherogenic risk. Given this evidence, parameters such as apoB or LDL particle concentration may be set as additional targets for many patients after lipoprotein cholesterol targets have been reached [21].

The current National Cholesterol Education Program Adult Treatment Panel III recommends LDL-C and non-HDL-C targets based on risk estimations. For diabetic patients, an LDL-C target of 100 mg/dL (non-HDL-C level of 130 mg/dL) has been recommended with an optional target of 70 mg/dL (non-HDL-C level of 100 mg/dL) for very high-risk patients such as those with established coronary artery disease, a recent acute coronary syndrome, or multiple poorly controlled components of the metabolic syndrome [18]. However, for the previously stated reasons, in diabetic patients, these targets may not adequately reflect the burden of atherogenic particles. With this in mind, the ADA and ACC released a consensus report recommending measurement of apoB in addition to LDL-C and non-HDL-C in patients on lipid-lowering therapy. Furthermore, they recommended apoB targets of <80 mg/dL in diabetic patients with an additional risk factor (i.e., smoking, hypertension, family history of premature CAD) and <90 mg/dL in diabetic subjects without additional risk factors; however, the rationale for these levels is not presented [22]. It remains unsettled whether more aggressive reduction of atherogenic particles, as measured by particle concentration or apoB, would more completely reduce residual risk [23]. However, given the known biology of atherosclerosis, there is a compelling scientific basis to research this question with observational evidence consistently showing risk reduction with progressive reduction in atherogenic apoB-containing lipoprotein concentration [13]. There is an association between the initiation of statin therapy and new-onset type 2 diabetes mellitus, which is modest, on the order of 1 new case per 1,000 patient years [24]. Patients who develop incident diabetes on statin therapy are frequently insulin resistant, so small incremental increases in glucose levels attributable to statin therapy may be sufficient to unmask a diagnosis of diabetes. The potential harm of new-onset diabetes is outweighed by concurrent reduction in cardiovascular morbidity and mortality on therapy, especially in high-risk patients. The epidemiologic link between statin initiation and type 2 diabetes mellitus should not substantially alter decision initiate statin therapy.

## Conclusions

In association with atherogenic lipoprotein reduction, there is robust evidence that statin therapy significantly lowers cardiovascular event rates in patients with diabetes mellitus. Multiple randomized clinical trials, spanning the last two decades, have consistently and unequivocally made this case. The beneficial impact of statins on cardiovascular events includes reductions in myocardial infarction, need for coronary revascularization, strokes, and cardiovascular mortality. The evidence supports a class effect as a number of statins have been tested. Regarding individual statins, atorvastatin, simvastatin, and pravastatin have been clinically tested in the largest number of diabetic patients. The tens of thousands of diabetic patients who have participated in randomized clinical statin trials have taught us that the proportional benefit of therapy, or relative risk reduction, is relatively constant across a wide array of diabetic patient subgroups and predictably related to the proportion of LDL-C lowering. With this wealth of data, we have witnessed a paradigm shift, dating back to the publication of the Heart Protection Study, in the way we manage cardiovascular risk in diabetic patients. Statins are now justifiably commonplace in the management of diabetic patients at various levels of risk. Further reduction of risk with statins may be achieved with more aggressive targets based on more accurate metrics of atherogenic burden, such as apoB or LDL particle concentration.

## References

1. Skalen K, Gustafsson M, Rydberg EK, Hulten LM, Wiklund O, Innerarity TL, et al. Subendothelial retention of atherogenic lipoproteins in early atherosclerosis. Nature. 2002;417(6890):750–4.
2. Tabas I, Williams KJ, Boren J. Subendothelial lipoprotein retention as the initiating process in atherosclerosis: update and therapeutic implications. Circulation. 2007;116(16):1832–44.
3. Fruchart JC, Sacks F, Hermans MP, Assmann G, Brown WV, Ceska R, et al. The residual risk reduction initiative: a call to action to reduce residual vascular risk in patients with dyslipidemia. Am J Cardiol. 2008;102(10 Suppl):1K–34.
4. Sniderman A, Williams K, de Graaf J. Non-HDL C equals apolipoprotein B: except when it does not! Curr Opin Lipidol. 2010;21(6):518–24.
5. Kastelein JJ, van der Steeg WA, Holme I, Gaffney M, Cater NB, Barter P, et al. Lipids, apolipoproteins, and their ratios in relation to cardiovascular events with statin treatment. Circulation. 2008;117(23):3002–9.
6. Sniderman A, Solhpour A. Targeting targets for LDL-lowering therapy: lessons from the Collaborative Atorvastatin Diabetes Study (CARDS). Clin Chem. 2009;55(3):391–3.

7. Heart Protection Study Collaborative Group. MRC/BHF Heart Protection Study of cholesterol lowering with simvastatin in 20,536 high-risk individuals: a randomised placebo-controlled trial. Lancet. 2002; 360(9326):7–22.
8. Collins R, Armitage J, Parish S, Sleigh P, Peto R. MRC/BHF Heart Protection Study of cholesterol-lowering with simvastatin in 5963 people with diabetes: a randomised placebo-controlled trial. Lancet. 2003;361(9374):2005–16.
9. Sever PS, Dahlof B, Poulter NR, Wedel H, Beevers G, Caulfield M, et al. Prevention of coronary and stroke events with atorvastatin in hypertensive patients who have average or lower-than-average cholesterol concentrations, in the anglo-scandinavian cardiac outcomes trial-lipid lowering arm (ASCOT-LLA): a multicentre randomised controlled trial. Lancet. 2003;361(9364):1149–58.
10. Sever PS, Poulter NR, Dahlof B, Wedel H, Collins R, Beevers G, et al. Reduction in cardiovascular events with atorvastatin in 2,532 patients with type 2 diabetes: anglo-scandinavian cardiac outcomes trial–lipid-lowering arm (ASCOT-LLA). Diabetes Care. 2005;28(5):1151–7.
11. Colhoun HM, Betteridge DJ, Durrington PN, Hitman GA, Neil HA, Livingstone SJ, et al. Primary prevention of cardiovascular disease with atorvastatin in type 2 diabetes in the collaborative atorvastatin diabetes study (CARDS): multicentre randomised placebo-controlled trial. Lancet. 2004;364(9435):685–96.
12. ALLHAT Officers and Coordinators for the ALLHAT Collaborative Research Group. The Antihypertensive and Lipid-Lowering Treatment to Prevent Heart Attack Trial. Major outcomes in moderately hypercholesterolemic, hypertensive patients randomized to pravastatin vs usual care: the Antihypertensive and Lipid-Lowering Treatment to Prevent Heart Attack Trial (ALLHAT-LLT). JAMA. 2002;288(23):2998–3007.
13. Kearney PM, Blackwell L, Collins R, Keech A, Simes J, Peto R, et al. Efficacy of cholesterol-lowering therapy in 18,686 people with diabetes in 14 randomised trials of statins: a meta-analysis. Lancet. 2008; 371(9607):117–25.
14. Ridker PM, MacFadyen JG, Fonseca FA, Genest J, Gotto AM, Kastelein JJ, et al. Number needed to treat with rosuvastatin to prevent first cardiovascular events and death among men and women with low low-density lipoprotein cholesterol and elevated high-sensitivity C-reactive protein: justification for the use of statins in prevention: an intervention trial evaluating rosuvastatin (JUPITER). Circ Cardiovasc Qual Outcomes. 2009;2(6):616–23.
15. Mihaylova B, Briggs A, Armitage J, Parish S, Gray A, Collins R. Lifetime cost effectiveness of simvastatin in a range of risk groups and age groups derived from a randomised trial of 20,536 people. BMJ. 2006; 333(7579):1145.
16. Gaede P, Lund-Andersen H, Parving HH, Pedersen O. Effect of a multifactorial intervention on mortality in type 2 diabetes. N Engl J Med. 2008;358(6):580–91.
17. de Graaf J, Couture P, Sniderman A. A diagnostic algorithm for the atherogenic apolipoprotein B dyslipoproteinemias. Nat Clin Pract Endocrinol Metab. 2008;4(11):608–18.
18. Grundy SM, Cleeman JI, Merz CN, Brewer Jr HB, Clark LT, Hunninghake DB, et al. Implications of recent clinical trials for the National Cholesterol Education Program Adult Treatment Panel III guidelines. Circulation. 2004;110(2):227–39.
19. Otvos JD, Mora S, Shalaurova I, Greenland P, Mackey RH, Goff Jr DC. Clinical implications of discordance between low-density lipoprotein cholesterol and particle number. J Clin Lipidol. 2011;5(2):105–13.
20. Sniderman AD, Williams K, Contois JH, Monroe HM, McQueen MJ, de Graaf J, et al. A meta-analysis of low-density lipoprotein cholesterol, non-high-density lipoprotein cholesterol, and apolipoprotein B as markers of cardiovascular risk. Circ Cardiovasc Qual Outcomes. 2011;4(3):337–45.
21. Davidson MH, Ballantyne CM, Jacobson TA, Bittner VA, Braun LT, Brown AS, et al. Clinical utility of inflammatory markers and advanced lipoprotein testing: advice from an expert panel of lipid specialists. J Clin Lipidol. 2011;5(5):338–67.
22. Brunzell JD, Davidson M, Furberg CD, Goldberg RB, Howard BV, Stein JH, et al. Lipoprotein management in patients with cardiometabolic risk: consensus conference report from the American Diabetes Association and the American College of Cardiology Foundation. J Am Coll Cardiol. 2008;51(15):1512–24.
23. Gotto Jr AM, Whitney E, Stein EA, Shapiro DR, Clearfield M, Weis S, et al. Relation between baseline and on-treatment lipid parameters and first acute major coronary events in the Air Force/Texas Coronary Atherosclerosis Prevention Study (AFCAPS/TexCAPS). Circulation. 2000;101(5):477–84.
24. Sattar N, Preiss D, Murray HM, Welsh P, Buckley BM, de Craen AJ, Seshasai SR, et al. Statins and risk of incident diabetes: a collaborative meta-analysis of randomised statin trials. Lancet. 2010;375:735–42.

# The PPAR System in Diabetes

# 19

Jean Claude Ansquer and Christelle Foucher

## Introduction

Peroxisome proliferator-activated receptors (PPARs), a family of cell receptors, are closely involved in glucose and lipoprotein metabolism. As discussed elsewhere in this book, PPAR alpha (PPAR α) agonists, such as fenofibrate, have shown clinical benefit for cardiovascular disease in some subgroups and for the macrovascular and microvascular complications of type 2 diabetes mellitus. This chapter reviews the basic science of the PPAR system and summarizes some clinical PPAR modulating drug trials, with an emphasis on diabetes, lipoproteins, and vascular disease. The chapter is divided into five sections:

1. PPAR gene and gene variants, proteins, and natural ligands
2. Synthetic ligands: from PPAR activators to PPAR agonists
3. The PPAR machinery with subsections on:
   - Coactivators and corepressors
   - Metabolic modification (phosphorylation, ubiquitination, sumoylation, and acetylation)
   - Partial agonists or SPPARMs
4. Effect of PPAR agonists in diabetes:
   - Pharmacology, in particular, in the pancreas
   - Effects in type 1 diabetes
   - Effects in type 2 diabetes and/or dyslipidemia with products reaching clinical development
5. Conclusions and perspectives

## PPAR Gene and Gene Variants, Proteins, and Natural Ligands

Peroxisome proliferator-activated receptors (PPARs) belong to a subfamily of the nuclear receptors which includes the retinoic acid receptors, the thyroid hormone receptors, and the RevErbA-related orphan receptors [1]. The PPAR subfamily contains three isoforms, namely, PPAR α (PPARA, NR1C1), PPAR β/δ (NR1C2 identified here as PPAR δ), and PPAR γ (PPARG, NR1C3, PPAR γ1, and PPAR γ2 sub-isoforms), that are encoded by different genes on different chromosomes.

In humans, PPAR α is mapped on chromosome 22 on the regions 22q12-q13.1; 22q13.31 with a linkage group of six genes and genetic markers [2]. The human PPAR γ gene is located on chromosome 3 at position 3p25, close to the retinoic acid receptor beta (RAR β) and the thyroid hormone receptor beta genes [3–5]. Two different human PPAR γ transcripts are expressed in hematopoietic cells: a 1.85-kb transcript, which corresponds to the full-length mRNA (PPAR γ1), and a shorter 0.65-kb transcript (PPAR γ2) [5].

J.C. Ansquer, M.D. • C. Foucher, Ph.D. (✉)
ClinSciences, 10 avenue Victor Hugo,
21000 Dijon, France
e-mail: jean-claude.ansquer@clinsciences.fr

A.J. Jenkins et al. (eds.), *Lipoproteins in Diabetes Mellitus*, Contemporary Diabetes,
DOI 10.1007/978-1-4614-7554-5_19, © Springer Science+Business Media New York 2014

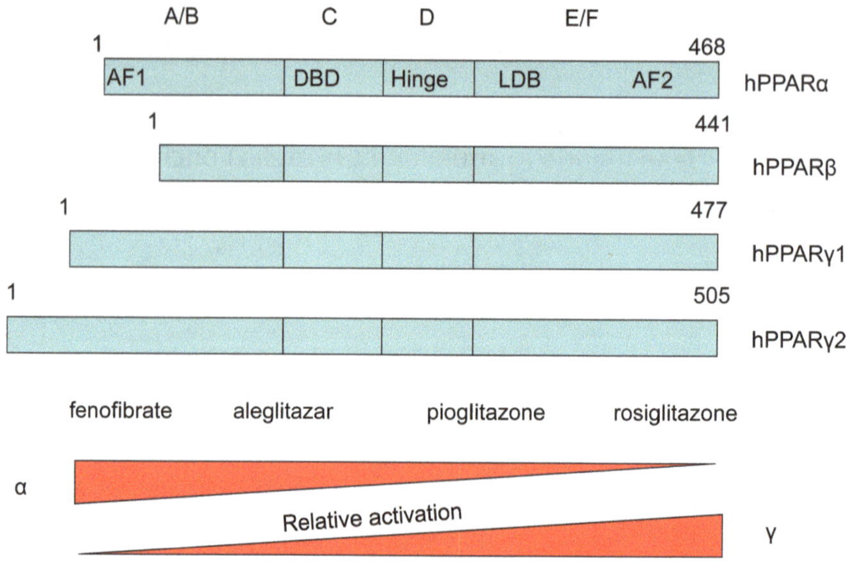


**Fig. 19.1** Structure of PPARs. In the *upper panel,* the structure of PPARs with their four domains: 1 is the NH2 terminal and 468 the COOH terminal for PPAR α. The *bottom panel* illustrates the relative activation for PPAR α and PPAR γ for major agonists with fenofibrate and rosiglitazone as behaving as specific activators and aleglitazar or pioglitazone with mixed effects

PPAR γ2 is mostly expressed in adipose tissue where the PPAR γ2/PPAR γ1 ratio of messenger RNA is directly correlated with body mass index and where a low-calorie diet downregulates PPAR γ2 messenger RNA in subcutaneous fat [6]. Several variants in the PPAR γ gene have been identified, with the Pro12Ala variant having been the most extensively examined in epidemiologic studies. A strong association between PPAR γ 12Ala polymorphism and a reduction in type 2 diabetes risk (odds ratio: 0.86, 95 % CI: 0.81–0.90) was described in an updated meta-analysis of 60 studies involving 32,849 subjects with type 2 diabetes mellitus (T2DM) and 47,456 control subjects evaluated by the Human Genome Epidemiology Network [7].

The human PPAR δ, which was cloned from a human osteosarcoma cell library, is located on chromosome 6 at position 6p21.1-p21.2 [8]. In the mouse, where the first PPAR, PPAR α, was identified in 1990 by Issemann and Green [9], PPAR α is found on chromosome 15, PPAR γ is located on chromosome 6 at position E3-F1, while PPAR δ is found on chromosome 17 [10]. In both human and mouse, the PPAR transcript is encoded by six exons (one in the A/B domain, two in the C domain, one for the hinge region, and two for the ligand binding domain).

PPAR isoforms share a common domain structure as shown in the schematic view in Fig. 19.1. Five domains designated A/B, C, D, E, and F are distinguishable, and each has a different function. The N-terminal A/B domain contains at least one constitutionally active transactivation region (AF-1) and several autonomous transactivation domains (AD) [1]. The specificity of gene transcription is granted by the isoform-specific sequence of the A/B domain of the receptor [11]. Chimeric proteins generated by fusion with the A/B domains of other receptor proteins attenuate the specificity of target gene activation [11]. The DNA binding domain (DBD, C domain) is the most conserved region, which contains a short motif responsible for DNA binding specificity (P-box) on sequences called peroxisome proliferator response elements (PPREs), typically containing the AGGTCA motif.

The D domain, called a hinge, permits the change in shape of PPARs. The C-terminal E/F domain contains the ligand binding domain (LBD) and the AF-2 region for binding coactivators and corepressors. When activated by ligands, PPARs heterodimerize with another nuclear receptor, the retinoid X receptor, and alter the transcription of target genes after binding to specific PPREs on target genes.

Natural ligands for PPARs are long chain fatty acids, saturated or not, and eicosanoids: 8-HETE (hydroxyeicosatetraenoic acid) and to some extent leukotriene B4 (LTB4) for PPAR α; 9- and 13-HODE (hydroxyoctadecadienoic acid), two 15 lipoxygenase metabolites of linoleic acid, and 15-deoxy PGJ2 for PPAR γ; and prostacyclin (PGI2) for PPAR δ [12–14]. However, tissue concentrations are probably too low for them being the active ligands [15]. A new candidate endogenous ligand for PPAR α in the liver is a glycerophosphocholine esterified with palmitic and oleic acids 16:0/18:1-GPC or POPC (1-palmitoyl,2-oleoyl-sn-glycero-3-phosphocholine hydroxyeicosatetraenoic acid), which was identified in the liver of mice by tandem mass spectrometry [16]. This phosphatidylcholine is displaced from PPAR α by the synthetic agonist Wy14643. Its portal infusion induces dependent gene expression of carnitine palmitoyltransferase I (CPT1) in wild-type mice, but not in PPAR α deficient mice. Recently, two other phosphatidylcholines, DLPC and DUPC (1,2-dilauroyl-sn-glycero-3-phospho-choline and 1,2-(cis-cis-9,12-octadecadienoyl)-sn-glycero-3-phosphatidylcholine, respectively), have been shown to improve glucose control in two mouse models of insulin resistance [17]; however, they did not affect rosiglitazone binding to PPAR γ, and their effects are linked to stimulation of another nuclear receptor liver receptor homologue (LRH)-1.

## Synthetic Ligands: From PPAR Activators to PPAR Agonists

PPAR α was first cloned from a mouse liver cDNA library at ICI, the pharmaceutical company which developed clofibrate, the first fibrate [9], and subsequently in humans [2, 18]. Fibrates, which were in clinical use as lipid-lowering agents for 20 years before this discovery, are weak PPAR α agonists, effective on human PPAR in the micromolar range, explaining the observation that they are given in the range of 100–1,200 mg per day. Fibrates, such as fenofibrate, mainly act via activation of PPAR α in the liver to regulate genes involved in fatty acid oxidation [19]. They were then called PPAR α activators, and their main laboratory effects are to reduce triglycerides and increase high-density lipoprotein (HDL) cholesterol levels. The first potent and selective PPAR α agonist acting in the nanomolar range with clinical data was LY518674, the development of which was stopped in 2007 when phase 2 studies showed no advantage over existing fenofibrate [20].

The link between PPAR γ activation and the thiazolidinedione insulin-sensitizing agents pioglitazone and rosiglitazone was established by researchers at Upjohn and Glaxo in 1994 and 1995, respectively [21, 22]. PPAR γ increases adipocyte differentiation and storage of fat. The short-term marker of PPAR γ activation in plasma is an increase in levels of the adipocytokine adiponectin, which increases insulin sensitivity in liver and muscle [23, 24]. The first animal results with PPAR δ agonists L165041 and GW501516 were reported in 1999 by researchers at Merck and in 2001 at Glaxo [25, 26].

## The PPAR Machinery

The PPAR machinery is similar to other nuclear receptors with sequential complexes of coactivators and corepressors with enzymatic activities (for review, see Rosenfeld 2006) [27] and a series of metabolic transformations that turn PPARs toward activation or direct them to degradation (Fig. 19.2). The role of these different proteins, their metabolic transformations, and the concept of selective PPAR modulator are summarized in the next sections. Without ligand the transcription of DNA into messenger RNA is usually repressed by the binding of corepressors on the heterodimer PPAR–RXR, and chromatin is compacted (Fig. 19.3). With the presence of ligand in the ligand binding domain, the structural changes in the AF-2 region permit to replace corepressors by coactivators, to associate remodeling of

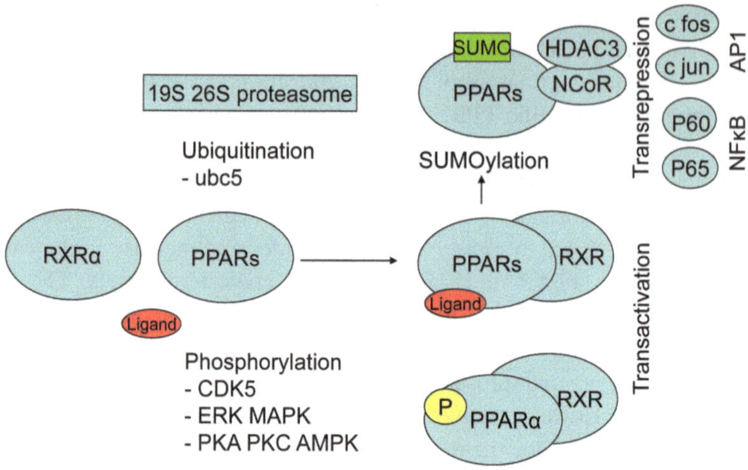


**Fig. 19.2** PPAR network. Upon activation with ligand, PPAR heterodimerizes with RXR α and activate target genes (transactivation). Phosphorylation has opposite effect transactivation for PPAR α or its inhibition for PPAR γ. Sumoylation of PPAR is associated with transrepression which prevents transcription of NFκB or AP-1-dependent inflammatory genes and with a reduction of degradation in the proteasome. CDK5, cyclin-dependent kinase 5; ERK MAPK, mitogen-activated kinase; PKA PKC AMPK, protein kinase A or C and AMP-activated kinase; NCoR, nuclear corepressor; HDAC3, histone deacetylase 3

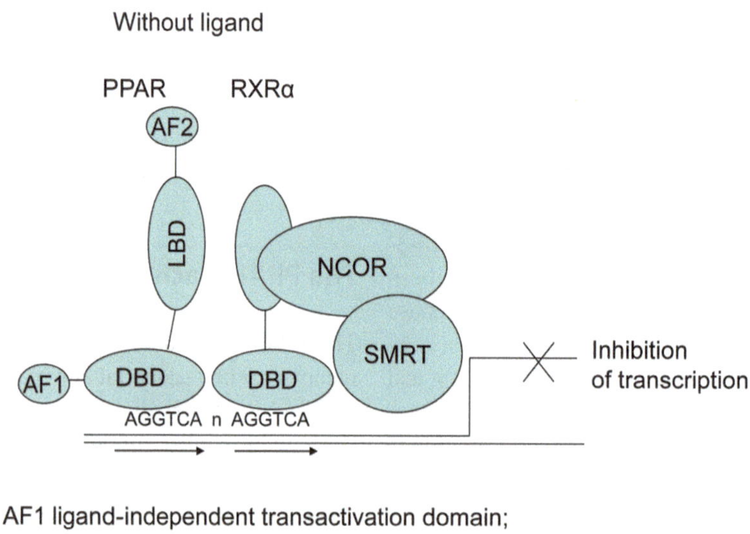


**Fig. 19.3** Corepressor complex: without ligand, PPAR and RXR α are linked to their PPRE direct repeat (AGGTCA n AGGTT) by the DNA binding domain; the corepressors NCoR and SMRT prevent DNA transcription. AF1 AF2 ligand-independent transactivation domains 1 and 2; DBD, DNA binding domain; LBD, ligand binding domain; NCoR, nuclear corepressor; SMRT, silencing mediator for retinoid and thyroid hormone

chromatin by acetylation of histones, in order for RNA polymerase to access the DNA and initiate transcription (Fig. 19.4). One important aspect common to PPAR activation is transrepression of inflammatory genes under the control of nuclear factor kappa B (NFκB) or activated protein (AP) 1. This transrepression is an indirect effect since there is no PPRE in the promoter. This was shown for PPAR γ on induction of tumor necrosis factor (TNF) α by phorbol myristate acetate in human

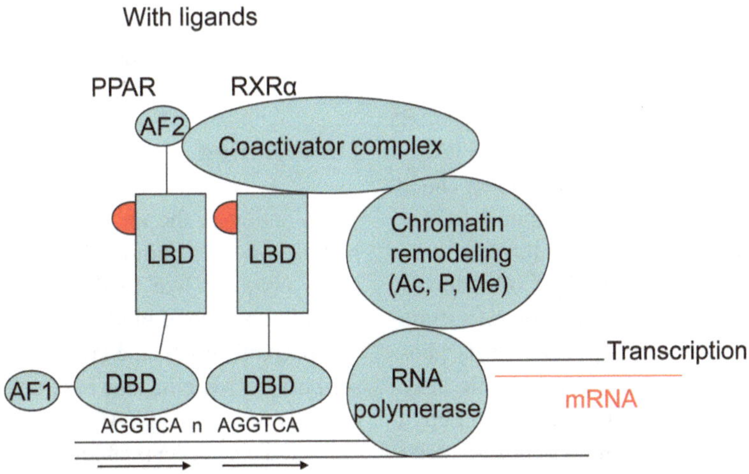


**Fig. 19.4** Coactivator complex: with fixation of ligands, conformational changes in ligand binding domain permit replacement of corepressors by coactivators, of which the enzymatic activities acetylate, phosphorylate, or methylate the chromatin allowing access to DNA or RNA polymerase and initiation of transcription into copies of messenger RNA

monocytes/macrophages [28], for PPAR α on human aortic smooth muscle cells and interleukin (IL)-1-induced IL6 expression [29, 30], and for PPAR δ with expression of monocyte chemoattractant protein (MCP)-1 [31]. In human endothelial cells, fenofibrate and L165041, but not rosiglitazone, inhibited TNF α-induced monocyte adhesion, vascular cell adhesion molecule-1 (VCAM-1) expression, and monocyte chemotactic protein-1 (MCP-1) secretion through inhibition of nuclear P65 translocation, necessary for NFκB activation [32].

## PPAR Coactivators and Corepressors

The main PPAR coactivator, or at least the best studied one, is peroxisome proliferator-activated receptor γ coactivator 1 α (PGC-1 α) [33]. Through a number of transcription factors, including PPARs, PGC-1 α modulates numerous metabolic pathways in the liver, skeletal and cardiac muscle, and adipose tissue, including gluconeogenesis and glycolysis, fatty acid synthesis, and oxidation. Indeed, PGC-1 α itself is subject to the same modulations as PPAR (see below through phosphorylation, ubiquitination, or sumoylation). Other PPAR coactivators are steroid receptor coactivator 1 (SRC1) and cyclic adenosine 5′-monophosphate (cAMP) response element binding protein (CBP/P300) which possess histone acetyltransferase activity, leading to the decondensation of chromatin which is necessary for gene transcription.

The main PPAR corepressors, nuclear receptor corepressor (NCoR) and silencing mediator for retinoid and thyroid hormone (SMRT), are associated with histone deacetylase activity which maintain chromatin in a compact state. The role of NCoR was studied by specifically knocking out its gene in mouse adipocytes (AKO) or muscle (MKO). MKO mice were able to run longer than normal mice [34]. AKO mice had higher insulin sensitivity in liver, muscle, and adipose tissue than normal mice, with limited additional effect of rosiglitazone since PPAR γ target genes were already derepressed by NCoR deletion [35]. The effects of rosiglitazone to cause hemodilution were the same in AKO and normal mice. In MKO mice, exercise capacity and mitochondrial oxidation are enhanced by the loss of a transcriptional cofactor in muscle cells through modulation of transcription factors that includes PPAR δ. SMRT is a protein structurally similar to NCoR, which possesses different receptor interaction domains (RID) for different nuclear receptors, called RID2 for PPAR or RXR or RID1 for retinoid acid receptor [36].

## Phosphorylation

Phosphorylation of PPAR γ by extracellular signal-related kinase (ERK) 1 at serine 112 inhibits adipogenesis [37]. Phosphorylation of PPAR α on serine residues in the ligand-independent transactivation domain AF-1 in response to insulin increases transcription activity through dissociation of corepressors [38]. HMG-CoA reductase inhibitors ("statins") have been shown to stimulate PPAR α transcription by reducing its phosphorylation in HepG2 cells, a synergistic effect with fenofibric acid [39]. Transcriptional activation of PPAR α by bezafibrate was dose-dependently increased by statins in human kidney 293T cells. In addition, concomitant administration of fenofibric acid and pitavastatin decreased the transactivation of NFκB induced by phorbol myristate acetate (PMA) [40]. Data on PPAR δ phosphorylation are limited to the location of predicted consensus phosphorylation sites and inhibition of PPAR δ activation by kinase inhibitors [41].

It was shown recently that phosphorylation of PPAR γ at serine 273 by activated CDK5 leads to a loss of transcription of PPAR γ in adipocytes [42]. The cyclin-dependent kinase (CDK) 5, which is present in the cytoplasm and the nucleus, is activated by phosphorylation at tyrosine 15 within a high glucose milieu and IL1β, by TNF α, or by high-fat diet. This finding permitted the same authors to discover new small molecules binding to PPAR γ blocking CDK5 serine 273 phosphorylation, like thiazolidinediones (TZDs), with potent antidiabetic activity in insulin-resistant mice fed with a high-fat, high-sugar diet, without causing fluid retention and weight gain [43].

## Ubiquitination

Proteins are degraded in the proteasome after fixation on lysine residues of repeated sequences of a small 76AA polypeptide called ubiquitin. In the absence of their ligands, PPARs are rapidly degraded by this process. The degradation of PPAR γ is increased by different TZD ligands [44]; conversely, ubiquitination of PPAR α is reduced transiently with different fibrate ligands [45], and ubiquitination of PPAR δ is markedly reduced by PPAR δ agonists [46].

## Sumoylation

Sumoylation is the attachment of another polypeptide of 101 amino acids called SUMO, for small ubiquitin-like modifier. Sumoylation at a lysine in the ligand binding domain of PPAR γ is the mechanism which converts activation of transcription by rosiglitazone into repression of NFκB or activator protein (AP) 1 in murine macrophages. This prevents ubiquitination of NCoR to maintain repression of inflammatory genes such as inducible NO synthase [47]. In adipose tissue, sumoylation of PPAR γ, which reduces the effect of rosiglitazone, is increased in the absence of the hepatokine fibroblast growth factor (FGF) 21 [48].

Similarly, sumoylation at lysine 185 has been identified in the hinge region of PPAR α [49]. To date, a potential sumoylation site for PPAR δ has been suggested on lysine 185, as for PPAR α.

Posttranslational regulation of PPARs by different patterns of mono- or polyubiquitination, as well as by mono- or polysumoylation, has been recently reviewed by Wadosky and Willis [50]. This review also reports that the coreceptor RXRα and the coactivators PGC-1α can be ubiquitinated or sumoylated, adding to the complexity of these regulatory processes.

## Acetylation

Acetylation and deacetylation of genes are major processes affecting gene expression through decondensation and recondensation of chromatin. It also affects proteins. The first nuclear receptors shown to be acetylated were the androgen–estrogen receptors; this has not been shown clearly for PPAR [51]. However, their key coactivator PGC-1 α is inactivated by acetylation in high-energy states or deacetylated by sirtuin 1 in low-energy states [52]. The nicotinamide adenine dinucleotide (NAD)-dependent histone deacetylases or sirtuins by interacting with PPARs and their coactivators thus provide a new level of complexity to the regulation of nuclear receptors [53].

## Partial Agonists or SPPARMs

A partial agonist is a ligand that induces a submaximal response even at full receptor occupancy. It can also reduce the full PPAR γ agonist response. For instance, in comparison with rosiglitazone, troglitazone is a full agonist on murine 3T3L1 adipocytes but a partial agonist in muscle C2C12 myotubes and HEK293T kidney cells [54]. Olefsky proposed to name selective PPAR modulators (SPPARMs); such products differ from full agonists by differential regulation of target genes [55]. SPPARMs are designed to separate efficacy and adverse effect dose–response curves. This concept was already developed in nuclear receptor pharmacology, with selective estrogen receptor modulators (SERMs), such as tamoxifen or raloxifene, which recruit corepressors such as NCoR to the AF-2 region, whereas estradiol recruits coactivators such as the glucocorticoid receptor-interacting protein 1 (GRIP1) [56] or with selective vitamin D modulators such as paricalcitol with differential recruitment of coactivators than calcitriol, the active form of vitamin D [57].

Increasing concentrations or doses with full PPAR γ agonists lead to greater efficacy but greater adverse events, such as weight gain and volume expansion.

PPAR γ partial agonists such as balaglitazone or INT131 displace a full agonist such as rosiglitazone. Metaglidasen, the (−) stereoisomer of halofenate, tested in the 1990s as a lipid-lowering agent, is another selective partial PPAR γ modulator and is still in clinical development for its uricosuric activity. They bind the same pocket as TZDs, which is required to block PPAR γ phosphorylation, but induce different conformational changes in PPAR γ, leading to different recruitment of coactivator/corepressor. As an example, INT131 induces less recruitment of DRIP205 (vitamin D-interacting protein 205), a coactivator involved in lipid accumulation than rosiglitazone or pioglitazone in HEK cells [58]. The same finding was reported with fibrates: gemfibrozil induced less recruitment of DRIP205 than fenofibrate and behaves as a partial agonist to increase apoA-I activation. This translated in a comparative trial in dyslipidemic patients to a larger increase in apoA-I levels, a protective apoprotein in HDL, with fenofibrate than with gemfibrozil [59].

## Effects of PPAR Agonists in Diabetes

This review is limited to PPAR activators or agonists which entered clinical development in diabetes and/or dyslipidemia (Table 19.1). Few PPAR antagonists were synthesized and they were not developed for the treatment of diabetes [60]. GW6471, a potent PPAR α antagonist, is used as a pharmacological agent to test whether an effect is PPAR dependent or PPAR independent. GW9662 is a PPAR γ antagonist which promotes the recruitment of NCoR. Finally, GSK0660 and GSK3787 are PPAR δ antagonists for pharmacological use.

The organs implicated in glucose control are listed in Table 19.2. With their direct effects on gene expression and their indirect effects on inflammation, and according to their tissue distribution, PPARs affect most of these organs, beyond the liver for PPAR α, the adipose tissue for PPAR γ, and the skeletal muscle for PPAR δ. In the kidney, they have different locations: PPAR α is located mainly in the proximal tubule, the medullary thick ascending limb, and in the mesangium; PPAR γ in the distal medullary collecting duct and glomeruli; and PPAR δ in a diffuse fashion as in other organs [62]. In the brain, the interplay of PPAR subtypes has been shown in cultures of astrocytes, where the three subtypes are present. Combined application of PPAR γ and PPAR δ activators increased cyclooxygenase 2 expression induced by lipopolysaccharide, whereas the additional application of a PPAR α agonist abolished this effect [63].

In the pancreas, the three PPARs are expressed in pancreatic β cells. PPAR α modulates fatty acid oxidation and PPAR γ directs them toward esterification. Although PPAR δ is the most abundant PPAR in the pancreas at the mRNA and the protein level, until recently its effects on fatty acid oxidation have been less well studied [64]. PPAR δ activation increases fatty acid oxidation and to a larger extent than PPAR α activation. In the pancreas, fatty acids acutely potentiate glucose-stimulated insulin secretion (GSIS), but

**Table 19.1** Phase of clinical development reached by PPAR agonists

| | PPAR α | PPAR γ | PPAR α/γ | PPAR δ | Pan-PPAR |
|---|---|---|---|---|---|
| Marketed | Bezafibrate<br>Ciprofibrate<br>Fenofibrate<br>Gemfibrozil<br>Clinofibrate<br>Etofibrate | Pioglitazone<br>Rosiglitazone | | | |
| No more marketed | Clofibrate | Troglitazone | | | |
| Phase 3 | | Balaglitazone<br>Metaglidasen[a]<br>Rivoglitazone[a]<br>Ciglitazone<br>Farglitazar[b] | Aleglitazard[d]<br>Lobeglitazone<br>Muraglitazar<br>Ragaglitazar<br>Tesaglitazar<br>Imiglitazar<br>MK767 | | |
| Phase 2 | K877<br>ZYH7<br>AVE8134<br>GW590735<br>KRP-105<br>LY518674<br>CP778875 | INT131<br>MBX2044<br>FK614 | Cevoglitazar<br>Naveglitazar<br>Sipoglitazar | MBX8025<br>GW501516<br>GW0742<br>L165041 | GFT505[c]<br>Chiglitazar<br>Indeglitazar<br>Sodelglitazar<br>Netoglitazone |

[a]Discontinued in diabetes
[b]Discontinued in hepatic fibrosis (McHutchison et al., 2010) [61]
[c]PPAR α/δ
[d]Withdrawn from clinical development in July 2013

**Table 19.2** Organs implicated in glucose control

| | PPAR α | PPAR γ | PPAR δ |
|---|---|---|---|
| Liver | Increase in fat oxidation and apoA-1 increase insulin sensitivity | Decrease in steatosis<br>Increase insulin sensitivity | |
| Skeletal muscle | | Increase insulin sensitivity | Increase in fat oxidation and energy expenditure |
| Adipose tissue | Reduction in inflammatory adipocytokines | Increase in adipocyte differentiation and adiponectin release | |
| Pancreas | | | Amplification of glucose-induced insulin secretion |
| Gut | | Anti-inflammatory | Increase in GLP1 production |
| Vascular wall | Increase in NO synthesis | | |

their chronic exposure elevates basal insulin secretion and alters GSIS, a phenomenon called lipotoxicity.

Discordant results are reported in the literature with PPAR α or PPAR γ agonists. PPAR α was described to potentiate and PPAR γ to attenuate GSIS in INS-1E cells, an immortalized insulinoma rat cell line [65]. On the contrary, in vivo, the PPAR α agonist fenofibrate impaired GSIS in neonatal rats receiving monosodium glutamate to induce obesity, while pioglitazone, a PPAR γ agonist, increased it in db/db mice [66, 67]. This discordance might be explained by the low expression level of PPAR γ in INS-1E cells.

Activation of PPAR δ by unsaturated FAs or a synthetic ligand enhanced GSIS in primary rat islets or INS-1E cells without affecting basal insulin secretion [64]. In order to maintain β cell function, PPAR δ would play a role of lipid sensor to adjust the mitochondrial fatty acid oxidation. It was recently suggested that 4-hydroxynonenal (4-HNE) was one endogenous activating ligand of PPAR δ [68]. The level of reactive oxygen species (ROS), such as 4-HNE, is essential to β cell function, as low-level ROS production increases glucose-induced insulin secretion, whereas high levels of ROS can induce β cell apoptosis.

GSIS is also linked to influx of calcium ions to the cytosol induced by depolarization from the voltage-dependent $Ca^{++}$ channel. In INS-1 cells, the sarco-endoplasmic reticulum $Ca^{++}$ ATPase (SERCA2) pump maintains intracellular $Ca^{++}$ homeostasis, in particular, a high $Ca^{++}$ level in the endoplasmic reticulum. The expression of this pump is decreased in animal models of diabetes and in diabetic human islets. Pioglitazone directly increases expression of SERCA2 through transcription of the gene and indirectly through prevention of CDK5-induced phosphorylation of PPAR γ [69]. This experiment suggests that blocking CDK5 could permit to dissociate positive effects on glucose homeostasis from other effects from PPAR γ agonists.

## Effects of PPAR Agonists in Type 1 Diabetes

Clinical studies with PPAR agonists in type 1 diabetes (T1DM) are limited to their effects on lipid or glucose markers. One placebo-controlled randomized study was conducted with fenofibrate in 44 patients with T1DM to assess its effect alone or in combination with vitamin E for 8 weeks on copper-induced oxidation of LDL and VLDL particles [70]. The lag time of oxidation was significantly prolonged by fenofibrate 200 mg + vitamin E 400 IU. A placebo-controlled randomized study is in the planning stage to evaluate the effects of fenofibrate on progression of diabetic retinopathy in 400 adults with T1DM (http://clinicaltrials.gov/ct2/show/NCT01320345) [71]. The lipid-modifying effects of bezafibrate in T1DM were evaluated in earlier placebo-controlled studies [72, 73]. Of note, this fibrate, now considered as an archetype pan-PPAR agonist in transactivation assays, did not improve HbA1c after 3 months of treatment [40, 74].

Three placebo-controlled randomized studies have been reported with TZDs in T1DM patients on insulin therapy, with modest insulin-sparing effects as compared to those observed in T2DM. In 50 overweight adults with T1DM, an 8-month intervention to achieve glycated hemoglobin level of 7.0 % required an 11 % increase in the daily dose of insulin in the placebo group, but no change in the rosiglitazone group [75]. In 36 T1DM adolescents aged 10–18 years, the dose of insulin was increased by 9 % with placebo and reduced by 6 % with rosiglitazone after 6 months of treatment, with HbA1c remaining stable around 8.5 % [76]. In 60 lean T1DM patients aged 14 years or more, 6-month treatment with pioglitazone was associated with a significant decrease in HbA1c (0.2 %) and in postprandial glucose levels (0.7 mmol/L) in the intervention group only, with no changes in insulin doses [77]. In patients with slowly progressive T1DM, diagnosed by the presence of glutamic acid decarboxylase (GAD) antibodies, an insulin-requiring state defined by HbA1c and post-glucose C-peptide levels was reached at 4 years in 4/4 subjects randomized to pioglitazone as compared to 1/5 subjects randomized to metformin [78]. Thus, the effects of TZD in T1DM sharply differ from those reported for T2DM prevention with troglitazone in TRIPOD [79], rosiglitazone in DREAM [80], and, more recently, pioglitazone in ACT-NOW [81] and from their effects on glucose control in people with established T2DM.

## Effects of PPAR Agonists in Type 2 Diabetes and Dyslipidemia

For the treatment of T2DM, the first TZD PPAR γ agonist troglitazone was introduced in the USA in October 1997 and was withdrawn in March 2000 for hepatic toxicity. Rosiglitazone and pioglitazone were introduced in the USA in 1999 and in Europe in 2000. In Japan, pioglitazone was introduced in 1999 and rosiglitazone in 2003. The effects of pioglitazone on macrovascular events in 5,238 T2DM patients were reported in 2005 [82]. Although the study primary end point was not reached, there was a significant 16 % reduction in the main secondary end point, which included death from any cause, acute nonfatal myocardial infarction, or stroke. The effect of TZDs on diabetes control and the controversy about their hazard on cardiovascular events have been the subject of numerous reviews in the last 5 years [83–85].

The first request for approval of a PPAR α/γ dual agonist, muraglitazar, was submitted to the Food and Drug Administration (FDA) for registration but was withdrawn in May 2006 after a combined analysis of clinical studies indicated an increased cardiovascular risk [86]. Such an increase in cardiovascular risk led to the suspension of registration of rosiglitazone in Europe in September 2010 and severe limitations to its use in the USA. Finally, in June 2011, pioglitazone was withdrawn from some European markets due to increased risk of bladder tumors, a decision not endorsed by the European Medicines Agency.

Discontinuation of the development of PPAR agonists occurred for multiple reasons: toxicity of the compound (vascular or bladder tumors in rodents with MK767 or ragaglitazar, respectively), long duration of development, clinical adverse events, expectation not to be better than existing drugs, and stopping of development efforts in the cardiometabolic domain. In particular, the FDA requested in July 2004 that 2-year rodent carcinogenicity studies be completed and reviewed before proceeding to phase 3 studies of more than 6-month duration. This decision was made after the evaluation of carcinogenicity in rodents for 11 PPAR agonists, with the observation of hemangioma/hemangiocarcinoma with 8/11 compounds and urinary bladder/renal pelvic transitional cell carcinomas with 5/6 PPAR α/γ dual agonists and pioglitazone (www.fda.gov/downloads/Drugs/Guidance ComplianceRegulatoryInformation/Guidances/UCM071624.pdf) [87]. In addition, the FDA requested in December 2008 that new antidiabetic agents had to demonstrate through randomized, prospective clinical trials that they do not increase risk for cardiovascular events (www.fda.gov/downloads/Drugs/Guidance Compliance RegulatoryInformation/Guidances/UCM071627.pdf) [88]. The thiazolidinedione intervention with vitamin D evaluation (TIDE) study, a large intervention study to assess the effect of the existing TZDs pioglitazone and rosiglitazone on cardiovascular events, planned in 16,000 T2DM patients at risk of CVD events was initiated in 2009 but stopped by the FDA 1 year later leaving uncertainty about the risks and benefits from TZDs (TIDE 2012) [89]. The authors stated that, had this study been initiated earlier, it would have provided clear evidence regarding the efficacy and safety of rosiglitazone and pioglitazone.

Currently the number of PPAR agonists in phase 2 or phase 3 of clinical development in diabetes and/or dyslipidemia has been markedly reduced as compared to the mid-2000s (Table 19.3).

The most promising was aleglitazar, a PPAR α/γ dual agonist with a large intervention study ALECARDIO underway in 7,000 T2DM patients with a recent acute coronary syndrome. They will be randomized to aleglitazar 150 μg or placebo and followed until there have been 950 primary events (cardiovascular death, nonfatal myocardial infarction, and nonfatal stroke) and for a minimum of 2.5 years for each participant (http://clinicaltrials.gov/ct2/show/NCT01042769) [90]. The dose of 150 μg was thought to offer glycemic control equal to pioglitazone and a more favorable effect on the lipid profile. The PPAR α component is responsible for a dose-related increase in circulating creatinine levels, with a 17 % reduction in measured glomerular filtration rate at the 600 μg dose [91, 92]. Another PPAR α/γ dual agonist, lobeglitazone or CKD-501, is currently recruiting T2DM patients in a 6-month comparative trial with pioglitazone (http://clinicaltrials.gov/ct2/show/NCT01106131) [93].

Two PPAR α agonists are in phase 2 of development for treatment of dyslipidemia in comparison with fenofibrate (K877 Kowa and ZYH7 Zydus http://clinicaltrials.gov/ct2/results?term=01539616) [94]. The PPAR γ SPPARMs balaglitazone and INT131 appear to be as effective as pioglitazone on HbA1c levels but cause less weight gain in 6-month trials (http://clinicaltrials.gov/ct2/show/NCT00631007) [95, 96].

Clinical studies with PPAR δ activators have been limited to short-term mechanistic studies. In healthy volunteer and in moderately obese subjects with dyslipidemia, GW501516 10 mg once daily (od) for 2 weeks reduced fasting and postprandial triglyceride (TG) levels by 30 %, liver fat measured by magnetic resonance imaging by 20 %, and urinary isoprostane levels, a marker of

**Table 19.3** Effects of recent PPAR agonists on lipids, glycated hemoglobin, and weight

| | Design/PPAR agonist | Study groups | HDL-C %change | TG %change | HbA1c %change | Weight change |
|---|---|---|---|---|---|---|
| Nissen [20] | R,DB,6PG, 12 weeks | Placebo | −1 % | +1 % | N/A | N/A |
| | *N*=309 dyslipidemic | Feno 200 mg | +14 % | −33 % | | |
| | LY518674 | LY 10 μg | +10 % | −36 % | | |
| | PPAR α | LY 25 μg | +16 % | −41 % | | |
| | | LY 50 μg | +11 % | −42 % | | |
| | | LY 100 μg | +2 % | −35 % | | |
| NCT00631007 [96] | R,DB,6PG, 24 weeks | Placebo | N/A | N/A | −0.1 % | 0/61 |
| | *N*=367 T2DM on | Pio 45 mg | | | −0.9 % | 6/60 |
| | metformin/sulfonylurea | 0.5 mg | | | −0.3 % | 0/60 |
| | INT-131 | 1 mg | | | −0.6 % | 2/61 |
| | PPAR γ | 2 mg | | | −0.9 % | 1/63 |
| | | 3 mg | | | −1.0 % | 4/61 |
| Henriksen [95] | R,DB,4PG, 26 weeks | Placebo | N/A | N/A | +0.7 % | +0.5 kg |
| | *N*=409 T2DM on insulin | Pio 45 mg | | | −0.5 % | +5 kg |
| | Balaglitazone | Bala 10 mg | | | −0.3 % | +3.5 kg |
| | Partial PPAR γ | Bala 20 mg | | | −0.4 % | +5 kg |
| Henry [91] | R,DB,6PG, 16 weeks | Placebo | + 4 % | +15 % | +0.4 % | −0.8 kg |
| | *N*=332 T2DM | Pio 45 mg | +16 % | −10 % | −0.3 % | +1.1 kg |
| | Aleglitazar | Ale 50 μg | +12 % | −15 % | 0.0 % | −0.2 kg |
| | PPAR α/γ | Ale 150 μg | +25 % | −30 % | −0.45 % | +0.5 kg |
| | SYNCHRONY | Ale 300 μg | +28 % | −35 % | −0.7 % | +1.2 kg |
| | | Ale 600 μg | +27 % | −40 % | −1.1 % | +2.7 kg |
| Sanwald-Ducray [102] | R,DB,7PG, 6 weeks | Placebo | +3 % | +10 % | N/A | −0.2 kg |
| | *N*=65 T2DM | Ale 20 μg | −3 % | −5 % | | 0.0 kg |
| | Aleglitazar | Ale 50 μg | +15 % | −15 % | | −0.2 kg |
| | PPAR α/γ | Ale 100 μg | +25 % | −20 % | | −0.7 kg |
| | | Ale 300 μg | +18 % | −35 % | | −0.2 kg |
| | | Ale 600 μg | +20 % | −25 % | | +1.1 kg |
| | | Ale 900 μg | +15 % | −35 % | | +1.5 kg |
| NCT00196989 GSK [101] | R,DB,7PG, 16 weeks | Placebo | −0.5 % | −9 % | −0.4 % | N/A |
| | *N*=352 T2DM on diet | Pio 30/45 mg | +10 % | −10 % | −1.1 % | |
| | and/or metformin | GW 2.5 mg | +11 % | −12 % | −0.35 % | |
| | GW677954 | GW 5 mg | +15 % | −27 % | 0.0 % | |
| | Sodelglitazar | GW 10 mg | +18 % | −34 % | −0.3 % | |
| | PPAR α/γ/δ | GW 15 mg | +16 % | −26 % | −0.2 % | |
| | | GW 20 mg | +18 % | −25 % | −0.2 % | |
| Bays [99] | R,DP,6PG, 8 weeks | Placebo | +1 % | −5 % | N/A | Unchanged |
| | *N*=181 dyslipidemia | Atorva 20 mg M 50 mg | +2 % | −18 % | | |
| | MBX-8025 | M 100 mg | +10 % | −32 % | | |
| | PPAR δ | A20+M 50 mg | +13 % | −33 % | | |
| | | A20+M 100 mg | +13 % | −35 % | | |
| | | | +2 % | −31 % | | |
| Cariou [100] | R,DB, 2PG, 5 weeks | Placebo | −3 % | −4 % | N/A | N/A |
| | *N*=47 prediabetes | GFT505 80 mg | +7 % | −32 % | | |
| | GFT505 | | | | | |
| | PPAR α/δ | | | | | |

*R* randomized, *DB* double blind, *PG* parallel group, *Atorva* atorvastatin, *Feno* fenofibrate, *N/A* not available, *Pio* pioglitazone, *T2DM* type 2 diabetes. If not provided, percent changes are estimated from figures or calculated from actual means before and after treatment

oxidative stress, by 30 %. In a skeletal muscle biopsy of the thigh, the expression of carnitine palmitoyltransferase 1b, which permits fatty acid to enter the mitochondria, was increased suggesting increased fat oxidation [97]. In a randomized, placebo-controlled, crossover trial,

13 obese dyslipidemic subjects received GW501516 2.5 mg once daily for 6 weeks. The GW501516 reduced apoC-III production, increased VLDL-apoB catabolism, and increased apoA-II production and HDL-cholesterol (HDL-C) levels [98]. MBX8025, another specific PPAR δ agonist, was recently reported to reduce TG and increase HDL-C levels alone or in combination with a statin in 181 dyslipidemic patients treated for 8 weeks [99]. GFT505 is a PPAR α/δ currently in phase 2 with a recently completed 3-month study in T2DM [100]. The first pan-PPAR agonist advanced to phase 2 was GW677954 or sodelglitazar which was discontinued from clinical development due to safety concerns. Chiglitazar is another pan-PPAR agonist in development in China.

## Conclusion and Perspectives

The pharmacology of PPARs, one family of nuclear receptors, is extremely complex as it regulates energy stores in major organs through modulation of genes in lipid and carbohydrate metabolism as well as adaptation to stress, fasting, and feeding. The natural ligands for PPARs are fatty acids and prostaglandins. Their first synthetic ligands are fibrates for PPAR α; thiazolidinediones for PPAR γ; within the last 10 years description of few PPAR δ agonists; and then dual and pan-PPAR agonists. Most of these well-designed products have been discontinued from clinical development for various reasons from animal toxicity and clinical safety to no advantage over existing drugs or hurdles to substantiate it. Currently, the most advanced new PPAR agonist is aleglitazar, a dual PPAR α/γ agonist, which is being evaluated for the prevention of cardiovascular events in people with type 2 diabetes and a recent acute coronary syndrome. The prevention and treatment of microvascular events, as shown with fenofibrate, now in clinical use for 40 years, should represent another area of research for new products. The anti-inflammatory effects of PPAR agonists have been well documented in animal experiments, although their potential in human disease is yet to be demonstrated. The search for natural PPAR ligands has been encouraged by the recent discovery that phosphatidylcholine derivatives can activate PPAR α and should continue for other PPARs and orphan nuclear receptors.

## References


1. Desvergne B, Wahli W. Peroxisome proliferator-activated receptors: nuclear control of metabolism. Endocr Rev. 1999;20:649–88.
2. Sher T, Yi HF, McBride OW, Gonzalez FJ. cDNA cloning, chromosomal mapping and functional characterization of the human peroxisome proliferator activated receptor. Biochemistry. 1993;32:5598–604.
3. Lazar MA, Chin WW. Nuclear thyroid hormone receptors. J Clin Invest. 1990;86:1777–82.
4. Mattei MG, Rivière M, Krust A, Ingvarsson S, Vennström B, Islam MQ, et al. Chromosomal assignment of retinoic acid receptor (RAR) genes in the human, mouse, and rat genomes. Genomics. 1991; 10:1061–9.
5. Greene ME, Blumberg B, McBride OW, Yi HF, Kronquist K, Kwan K, Hsieh L, Greene G, Nimer SD. Isolation of the human peroxisome proliferator activated receptor gamma cDNA: expression in hematopoietic cells and chromosomal mapping. Gene Expr. 1995;4:281–99.
6. Vidal-Puig AJ, Considine RV, Jimenez-Linan M, Werman A, Pories WJ, Caro JF, Flier JS. Peroxisome proliferator-activated receptor gene expression in human tissues. J Clin Invest. 1997;99:2416–22.
7. Gouda HN, Sagoo GS, Harding AH, Yates J, Sandhu MS, Higgins JP. The association between the peroxisome proliferator-activated receptor-gamma2 (PPARG2) Pro12Ala gene variant and type 2 diabetes mellitus: a HuGE review and meta-analysis. Am J Epidemiol. 2010;171:645–55.
8. Schmidt A, Endo N, Rutledge SJ, Vogel R, Shinar D, Rodan GA. Identification of a new member of the steroid hormone receptor superfamily that is activated by a peroxisome proliferator and fatty acids. Mol Endocrinol. 1992;6:1634–41.
9. Issemann I, Green S. Activation of a member of the steroid hormone receptor superfamily by peroxisome proliferators. Nature. 1990;347:645–50.
10. Youssef J, Badr M. Role of peroxisome proliferator-activated receptors in inflammation control. J Biomed Biotechnol. 2004;3:156–66.
11. Hummasti S, Tontonoz P. The peroxisome proliferator-activated receptor N-terminal domain controls isotype-selective gene expression and adipogenesis. Mol Endocrinol. 2006;20:1261–75.
12. Devchand P, Keller H, Peters H, Vasquze M, Gonzalez F, Wahli W. The PPAR alpha-leukotriene B4 pathway to inflammation control. Nature. 1996;384:39–43.

13. Kliewer SA, Sundseth SS, Jones SA, Brown PJ, Wisely GB, Koble CS. Fatty acids and eicosanoids regulate gene expression through direct interactions with peroxisome proliferator-activated receptors α and γ. Proc Natl Acad Sci USA. 1997;94:4318–23.
14. Forman BM, Chen J, Evans RM. Hypolipidemic drugs, polyunsaturated fatty acids, and eicosanoids are ligands for peroxisome proliferator-activated receptors α and δ. Proc Natl Acad Sci USA. 1997;94:4312–7.
15. Willson TM, Brown PJ, Sternbach DD, Henke BR. The PPARs: from orphan receptors to drug discovery. J Med Chem. 2000;43:527–50.
16. Chakravarthy MV, Lodhi IJ, Yin L, Malapaka RV, Xu HE, Turk J, Semenkovich CF. Identification of a physiologically relevant endogenous ligand for PPAR α in liver. Cell. 2009;138:476–88.
17. Lee JM, Lee YK, Mamrosh JL, Busby SA, Griffin PR, Pathak MC, et al. A nuclear-receptor-dependent phosphatidylcholine pathway with antidiabetic effects. Nature. 2011;474:506–12.
18. Mukherjee R, Jow L, Noonan D, McDonnell DP. Human and rat peroxisome proliferator activated receptors (PPARs) demonstrate similar tissue distribution but different responsiveness to PPAR activators. J Steroid Biochem Mol Biol. 1994;51:157–66.
19. Schoonjans K, Staels B, Auwerx J. The peroxisome proliferator activated receptors (PPARs) and their effects on lipid metabolism and adipocyte differentiation. Biochim Biophys Acta. 1996;1302:93–109.
20. Nissen SE, Nicholls SJ, Wolski K, Howey DC, McErlean E, Wang MD, et al. Effects of a potent and selective PPAR-alpha agonist in patients with atherogenic dyslipidemia or hypercholesterolemia: two randomized controlled trials. JAMA. 2007;297:1362–73.
21. Harris PK, Kletzien RF. Localization of a pioglitazone response element in the adipocyte fatty acid-binding protein gene. Mol Pharmacol. 1994;45: 439–45.
22. Lehmann JM, Moore LB, Smith-Oliver TA, Wilkison WO, Willson TM, Kliewer SA. An antidiabetic thiazolidinedione is a high affinity ligand for peroxisome proliferator-activated receptor gamma (PPAR gamma). J Biol Chem. 1995;270:12953–6.
23. Matsuzawa Y, Funahashi T, Nakamura T. Molecular mechanism of metabolic syndrome X: contribution of adipocytokines adipocytes-derived bioactive substances. Ann N Y Acad Sci. 1999;892:146–54.
24. Wagner JA, Wright EC, Ennis MM, Prince M, Kochan J, Nunez DJ, et al. Utility of adiponectin as a biomarker predictive of glycemic efficacy is demonstrated by collaborative pooling of data from clinical trials conducted by multiple sponsors. Clin Pharmacol Ther. 2009;86:619–25.
25. Berger J, Leibowitz MD, Doebber TW, Elbrecht A, Zhang B, Zhou G, et al. Novel peroxisome proliferator-activated receptor (PPAR) γ and PPAR δ ligands produce distinct biological effects. J Biol Chem. 1999;274:6718–25.
26. Oliver WR, Shenk JL, Snaith MR, Russell CS, Plunket KD, Bodkin NL, et al. A selective peroxisome proliferator-activated receptor δ agonist promotes reverse cholesterol transport. Proc Natl Acad Sci USA. 2001;98:5306–11.
27. Rosenfeld MG, Lunyak VV, Glass CK. Sensors and signals: a coactivator/corepressor/epigenetic code for integrating signal-dependent programs of transcriptional response. Genes Dev. 2006;20:1405–28.
28. Jiang C, Ting AT, Seed B. PPAR-γ agonists inhibit production of monocyte inflammatory cytokines. Nature. 1998;391:82–6.
29. Staels B, Koenig W, Habib A, Merval R, Lebret M, Torra IP, et al. Activation of human aortic smooth-muscle cells is inhibited by PPAR alpha but not by PPAR gamma activators. Nature. 1998;393:790–3.
30. Delerive P, De Bosscher K, Besnard S, Vanden Berghe W, Peters JM, Gonzalez FJ, et al. Peroxisome proliferator-activated receptor alpha negatively regulates the vascular inflammatory gene response by negative cross-talk with transcription factors NF-kappa B and AP-1. J Biol Chem. 1999;274:32048–54.
31. Lee C-H, Chawla A, Urbiztondo N, Liao D, Boisvert WA, Evans RM. Transcriptional repression of atherogenic inflammation: modulation by PPAR delta. Science. 2003;302:453–7.
32. Rival Y, Benéteau N, Taillandier T, Pezet M, Dupont-Passelaigue E, Patoiseau JF, et al. PPARalpha and PPARdelta activators inhibit cytokine-induced nuclear translocation of NF-kappaB and expression of VCAM-1 in EAhy926 endothelial cells. Eur J Pharmacol. 2002;435:143–51.
33. Fernandez-Marcos PJ, Auwerx J. Regulation of PGC-1α, a nodal regulator of mitochondrial biogenesis. Am J Clin Nutr. 2011;93:884S–90.
34. Yamamoto H, Williams EG, Mouchiroud L, Cantó C, Fan W, Downes M, et al. NCoR1 is a conserved physiological modulator of muscle mass and oxidative function. Cell. 2011;147:827–39.
35. Li P, Fan W, Xu J, Lu M, Yamamoto H, Auwerx J. Adipocyte NCoR knockout decreases PPARγ phosphorylation and enhances PPARγ activity and insulin sensitivity. Cell. 2011;147:815–26.
36. Reilly SM, Bhargava P, Liu S, Gangl MR, Gorgun C, Nofsinger RR, et al. Nuclear receptor corepressor SMRT regulates mitochondrial oxidative metabolism and mediates aging-related metabolic deterioration. Cell Metab. 2010;12:643–53.
37. Hu E, Kim JB, Sarraf P, Spiegelman BM. Inhibition of adipogenesis through MAP kinase-mediated phosphorylation of PPAR gamma. Science. 1996;274:2100–3.
38. Juge-Aubry CE, Hammar E, Siegrist-Kaiser C, Pernin A, Takeshita A, Chin WW, et al. Regulation of the transcriptional activity of the peroxisome proliferator-activated receptor alpha by phosphorylation of a ligand-independent trans-activating domain. J Biol Chem. 1999;274:10505–10.

39. Martin G, Duez H, Blanquart C, Berezowski V, Poulain P, Fruchart JC, et al. Statin-induced inhibition of the Rho-signaling pathway activates PPARalpha and induces HDL apoA-I. J Clin Invest. 2001;107:1423–32.
40. Inoue I, Itoh F, Aoyagi S, Tazawa S, Kusama H, Akahane M, Mastunaga T, et al. Fibrate and statin synergistically increase the transcriptional activities of PPARα/RXRα and decrease the transactivation of NFκB. Biochem Biophys Res Commun. 2002;290: 131–9.
41. Burns KA, Vanden Heuvel JP. Modulation of PPAR activity via phosphorylation. Biochim Biophys Acta. 2007;1771:952–60.
42. Choi JH, Banks AS, Estall JL, Kajimura S, Bostrom P, Laznik D, et al. Anti-diabetic drugs inhibit obesity-linked phosphorylation of PPARγ by Cdk5. Nature. 2010;466:451–7.
43. Choi JH, Banks AS, Kamenecka TM, Busby SA, Chalmers MJ, Kumar N, et al. Antidiabetic actions of a non-agonist PPARγ ligand blocking Cdk5-mediated phosphorylation. Nature. 2011;477:477–81.
44. Hauser S, Adelmant G, Sarraf P, Wright HM, Mueller E, Spiegelman BM. Degradation of the peroxisome proliferator-activated receptor gamma is linked to ligand-dependent activation. J Biol Chem. 2000;275:18527–33.
45. Blanquart C, Barbier O, Fruchart JC, Staels B, Glineur C. Peroxisome proliferator-activated receptor alpha (PPARalpha) turnover by the ubiquitin-proteasome system controls the ligand-induced expression level of its target genes. J Biol Chem. 2002;277:37254–9.
46. Genini D, Catapano CV. Block of nuclear receptor ubiquitination. A mechanism of ligand-dependent control of peroxisome proliferator-activated receptor δ activity. J Biol Chem. 2007;282:11776–85.
47. Pascual G, Fong AL, Ogawa S, Gamliel A, Li AC, Perissi V, et al. A SUMOylation-dependent pathway mediates transrepression of inflammatory response genes by PPAR-gamma. Nature. 2005;437:759–63.
48. Dutchak PA, Katafuchi T, Bookout AL, Choi JL, Yu RT, Mangelsdorf DJ, Kliewer SA. Fibroblast growth factor-21 regulates PPAR γ activity and the antidiabetic actions of thiazolidinediones. Cell. 2012;148:556–67.
49. Pourcet B, Pineda-Torra I, Derudas B, Staels B, Glineur C. SUMOylation of human peroxisome proliferator-activated receptor alpha inhibits its transactivity through the recruitment of the nuclear corepressor NCoR. J Biol Chem. 2010;285:5983–92.
50. Wadosky KM, Willis MS. The story so far: post translational regulation of peroxisome proliferator-activated receptors by ubiquitination and SUMOylation. Am J Physiol Heart Circ Physiol. 2011;302:H515–26.
51. Wang C, Powell MJ, Popov VM, Pestell RG. Acetylation in nuclear receptor signaling and the role of sirtuins. Mol Endocrinol. 2008;22:539–45.
52. Lerin C, Rodgers JT, Kalume DE, Kim SH, Pandey A, Puigserver P. GCN5 acetyltransferase complex controls glucose metabolism through transcriptional repression of PGC-1alpha. Cell Metab. 2006;3: 429–38.
53. Finkel T, Deng CX, Mostoslavsy P. Recent progress in the biology and physiology of sirtuins. Nature. 2009;460:587–91.
54. Camp HS, Li O, Wise SC, Hong YH, Frankowski CL, Shen X, et al. Differential activation of peroxisome proliferator-activated receptor-[gamma] by troglitazone and rosiglitazone. Diabetes. 2000;49: 539–47.
55. Olefsky JM. Treatment of insulin resistance with peroxisome proliferator-activated receptor gamma agonists. J Clin Invest. 2000;106:467–72.
56. Shang Y, Hu X, DiRenzo J, Lazar MA, Brow M. Cofactor dynamics and sufficiency in estrogen receptor-regulated transcription. Cell. 2000;103:843–52.
57. Issa LL, Leong GM, Sutherland RL, Eisman JA. Vitamin D analogue-specific recruitment of vitamin D receptor coactivators. J Bone Miner Res. 2002;17: 879–90.
58. Higgins LS, Mantzoros CS. The development of INT131 as a selective PPAR γ modulator: approach to a safer insulin sensitizer. PPAR Res. 2008. doi:10.1155/2009/936906.
59. Duez H, Lefebvre B, Poulain P, Pineda Torra I, Percevault F, Luc G, et al. Regulation of human ApoA-I by gemfibrozil and fenofibrate through selective peroxisome proliferator-activated receptor α modulation. Arterioscler Thromb Vasc Biol. 2005;25:1–7.
60. Pirat C, Farce A, Lebegue N, Renault N, Furman C, Millet R, et al. Targeting peroxisome proliferator-activated receptors (PPARs): development of modulators. J Med Chem. 2012 Jan 19. doi:10.1021/jm101360s.
61. McHutchison J, Goodman Z, Patel K, Makhlouf H, Rodriguez-Torres M, Shiffman M. Farglitazar lacks antifibrotic activity in patients with chronic hepatitis C infection. Gastroenterology. 2010;138:1365–73.
62. Guan Y, Breyer MD. Peroxisome proliferator-activated receptors (PPARs): novel therapeutic target in renal disease. Kidney Int. 2001;60:14–30.
63. Aleshin S, Grabeklis S, Hanck T, Sergeeva M, Reiser G. Peroxisome proliferator-activated receptor (PPAR)-gamma positively controls and PPARalpha negatively controls cyclooxygenase-2 expression in rat brain astrocytes through a convergence on PPARbeta/delta via mutual control of PPAR expression levels. Mol Pharmacol. 2009;76:414–24.
64. Ravnskjaer K, Frigerio F, Boergesen M, Nielsen T, Maechler P, Mandrup S. PPAR delta is a fatty acid sensor that enhances mitochondrial oxidation in insulin-secreting cells and protects against fatty acid-induced dysfunction. J Lipid Res. 2010;51:1370–9.
65. Ravnskjaer K, Boergesen M, Rubi B, Larsen JK, Nielsen T, Fridriksson J, et al. Peroxisome

proliferator-activated receptor α (PPARα) potentiates, whereas PPAR γ attenuates, glucose-stimulated insulin secretion in pancreatic β cells. Endocrinology. 2005;146:3266–76.
66. Liu S, Lui Q, Li L, Huan Y, Sun S, Shen Z. Long-term fenofibrate treatment impaired glucose-stimulated insulin secretion and up-regulated pancreatic NF-kappa B and iNOS expression in monosodium glutamate-induced obese rats: is it a latent disadvantage? J Transl Med. 2011;9:176.
67. Yajima K, Hirose H, Fujita H, Seto Y, Fujita H, Ukeda K, et al. Combination therapy with PPAR γ and PPAR α agonists increases glucose-stimulated insulin secretion in db/db mice. Am J Physiol Endocrinol Metab. 2003;284:E966–71.
68. Cohen G, Riahi Y, Shamni O, Guichardant M, Chatgilialoglu C, Ferreri C, et al. Role of lipid peroxidation and PPAR-δ in amplifying glucose-stimulated insulin secretion. Diabetes. 2011;60:2830–42.
69. Kono T, Ahn G, Moss DR, Gann L, Zarain-Herzberg A, Nishiki Y, et al. PPAR γ activation restores pancreatic islet SERCA2 levels and prevents β-cell dysfunction under conditions of hyperglycaemic and cytokine stress. Mol Endocrinol. 2012;26:257–71.
70. Engelen W, Manuel-y-Keenoy B, Vertommen J, De Leeuw I, Van Gaal L. Effects of micronized fenofibrate and vitamin E on in vitro oxidation of lipoproteins in patients with type 1 diabetes mellitus. Diabetes Metab. 2005;31:197–204.
71. A trial in adults with type 1 diabetes mellitus evaluating the effects of fenofibrate versus placebo on macular thickness and volume (FAME 1 EYE). Available from: http://clinicaltrials.gov/ct2/show/NCT01320345. Last Accessed 8 Mar 2012.
72. Winocour PH, Durrington PN, Bhatagnar D, Ishola M, Arrol S, Lahor BC, Anderson DC. Double-blind placebo-controlled study of the effects of bezafibrate on blood lipids, lipoproteins and fibrinogen in hypercholipidaemic type 1 diabetes. Diabet Med. 1990;7:736–43.
73. Winocour PH, Durrington PN, Bhatagnar D, Ishola M, Mackness M, Arrol S, Anderson DC. The effect of bezafibrate on very low density lipoprotein (VLDL), intermediate density lipoprotein (IDL), and low density lipoprotein (LDL) composition in type 1 diabetes associated with hypercholesterolaemia or combined hyperlipidaemia. Atherosclerosis. 1992;93:83–94.
74. Tenenbaum A, Motro M, Fisman EZ. Dual and pan-peroxisome proliferator-activated receptors (PPAR) co-agonism: the bezafibrate lessons. Cardiovasc Diabetol. 2005;4:14. doi:10.1186/475-2840-4-14.
75. Strowig SM, Raskin P. The effect of rosiglitazone on overweight subjects with type 1 diabetes. Diabetes Care. 2005;28:1562–7.
76. Stone ML, Walker JL, Chisholm D, Craig ME, Donaghue KC, Crock P, et al. The addition of rosiglitazone to insulin in adolescents with type 1 diabetes and poor glycaemic control: a randomized-controlled trial. Pediatr Diabetes. 2008;9(part 1):326–34.
77. Bhat R, Bhansali A, Bhadada S, Sialy R. Effect of pioglitazone therapy in lean type 1 diabetes mellitus. Diabetes Res Clin Pract. 2007;78:349–54.
78. Shimada A, Shigihara T, Okubo Y, Katsuki T, Yamada Y, Oikawa Y. Pioglitazone may accelerate disease course of slowly progressive type 1 diabetes. Diabetes Metab Res Rev. 2011;27:951–3.
79. Buchanan TA, Xiang AH, Peters RK, Kjos SL, Marroquin A, Goico J, et al. Preservation of pancreatic beta-cell function and prevention of type 2 diabetes by pharmacological treatment of insulin resistance in high-risk Hispanic women. Diabetes. 2002;51:2796–803.
80. Gerstein HC, Yusuf S, Bosch J, Pogue J, Sheridan P, Dinccag N, et al. Effect of rosiglitazone on the frequency of diabetes in patients with impaired glucose tolerance or impaired fasting glucose. Lancet. 2006;368:1096–105.
81. DeFronzo RA, Tripathy D, Schwenke DC, Banerji M, Bray GA, Buchanan TA. Pioglitazone for diabetes prevention in impaired glucose tolerance. N Engl J Med. 2011;364:1104–15.
82. Dormandy JA, Charbonnel B, Eckland DJ, Erdmann E, Massi-Benedetti M, Moules IK, et al. Secondary prevention of macrovascular events in patients with type 2 diabetes in the PROactive Study (PROspective pioglitAzone Clinical Trial in macroVascular Events): a randomised controlled trial. Lancet. 2005;366:1279–89.
83. Derosa G. Efficacy and tolerability of pioglitazone in patients with type 2 diabetes mellitus: comparison with other oral antihyperglycaemic agents. Drugs. 2010;70:1945–61.
84. Krentz AJ. Rosiglitazone: trials, tribulations and termination. Drugs. 2011;71:123–30.
85. Friedland SN, Leong A, Filion KB, Genest J, Lega IC, Mottillo S, et al. The cardiovascular effects of peroxisome proliferator-activated receptor agonists. Am J Med. 2012;125:126–33.
86. Nissen SE, Wolski K, Topol EJ. Effect of muraglitazar on death and major adverse cardiovascular events in patients with type 2 diabetes mellitus. JAMA. 2005;294:2581–6.
87. FDA guidance for the industry. Diabetes mellitus. Developing drugs and therapeutic biologics for treatment and prevention. www.fda.gov/downloads/Drugs/GuidanceComplianceRegulatoryInformation/Guidances/UCM071624.pdf. Accessed 17 Feb 2012.
88. FDA guidance for industry. Diabetes Mellitus. Evaluating cardiovascular risk in new antidiabetic therapies to treat type 2 Diabetes. www.fda.gov/downloads/Drugs/GuidanceComplianceRegulatoryInformation/Guidances/UCM071627.pdf. Accessed 17 Feb 2012.
89. The TIDE Trial Investigators. Design, history and results of the thiazolidinedione intervention with

vitamin D evaluation (TIDE) randomised controlled trial. Diabetologia. 2012;55:36–45.
90. A study with aleglitazar in patients with a recent acute coronary syndrome and type 2 diabetes. Available from: http://clinicaltrials.gov/ct2/show/NCT01042769. Last Accessed 8 Mar 2012.
91. Henry RR, Lincoff AM, Mudaliar S, Rabbia M, Chognot C, Herz M. Effect of the dual peroxisome proliferator-activated receptor-alpha/gamma agonist aleglitazar on risk of cardiovascular disease in patients with type 2 diabetes (SYNCHRONY): a phase II, randomised, dose-ranging study. Lancet. 2009;374:126–35.
92. Herz M, Gaspari F, Perico N, Viberti G, Urbanowska T, Rabbia M, et al. Effects of high dose aleglitazar on renal function in patients with type 2 diabetes. Int J Cardiol. 2011;151(2):136–42.
93. Efficacy and safety of CKD-501 versus pioglitazone when added to metformin. Available from: http://clinicaltrials.gov/ct2/show/NCT01106131. Last Accessed 8 Mar 2012.
94. A clinical trial to evaluate the safety and efficacy of ZYH7 compared with fenofibrate in patients with dyslipidemia. Available from: http://clinicaltrials.gov/ct2/results?term=01539616. Last Accessed 1 Mar 2012.
95. Henriksen K, Byrjalsen I, Qvist P, Beck-Nielsen H, Hansen G, Riis BJ. Efficacy and safety of the PPARγ partial agonist balaglitazone compared with pioglitazone and placebo: a phase III, randomized, parallel-group study in patients with type 2 diabetes on stable insulin therapy. Diabetes Metab Res Rev. 2011;27:392–401.
96. A placebo-controlled safety and efficacy study of INT131 besylate in type 2 diabetes with an active comparator. Available from: http://clinicaltrials.gov/ct2/results?term=00631007. Last Accessed 1 Mar 2012.
97. Risérus U, Sprecher D, Johnson T, Olson E, Hirschberg S, Liu A, et al. Activation of peroxisome proliferator-activated receptor (PPAR)delta promotes reversal of multiple metabolic abnormalities, reduces oxidative stress, and increases fatty acid oxidation in moderately obese men. Diabetes. 2008;57:332–9.
98. Ooi EM, Watts GF, Sprecher DL, Chan DC, Barrett PH. Mechanism of action of a peroxisome proliferator-activated receptor (PPAR)-delta agonist on lipoprotein metabolism in dyslipidemic subjects with central obesity. J Clin Endocrinol Metab. 2011;96:E1568–76.
99. Bays HE, Schwartz S, Littlejohn T 3rd, Kerzner B, Krauss RM, Karpf DB. MBX-8025, a novel peroxisome proliferator receptor-delta agonist: lipid and other metabolic effects in dyslipidemic overweight patients treated with and without atorvastatin. J Clin Endocrinol Metab. 2011;96:2889–97.
100. Cariou B, Zaïr Y, Staels B, Bruckert E. Effects of the new dual PPAR α/δ agonist GFT505 on lipid and glucose homeostasis in abdominally obese patients with combined dyslipidemia or impaired glucose metabolism. Diabetologia. 2011;34:2008–14.
101. A multicenter, randomized, double-blind, double-dummy, parallel-group, placebo-controlled, Study to Evaluate Efficacy, Safety and Tolerability of Oral GW677954 Capsules (2.5, 5, 10, 15 And 20 mg Once A Day) as a Monotherapy (Diet and/or exercise treated) or as an Add-On to Metformin for 16 Weeks Duration in Subjects with Type 2 Diabetes Mellitus. Study No.: ADG20001, available on: gsk-clinicalstudyregister.com/files/20462.pdf - 2010-.
102. Sanwald-Ducray P, Liogier D'ardhuy X, Jamois C, Banken L. Pharmacokinetics, pharmacodynamics, and tolerability of aleglitazar in patients with type 2 diabetes: results from a randomized, placebo-controlled clinical study. Clin Pharmacol Ther. 2010;88:197–203.

# Fibrate Therapy: Impact on Dyslipidemia and Cardiovascular Events in Diabetic Patients

# 20

Eliot A. Brinton

## Introduction

Coronary heart disease (CHD) and ischemic stroke are both primarily due to atherosclerosis. Due to their common pathophysiology, they are often considered together under the term of cardiovascular disease (CVD). CVD is the leading cause of morbidity and mortality in the United States [1], with over three-quarters of a million new cases of CHD and a similar number of strokes each year. Lowering of levels of low-density lipoprotein-cholesterol (LDL-C) with statin monotherapy is well proven to reduce CVD events by about 20–50 % [2]. Importantly, the degree of risk reduction is proportional to the degree of LDL-C decrease—21 % CVD event decrease per 39 mg/dL (1 mmol/L) LDL-C decrease [2]—and an identical 21 % decrease per 39 mg/dL decrease is seen in patients with diabetes mellitus type 2 (DM-2) [3]. Due to higher overall CVD risk in DM-2 (other risk factors being equal), the absolute risk reduction is greater than in those without DM-2, and only 24 patients with DM-2 would need a statin-induced 39 mg/dL decrease in LDL-C for 5 years to prevent one major CVD event. Although such treatment is clinically useful and generally cost-effective, it is important to note that the majority of CVD events, roughly 50–80 %, still occur despite statin treatment [4–7]. Of course, there is considerable interest in learning how to reduce this large residual risk. This is especially true in patients with high CVD risk due to strong risk factors such as DM-2, among whom the 50–80 % residual CVD risk is thus larger in absolute terms.

Much of the excess CVD risk in DM-2 appears to come from the characteristic "atherogenic dyslipidemia" often seen with this disorder. It consists of high plasma triglyceride (TG) levels, low HDL-C levels, and an increased number of smaller, denser LDL particles and usually without elevated LDL-C levels. Importantly, this classic diabetic dyslipidemia is not well addressed by statin treatment. Instead, it is well treated by a class of peroxisome proliferator activator receptor (PPAR)-alpha agonists called fibrates. The impact of fibrates on dyslipidemia and related CVD risk factors, and on CVD risk itself, in patients with DM-2 is the focus of this chapter.

E.A. Brinton, M.D., FAHA., FNLA. (✉)
Cardiovascular Genetics, University of Utah School of Medicine, 30 N. 1900 E., Salt Lake City, UT, USA

Utah Lipid Center, Salt Lake City, UT, USA

Utah Foundation for Biomedical Research, Salt Lake City, UT, USA
e-mail: eliot.brinton@utahresearch.org; eliot.brinton@utahlipidcenter.com; eliot.brinton@utah.edu

A.J. Jenkins et al. (eds.), *Lipoproteins in Diabetes Mellitus*, Contemporary Diabetes,
DOI 10.1007/978-1-4614-7554-5_20, © Springer Science+Business Media New York 2014

## Pathophysiology of the Atherogenic (Diabetic) Dyslipidemia and Atherosclerosis

Epidemiological studies consistently show that HDL-C levels are inversely associated with atherosclerosis, and CVD risk [8–11], and that low HDL-C is particularly prevalent in patients with DM-2 [12]. Importantly, even with aggressive statin therapy and the achievement of low LDL-C levels, low HDL-C levels remain an independent cardiovascular risk factor, appearing to account for a significant percentage of the residual CVD event risk in this setting [13–15].

High residual CVD risk related to low HDL-C despite statin treatment was recently confirmed in a clinical trial, Atherothrombosis Intervention in Metabolic Syndrome with Low HDL/High Triglycerides: Impact on Global Health Outcomes (AIM-HIGH), which recruited subjects primarily for prior CVD and low HDL-C levels [16]. The vast majority of subjects had been on statin therapy prior to study entry, and as a part of the study protocol, all were treated with aggressive statin-based treatment to an LDL-C goal of less than 80 mg/dL (median on-study LDL-C levels were 67 or 62 mg/dL, depending on study arm, decreased from baseline median of 74). Although HDL-C levels increased with varying degrees of niacin treatment in both study arms, on-study HDL-C remained low (median 38 and 42 mg/dL, depending on study arm, increased from baseline median 35). In this setting of persistent low HDL-C despite extensive statin-based LDL-C lowering, a staggering 5.4 % of the overall subject population had a major CVD event per year during the 3 years average follow-up (with or without added high-dose niacin treatment) [16]. Fully one-third of the subjects had DM-2 at study entry [16]. It is likely, although as yet unreported, that many of the two-thirds of subjects without DM-2 had insulin resistance and that both these and subjects with DM-2 also had persistently high CVD rates despite aggressive study-related statin treatment.

In discussing the relationship between HDL levels and CVD risk, it is well to consider HDL composition and function. Plasma steady-state HDL-C levels do not directly reflect the antiatherogenic and vascular protective effects of HDL particles. Measurement of one particular antiatherogenic HDL function, such as its capacity to promote cholesterol efflux or to inhibit LDL oxidation, can be made in cell culture systems and have been proposed to be more effective than HDL-C levels in assessing CVD risk [17]. Despite such promise, however, there are only very limited data regarding how well any particular assay of HDL function may predict atherosclerosis or CVD risk, and so there is no consensus regarding which measurement to use [18, 19]. Further, any measurement of HDL function will likely be very cumbersome for clinical use. In this context it is well to remember that the composition of a given HDL particle must determine its function(s), and thus, the appropriate HDL compositional assay could prove to be a good surrogate for measurement of HDL function. Complicating this, however, is a relative lack of data regarding advanced parameters of HDL composition, beyond total HDL-C, for CVD risk prediction, and the resulting lack of consensus regarding the HDL composition assay of choice. In addition to the fact that an advanced parameter of HDL composition is likely to be more difficult to assay than HDL-C, the relationship between HDL composition and function is likely complicated as being not only a determinant of future function but also a reflection of prior function. Thus, parameters of HDL composition, such as particle size or apolipoprotein content, are likely reasonable surrogates of HDL function, but they require further validation in general and also in the particular setting of fibrate treatment in DM-2.

High TG (HTG) levels are another dyslipidemia commonly found in DM-2 and associated with increased atherosclerosis and CVD risk [20]. For example, studies have shown substantial increases in CVD risk above a TG of 200 mg/dL [21, 22]. Further, a meta-analysis of observational studies found a 32 % and 76 % increased risk of CVD in men and women, respectively, for each 88 mg/dL increase in TG independent of HDL-C levels [23]. Since fibrate treatment exerts its most prominent lipid effect on TG levels, it is of key importance in the considerations of this chapter to realize that plasma TG predicts CVD risk even in the setting of aggressive statin-based LDL-C lowering [24–27]. The association of HTG with CVD may be especially strong with non-fasting TG levels, especially in women [28, 29].

Despite the strength and consistency of these observational associations, by themselves they do not establish that either HTG or low HDL-C is a causal factor in atherosclerosis. There are many biological mechanisms, however, by which HDL may be able to prevent atherosclerosis or promote its stabilization or regression, and some of these have been shown to operate in human subjects. This interesting and much-studied topic has been the object of recent reviews [30–33].

Although there is less evidence for mechanisms by which HTG could contribute directly to atherogenesis, compared to that for low HDL levels, there are at least two ways in which TG levels may have direct causal effects. First, several types of TG-rich lipoproteins are directly atherogenic [34], and their excess is largely signaled by high plasma TG levels. Second, artery wall macrophages can readily lipolyze TG from TG-rich lipoproteins, and the products of that lipolysis can be pro-inflammatory and pro-atherogenic [35]. A third likely contribution of HTG to atherogenesis is less direct. HTG is strongly associated with small, dense (SD) LDL particles due to exchange of TG for CE in the core of LDL via CETP. Although this initial exchange does not reduce core size, subsequent lipolysis of LDL TG results in decreased core lipid, resulting in SD LDL particles [36]. In HTG patients, a similar effect on HDL particles results in smaller, denser HDL and in accelerated renal clearance of apo A-I which is lost from HDL as it shrinks [34, 37, 38]. The conjunction of these three lipid abnormalities, HTG, SD LDL, and low HDL-C levels, is termed "the atherogenic dyslipidemia," which is relatively common in insulin resistance and DM-2 [39].

SD LDL is associated with increased risk of CVD compared to larger, normal-sized LDL particles [40–43]. The mechanisms by which SD LDL appear to be more atherogenic include (1) increased penetration of smaller LDL from plasma through the endothelium into the subendothelial space, (2) greater adhesion to the subendothelial matrix, (3) greater susceptibility to become oxidized, and (4) less binding to and clearance by the LDL receptor [44].

## Fibrate Effects on Lipoprotein Levels

Several studies have reported the lipid effects of gemfibrozil and fenofibrate (the two fibrates clinically available in the USA), as outlined in two recent reviews, the data from which are summarized in Table 20.1 [45] and Fig. 20.1 [46]. The greatest and most consistent effect of fibrates on a major lipid parameter is a decrease in TG levels. In contrast with the variable changes in LDL-C and HDL-C levels (see below), fibrates always cause substantial decreases in TG levels, although the degree of decrease varies directly according to the baseline TG level (Table 20.1) [45, 46]. The effect of fenofibrate to reduce plasma TG levels is related to a significant reduction in the large buoyant VLDL1 (−46.5 %; $P<0.001$) which appears to be greater than in the smaller, denser VLDL2 (−33.3 %; $P<0.001$) [44]. VLDL1-TG levels are primary determinants of plasma TG and are related to SD LDL particles (see below).

Fibrates may decrease, increase, or have a neutral effect on LDL-C levels, and baseline TG can be a very strong positive determinant of these changes (Fig. 20.2) [45]. The increase in LDL-C seen with fibrate use in the setting of a high baseline TG level likely relates to an increase in average LDL particle size ($P<0.001$) [47–49], rather than due to an increase in LDL particle concentration. This is strongly suggested by the decrease in plasma apo B levels ($P<0.001$), even when baseline TG is low [48], since there is one apo B molecule per VLDL, IDL, and LDL particle, and the vast majority of apo B-containing particles are LDL. Importantly, TG content of the large VLDL1 particles, which is a primary determinant of total plasma TG levels, is also directly related to the prevalence of SD LDL particles. This could be because large VLDL1 are direct precursors of SD LDL. More likely, however, it is because

**Table 20.1** Effects of fenofibrate and gemfibrozil on TG, LDL-C, and HDL-C in published randomized placebo-controlled trials (adapted from Abourbih et al. [45])

| | | | | TG | | LDL-C | | HDL-C | |
|---|---|---|---|---|---|---|---|---|---|
| First author (ref. #) | Year published | *N* | Duration | Baseline TG | Placebo-corrected % change TG | Baseline LDL-C | Placebo-corrected % change LDL-C | Baseline HDL-C | Placebo-corrected % change HDL-C |
| *Fenofibrate* | | | | | | | | | |
| Keech | 2005 | 9,795 | 260 | 153.5 | −23 % | 118.5 | −6 % | 42.5 | 1 % |
| Vakkilainen | 2003 | 405 | 172 | 225.6 | −24 % | 130.5 | −9 % | 39.6 | 3 % |
| Farnier[a] | 2005 | 253 | 12 | 276.5 | −26 % | 165 | −3 % | 42.5 | 16 % |
| Farnier[a] | 2005 | 372 | 12 | 274.3 | −33 % | 160.2 | −5 % | 42.5 | 15 % |
| Farnier[a] | 2007 | 244 | 12 | 231.1 | −38 % | 162.6 | −11 % | 45.3 | 19 % |
| Farnier[a] | 2007 | 367 | 12 | 226.4 | −20 % | 162.1 | −1 % | 44.7 | 1 % |
| Knopp | 1987 | 227 | 24 | 193.1 | −44 % | NR | NA | 47.5 | 21 % |
| Davidson | 2006 | 146 | 8 | 479.7 | −37 % | 119.3 | 16 % | 35.7 | 16 % |
| Krempf | 2000 | 138 | 13 | 127.9 | −40 % | 225.7 | −33 % | 56.8 | 4 % |
| Seidehamel | 1989 | 147 | 8 | 614.6 | −56 % | 109.9 | 34 % | 30.8 | 22 % |
| Nissen | 2007 | 102 | 12 | 246 | −37 % | NR | NA | 37.4 | 15 % |
| *Gemfibrozil* | | | | | | | | | |
| Frick | 1987 | 4,081 | 262 | 176 | −36 % | 188.7 | −9 % | 47.3 | 9 % |
| Rubins | 1999 | 2,531 | 52 | 160.5 | −32 % | 111.5 | 0 % | 32 | 6 % |
| Frick | 1993 | 628 | 260 | 183.2 | −41 % | 188.1 | −11 % | 46.3 | 10 % |
| Vinik | 1993 | 442 | 20 | 272.3 | −32 % | NR | NA | NR | NA |
| Schaeffer | 1996 | 305 | 13 | 177.2 | −42 % | 206.5 | −10 % | 34.8 | 10 % |
| Avogaro | 1999 | 217 | 20 | 317 | −52 % | NR | NA | NR | NA |
| Wiklund | 1993 | 137 | 12 | 159.8 | −44 % | 198.8 | −14 % | 46.3 | 19 % |

[a]These studies had separate study arms which tested fenofibrate against different background treatments and so are divided

| | Drug | Fibrate | | | Control | | | Weight | Mean difference IV, random, 95% CI |
|---|---|---|---|---|---|---|---|---|---|
| | | Mean | SD | Total | Mean | SD | Total | | |
| **LDL** | | | | | | | | | |
| LOCAT (1997)[27] | Gemfibrozil | 3·39 | 0·56 | 197 | 3·83 | 0·59 | 198 | 31·8% | −0·45 (−0·56 to −0·34) |
| Helsinki Heart (1987)[26] | Gemfibrozil | 4·48 | 0·79 | 2046 | 4·95 | 0·79 | 2035 | 33·9% | −0·47 (−0·52 to −0·42) |
| FIELD (2005)[16] | Fenofibrate | 2·43 | 0·65 | 4895 | 2·6 | 0·78 | 4900 | 34·2% | −0·17 (−0·20 to −0·14) |
| **Total (95% CI)** | | | | **7138** | | | **7133** | **100·0%** | **−0·36 (−0·59 to −0·13)** |
| Heterogeneity: $\tau^2$=0·04; $\chi^2$=120·85, df=2 (p<0·00001); $I^2$=98% | | | | | | | | | |
| Test for overall effect: Z=3·03 (p=0·002) | | | | | | | | | |
| **HDL** | | | | | | | | | |
| LOCAT (1997)[27] | Gemfibrozil | 0·98 | 0·17 | 197 | 0·88 | 0·15 | 198 | 31·0% | 0·10 (0·07 to 0·13) |
| Helsinki Heart (1987)[26] | Gemfibrozil | 1·32 | 0·3 | 2046 | 1·26 | 0·27 | 2035 | 34·1% | 0·06 (0·04 to 0·08) |
| FIELD (2005)[16] | Fenofibrate | 1·13 | 0·3 | 4895 | 1·12 | 0·29 | 4900 | 34·9% | 0·01 (−0·00 to 0·02) |
| **Total (95% CI)** | | | | **7138** | | | **7133** | **100·0%** | **0·05 (0·01 to 0·10)** |
| Heterogeneity: $\tau^2$=0·00; $\chi^2$=41·20, df=2 (p<0·00001); $I^2$=95% | | | | | | | | | |
| Test for overall effect: Z=2·22 (p=0·03) | | | | | | | | | |
| **Triglyceride** | | | | | | | | | |
| LOCAT (1997)[27] | Gemfibrozil | 1·02 | 0·37 | 197 | 1·69 | 0·68 | 198 | 25·2% | −0·67 (−0·78 to −0·56) |
| Helsinki Heart (1987)[26] | Gemfibrozil | 1·3 | 0·76 | 2046 | 2·0 | 1·06 | 2035 | 26·4% | −0·70 (−0·76 to −0·64) |
| FIELD (2005)[16] | Fenofibrate | 1·47 | 0·78 | 4895 | 1·87 | 0·96 | 4900 | 26·8% | −0·40 (−0·43 to −0·37) |
| Hanefeld (1991)[30] | Clofibrateil | 1·98 | 1·54 | 379 | 2·09 | 1·25 | 382 | 21·6% | −0·11 (−0·31 to 0·09) |
| **Total (95% CI)** | | | | **7517** | | | **7515** | **100·0%** | **−0·48 (−0·69 to −0·28)** |
| Heterogeneity: $\tau^2$=0·04; $\chi^2$=103·39, df=3 (p<0·00001); $I^2$=97% | | | | | | | | | |
| Test for overall effect: Z=4·54 (p<0·00001) | | | | | | | | | |
| **Total cholesterol** | | | | | | | | | |
| LOCAT (1997)[27] | Gemfibrozil | 4·83 | 0·63 | 197 | 5·48 | 0·68 | 198 | 24·7% | −0·65 (−0·78 to −0·52) |
| Helsinki Heart (1987)[26] | Gemfibrozil | 6·38 | 0·88 | 2046 | 7·04 | 0·82 | 2035 | 26·4% | −0·66 (−0·71 to −0·61) |
| FIELD (2005)[16] | Fenofibrate | 4·23 | 0·78 | 4895 | 4·56 | 0·9 | 4900 | 26·6% | −0·33 (−0·36 to −0·30) |
| Hanefeld (1991)[30] | Clofibrateil | 5·96 | 1·41 | 379 | 6·06 | 1·4 | 382 | 22·3% | −0·10 (−0·30 to 0·10) |
| **Total (95% CI)** | | | | **7517** | | | **7515** | **100·0%** | **−0·44 (−0·67 to −0·22)** |
| Heterogeneity: $\tau^2$=0·05; $\chi^2$=130·77, df=3 (p<0·00001); $I^2$=98% | | | | | | | | | |
| Test for overall effect: Z=3·80 (p=0·0001) | | | | | | | | | |

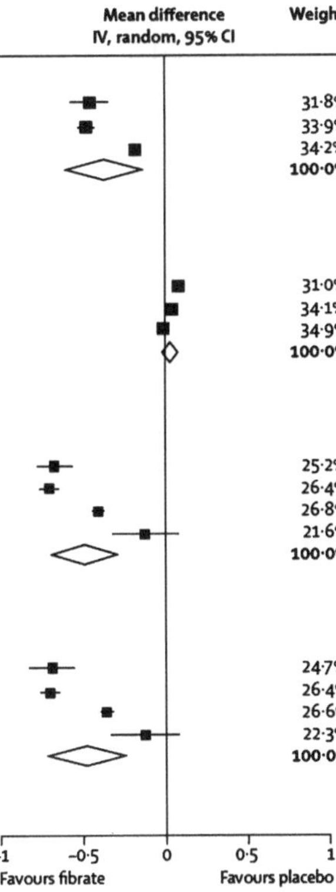


**Fig. 20.1** Effects of gemfibrozil, fenofibrate, and clofibrate on major lipid parameters from a meta-analysis of several large randomized controlled fibrate trials. The name of the study or of the first author and the publication year are noted (the numbered references are from the publication by Jun et al. [46])

VLDL1 drives CE depletion and TG enrichment of the LDL core, followed by rapid lipolysis of that TG, resulting in a net shrinkage of the core, and of the entire LDL particle [44]. Thus, the ability of fibrates to reduce levels of plasma TG in general and VLDL1 in particular appears to correct two major aspects of the so-called atherogenic dyslipidemia common in DM-2: high TG levels and SD LDL [44].

Low levels of HDL-C and of apo A-I clearly can result from HTG, by mechanisms similar to those for LDL size, noted above. That is, loss of CE and gain of TG by the HDL core is followed by rapid lipolysis of that TG, resulting in a net shrinkage of the core and of the entire HDL particle. Shrinkage of HDL results in exit of apo A-I from the particle, leading to rapid glomerular filtration and permanent catabolic loss of apo A-I from the plasma [38, 50]. Interestingly, however, the changes in HDL composition related to lower TG levels [38], and for that matter, niacin treatment [51, 52], which are larger particles, increased apo A-I and increased Lp A-I, are the opposite of those seen with fibrate use, as noted below. This suggests that fibrate-induced lowering of TG levels is not the mechanism by which fibrates raise HDL levels.

In addition to the strong impact of baseline TG levels on fibrate lipid effects, baseline HDL-C levels also may alter effects of fibrate treatment on major lipid parameters and HDL composition. Fenofibrate (160 mg/day) and simvastatin (40 mg/day) were given for 8 weeks in 52 patients, with moderate to very high CHD risk, selected for HDL-C levels <40 mg/dL [49]. Fenofibrate had dramatic effects on TG and HDL-C, with a 43 % decrease and 22 % increase, respectively, and baseline HDL-C was a strong inverse predictor of the HDL-C increase ($R$=−0.56, $P$=0.003). Despite the large increase in HDL-C with fenofibrate, plasma levels of the major HDL protein, apo A-I, did not change. In the same study, plasma

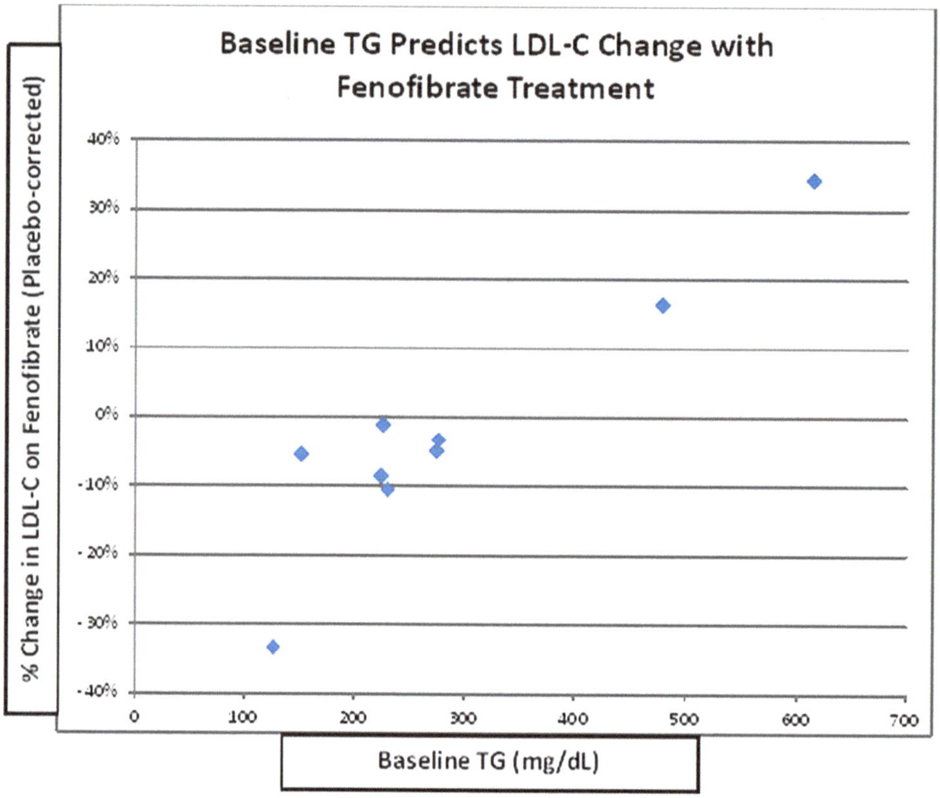


**Fig. 20.2** Baseline TG predicts change in LDL-C with fenofibrate. Data from published randomized clinical trials analyzed by Abourbih et al. [45]

levels of Lp A-I particles (HDL with apo A-I but lacking apo A-II) actually decreased following fenofibrate treatment but were unchanged after simvastatin treatment. The HDL subclass distribution shifted towards smaller particles (significant increase in small HDL and decrease in large HDL) with fenofibrate treatment, but no changes in HDL size distribution were observed with simvastatin [49]. Other studies have confirmed these results that fibrate treatment causes a decrease in average HDL size and primarily an increase in apo A-II content [48, 49, 53].

## Long-Term Effects of Fibrates on Lipids and Lipoproteins

An interesting paradox of fibrate therapy is a general lack of connection between lipid effects and CVD benefits. One manifestation is the lack of ability of lipid changes directly to predict reduction in CVD risk, as noted in the last section of this chapter. Another manifestation is that although lipid effects of fibrates may not be fully maintained throughout long-term clinical trials (see below), CVD effects tend to continue and even may increase with long-term treatment [54].

In the Fenofibrate Intervention and Event Lowering in Diabetes (FIELD) trial, in patients with diabetes, fenofibrate increased HDL-C levels modestly for the first 2–3 years after the start of treatment and then returned to near baseline levels by the end of the study [55]. There was a similar result of only partial long-term persistence of the initial HDL-C increase and TG reduction in the ACCORD-Lipid trial [56]. Interestingly, there appeared to be somewhat better preservation of HDL-C effects in the Helsinki Heart Study (HHS) with an average 11 % increase over the several years of the study [57]. Unfortunately, obvious possible explanations of the differences in persistence in long-term lipid effects among these studies, such as differences in patient compliance, do not appear to explain the discrepancies in degree and durability of lipid effects.

## Lipid and Lipid-Related Effects of Fibrates vs. Statins or in Combination with Them

The lipid effects of fibrates tend to be complementary to those of statins, as has been noted in prior reviews of various studies [58, 59]. For example, lipid effects of fenofibrate (160 mg/day) were compared with those of simvastatin (40 mg/day), as noted above [49]. Fenofibrate had dramatic effects on TG and HDL-C, with a 43 % decrease and 22 % increase, respectively. In contrast, the TG and HDL-C changes were far less with simvastatin (−15 % and +6 %, respectively). Conversely, simvastatin significantly reduced LDL-C and total cholesterol levels (−28 % and −19 %, respectively) whereas fenofibrate did not significantly affect these parameters [49].

Since the majority of dyslipidemic patients are treated with statins, the question of the additivity of fibrate effects on lipids to those of a statin is of great clinical importance. As noted in several studies and reviews [58–60], the lipid effects of fibrates tend to be additive (as well as complementary, as noted above) to those of statins. A special case of fibrate-statin interaction is the FIELD study, in which half the patients were randomized to double-blind fenofibrate treatment while statins, excluded at baseline, were given to a moderate number of subjects in a non-blinded "drop-in" fashion by non-study physicians as desired on clinical grounds. To attempt to assess lipid effects of fenofibrate monotherapy in FIELD, Hiukka et al. examined lipid parameter changes with fenofibrate treatment among subjects followed at the Helsinki site who did not have drop-in statin treatment during the 5 years of the study [48]. Mean age of these subjects was 62 ± 5.7 years and duration of diabetes averaged 6 years. Differences were noted between fenofibrate and placebo groups for total cholesterol (−18.7 %; $P<0.001$), TG (−25.8 %; $P<0.001$), and LDL-C (−20.5 %; $P<0.001$). No significant differences were observed between fenofibrate and placebo groups for HDL-C levels. Part of the explanation for the lack of HDL-C increase may lie in the fact that the mean baseline levels of HDL-C for both fenofibrate and placebo groups (42.9 mg/dL) were already above the NCEP ATP-III cutoff for low HDL-C (<40 mg/dL) [61] and the fact that HDL-C increases with any agent are generally inversely related to baseline HDL-C. It must be remembered that due to the nonrandom nature of the statin drop-in treatment in FIELD, these subjects are likely not representative of FIELD subjects in general, and so interpretation of lipid effects of fenofibrate in FIELD is unavoidably problematic.

## Effects of Fibrates on Lipoprotein-Related Factors of Cholesterol Transport

A major function of HDL appears to be the promotion of cholesterol removal or efflux from extrahepatic cells and then delivery of that cholesterol to the liver, where it can be excreted from the body, a process called reverse cholesterol transport. The initial step in this process appears to be through interaction of HDL with specific cell membrane transport proteins such as the ATP-binding cassette transporter (ABCA1) [62]. In contrast, the scavenger receptor B1 (SR-B1) is believed to play an important role in cholesterol transport from HDL to the liver as a last step of reverse cholesterol transport [18]. Using plasma from patients treated with fenofibrate or simvastatin (as a source of HDL), cholesterol flux between cells and lipoproteins was determined in macrophages for ABCA1-mediated efflux and in hepatoma cells for SR-B1-mediated flux (measured as efflux but presumably also reflecting the ability of HDL to mediate influx). ABCA1-mediated cholesterol efflux to plasma and HDL was significantly increased with plasma from fenofibrate—but not simvastatin-treated patients (Fig. 20.3) [49]. Conversely, SR-BI-mediated cholesterol flux was significantly increased with

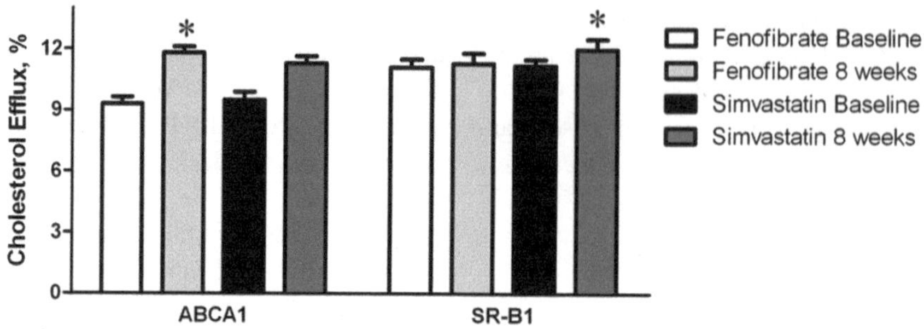


**Fig. 20.3** Efflux of cholesterol through the ABCA1-mediated and SR-B1-mediated pathways to plasma from low HDL-C patients treated with fenofibrate or simvastatin. Asterisk denotes $P = 0.015$ for fenofibrate increase on ABCA1 from baseline and $P = 0.016$ for simvastatin increase on SR-B1 from baseline (figure is adapted from Franceschini, et al. [49])

plasma from simvastatin—but not fenofibrate-treated patients (Fig. 20.3) [49]. Thus, a combination fenofibrate and statin therapy may be better than either drug alone to enhance the full process of reverse cholesterol transport from the periphery to the liver.

Two additional factors related to HDL metabolism, concentration, composition, and particle size distribution and to reverse cholesterol transport are cholesteryl ester transfer protein (CETP) and lecithin cholesterol acyl transferase (LCAT). Fenofibrate and simvastatin are reported to significantly increase CETP by 17 % and 9 %, respectively [49]. In contrast, another study reported decreased CETP activity with fenofibrate and found that the decrease was related to increased LDL particle size and decreased coronary intimal hyperplasia after angioplasty and stent placement [63]. An explanation for the contrast between the two studies in the findings on fenofibrate effects on CETP activity is not readily available. LCAT may trend slightly, but nonsignificantly upward with fenofibrate and simvastatin therapy, by 7 % and 6 %, respectively [49].

## Effects of Fibrates on Factors Related to Inflammation and Insulin Resistance

Increased inflammation is common in diabetes and appears to contribute to the excess CVD risk seen in this disorder. Several lines of evidence suggest that the inverse relationship between HDL-C levels and atherosclerosis may be mediated in part by an anti-inflammatory effect of HDL particles [64]. Thus, the low HDL-C levels often seen in DM-2 may be expected to contribute to the increased inflammation seen in this disorder. Further, the increase in HDL-C levels seen with fibrate therapy might be anticipated to have an anti-inflammatory effect in diabetes, as well as generally.

In addition to frequent low HDL-C levels, DM-2 is directly associated with increased levels of inflammatory biomarkers, including C-reactive protein (CRP) and lipoprotein-associated phospholipase $A_2$ (Lp-PLA$_2$) [65, 66]. Importantly, fibrate therapy can reduce levels of CRP and Lp-PLA$_2$ [66, 67], as well as VCAM-1 and other inflammatory factors (see a recent review by Elkeles [68]), which presumably is a reflection of its anti-inflammatory effects. The effects of fibrate or statin monotherapy vs. their combination on inflammatory biomarkers in patients with DM-2 has been reported by Muhlestein et al., who studied 300 patients with diabetes and mixed dyslipidemia [60]. Treatment with fenofibrate, simvastatin, or combined therapy reduced hs-CRP by 14.1 % ($P = 0.17$), 16 % ($P = 0.04$), or 15.9 % ($P = 0.01$), respectively (Fig. 20.4) and significantly decreased Lp-PLA$_2$ by 26.9 %, 34.5 %, and 36.2 %, respectively (all $P < 0.001$, Fig. 20.4). Interestingly, combination therapy of fenofibrate with simvastatin had no additive effects on these markers despite the tendency towards additive effects (noted above) on lipid and lipoprotein parameters [60].

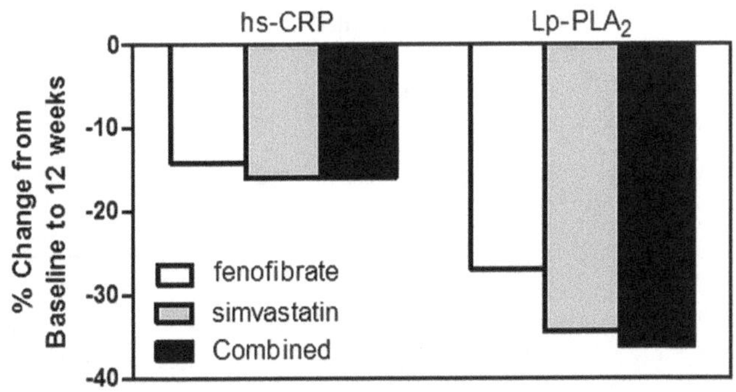


**Fig. 20.4** Comparison of treatment with fenofibrate, simvastatin, and combined therapy on inflammatory biomarkers high-sensitivity C-reactive protein (hs-CRP) and lipoprotein phospholipase $A_2$ ($Lp\text{-}PLA_2$) after 12 weeks. Adapted from Muhlestein et al. [60]

Another effect of fibrates which is likely of clinical importance in treatment of patients with diabetes is their tendency to reduce insulin resistance, particularly in patients with high TG, low HDL-C, and other elements of the metabolic syndrome [69] (see also a recent review by Elkeles [68]), and it has even been suggested that fibrates be tested for a possible ability to prevent new-onset DM-2 [68]. Of equal or greater importance, the ability of fibrate therapy to reduce CVD risk may relate directly to the degree of baseline insulin resistance, as discussed below.

## Effects of Fibrates on Microvascular Disease

Effects of fenofibrate on microvascular disease end points common in patients with diabetes have been explored in a meta-analysis [46] which included three recent trials of fenofibrate, the Diabetes Atherosclerosis Intervention Study (DAIS) [70], FIELD [55], and ACCORD-Lipid [56], as well as a small trial of etofibrate [71].

Beneficial effects of fenofibrate on certain aspects of diabetic retinopathy were reported in FIELD [72]. Although the pre-study primary end point of 2-step progression of retinopathy grade was not significantly reduced in the overall subject population (9.6 % with fenofibrate vs. 12.3 % with placebo; $p=0.19$) or in those without pre-existing retinopathy (11.4 % vs. 11.7 %; $p=0.87$), it was reduced substantially in patients with pre-existing retinopathy (3.1 % vs. 14.6 %; $p=0.004$) [72]. First laser treatment for retinopathy was required less often with fenofibrate than placebo (164 [3.4 %] vs. 238 [4.9 %] in placebo patients, respectively; hazard ratio [HR] 0.69, 95 % CI 0.56–0.84; $p=0.0002$; absolute risk reduction 1.5 % [0.7–2.3]) [72]. Of likely importance, these effects were independent of traditional retinopathy risk factors of glycemia and blood pressure and, curiously, were also independent of on-study lipid levels. Also, a small trial of etofibrate (which has never been available in the USA), reported only in a German-language publication, showed reduced retinopathy [71]. A meta-analysis of the results of this trial and FIELD showed a highly statistically significant 47 % decrease in retinopathy (Fig. 20.5).

Regarding renal function, in a meta-analysis of three trials of fenofibrate, there was a statistically significant 14 % reduction in the risk of albuminuria progression (95 % CI 2–25 %; $p=0.028$, see Fig. 20.5) [46]. Although the frequency of increased serum creatinine concentrations doubled ($p<0.0001$), the absolute degree of increase was almost invariably modest in size and appears to be completely and rapidly reversible upon discontinuation of the medication, even after long-term use [46]. In FIELD, the largest of the three trials in this meta-analysis, there were 14 % fewer fenofibrate-treated subjects who had progression and 18 % more with regression of albuminuria vs. those on placebo ($p<0.001$) [73]. Although plasma creatinine remained higher on fenofibrate than on placebo throughout the study, the chronic rate of rise was significantly slower (1.62 vs. 1.89 μmol/L annually, $p=0.01$), with far less estimated age-related GFR loss (1.19 vs. 2.03 mL/min per 1.73 $m^2$ annually, $p<0.001$). Further, after fenofibrate washout at the end of the study, estimated GFR had fallen 72 % less from baseline on fenofibrate (1.9 mL $min^{-1}$

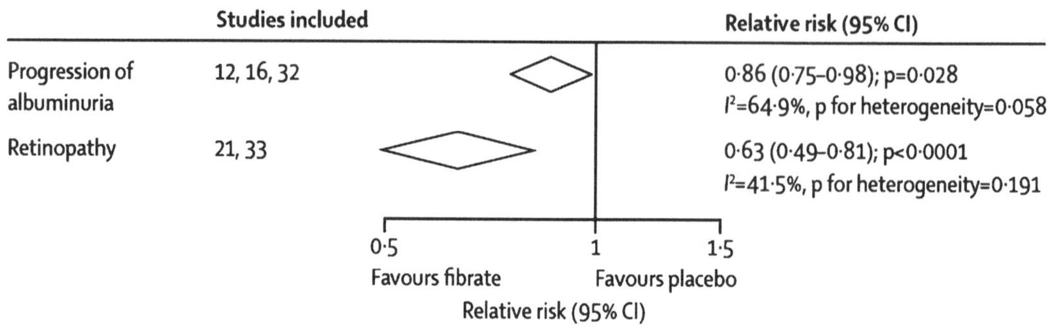


**Fig. 20.5** Decreases in the microvascular end points of albuminuria and retinopathy with fibrate treatment. Adapted from a figure in a recent meta-analysis by Jun et al. [46]. Study references in the figure are as follows: "12" is ACCORD-Lipid [56], "16" is FIELD [55], "32" is DAIS [91], "21" is Emmerich [71], and "33" is a substudy of FIELD [72]

1.73 $m^{-2}$, $p=0.065$) than on placebo (6.9 mL/min per 1.73 $m^2$, $p<0.001$), sparing 5.0 mL/min per 1.73 $m^2$ (95 % CI 2.3–7.7, $p<0.001$) [73]. Of particular interest, this greater preservation of estimated GFR with fenofibrate was seen primarily in subjects with either (1) baseline-high TG levels alone, (2) with baseline-high TG and low HDL-C together, or (3) TG reductions of ≥43 mg/dL on study drug. Curiously, however, progression to end-stage renal disease was not significantly reduced, occurring in 21 vs. 26 subjects with fenofibrate vs. placebo, respectively ($p=0.48$) [73]. Thus, the overall net effect of fenofibrate on renal function in DM-2 appears to be at least modestly favorable. Of likely clinical importance and possible mechanistic meaning, these benefits are predicted by the same baseline lipid levels and on-treatment lipid changes as are the CVD effects (see below).

Lower extremity amputation is devastating complication of diabetes, which appears to be a result both of microvascular and macrovascular disease. In FIELD, any lower-extremity amputation was less often needed with fenofibrate than with placebo (45 vs. 70 events; hazard ratio HR 0.64, 95 % CI 0.44–0.94; $p=0.02$, see Fig. 20.6) [74]. This finding was driven entirely by fewer "minor" (below the ankle) amputations (18 vs. 34 events; 0.53, 0.30–0.94; $p=0.027$) with no difference between groups in "major" (ankle or above) amputations (24 vs. 26 events; 0.93, 0.53–1.62; $p=0.79$, see Fig. 20.6) [74]. Interestingly, these effects of fenofibrate were seen primarily among patients without known large-vessel lower-extremity disease, and the benefits were unrelated to on-study lipid levels.

## Effects of Fibrates on Atherosclerosis

At least six studies have assessed effects of fibrate treatment on atherosclerosis. Three trials (two with fenofibrate and one with bezafibrate) have used carotid ultrasound for the measurement of carotid intima-media thickness (CIMT). In the St. Mary's, Ealing, Northwick Park Diabetes Cardiovascular Disease Prevention (SENDCAP) Study, bezafibrate showed no effect on CIMT [75]. A similar lack of efficacy on carotid atherosclerosis was found with fenofibrate in the Helsinki cohort of the FIELD study [76]. A third study, however, found that over the 24-month study period, carotid wall thickness did not progress with fenofibrate, but did progress in the control group [77]. Of potential clinical relevance in explaining the differences among these studies, the two without evident carotid atherosclerosis benefit were exclusively in patients with DM-2, while the study showing a beneficial effect excluded DM-2 patients.

In contrast with the frequently negative findings in carotid atherosclerosis, particularly in

| | Fenofibrate (n=4895) n (%) | Placebo (n=4900) n (%) | HR (95% CI) | p value |
|---|---|---|---|---|
| **First amputation*** | | | | |
| Minor | 28 (0·6%) | 52 (1·1%) | 0·54 (0·34–0·85) | 0·007 |
| Major | 24 (0·5%) | 26 (0·5%) | 0·93 (0·53–1·62) | 0·79 |
| Minor, without large-vessel disease | 18 (0·4%) | 34 (0·7%) | 0·53 (0·30–0·94) | 0·027 |
| Major or minor, with large-vessel disease | 34 (0·7%) | 42 (0·9%) | 0·81 (0·52–1·28) | 0·37 |
| Any amputation | 45 (0·9%) | 70 (1·4%) | 0·64 (0·44–0·94) | 0·02 |
| **Multiple events analysis†** | | | | |
| All amputations | 73 | 117 | 0·63 (0·40–0·97) | 0·04 |

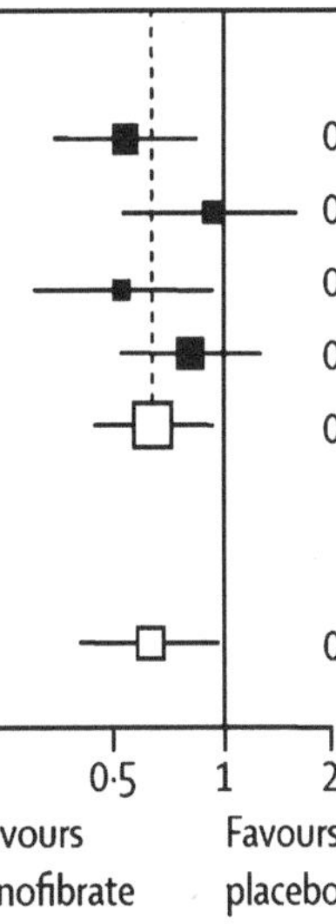


**Fig. 20.6** Changes in frequency of lower-extremity amputations with fenofibrate in the FIELD study. For "first amputation," patients are counted only once in each category. For the "multiple events analysis," all amputations for each category are counted (Poisson method). "Minor" means amputations below the ankle; "major" means at or above the ankle. The figure is taken from Rajamani et al. [74]

patients with DM-2, fibrates consistently have been found to reduce atherosclerosis in the coronary arterial tree. Three published trials have studied the effects of fibrates on coronary atherosclerosis by quantitative angiography, with minimum lumen diameter (MLD) as the primary end point, and all three have reported favorable results. The first of these was a trial using bezafibrate [78] which found improvement in coronary lumen diameter, by quantitative coronary angiography, in young men after a myocardial infarction. The second study, the Lopid Coronary Angiography Trial (LOCAT) used gemfibrozil and found similar benefits [79]. The third trial, Diabetes Atherosclerosis Intervention Study (DAIS), used fenofibrate and also found improved coronary atherosclerosis [70]. It is of interest to note that this beneficial effect of fenofibrate on coronary atherosclerosis in DAIS was strongly related to its capacity to increase LDL particle size [47].

The mechanisms by which fibrates might tend to lack beneficial effects on carotid atherosclerosis, while in contrast, reproducibly reduce coronary atherosclerosis, are unknown. Interestingly, however, these regional differences in effects on atherosclerosis per se do correspond with a difference in regional effect on clinical events. That is, fibrates consistently reduce coronary heart disease events, but have little if any favorable effect on the cerebrovascular event of stroke, as discussed below. Curiously, in this regard, the one study showing reduced progression of carotid atherosclerosis is the only clinical trial of a fibrate to report reduction in stroke in an overall study population [77].

## Fibrate Effects on Macrovascular CVD Events in General Study-Subject Populations

There has been no single randomized clinical trial of sufficient size and power to provide definitive data regarding effects of fibrate treatment on cardiovascular events. Consideration of individual

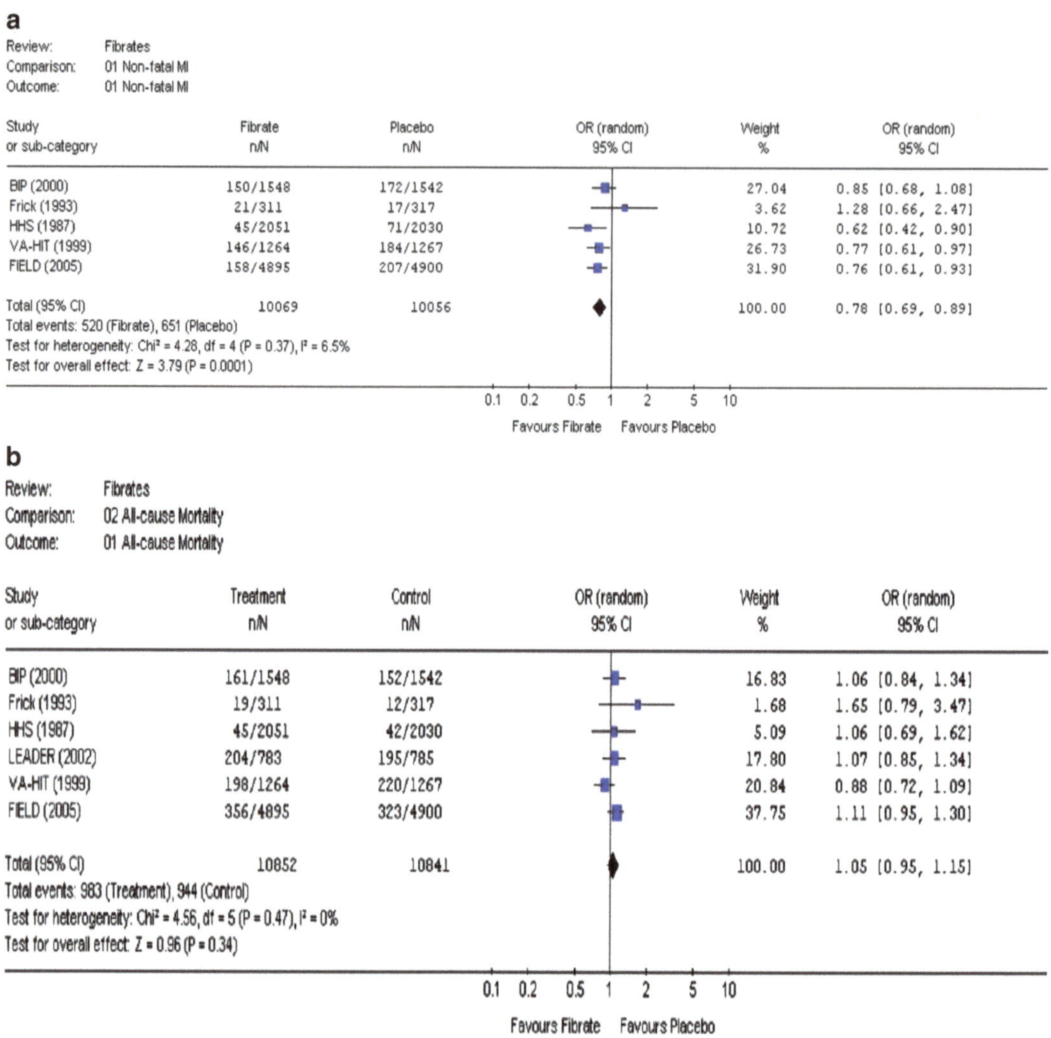


**Fig. 20.7** Effects of fibrate treatment on the incidence of major clinical events: (**a**) nonfatal myocardial infarction (MI) and (**b**) all-cause mortality. The name of the study or first author and the publication year are noted. The figures are taken from the meta-analysis of Abourbih et al. [45]. *OR* odds ratio, *CI* confidence interval

trials can be instructive regarding certain specific aspects of this question, and some discussion of data from larger individual trials is included below, but the best assessment of the ability of fibrates to reduce CVD in general or any specific CVD end point comes from meta-analyses of available trials. Although trials can be difficult to pool due to differences in patient population, drug intervention, end points, etc., effective meta-analyses can be very instructive for the drawing of clinically relevant conclusions.

One large and fairly recent meta-analysis, by Abourbih and coworkers [45], looked at a total of 20 trials, using bezafibrate, fenofibrate, and gemfibrozil, with 25,655 subjects in nine and seven trials and 12,398 and 8,273 subjects using fenofibrate and gemfibrozil, respectively. Focusing on five trials with MI data, they found a significant 22 % decrease in nonfatal MI (Fig. 20.7a). In sharp contrast, focusing on six trials with mortality data, they found a nonsignificant trend towards a 5 % increase in all-cause mortality (Fig. 20.7b) [45].

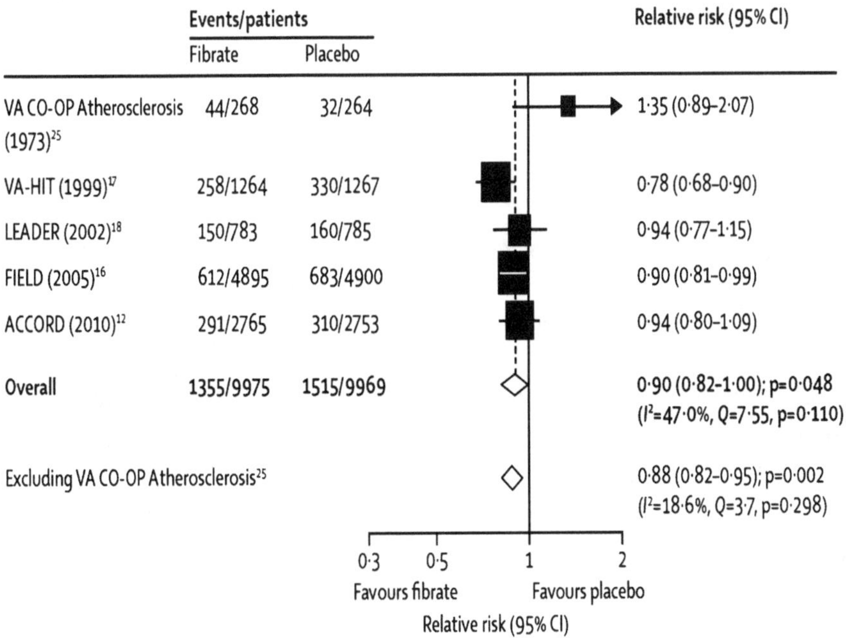


**Fig. 20.8** Effects of fibrate treatment on major cardiovascular events. The studies are noted by study name and year of publication. The figure is taken from the meta-analysis of Jun et al. [46]. *CI* confidence interval

Another, more recent, meta-analysis, by Jun et al. [46], was the first (and only comprehensive one so far) to include the most recent and arguably most important trial of fibrate effects on CVD events, the ACCORD-Lipid study [56]. Due to differing trial selection methodology, some trials from the Abourbih meta-analysis were not included in the one by Jun, so both are discussed here. The Jun meta-analysis focused on studies selected for presenting CVD event data in at least 100 patient-years follow-up. These 18 trials included 45,058 subjects who had 2,870 major CVD events and 3,880 deaths [46]. Among five major trials with relevant data (two with fenofibrate and one each with clofibrate, gemfibrozil, and bezafibrate), there was a borderline significant ($p=0.048$) 10 % decrease (relative risk, RR, of 0.90) in major cardiovascular outcomes, which became a highly significant 12 % decrease ($p=0.002$) after exclusion of the one small clofibrate trial (see Fig. 20.8) [46]. Further, among 16 trials (six using clofibrate, three with gemfibrozil, four with bezafibrate, and three with fenofibrate), there was a highly significant 13 % decrease in coronary events, without evidence for heterogeneity among trials ($p<0.001$, see Fig. 20.9) [46]. In further analyses of various cardiovascular events and other major end points, as noted in Fig. 20.10, pooled analysis of all studies with available data for each end point showed a highly significant 19 % decrease in nonfatal coronary events ($p<0.0001$), but only nonsignificant trends towards reductions in sudden death and cardiovascular death (11 % and 7 % decreases and $p=0.2$ and 0.1, respectively, Fig. 20.10). Similarly, there was a modest, borderline statistically significant trend towards a 10 % increase in nonvascular death (RR 1.10, $p=0.06$), but there was no evidence for any benefit on total stroke (RR 1.03, Fig. 20.10) [46]. Curiously, with regard to stroke, one small clinical trial did report a statistically significant reduction in stroke with fenofibrate therapy [77]. Oddly, this trial does not appear in the Jun meta-analysis, an omission which may well have been inadvertent since it seems to have met the inclusion criteria [46].

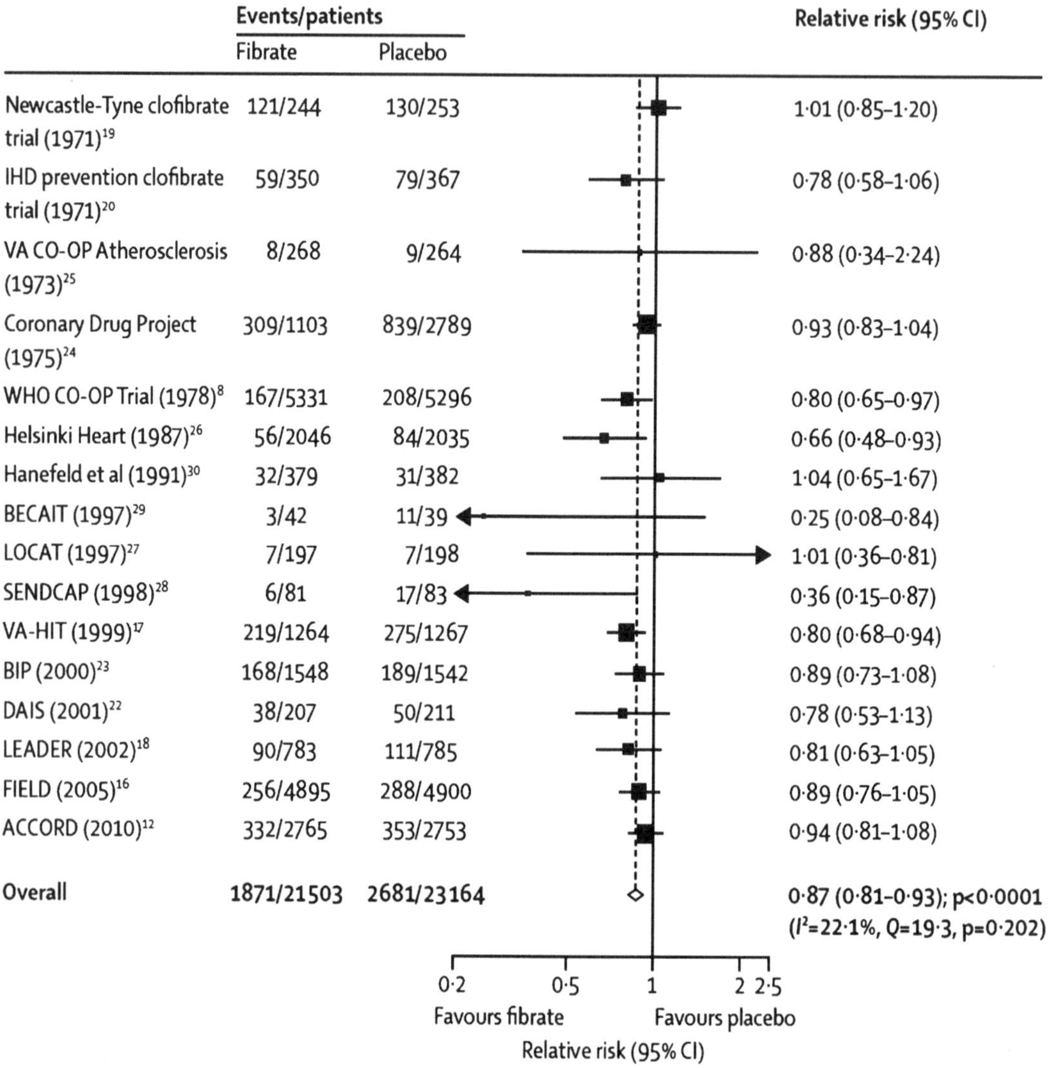


**Fig. 20.9** Effects of fibrate treatment on coronary events. The studies are noted by name of the study or first author and year of publication. The figure is taken from the meta-analysis of Jun et al. [46]. *CI* confidence interval

Patient subgroup analyses were also performed using a composite of all coronary events, the broad end point most clearly reduced by fibrates (Fig. 20.11). There was a suggestion of much greater benefit in treatment of patients without prior cardiovascular disease vs. those with a prior history (primary prevention vs. secondary prevention, RR 0.75 vs. 0.90, respectively, $p$ value for heterogeneity 0.07, Fig. 20.11). No other subgroup analysis approached statistical significance, except for baseline TG levels, which difference is discussed below. Interestingly, however, intercomparison among studies by the specific fibrate used suggested greater benefit with gemfibrozil (RR 0.78, 95 % CI 0.67–0.89) than with fenofibrate (RR 0.91, 95 % CI 0.82–1.00), even though the overall heterogeneity among trials of the four fibrates had a $p$ value of only 0.6 (Fig. 20.11) [46].

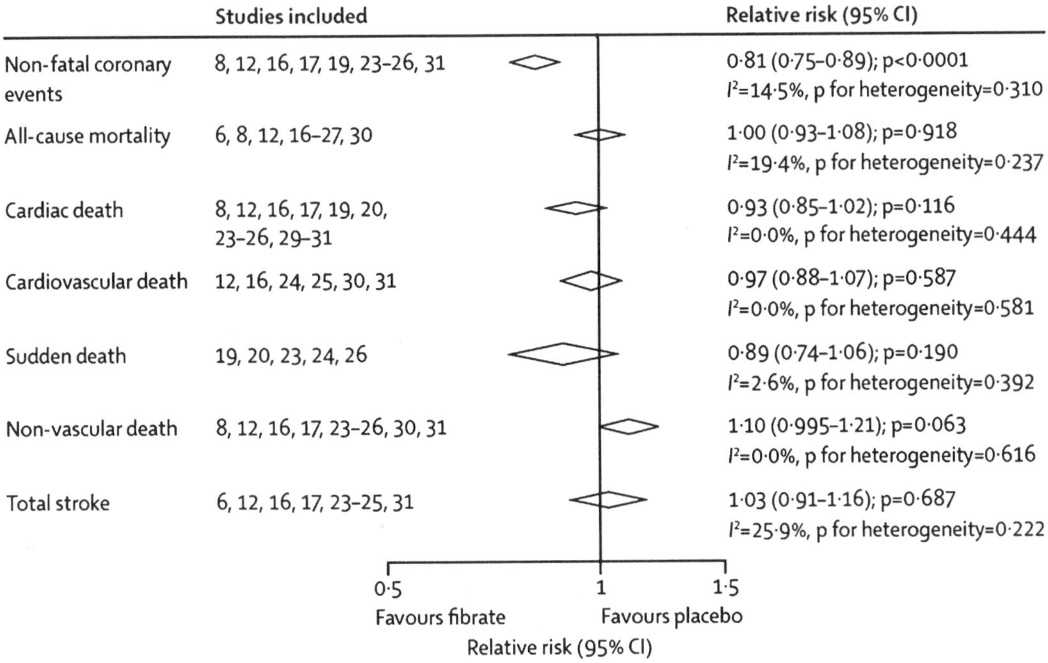


**Fig. 20.10** Effects of fibrate treatment on various cardiovascular and other major clinical events. Study references are as given in the meta-analysis of Jun et al., from which this figure is adapted [46]. *CI* confidence interval

## CVD Effects in Insulin-Resistant or "Prediabetic" Patients

The Veterans Affairs High Density Lipoprotein Intervention Trial (VA-HIT) study recruited subjects mainly on the basis of a low HDL-C level, and it was not primarily designed to test gemfibrozil effects in the insulin-resistant state. Due, however, to the strong relationship between low HDL-C and disorders of glucose and insulin metabolism, 43 % of VA-HIT patients had one or another insulin-resistant state: either impaired fasting glucose (13 %) or DM-2, whether newly diagnosed at the time of study entry (6 %) or previously diagnosed (25 %) [80]. A key subgroup analysis was performed among all subjects without DM-2, whether with or without impaired fasting glucose, to exclude use of diabetes medications which would likely alter fasting plasma insulin levels. Among these patients, the quartile of fasting insulin level (a good surrogate for degree of insulin resistance) was a strong direct predictor of CVD risk ($P=0.02$) [80]. Importantly, CVD reduction with gemfibrozil increased progressively across quartiles of baseline fasting insulin levels, from a possible 15 % increase in the lowest quartile to reductions of 20, 22, and 35 % in the second through fourth quartiles (Fig. 20.12), and this benefit remained after adjustment for other risk factors [80]. This finding is important due to the high and rising prevalence of insulin resistance throughout the world and due to its strength as a CVD risk factor. It is also intriguing since, paradoxically, both the decrease in TG and the increase in HDL-C were blunted with increasing insulin resistance, as discussed further below (Fig. 20.15) [81].

## CVD Effects of Fibrates in Patients With Diabetes Mellitus-2

With regard to the ability of fibrates to reduce CVD in patients with DM-2, three of the 17 relevant studies analyzed by Jun et al. did not report subjects' diabetes status [46]. In nine of the remaining studies, between 0 and 66 % of subjects had diabetes, while in the remaining five, all had DM-2. Importantly, coronary event reduction

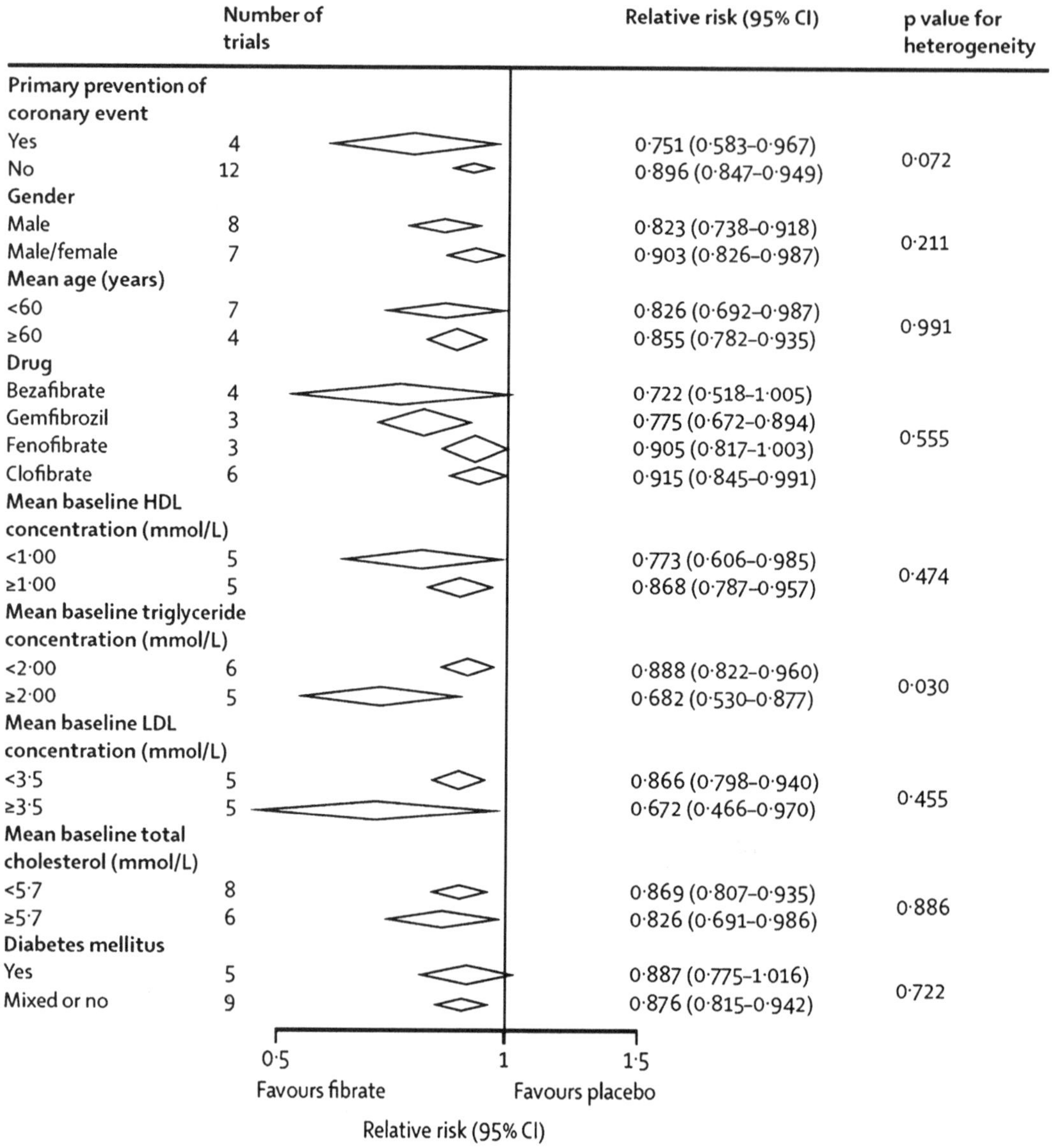


**Fig. 20.11** Effects of fibrate treatment on coronary events, divided by subgroups of fibrate study subjects. The figure is adapted from the meta-analysis of Jun et al. [46]. *CI* confidence interval

in studies exclusively in patients with DM-2 tended to be very similar to that in studies with mixed or non-DM-2 patient populations (RR 0.89 vs. 0.88, *p* value for heterogeneity 0.7, Fig. 20.11) [46]. In light of the uncertainties of cross-study comparisons, however, it is instructive to note within-study results from the VA-HIT. This study had a relatively large DM-2 subgroup, 769 or 31 % of total subjects, and is one of few trials to publish substantial within-study comparisons between patients with and without DM-2. As expected, those with established or newly diagnosed DM-2 had 87 % and 72 %, respectively, more total CVD events than those with normal fasting glucose [80]. The percent reduction of the primary combined CVD end point with gemfibrozil was nearly twice as great in those with DM-2 as in those without it (32 %

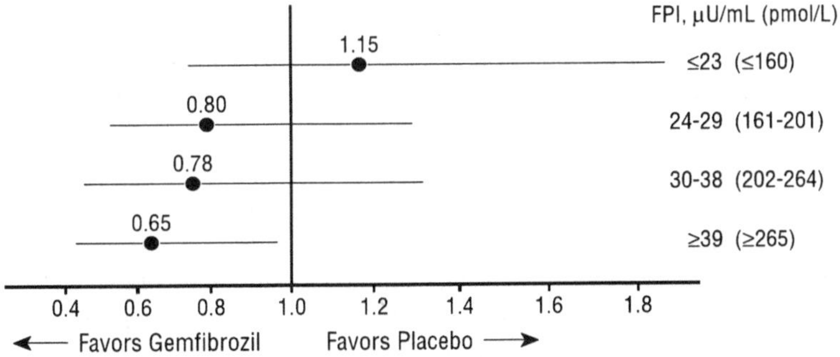


**Fig. 20.12** Hazard ratios (HR), from Cox models, for major cardiovascular events by quartile of fasting plasma insulin (FPI) level in VA-HIT subjects without diabetes. The figure is taken from Rubins et al. [80]

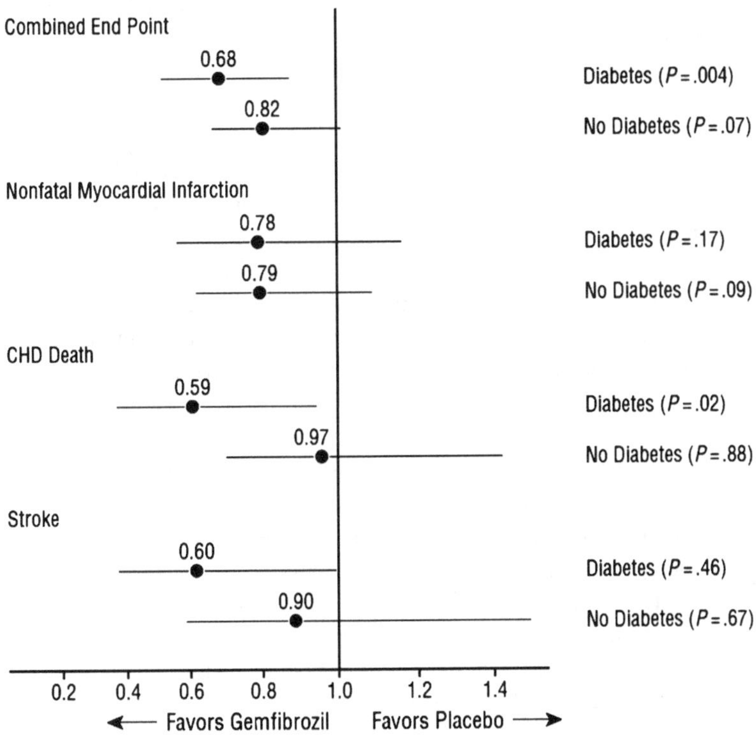


**Fig. 20.13** Hazard ratios (HR), from Cox models, for major cardiovascular events in VA-HIT subjects with or without diabetes. Please note that the *p* value second from *bottom* (stroke in patients with diabetes) is in error and should read "0.046" rather than "0.46." The figure is taken from Rubins et al. [80]

vs. 18 %, Fig. 20.13), although the difference was not statistically significant. Further, the absolute risk reduction was extremely high at 10 %, suggesting that only ten patients with DM-2 would need to be treated with gemfibrozil for five years to prevent one event [80]. Of interest and possible clinical significance, two individual components of the composite CVD end point which had not been found to be reduced by fibrates in the large meta-analyses, CHD death and stroke, were both shown to be reduced by gemfibrozil in subjects with DM-2 in VA-HIT (HR 0.59, $p=0.02$ and HR 0.60, $p=0.046$, Fig. 20.13) [80]. Paradoxically running somewhat counter to this observation of a decrease in stroke in DM-2, but lack of stroke benefit in subjects without DM-2 is the finding in the small open-label single-center study of Zhu et al. [77], in which Chinese subjects with hypertension but without DM-2 were found to have a statistically significant 48 % decrease in total stroke. Although the Chinese study was much smaller and shorter than the mainly Caucasian VA-HIT, the total number of strokes in patients without DM-2 in the latter, although not directly reported, was probably not more than twice the number reported in the Chinese study. Thus, the potential for reduction of stroke risk with fibrate treatment, whether with gemfibrozil or fenofibrate, whether in patients with or without DM-2, or whether population specific, remains unclear.

As an interesting contrast to the robust CVD benefit seen in patients with gemfibrozil in DM-2 patients in VA-HIT, the nearly 10,000 FIELD subjects, all with DM-2, had only a nonsignificant trend towards reduction of the primary study end point of pooled major cardiovascular events [55]. There was a statistically significant reduction in the rate of nonfatal myocardial infarctions and coronary revascularizations, but these were secondary end points [55]. The apparent benefit afforded by fenofibrate treatment in FIELD may have been reduced, however, by some key aspects of this study. First, many more patients randomized to blinded placebo therapy ended up receiving off-study statin therapy than did those in the fenofibrate arm [55]. This imbalance probably occurred because primary care physicians, who were not blinded to the lipid benefits of fenofibrate during the trial, saw more residual dyslipidemia in the placebo-treated patients and therefore were more likely to choose to add statin treatment in them. Perhaps of greater importance, no particular effort was made to focus on patients with high TG and/or low HDL-C [82], despite the fact that an analysis of the HHS, published years earlier [83], had shown strong evidence that these patients had far greater CVD reduction with fibrate therapy than did those with other dyslipidemias. As noted below, the relatively small numbers of FIELD patients with high TG and/or low HDL-C later proved to have substantially greater CVD benefit than the overall study population [84].

## Prediction of Fibrate CVD Effects by Baseline Lipids and On-Treatment Lipid Effects

Beginning with some of the earlier clinical trials, baseline lipid levels have been found to help predict CVD benefit of fibrate treatment. For example, post hoc analysis of the HHS showed considerable CVD benefit of gemfibrozil in patients with high TG levels and low HDL-C at baseline [83]. A similar analysis of FIELD reported that study subjects with either TG > 200 mg/dL, HDL-C < 40 mg/dL, or both achieved statistically and clinically significant reduction in the primary CVD end point (HR 0.77, 0.86, and 0.73, $p = 0.01$, 0.03 and 0.005, respectively) [84]. In the large and recent fibrate trial, meta-analysis of Jun et al. [46] lower (vs. higher) HDL-C, and higher (vs. lower) LDL-C tended to predict greater CVD benefit with fibrate treatment (RR 0.77 vs. 0.87 and 0.67 vs. 0.87, respectively), but the $p$ value for heterogeneity did not approach significance (0.5 for both, Fig. 20.11). In contrast, baseline-high TG significantly predicted greater CVD reduction (RR 0.89 vs. 0.68, $p$ value for heterogeneity 0.03, Fig. 20.11). The most recent meta-analysis of fibrate effects on CVD events focused primarily on the question of the prediction of CVD benefit by baseline lipid levels. In the five fibrate trials which reported both baseline TG and HDL-C levels, having either a high TG or a low HDL-C, or both strongly predicted CVD reduction (Fig. 20.14) [85]. High TG was strongly and consistently associated with a favorable CVD risk ratio of 0.75 (95 % CI 0.65–0.85). Low-baseline HDL-C had a somewhat smaller but still robust beneficial association with a risk ratio of 0.84 (0.77–0.91). Having both conditions appeared even more favorable with a risk ratio of 0.71 (0.62–0.82). In sharp contrast, having neither high TG nor low HDL-C predicted a lack of CVD benefit, the risk ratio being 0.94 (0.82–1.08, Fig. 20.14) [85]. In further analysis, other factors appeared to interact with these findings (Table 20.2) [85]. That is, high TG appeared to have a greater impact in patients without DM-2

| Study or Subgroup | Fibrates Events | Fibrates Total | Control Events | Control Total | Weight | Risk Ratio M-H, Random, 95% CI |
|---|---|---|---|---|---|---|
| **6.1.1 High triglycerides** | | | | | | |
| ACCORD 2010[12] | 104 | 934 | 114 | 888 | 22.9% | 0.87 [0.68, 1.11] |
| BIP 2005[23] | 28 | 234 | 44 | 225 | 9.2% | 0.61 [0.40, 0.95] |
| FIELD 2009[14] | 173 | 1295 | 210 | 1222 | 33.8% | 0.78 [0.65, 0.94] |
| HHS 1992[24] | 15 | 540 | 32 | 506 | 5.1% | 0.44 [0.24, 0.80] |
| VA HIT 2001[11] | 118 | 590 | 159 | 595 | 29.1% | 0.75 [0.61, 0.92] |
| **Subtotal (95% CI)** | | **3593** | | **3436** | **100.0%** | **0.75 [0.65, 0.86]** |
| Total events | 438 | | 559 | | | |
| Heterogeneity: Tau² = 0.01; Chi² = 5.30, df = 4 (P = 0.26); I² = 24% | | | | | | |
| Test for overall effect: Z = 4.04 (P < 0.0001) | | | | | | |
| **6.1.2 Low HDL cholesterol** | | | | | | |
| ACCORD 2010[12] | 205 | 1824 | 223 | 1772 | 19.5% | 0.89 [0.75, 1.07] |
| BIP 2005[23] | 129 | 798 | 144 | 818 | 13.5% | 0.92 [0.74, 1.14] |
| FIELD 2009[14] | 379 | 2924 | 437 | 2896 | 35.0% | 0.86 [0.76, 0.98] |
| HHS 1992[24] | 22 | 694 | 39 | 651 | 2.6% | 0.53 [0.32, 0.88] |
| LOCAT 1997[10] | 7 | 197 | 7 | 198 | 0.6% | 1.01 [0.36, 2.81] |
| VA HIT 2001[11] | 258 | 1264 | 330 | 1267 | 28.8% | 0.78 [0.68, 0.90] |
| **Subtotal (95% CI)** | | **7701** | | **7602** | **100.0%** | **0.84 [0.77, 0.91]** |
| Total events | 1000 | | 1180 | | | |
| Heterogeneity: Tau² = 0.00; Chi² = 5.38, df = 5 (P = 0.37); I² = 7% | | | | | | |
| Test for overall effect: Z = 4.12 (P < 0.0001) | | | | | | |
| **6.1.3 Both high triglycerides and low HDL cholesterol** | | | | | | |
| ACCORD 2010[12] | 60 | 485 | 80 | 456 | 18.1% | 0.71 [0.52, 0.96] |
| BIP 2005[23] | 24 | 184 | 36 | 162 | 8.4% | 0.59 [0.37, 0.94] |
| FIELD 2009[14] | 141 | 1044 | 173 | 970 | 35.8% | 0.76 [0.62, 0.93] |
| HHS 1992[24] | 8 | 294 | 23 | 288 | 3.1% | 0.34 [0.15, 0.75] |
| VA HIT 2001[11] | 118 | 590 | 159 | 595 | 34.6% | 0.75 [0.61, 0.92] |
| **Subtotal (95% CI)** | | **2597** | | **2471** | **100.0%** | **0.71 [0.62, 0.82]** |
| Total events | 351 | | 471 | | | |
| Heterogeneity: Tau² = 0.00; Chi² = 4.58, df = 4 (P = 0.33); I² = 13% | | | | | | |
| Test for overall effect: Z = 4.76 (P < 0.00001) | | | | | | |
| **6.1.4 Neither high triglycerides nor low HDL cholesterol** | | | | | | |
| ACCORD 2010[12] | 42 | 492 | 53 | 549 | 12.7% | 0.88 [0.60, 1.30] |
| BIP 2005[23] | 78 | 700 | 80 | 661 | 22.1% | 0.92 [0.69, 1.23] |
| FIELD 2009[14] | 201 | 1720 | 209 | 1752 | 57.4% | 0.98 [0.82, 1.17] |
| HHS 1992[24] | 27 | 1111 | 36 | 1161 | 7.8% | 0.78 [0.48, 1.28] |
| **Subtotal (95% CI)** | | **4023** | | **4123** | **100.0%** | **0.94 [0.82, 1.08]** |
| Total events | 348 | | 378 | | | |
| Heterogeneity: Tau² = 0.00; Chi² = 0.84, df = 3 (P = 0.84); I² = 0% | | | | | | |
| Test for overall effect: Z = 0.92 (P = 0.36) | | | | | | |

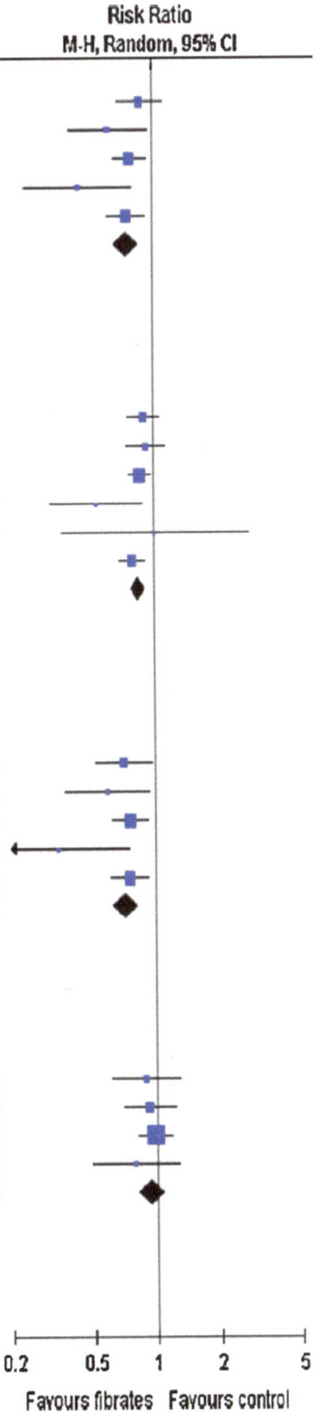


**Fig. 20.14** Effects of fibrate treatment on cardiovascular events by study and by baseline lipid values. The risk ratio was calculated using the Mantel-Haenszel random-effects model (M-H, Random). The studies are noted by study name and year of publication. The figure is taken from Lee et al. [85]. *CI* confidence interval, *df* degrees of freedom

**Table 20.2** The effects of fibrates on risk of CVD events in patients with elements of "the atherogenic dyslipidemia" (high TG and/or low HDL-C levels) from Lee et al. [85]

| | Triglyceride >200 mg/dL or nearest equivalent RR (95 % CI) | HDL cholesterol <40 mg/dL or nearest equivalent RR (95 % CI) |
|---|---|---|
| Population | | |
| Diabetes mellitus as an entry criteria | 0.81 (0.70–0.94) | 0.87 (0.78–0.97) |
| Diabetes mellitus not as an entry criteria | 0.65 (0.50–0.85) | 0.80 (0.68–0.95) |
| Prevention | | |
| Primary (<50 % people with CVD at entry) | 0.75 (0.59–0.96) | 0.84 (0.71–0.98) |
| Secondary | 0.72 (0.60–0.87) | 0.82 (0.73–0.93) |
| Treatment regimen | | |
| Gemfibrozil | 0.62 (0.37–1.02) | 0.74 (0.59–0.93) |
| Bezafibrate | 0.61 (0.40–0.95) | 0.92 (0.74–1.14) |
| Fenofibrate | 0.81 (0.70–0.94) | 0.87 (0.78–0.97) |
| Monotherapy vs. combination therapy | | |
| Fibrate alone | 0.72 (0.61–0.84) | 0.83 (0.75–0.92) |
| Fibrate + statin | 0.87 (0.68–1.11) | 0.89 (0.75–1.07) |
| End point used for analysis | | |
| CVD | 0.79 (0.70–0.89) | 0.84 (0.77–0.91) |
| CHD | 0.55 (0.38–0.78) | 0.78 (0.52–1.16) |

than in those with it. High TG also tended to be more important in patients taking gemfibrozil (vs. fenofibrate), in fibrate monotherapy (vs. statin combination), and in coronary events, vs. total cardiovascular events. Generally the same pattern held for the combination of high TG and low HDL-C. In partial contrast, low HDL-C appeared to better predict benefit only from gemfibrozil (vs. fenofibrate) but did not otherwise vary substantially with the above factors (Table 20.2) [85].

Intuitively, the degree of change in lipid levels with a lipid lowering agent, and/or the on-treatment lipid levels achieved, would be expected to predict the degree of CVD benefit. For example, the reduction in LDL-C during clinical trials of statins is a strong predictor of CVD reduction in general subjects [86] and in those with DM-2 [3]. Surprisingly, however, lipid changes from baseline with fibrates, and the separate but related parameter of on-study lipid levels during fibrate treatment, tend to be poor predictors of their CVD benefits. In the VA-HIT study, patients taking gemfibrozil had a 22 % reduction in major cardiovascular events ($P=0.006$) and a 24 % decrease in death from coronary disease, nonfatal myocardial infarction, and stroke ($P<0.001$) compared to patients receiving placebo. The patients receiving gemfibrozil had a modest 6 % increase in HDL-C levels compared to those receiving placebo ($P<0.001$) but a 31 % decrease in TG levels ($P<0.001$). Despite the fact that the HDL-C increase was much smaller than the TG decrease, the former predicted CVD risk reduction while the latter did not [81]. Related to this finding, fasting insulin levels (a surrogate for insulin resistance), which strongly predicted CVD benefit, were paradoxically a strong inverse predictor of both TG and HDL-C change. That is, VA-HIT patients with higher baseline insulin had less lipid change but greater CVD reduction on gemfibrozil (Fig. 20.15) [81].

Meta-regression analysis of on-treatment lipid levels in fibrate trials as predictors of CVD event reduction was performed as part of the meta-analysis of Jun et al. [46]. As was true for the analysis of change in levels, in ten trials, on-treatment TG levels significantly predicted CVD benefit ($p=0.026$) with a 5 % reduction per 88 mg/dL lower TG levels. There was also a possible suggestion in data from seven trials of a 2 % CVD reduction per 3.9 mg/dL lower on-treatment LDL-C and of a 3 % CVD reduction per 0.8 mg/dL higher

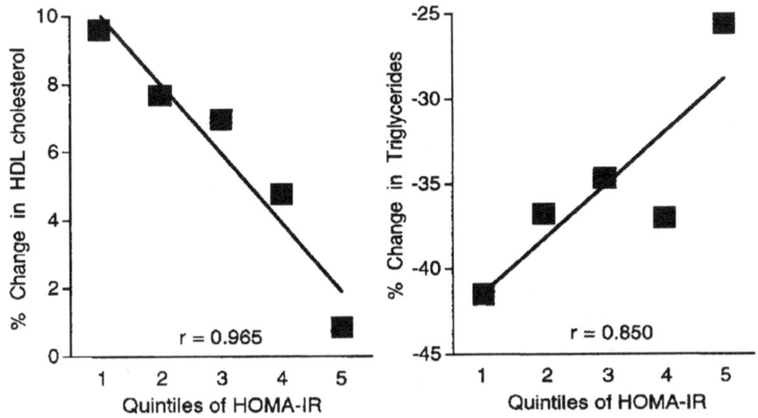


**Fig. 20.15** Relationship between % change in HDL-C or in triglycerides with quintiles of baseline insulin resistance calculated by the homeostasis model assessment (HOMA-IR) in VA-HIT subjects. The figure is from Robins et al. [81]

HDL-C (but neither of these reached statistical significance ($p=0.09$ and 0.13, respectively)) [46]. This is in partial contrast to the very robust data, in many more trial subjects, showing prediction of CVD reductions with statins by the degree of LDL-C lowering and on-study LDL-C [86].

Finally, analysis of lipoprotein particle concentrations by NMR in plasma samples from a nested case-control subgroup of the VA-HIT trial has suggested that both baseline and on-treatment levels of LDL-P and HDL-P predicted CVD events better than on-treatment apo B or HDL-C [53]. As pointed out, however, in an accompanying editorial [87], these observations raised more questions than they answered, and their interpretation is uncertain in light of larger data sets of more conventional lipoprotein measurements reviewed above.

## CVD Effects When Fibrates Are Added to Statins

Given the fact that statins are best proven among all classes of dyslipidemia medications for reducing CVD event rates, and indeed are widely recommended and used in patients with DM-2 [61], it is critical to ask whether fibrates can further reduce CVD risk when added to statin therapy. This question was addressed in the ACCORD-Lipid trial, in which all subjects received statin and half each were randomized to receive either fenofibrate or matching placebo [56]. Interestingly, in both ACCORD-Lipid [56] and FIELD [55], there was only a modest nonsignificant reduction in the overall population, while in both studies the CVD event reduction was much greater (and significant or near significant) in those with HTG and low HDL-C at baseline [85].

Intercomparison among studies according to the specific fibrate used has suggested greater benefit with gemfibrozil (RR 0.78, 95 % CI 0.67–0.89) than with fenofibrate (RR 0.91, 95 % CI 0.82–1.00), even though the overall heterogeneity among the four fibrates compared had a p value of 0.6 (Fig. 20.11). This suggested difference, however, may simply be an artifact of differential statin use. In the two largest gemfibrozil trials (HHS and VA-HIT), statins were scarcely or not at all yet available and so were not used by any subjects. In contrast, in the two largest fenofibrate trials (FIELD and ACCORD-Lipid), statins were used often in the placebo group (FIELD [55]) or were used in all subjects (ACCORD-Lipid [56]), thus likely making it much harder to see incremental fibrate benefits. Does this mean that fibrates cannot add to the CVD reduction obtained by statin monotherapy? Post hoc, subgroup analysis by baseline lipid levels (see above) suggests that fibrates may be beneficial when added to statin treatment in patients with baseline-high TG and low HDL-C.

These analyses, although remarkably consistent between these two large trials (and consistent with other fibrate trial data in the absence of statin use, see [85]), are not definitive. A trial of fibrate add-on to statin monotherapy in patients with the high TG and low HDL-C ("atherogenic dyslipidemia") is sorely needed, since this is a common condition in DM-2 and a setting in which fibrates are often used.

A key consideration in use of fibrates in combination with statins is the risk of myopathy, which is present with either agent alone, and which tends to be elevated in combination therapy [88]. Although FDA-approved labeling includes a similar precaution for statin use with both gemfibrozil and fenofibrate, the effect on statin levels, and thus on the potential for increased myopathy risk, is only about one-fifteenth as great with fenofibrate as with gemfibrozil [89]. Among the seven currently available statins, only fluvastatin (one of the least used statins) lacks this adverse interaction with gemfibrozil. Due to the relatively high risk of adverse interaction between gemfibrozil and statins, there is very little gemfibrozil use at present (except in monotherapy when a statin is not indicated or tolerated). Further, no large clinical trials using gemfibrozil in combination with statins have been, or are likely to be, conducted, and the general lack of gemfibrozil use seems unlikely to change in the future. In contrast, both FIELD [55] and ACCORD-Lipid [56] showed essentially no adverse safety signal for increased myopathy among thousands of patients taking fenofibrate with a statin. Even prior to the publication of the more robust of these two studies (ACCORD-Lipid [56]), fenofibrate has been widely considered as safe in combination use with statins [88].

## Guideline Recommendations for Fibrate Use

Fibrates have excellent overall safety in monotherapy, there being no increase in serious drug-related adverse events vs. placebo (RR 1.21, $p>0.2$), among a total of 17,413 participants in multiple trials [46]. As noted above, fenofibrate showed excellent safety in combination use with statins. There is also considerable evidence that fibrate monotherapy can reduce CVD events, although the effects appear to be relatively modest, as discussed above. Unfortunately, there are no data directly testing CVD effects and tolerability of fibrate monotherapy in statin-intolerant patients, where it might be of particular benefit. Most importantly, since the vast majority of patients with DM-2 and dyslipidemia already are, or should be, taking a statin, the lack of clear data for added CVD benefit when fibrates are added to a statin must temper enthusiasm for use of this combination.

Nevertheless, there is sufficient evidence for CVD reduction with fibrate monotherapy, and added to a statin, that the national cholesterol education program (NCEP) guidelines from the USA have suggested that fenofibrate (along with niacin) be considered for use in addition to a statin when high TG and/or low HDL-C persists after statin monotherapy [61]. Also, the European Atherosclerosis Society Consensus Panel has suggested that fibrates (and niacin) be considered as monotherapy for HTG (>150 mg/dL) and/or low HDL-C (<40 mg/dL) when diet and lifestyle are insufficient [90]. Given the evidence, but lack of certainty, for CVD benefit with fibrates when added to statins, the above suggestions seem to be both reasonable and appropriately tentative.

## Conclusions

Fibrates have been used extensively in clinical trials and clinical practice for more than four decades. They are the most effective medication class for reducing elevated TG levels and are primarily used for this indication. They are also moderately effective for increasing HDL-C levels and can increase LDL particle size. Since HTG, low HDL-C, and SD LDL (the so-called atherogenic dyslipidemia) are common in patients with insulin resistance and DM-2, much of fibrate use has been in patients with either or both of these conditions. In addition to their several lipid effects, fibrates may have other potentially antiatherogenic effects which may be especially important in DM-2, such as promotion of reverse cholesterol transport or reduction of inflammation. Further, the lack of adverse glycemic effects of fibrates also makes them an attractive choice for use in patients with diabetes. Also in this regard, the possibility that fibrates have greater CVD benefits in patients with DM-2 or insulin resistance makes them more attractive in these patients. Although the evidence is modest, at best, that fibrates can further reduce CVD events when added to statins, their lipid and non-lipid effects tend to be complimentary to each other. Randomized placebo-controlled clinical trials are sorely needed to test the CVD effects of fibrates added to statins in subject populations specifically recruited for moderate HTG and DM-2, possibly also with low HDL-C and other related CVD risk factors. Meanwhile, fenofibrate is quite safe in combination with statins, and given reasonable data regarding efficacy in reduction CVD risk, it can be considered as an adjunct to statin use (or as an alternative in statin-intolerant individuals) in patients with residual HTG and/or low HDL-C despite optimized statin monotherapy, with or without DM-2.

## References


1. Roger VL, Go AS, Lloyd-Jones DM, et al. Heart disease and stroke statistics—2012 update. Circulation 2012;125(22):e1002.
2. Baigent C, Keech A, Kearney PM, et al. Efficacy and safety of cholesterol-lowering treatment: prospective meta-analysis of data from 90,056 participants in 14 randomised trials of statins. Lancet. 2005;366:1267–78.
3. Kearney PM, Blackwell L, Collins R, et al. Efficacy of cholesterol-lowering therapy in 18,686 people with diabetes in 14 randomised trials of statins: a meta-analysis. Lancet. 2008;371:117–25.
4. Scandinavian Simvastatin Survival Study Group. Randomised trial of cholesterol lowering in 4444 patients with coronary heart disease: the Scandinavian Simvastatin Survival Study (4S). Lancet. 1994;344: 1383–9.
5. Downs JR, Clearfield M, Weis S, et al. Primary prevention of acute coronary events with lovastatin in men and women with average cholesterol levels. JAMA. 1998;279:1615–22.
6. Heart Protection Study Collaborative Group. MRC/BHF Heart Protection Study of antioxidant vitamin supplementation in 20536 high-risk individuals: a randomised placebo-controlled trial. Lancet. 2002;360:23–33.
7. Marschner IC, Colquhoun D, Simes RJ, et al. Long-term risk stratification for survivors of acute coronary syndromes. Results from the Long-term Intervention with Pravastatin in Ischemic Disease (LIPID) Study. LIPID Study Investigators. J Am Coll Cardiol. 2001;38:56–63.
8. Asztalos BF, Batista M, Horvath KV, et al. Change in alpha1 HDL concentration predicts progression in coronary artery stenosis. Arterioscler Thromb Vasc Biol. 2003;23:847–52.
9. Ballantyne CM, Herd JA, Ferlic LL, et al. Influence of low HDL on progression of coronary artery disease and response to fluvastatin therapy. Circulation. 1999;99:736–43.
10. Johnsen SH, Mathiesen EB, Fosse E, et al. Elevated high-density lipoprotein cholesterol levels are protective against plaque progression: a follow-up study of 1952 persons with carotid atherosclerosis the Tromso study. Circulation. 2005;112:498–504.
11. Despres JP, Lemieux I, Dagenais GR, Cantin B, Lamarche B. HDL-cholesterol as a marker of coronary heart disease risk: the Quebec cardiovascular study. Atherosclerosis. 2000;153:263–72.
12. Grant RW, Meigs JB. Prevalence and treatment of low HDL cholesterol among primary care patients with type 2 diabetes: an unmet challenge for cardiovascular risk reduction. Diabetes Care. 2007;30:479–84.
13. Bruckert E, Baccara-Dinet M, McCoy F, Chapman J. High prevalence of low HDL-cholesterol in a pan-European survey of 8545 dyslipidaemic patients. Curr Med Res Opin. 2005;21:1927–34.
14. Barter P, Gotto AM, LaRosa JC, et al. HDL cholesterol, very low levels of LDL cholesterol, and cardiovascular events. N Engl J Med. 2007;357:1301–10.
15. Di Angelantonio E, Sarwar N, Perry P, et al. Major lipids, apolipoproteins, and risk of vascular disease. JAMA. 2009;302:1993–2000.
16. Boden WE, Probstfield JL, Anderson T, et al. Niacin in patients with low HDL cholesterol levels receiving intensive statin therapy. N Engl J Med. 2011;365: 2255–67.
17. Khera AV, Cuchel M, de la Llera-Moya M, et al. Cholesterol efflux capacity, high-density lipoprotein function, and atherosclerosis. N Engl J Med. 2011; 364:127–35.
18. Cavigiolio G, Shao B, Geier EG, Ren G, Heinecke JW, Oda MN. The interplay between size, morphology, stability, and functionality of high-density lipoprotein subclasses. Biochemistry. 2008;47:4770–9.
19. von Eckardstein A. Implications of torcetrapib failure for the future of HDL therapy: is HDL-cholesterol the right target? Expert Rev Cardiovasc Ther. 2010;8: 345–58.
20. Hokanson JE, Austin MA. Plasma triglyceride level is a risk factor for cardiovascular disease independent of high-density lipoprotein cholesterol level: a meta-analysis of population-based prospective studies. J Cardiovasc Risk. 1996;3:213–9.
21. Hopkins PN, Wu LL, Hunt SC, Brinton EA. Plasma triglycerides and type III hyperlipidemia are

independently associated with premature familial coronary artery disease. J Am Coll Cardiol. 2005;45: 1003–12.
22. Yuan G, Al-Shali KZ, Hegele RA. Hypertriglyceridemia: its etiology, effects and treatment. CMAJ. 2007;176:1113–20.
23. Austin MA, Hokanson JE, Edwards KL. Hypertriglyceridemia as a cardiovascular risk factor. Am J Cardiol. 1998;81:7B–12.
24. Sacks FM, Tonkin AM, Shepherd J, et al. Effect of pravastatin on coronary disease events in subgroups defined by coronary risk factors: the Prospective Pravastatin Pooling Project. Circulation. 2000;102: 1893–900.
25. Sacks FM, Alaupovic P, Moye LA, et al. VLDL, apolipoproteins B, CIII, and E, and risk of recurrent coronary events in the Cholesterol and Recurrent Events (CARE) trial. Circulation. 2000;102:1886–92.
26. Miller M, Cannon CP, Murphy SA, Qin J, Ray KK, Braunwald E. Impact of triglyceride levels beyond low-density lipoprotein cholesterol after acute coronary syndrome in the PROVE IT-TIMI 22 trial. J Am Coll Cardiol. 2008;51:724–30.
27. Drexel H, Aczel S, Marte T, Vonbank A, Saely CH. Factors predicting cardiovascular events in statin-treated diabetic and non-diabetic patients with coronary atherosclerosis. Atherosclerosis. 2010;208:484–9.
28. Langsted A, Freiberg JJ, Tybjaerg-Hansen A, Schnohr P, Jensen GB, Nordestgaard BG. Nonfasting cholesterol and triglycerides and association with risk of myocardial infarction and total mortality: the Copenhagen City Heart Study with 31 years of follow-up. J Intern Med. 2011;270:65–75.
29. Langsted A, Nordestgaard BG. Nonfasting lipids, lipoproteins, and apolipoproteins in individuals with and without diabetes: 58 434 individuals from the Copenhagen General Population Study. Clin Chem. 2011;57:482–9.
30. Rader DJ. Mechanisms of disease: HDL metabolism as a target for novel therapies. Nat Clin Pract Cardiovasc Med. 2007;4:102–9.
31. Vergeer M, Holleboom AG, Kastelein JJ, Kuivenhoven JA. The HDL hypothesis: does high-density lipoprotein protect from atherosclerosis? J Lipid Res. 2010;51:2058–73.
32. Brewer Jr HB. Clinical review: the evolving role of HDL in the treatment of high-risk patients with cardiovascular disease. J Clin Endocrinol Metab. 2011;96:1246–57.
33. Navab M, Reddy ST, Van Lenten BJ, Fogelman AM. HDL and cardiovascular disease: atherogenic and atheroprotective mechanisms. Nat Rev Cardiol. 2011;8: 222–32.
34. Ginsberg HN. New perspectives on atherogenesis: role of abnormal triglyceride-rich lipoprotein metabolism. Circulation. 2002;106:2137–42.
35. Wang L, Gill R, Pedersen TL, Higgins LJ, Newman JW, Rutledge JC. Triglyceride-rich lipoprotein lipolysis releases neutral and oxidized FFAs that induce endothelial cell inflammation. J Lipid Res. 2009;50:204–13.
36. Austin MA, King MC, Vranizan KM, Krauss RM. Atherogenic lipoprotein phenotype. A proposed genetic marker for coronary heart disease risk. Circulation. 1990;82:495–506.
37. Brinton EA, Eisenberg S, Breslow JL. Increased apo A-I and apo A-II fractional catabolic rate in patients with low high density lipoprotein-cholesterol levels with or without hypertriglyceridemia. J Clin Invest. 1991;87:536–44.
38. Brinton EA, Eisenberg S, Breslow JL. Human HDL cholesterol levels are determined by apoA-I fractional catabolic rate, which correlates inversely with estimates of HDL particle size. Effects of gender, hepatic and lipoprotein lipases, triglyceride and insulin levels, and body fat distribution. Arterioscler Thromb. 1994;14:707–20.
39. Taskinen MR. Diabetic dyslipidaemia: from basic research to clinical practice. Diabetologia. 2003;46: 733–49.
40. Lamarche B, Tchernof A, Moorjani S, et al. Small, dense low-density lipoprotein particles as a predictor of the risk of ischemic heart disease in men. Prospective results from the Quebec Cardiovascular Study. Circulation. 1997;95:69–75.
41. St-Pierre AC, Ruel IL, Cantin B, et al. Comparison of various electrophoretic characteristics of LDL particles and their relationship to the risk of ischemic heart disease. Circulation. 2001;104:2295–9.
42. Hirano T, Ito Y, Koba S, et al. Clinical significance of small dense low-density lipoprotein cholesterol levels determined by the simple precipitation method. Arterioscler Thromb Vasc Biol. 2004;24:558–63.
43. Rizzo M, Pernice V, Frasheri A, et al. Small, dense low-density lipoproteins (LDL) are predictors of cardio- and cerebro-vascular events in subjects with the metabolic syndrome. Clin Endocrinol (Oxf). 2009;70:870–5.
44. Taskinen MR. LDL-cholesterol, HDL-cholesterol or triglycerides–which is the culprit? Diabetes Res Clin Pract. 2003;61 Suppl 1:S19–26.
45. Abourbih S, Filion KB, Joseph L, et al. Effect of fibrates on lipid profiles and cardiovascular outcomes: a systematic review. Am J Med. 2009;122:962 e1–8.
46. Jun M, Foote C, Lv J, et al. Effects of fibrates on cardiovascular outcomes: a systematic review and meta-analysis. Lancet. 2010;375:1875–84.
47. Vakkilainen J, Steiner G, Ansquer JC, et al. Relationships between low-density lipoprotein particle size, plasma lipoproteins, and progression of coronary artery disease: the Diabetes Atherosclerosis Intervention Study (DAIS). Circulation. 2003;107: 1733–7.
48. Hiukka A, Leinonen E, Jauhiainen M, et al. Long-term effects of fenofibrate on VLDL and HDL subspecies in participants with type 2 diabetes mellitus. Diabetologia. 2007;50:2067–75.
49. Franceschini G, Calabresi L, Colombo C, Favari E, Bernini F, Sirtori CR. Effects of fenofibrate and simvastatin on HDL-related biomarkers in low-HDL patients. Atherosclerosis. 2007;195:385–91.

50. Ginsberg HN. Insulin resistance and cardiovascular disease. J Clin Invest. 2000;106:453–8.
51. Atmeh RF, Shepherd J, Packard CJ. Subpopulations of apolipoprotein A-I in human high-density lipoproteins. Their metabolic properties and response to drug therapy. Biochim Biophys Acta. 1983;751:175–88.
52. Toth PP, Thakker KM, Jiang P, Padley RJ. Niacin extended-release/simvastatin combination therapy produces larger favorable changes in high-density lipoprotein particles than atorvastatin monotherapy. Vasc Health Risk Manag. 2012;8:39–44.
53. Otvos JD, Collins D, Freedman DS, et al. Low-density lipoprotein and high-density lipoprotein particle subclasses predict coronary events and are favorably changed by gemfibrozil therapy in the Veterans Affairs High-Density Lipoprotein Intervention Trial. Circulation. 2006;113:1556–63.
54. Tenkanen L, Manttari M, Kovanen PT, Virkkunen H, Manninen V. Gemfibrozil in the treatment of dyslipidemia: an 18-year mortality follow-up of the Helsinki Heart Study. Arch Intern Med. 2006;166:743–8.
55. Keech A, Simes RJ, Barter P, et al. Effects of long-term fenofibrate therapy on cardiovascular events in 9795 people with type 2 diabetes mellitus (the FIELD study): randomised controlled trial. Lancet. 2005;366: 1849–61.
56. Ginsberg HN, Elam MB, Lovato LC, et al. Effects of combination lipid therapy in type 2 diabetes mellitus. N Engl J Med. 2010;362:1563–74.
57. Manninen V, Elo MO, Frick MH, et al. Lipid alterations and decline in the incidence of coronary heart disease in the Helsinki Heart Study. JAMA. 1988;260:641–51.
58. Farnier M. Combination therapy with an HMG-CoA reductase inhibitor and a fibric acid derivative: a critical review of potential benefits and drawbacks. Am J Cardiovasc Drugs. 2003;3:169–78.
59. Brinton EA. Does the addition of fibrates to statin therapy have a favorable risk to benefit ratio? Curr Atheroscler Rep. 2008;10:25–32.
60. Muhlestein JB, May HT, Jensen JR, et al. The reduction of inflammatory biomarkers by statin, fibrate, and combination therapy among diabetic patients with mixed dyslipidemia: the DIACOR (Diabetes and Combined Lipid Therapy Regimen) study. J Am Coll Cardiol. 2006;48:396–401.
61. Expert Panel on Detection, Evaluation, and Treatment of High Blood Cholesterol in Adults (Adult Treatment Panel III). Executive summary of the third report of the national cholesterol education program (NCEP) expert panel on detection, evaluation, and treatment of high blood cholesterol in adults (adult treatment panel III). JAMA. 2001;285:2486–97.
62. van Eck M, Bos IS, Kaminski WE, et al. Leukocyte ABCA1 controls susceptibility to atherosclerosis and macrophage recruitment into tissues. Proc Natl Acad Sci USA. 2002;99:6298–303.
63. Miyazaki T, Shimada K, Miyauchi K, et al. Effects of fenofibrate on lipid profiles, cholesterol ester transfer activity, and in-stent intimal hyperplasia in patients after elective coronary stenting. Lipids Health Dis. 2010;9:122.
64. Navab M, Yu R, Gharavi N, et al. High-density lipoprotein: antioxidant and anti-inflammatory properties. Curr Atheroscler Rep. 2007;9:244–8.
65. Schaefer EJ, McNamara JR, Asztalos BF, et al. Effects of atorvastatin versus other statins on fasting and postprandial C-reactive protein and lipoprotein-associated phospholipase A2 in patients with coronary heart disease versus control subjects. Am J Cardiol. 2005;95:1025–32.
66. Ridker PM, Cook N. Clinical usefulness of very high and very low levels of C-reactive protein across the full range of Framingham Risk Scores. Circulation. 2004;109:1955–9.
67. Albert MA, Danielson E, Rifai N, Ridker PM. Effect of statin therapy on C-reactive protein levels: the pravastatin inflammation/CRP evaluation (PRINCE): a randomized trial and cohort study. JAMA. 2001;286:64–70.
68. Elkeles R. Fibrates: old drugs with a new role in type 2 diabetes prevention? Br J Diabetes Vasc Dis. 2011;11:4–9.
69. Tenenbaum A, Fisman EZ, Boyko V, et al. Attenuation of progression of insulin resistance in patients with coronary artery disease by bezafibrate. Arch Intern Med. 2006;166:737–41.
70. Steiner G. Effect of fenofibrate on progression of coronary-artery disease in type 2 diabetes: the Diabetes Atherosclerosis Intervention Study, a randomised study. Lancet 2001;357:905–10.
71. Emmerich KH, Poritis N, Stelmane I, et al. Efficacy and safety of etofibrate in patients with non-proliferative diabetic retinopathy. Klin Monbl Augenheilkd. 2009;226:561–7.
72. Keech AC, Mitchell P, Summanen PA, et al. Effect of fenofibrate on the need for laser treatment for diabetic retinopathy (FIELD study): a randomised controlled trial. Lancet. 2007;370:1687–97.
73. Davis TM, Ting R, Best JD, et al. Effects of fenofibrate on renal function in patients with type 2 diabetes mellitus: the Fenofibrate Intervention and Event Lowering in Diabetes (FIELD) Study. Diabetologia. 2011;54:280–90.
74. Rajamani K, Colman PG, Li LP, et al. Effect of fenofibrate on amputation events in people with type 2 diabetes mellitus (FIELD study): a prespecified analysis of a randomised controlled trial. Lancet. 2009; 373:1780–8.
75. Elkeles RS, Diamond JR, Poulter C, et al. Cardiovascular outcomes in type 2 diabetes. A double-blind placebo-controlled study of bezafibrate: the St. Mary's, Ealing, Northwick Park Diabetes Cardiovascular Disease Prevention (SENDCAP) Study. Diabetes Care. 1998;21:641–8.
76. Hiukka A, Westerbacka J, Leinonen ES, et al. Long-term effects of fenofibrate on carotid intima-media thickness and augmentation index in subjects with type 2 diabetes mellitus. J Am Coll Cardiol. 2008;52: 2190–7.

77. Zhu S, Su G, Meng QH. Inhibitory effects of micronized fenofibrate on carotid atherosclerosis in patients with essential hypertension. Clin Chem. 2006;52: 2036–42.
78. Ericsson CG, Hamsten A, Nilsson J, Grip L, Svane B, de Faire U. Angiographic assessment of effects of bezafibrate on progression of coronary artery disease in young male postinfarction patients. Lancet. 1996; 347:849–53.
79. Frick MH, Syvanne M, Nieminen MS, et al. Prevention of the angiographic progression of coronary and vein-graft atherosclerosis by gemfibrozil after coronary bypass surgery in men with low levels of HDL cholesterol. Lopid Coronary Angiography Trial (LOCAT) Study Group. Circulation. 1997;96: 2137–43.
80. Rubins HB, Robins SJ, Collins D, et al. Diabetes, plasma insulin, and cardiovascular disease: subgroup analysis from the Department of Veterans Affairs high-density lipoprotein intervention trial (VA-HIT). Arch Intern Med. 2002;162:2597–604.
81. Robins SJ, Rubins HB, Faas FH, et al. Insulin resistance and cardiovascular events with low HDL cholesterol: the Veterans Affairs HDL Intervention Trial (VA-HIT). Diabetes Care. 2003;26:1513–7.
82. FIELD Study Investigators. The need for a large-scale trial of fibrate therapy in diabetes: the rationale and design of the Fenofibrate Intervention and Event Lowering in Diabetes (FIELD) study. [ISRCTN64783481]. Cardiovasc Diabetol. 2004;3:9.
83. Manninen V, Tenkanen L, Koskinen P, et al. Joint effects of serum triglyceride and LDL cholesterol and HDL cholesterol concentrations on coronary heart disease risk in the Helsinki Heart Study. Implications for treatment. Circulation. 1992;85:37–45.
84. Scott R, O'Brien R, Fulcher G, et al. Effects of fenofibrate treatment on cardiovascular disease risk in 9,795 individuals with type 2 diabetes and various components of the metabolic syndrome: the Fenofibrate Intervention and Event Lowering in Diabetes (FIELD) study. Diabetes Care. 2009;32:493–8.
85. Lee M, Saver JL, Towfighi A, Chow J, Ovbiagele B. Efficacy of fibrates for cardiovascular risk reduction in persons with atherogenic dyslipidemia: a meta-analysis. Atherosclerosis. 2011;217:492–8.
86. Baigent C, Blackwell L, Emberson J, et al. Efficacy and safety of more intensive lowering of LDL cholesterol: a meta-analysis of data from 170,000 participants in 26 randomised trials. Lancet. 2010;376: 1670–81.
87. Barter PJ, Rye KA. Cardioprotective properties of fibrates: which fibrate, which patients, what mechanism? Circulation. 2006;113:1553–5.
88. Davidson MH, Armani A, McKenney JM, Jacobson TA. Safety considerations with fibrate therapy. Am J Cardiol. 2007;99:3C–18.
89. Jones PH, Davidson MH. Reporting rate of rhabdomyolysis with fenofibrate+statin versus gemfibrozil+any statin. Am J Cardiol. 2005;95:120–2.
90. Chapman MJ, Ginsberg HN, Amarenco P, et al. Triglyceride-rich lipoproteins and high-density lipoprotein cholesterol in patients at high risk of cardiovascular disease: evidence and guidance for management. Eur Heart J. 2011;32:1345–61.
91. Ansquer JC, Foucher C, Rattier S, Taskinen MR, Steiner G. Fenofibrate reduces progression to microalbuminuria over 3 years in a placebo-controlled study in type 2 diabetes: results from the Diabetes Atherosclerosis Intervention Study (DAIS). Am J Kidney Dis. 2005;45:485–93.

# Niacin Therapy: Impact on Dyslipidemia and Cardiovascular Events in Diabetic Patients

21

Henry A. Tran, Arthur Z. Schwartzbard, and James A. Underberg

## Introduction

Niacin (nicotinic acid or vitamin B3) was the first pharmacologic agent identified to lower serum cholesterol levels in humans. To date it remains the most effective currently available medication to increase high-density lipoprotein cholesterol (HDL-C) levels. In typical pharmacologic doses (2–3 g/day), niacin usually increases HDL-C by 15–35 %, decreases low-density lipoprotein cholesterol (LDL-C) by 5–25 %, and reduces levels of triglycerides (TGs) by 20–50 % [1]. Although these beneficial effects were first discovered more than 50 years ago, its true clinical efficacy in the reduction of cardiovascular events remains a promising but somewhat unproven proposition in the era of HMG-CoA reductase inhibitors ("statin") therapy. Niacin's usage has been hindered by its side effect profile. Flushing is a common symptom, especially with crystalline or immediate-release niacin (niacin IR). Furthermore, concerns of niacin-induced hyperglycemia have limited its use in patients with diabetes mellitus. Statins, in addition to being better tolerated lipid-lowering drugs, consistently have been shown to reduce cardiovascular (CV) events and are the cornerstone of modern lipid-lowering therapy.

A significant residual risk of CV events remains despite effective LDL-C lowering, and strong epidemiologic data support a robust inverse relationship between HDL-C levels and CV events. For these reasons, there has been a persistent interest in niacin either as adjunctive therapy to statins or as primary therapy in statin-intolerant patients. Additionally, patients with diabetes and cardiometabolic risk (CMR) frequently have comorbid dyslipidemia, characteristically marked by low HDL-C and elevated triglycerides (TGs), which makes niacin therapy particularly attractive.

This chapter will review the history, pharmacokinetics, side effects, and clinical trial data supporting the use of niacin to treat CV disease, with specific emphasis on patients with diabetes.

H.A. Tran, M.D., M.Sc.
Greenberg Division of Cardiology, Weill Cornell Medical College, 520 East 70th St, Starr 427, New York, NY 10021, USA

New York University Langone School of Medicine, New York City, NY, USA

A.Z. Schwartzbard, M.D., F.A.C.C.
Leon H. Charney Division of Cardiology, Department of Medicine, Veteran's Administration, New York Harbor Healthcare System, New York, NY, USA

University Langone School of Medicine, 423 East 23rd St, New York, NY 10016, USA

J.A. Underberg, M.D., M.S., F.A.C.P.M., F.A.C.P., F.A.S.H., F.N.L.A. (✉)
Department of Medicine, New York University School of Medicine, 317 East 34th St., 7th Floor, New York, NY 10016, USA
e-mail: james.underberg@nyumc.org

A.J. Jenkins et al. (eds.), *Lipoproteins in Diabetes Mellitus*, Contemporary Diabetes,
DOI 10.1007/978-1-4614-7554-5_21, © Springer Science+Business Media New York 2014

## History

The story of the discovery and development of niacin as a lipid-altering medication is interesting and convoluted. Due to changes in the processing of corn from traditional methods, the nutritional bioavailability of niacin was reduced. Populations which subsisted heavily on corn and cereal diets experienced endemic outbreaks of pellagra due to niacin deficiency. This syndrome is characterized by photosensitive dermatitis, dementia, and diarrhea. In the early twentieth century, it was discovered that supplemental niacin (15–20 mg/day) effectively treated pellagra in humans. Unfortunately, even in small doses of niacin, intense cutaneous flushing can occur, and this limits its use and tolerability. For this reason, related vitamin B compounds, such as nicotinamide, were used as they were equally efficacious in treating pellagra but did not induce significant flushing [2]. In the early 1950s, before Thorazine had revolutionized pharmacotherapy for psychiatric disease, niacin in large, supraphysiologic doses (1–3 g/days) was used to treat patients institutionalized for schizophrenia. In an effort to understand the flushing side effects, Canadian psychiatrist Dr. Hoffer started taking large doses of niacin and made the curious observation that it improved his gingival bleeding. This was mentioned in passing to his former professor, pathologist Rudolf Altschul who theorized at the time that hypercholesterolemia was related to impaired repair of vascular intimal damage [3]. A few months after this chance conversation, Rudolf Altschul et al. demonstrated that niacin reduced serum cholesterol levels in human subjects [4]. Altschul administered 4 g of niacin IR to 11 medical students and observed an 8.4 % decrease in serum cholesterol within 24 h. Later, he was able to demonstrate regression of atherosclerotic plaque in a rabbit model [5]. This discovery of the first therapeutic agent that reduced serum cholesterol in humans remained mostly unnoticed by the medical community. It was not until a randomized trial conducted by Parsons et al. at the Mayo Clinic confirmed these findings that niacin usage becomes more widely adopted [3].

## Mechanism of Lipid-Altering Effects

Beyond being the most effective clinically available drug to increase HDL-C and apolipoprotein A-I (apoA-1) levels [6, 7], niacin also induces favorable changes in the lipid profile by decreasing levels of LDL-C, triglycerides (TGs), very low-density lipoproteins (VLDL), and lipoprotein(a) [Lp(a)] [8]. There is emerging evidence that niacin also modulates lipoprotein particle size and number which may impact their atherogenic potential. Niacin decreases small-dense LDL particle number (LDL-P) and ApoB levels when added to a statin as compared to statin monotherapy [9–12]. Since patients with diabetes and CMR have a high incidence of elevated non-HDL cholesterol, ApoB, or LDL-P, the use of niacin in these populations would seem to be beneficial. The manner by which niacin induces changes in lipoproteins is incompletely understood, but recent discoveries have elucidated several potential mechanisms of action.

## The Niacin Receptor

Upon oral administration of niacin, it quickly exits the plasma and is sequestered in adipose tissue. The initial effect of niacin is a rapid decrease in plasma free fatty acid (FFA) followed by a delayed decrease in circulating TG and LDL-C levels. With niacin IR (crystalline niacin), this effect is transient, and there is a large rebound increase of plasma FFA within an hour [13]. However, extended-release niacin (ERN) is more effective at sustaining reduced FFA levels with an attenuated rebound in FFA [14].

Based on several early studies, niacin was hypothesized to exert its effects as a hormone activating a $G_i$-coupled receptor [15, 16]. In 2003, a formerly orphan receptor that binds with high affinity to nicotinic acid was identified [17–19]. Initially called GPR109A (HM74A) in humans and PUMA-G in mice, this $G_i$-coupled receptor is abundantly expressed in adipocytes and immune cells. The receptor has been renamed hydroxy-carboxylic acid (HCA) receptor ($HCA_2$). It is encoded on the human chromosome 12q24.31 [20]. Nicotinamide, which does not induce any significant changes in serum lipoprotein levels, binds very weakly to the $HCA_2$ receptor.

When nicotinic acid binds to $HCA_2$, it inhibits adenylyl cyclase, and, consequently, cyclic adenosine monophosphate (cAMP) is downregulated. cAMP is the primary second messenger regulating lipolysis via protein kinase A (PKA) [21]. PKA downregulates mRNA expression of hormone-sensitive lipase and its activity [22, 23]. The essential role of $HCA_2$ in the antilipolytic effects of niacin was confirmed in a murine model lacking PUMA-G. Niacin administration in these mice did not reduce FFA or TG [18].

In vitro studies have shown that nicotinic acid also noncompetitively inhibits hepatic diacylglycerol acyltransferase 2 (DGAT2) [24]. DGAT2 catalyzes the final and rate-limiting step in hepatic synthesis of TG. The inhibition of lipolysis in adipocytes deprives the liver of FFA substrate to generate TGs [25]. In the setting of reduced plasma FFA, decreased DGAT2 expression may explain the niacin-induced alterations in hepatic VLDL secretion and plasma lipoprotein levels [26]. However, recent data from transgenic mice expressing human CETP cast serious doubt on a direct relationship between FFA suppression and beneficial antidyslipidemic effects (↑HDL-C, ↓LDL-C) [27]. Niacin administration to these transgenic mice significantly increased HDL-C levels. Importantly though, the absence of the $HCA_2$ receptor did not affect niacin-induced changes in HDL-C or LDL-C, but did block the reduction of plasma FFA [28].

## Elevation of HDL-C

In contrast to the current understanding of niacin's mechanism of action on TG and LDL-C, niacin-induced HDL-C elevation is less well characterized. Normally, HDL-cholesteryl esters are removed from plasma by selective hepatic uptake up via the HDL receptor scavenger receptor class B type I (SR-BI), without lipoprotein particle uptake and degradation [29, 30]. Niacin-induced HDL-C elevation appears to result in large part due to decreased hepatic uptake of HDL particles from the plasma [31]. It is believed that niacin modulates hepatic uptake of HDL-C through a pathway independent of SR-BI as it does not affect SR-BI expression or function [32, 33]. One potential alternative hepatic receptor is the ATP synthase β-chain, which is known to act as an apoA-I/HDL receptor [34]. Niacin (but not nicotinamide) decreases the surface expression of this moiety in cultured HepG2 cells and decreased $I^{125}$-labeled HDL uptake by ~35 % [35]. Thus, decreased holoparticle removal of HDL may lead to higher plasma levels of apoA-I and HDL-C.

Another putative mechanism is that niacin acts either directly or indirectly as a CETP inhibitor. Niacin causes decreased hepatic production of VLDL which reduces CETP-mediated exchange of TG in VLDL particles for cholesteryl esters in HDL particles. The essential role for CETP in this process was supported by an experiment using transgenic mice. Wild-type mice do not normally express CETP. In transgenic mice expressing human CETP, niacin in a dose-dependent fashion increased levels of HDL-C while at the same time reduced both plasma TG and VLDL-C concentrations. However, wild-type mice did not have an increase in HDL-C levels when niacin was administered. CETP mass, activity, and expression were also reduced by niacin treatment in the transgenic mice [36, 37]. This mechanism is independent of the nicotinic acid receptor as hepatocytes do not express $HCA_2$.

## Pharmacokinetics and Metabolism

There are many different formulations of niacin with varying rates of absorption. The safety, tolerability, and efficacy profile of niacin are primarily determined by the rate of absorption from the gastrointestinal tract. To understand this relationship, it must also be recognized that niacin is metabolized by the liver through two separate and distinct pathways. One is a high-affinity, low-capacity oxidative (nonconjugative) pathway which leads to the formation of nicotinamide (which has lipoprotein-modifying effects) and pyridine metabolites, which are associated with hepatotoxicity. The second is a low-affinity, high-capacity conjugative pathway associated with flushing which leads to the formation of nicotinuric acid [38, 39]. The absorption kinetics of niacin determines the relative saturation of the slower oxidative pathway and shunting towards the faster conjugative pathways. Niacin IR (crystalline niacin) is rapidly absorbed and saturates the high-affinity but low-capacity pathway. This leads to the increased incidence of flushing. Alternatively, sustained-release formulations (slow release, long acting) have a delayed absorption, developed in an effort to reduce cutaneous flushing. However, these formulations are also associated with higher incidence of hepatotoxicity and reduced effect on HDL due to greater metabolism by the oxidative pathway [40]. Therefore, an optimal balance between the reduction in cutaneous flushing while limiting hepatotoxicity may best be achieved with ERN. ERN has absorption characteristic between niacin IR and sustained-release formulations. The only FDA-approved ERN is Niaspan© (Abbott Laboratories; Abbott Park, IL). Niaspan© is not recommended in doses greater than 2,000 mg/day [41].

## Hyperglycemia

Given the dyslipidemic profile often seen in patients with diabetes, in particular Type 2 diabetes, niacin may offer unique benefits by targeting TGs, HDL-C, LDL-C, and other lipoproteins. Unfortunately, for many years, niacin usage in diabetic patients was very limited partly due to safety concerns of niacin-induced hyperglycemia and insulin resistance (which can occur in patients without as well) [42, 43]. At one time, even the American Diabetes Association (ADA) guidelines discouraged the use of niacin [44]. However, data from randomized trials and observational studies demonstrate that niacin induces only mild elevations of fasting glucose levels (usually 4–5 %) and that its overall impact on the control of hyperglycemia is likely minimal [45–48].

It is well understood that niacin can worsen insulin sensitivity. In small short-term, placebo-controlled studies using the hyperinsulinemic–euglycemic clamp method in nondiabetic volunteers, niacin IR modestly decreases insulin sensitivity by 18 %. However, mean 24-h blood pressure, fasting glucose, FFA, and fasting serum insulin levels were not significantly changed after 2 weeks of treatment [49, 50]. At least in nondiabetic subjects, decreased insulin sensitivity may be offset by increased β-cell secretory activity. In one study with 11 healthy volunteers treated with niacin IR (up to 2 g/day) for 2 weeks, fasting glucose levels were not significantly changed ($p<0.10$). However, there was a marked drop in insulin sensitivity accompanied by significantly increased β-cell secretory activity as marked by levels of acute insulin and pro-insulin ($p<0.05$) [51].

A post hoc analysis of the Coronary Drug Project (CDP) trial showed that subjects with diabetes or impaired fasting glucose had the same cardiovascular benefit as subjects with normal fasting glucose. Compared to the control group, nonfatal myocardial infarction (MI) (at 6 months) and total mortality at 15-year follow-up was significantly reduced in niacin-treated patients across the spectrum of fasting glucose values after 1 year. Interestingly, there was a nonsignificant inverse correlation between 15-year mortality and fasting glucose at 1 year. Mortality actually decreased across the tertiles of elevated fasting glucose [52]. In the HDL-Atherosclerosis Treatment Study (HATS) trial, 25 type 2 diabetic patients were randomized to receive one of four factorial combinations therapies. In the simvastatin–niacin group, glycemic control did decline initially, and the titration of hypoglycemic medications was more common. However, after 8 months, glucose levels returned to pretreatment levels and remained stable for the remainder of the 3-year trial [53].

A caveat is that in many of the early clinical trials involving niacin, fasting glucose levels were not systematically monitored. The reporting of new onset diabetes was incumbent on the clinical investigators and not a prespecified clinical end point. This could have led to significant underreporting of the hyperglycemic and pro-diabetic effects of niacin. Reassuringly, more recent studies have shown only mild increases

(2–4 mg/dL) of fasting glucose in niacin patients with diabetes or metabolic syndrome [54].

Data from two randomized trials comparing niacin vs. placebo using hemoglobin A1c ($Hb_{A1c}$) levels further support the safety of niacin in people with diabetes. The Arterial Disease Multiple Intervention Trial (ADMIT) randomized subjects (125 with type 2 diabetes) to niacin IR (up to 3 g/day) or placebo. At 60-week follow-up, participants with diabetes who were randomized to niacin IR had modestly elevated fasting glucose but had no significant change in HbA1c [55].

Concordant with these findings, the Assessment of Diabetes Control and Evaluation of the Efficacy of Niaspan Trial (ADVENT), patients with type 2 diabetes were treated with either placebo, ERN 1,000 mg/day, or ERN 1,500 mg/day. After 16 weeks, HbA1c increased 0.19 % in the ERN 1,000 mg/day group, which was not significantly different than placebo. In the ERN 1,500 mg/day group, $Hb_{A1c}$ mildly increased 0.29 %, which just met statistical significance ($p=0.048$) compared to placebo [56].

Therefore, while niacin may elevate fasting glucose and worsen insulin resistance, even in patients without diabetes, clinical trial data demonstrate that absolute changes in HbA1c are often small and modest. With careful monitoring of glucose and appropriate management of hypoglycemic medications, the CV benefits of niacin can be achieved without significantly worsened glycemic control in patients with type 2 diabetes. Of note, there has not been any published data regarding niacin's dyslipidemic or hyperglycemic effects in patients with type I diabetes mellitus [48].

## Flushing

Niacin is well known to cause cutaneous flushing. In addition, patients may feel pruritus, burning, warmth, and tingling which starts in the face and extends towards the torso and arms. Generally flushing begins 20–60 min after administration and lasts usually for 1 h [57]. Though tolerance to flushing often develops within 1–2 weeks of usage, it still leads to discontinuation in 10–50 % of patients [58].

This side effect is highly dependent on its rate of absorption from the gastrointestinal tract. Flushing occurs most intensely with immediate-release formulations of niacin, which has led to the development of formulations with slower absorption. Flushing is less common with ERN (absorption time 8–12 h) and slow-release niacin (absorption time over 12 h). Slow-release formulations have a higher risk of liver toxicity in doses greater than 1,500 mg/day [47].

Niacin-induced flushing is caused by prostaglandin D2 (PGD2), released from Langerhans cells, which stimulate the PGD2 receptor-1 (DP1 receptors) on dermal vascular smooth muscle cells. This is turn induces vasodilation of dermal arterioles, thereby increasing blood flow to cutaneous tissues and inducing the flushing phenomenon.

Niacin-induced flushing can be reduced with pretreatment using prostaglandin inhibitors such aspirin 325 mg or ibuprofen 200 mg min prior to niacin ingestion [59, 60]. Other strategies to manage flushing effects and improve adherence is to dose niacin at bedtime along with avoiding alcohol, hot beverages, or spicy foods [61].

Another potentially effective medication is laropiprant (LRPT), a highly selective DP1-receptor antagonist that effectively reduces niacin-induced flushing. Trials using ERN/LPRT combination formulations demonstrated the combination reduced flushing but conserve the lipid-lowering effects of niacin [62]. A large-scale trial of ERN/LPRT vs. placebo (see HPS-THRIVE) is underway. This trial is a multicenter, randomized, double-blind, placebo-controlled trial which enrolled over 25,000 patients (7,000 with diabetes) with CAD, cerebrovascular disease, and peripheral arterial disease from the UK, Scandinavia, and China. Enrollment in HPS2-THRIVE was completed in June 2010, and preliminary results are anticipated in 2013.

## Pleiotropic Effects

Beyond its lipid-altering effects, niacin may have other properties which reduce inflammation, improve endothelial function, and reduce the progression of atherosclerosis. Adiponectin is a hormone synthesized and secreted by adipocytes which modulates a variety of metabolic processes, such as glucose and fatty acid catabolism, the regulation of serum glucose levels, and is believed to have anti-inflammatory and antiatherogenic properties. Niacin treatment markedly increases serum levels of adiponectin and decreases levels of nonesterified fatty acids (NEFAs) via the $HCA_2$ receptor in humans and mice [63, 64]. In vivo, it has also been shown to reduce proinflammatory chemokines (fractalkine, monocyte chemotactic protein-2) in adipocytes [65]. Niacin has been shown to reduce markers of inflammation such as high-sensitivity C-reactive protein (hs-CRP), lipoprotein-associated phospholipase A2, and tumor necrosis factor-α [10, 11].

## Clinical Trial Data (Table 21.1)

### Coronary Drug Project

This landmark and pioneering study sponsored by the US National Heart Lung and Blood Institute (NHLBI) evaluated the mortality benefits of four different therapies in male survivors of MI. The trial is also notable for being the only trial to ever have evaluated the cardiovascular outcomes of niacin as monotherapy. Eleven years after Altschul's seminal publication, the CDP group randomized 8,341 men with a history of MI, including type 2 diabetes, to one of six treatment groups: conjugated estrogen (high or lose dose), dextrothyroxine sodium, clofibrate (1.8 g/day), niacin IR (3 g/day), or lactose placebo. The trial began enrollment in March 1966 and randomized the last patient in October 1969. Follow-up data was censored in February 1975, and 95 % of patients were followed for at least five years.

Although the inclusion criteria targeted a high-risk population for secondary prevention, patients with insulin-dependent diabetes mellitus were specifically excluded. The majority of patients had angina and nearly one-half of the niacin-treated patients had a serum cholesterol >250 mg/dL. Nonetheless, there was still a large group of patients with diabetes or prediabetes, and 5.4 % of patients randomized to niacin were concomitantly treated with oral hypoglycemic medications at enrollment. Nearly 40 % of niacin-treated patients had evidence of abnormal fasting glucose (>100 mg/dL) and/or impaired glucose tolerance (≥180 mg/100 mL) after an oral glucose test.

Among the significant findings of this trial was the excess mortality of patients randomized to either estrogen or dextrothyroxine. Due to the increased risk of death, high-dose estrogen therapy (5.0 mg/day) was discontinued in 1970 and low-dose estrogen (2.5 mg/day) and dextrothyroxine stopped in 1971. Clofibrate, niacin, and placebo groups were continued in the trial as originally planned.

Despite significant reductions in total serum cholesterol and triglycerides, there was no significant difference between the active treatment groups and placebo in terms of the primary end point of all-cause mortality. All-cause mortality in niacin-treated patients was not significantly different compared to placebo (24.4 % vs. 25.4 %). The survival curves for niacin, clofibrate, and placebo were virtually superimposable during the first 68 months of follow-up. An adjusted analysis of all-cause mortality failed to find a benefit of niacin in 5-year mortality either. A subgroup analysis of patients being treated with oral hypoglycemic agents found no significant difference in 5-year mortality between niacin and placebo (32.8 % vs. 32.5 %, $Z_N = 0.05$). $Z_N$ values between −1.96 and 1.96 indicate homogeneity or no statistically significant difference between groups ($p > 0.05$). With regard to lipoprotein effects, the mean total cholesterol decreased by −9.8 % and TG decreased by 26.1 %. These improvements in cholesterol and triglycerides were slightly more robust than with clofibrate. There was no specific HDL-C or LDL-C measurement.

Though the CDP was a negative trial based on the initial analyses, several secondary end points suggested cardiovascular benefit with niacin. The combined end point of CHD death/nonfatal MI was lower in the niacin group, primarily driven by a significantly reduced incidence of nonfatal MI, which was 27 % lower in the niacin group (8.9 %

**Table 21.1** Summary of selected randomized trials examining niacin

| | No. of patients | | No. of patients with DM | | Changes in lipids in treatment group compared to control | | | | |
|---|---|---|---|---|---|---|---|---|---|
| Trial name | Niacin | Placebo | Niacin | Placebo | TC | TGs | LDL-C | HDL-C | Outcome |
| Coronary Drug project (1975) | 1,119 | 2,789 | (5.2 %); insulin users excluded | | ↓10 | ↓26 | NR | NR | All-cause mortality: 24.8 % vs. 25.9 %, $p=NS$ |
| | | | | | | | | | Nonfatal MI: 10.7 % vs. 14.8 %, $p=0001$ |
| Stockholm (1988) | 279 | 276 | 3.0 % | 3.6 % | ↓13 | ↓19 | NR | NR | Mortality decreased 26.6 % |
| | | | | | | | | | CV death dec 36 % |
| | | | | | | | | | Serum cholesterol decreased 13 % |
| | | | | | | | | | Serum Trig dec 19 % |
| FATS (1990) | 48 | 52 | Excluded patients with diabetes | | ↓23 | ↓29 | ↓32 | ↑43 | ↓80% clinical events (<0.01) |
| | | | | | | | | | Significant angiographic regression |
| CLAS (1987) | 80 | 82 | Excluded patients with diabetes | | ↓26 | ↓22 | ↓43 | ↑37 | Significantly less angiographic progression |
| | | | | | | | | | No difference in clinical events |
| HATS (2001) | 73 | 73 | 16 %; uncontrolled diabetes excluded | | ↓29 | ↓34 | ↓48 | ↑18 | ↓60% clinical events ($p<0.02$) in simvastatin–niacin |
| | | | | | | | | | Significant angiographic regression |
| ARBITER-2 (2004) | 87 | 80 | 22 | 24 | NC | ↓13 | ↓2 | ↑21 | No significant difference of CIMT |
| ARIBITER-6 (2009)[a] | 97 | 111 | 31 | 44 | ↓6 | ↓16 | ↓12 | ↑18 | Mean CIMT significantly reduced |
| | | | | | | | | | MACE: 1 % vs. 5 %, $p=0.04$ |
| AIM-HIGH (2011) | 1,718 | 1,696 | 588 | 570 | NR | ↓26 | ↓16 | ↑20 | No difference in MACE |
| HPS2-THRIVE | 25,673 | | 7,000+ | | | | | | Expected 2013 |

*NR* not reported, *NC* no significant change

[a]Active comparator group treated with ezetimibe 10 mg

vs. 12.2 %, $Z_N = -2.88$). The niacin group also had a 24 % lower incidence of CVA (8.5 % vs. 11.2 %, $Z_N = -2.46$). This reduction is particularly important given that compared to placebo, a slightly higher incidence of atrial fibrillation (4.7 vs. 2.9, $Z_N = 2.63$) and other arrhythmias (32.7 vs. 28.2 %, $Z_N = 2.74$) was noted in niacin-treated patients.

At 5-year follow-up, measurements of serum glucose demonstrated that niacin did worsen hyperglycemia mildly. Mean fasting glucose increased 8.0 % from baseline in the niacin group vs. 5.0 % in the placebo group ($Z_N = 2.52$). The 5-year incidence of elevated fasting glucose (>120 mg/dL) in niacin-treated patients was also significantly increased compared to placebo: 23.8 % vs. 15.9 % ($Z_N = 5.23$). However, the incidence of glucosuria was not significantly different. At five years, there was no significant difference in the prevalence of insulin or oral hypoglycemic medication use in niacin-treated patients compared to placebo: 4.6 % vs. 5.4 %.

Based on the initial follow-up of CDP results, it was concluded that despite the reduction of total cholesterol and lower morbidity (nonfatal MI's, fatal/nonfatal CVA) in niacin-treated patients, there was no mortality benefit to niacin treatment. The authors also cautioned against the use of niacin treatment in patients with diabetes.

## Coronary Drug Project 15-Year Mortality

Due to the possible excess cancer mortality of patients randomized into the low-dose estrogen group and concerns of clofibrate safety from the World Health Organization Trial, the NHLBI sponsored a long-term follow-up study of all patients who were randomized in the CDP [46]. The primary goal of the study was to determine the vital status of 6,008 patients who were alive at the initial data censure in February 1975. The mean follow-up was 15 years (6.2 years during treatment and 8.8 after termination of the study).

Unexpectedly and discordant with the original CDP trial, the all-cause mortality of the niacin-treated patients was 6.2 % lower than placebo (52.0 % vs. 58.2 %, $p = 0.0004$). The main difference in overall mortality was a significant reduction of cardiovascular mortality; however, there was a trend towards reduced mortality due to cerebrovascular, cancer, and noncancer causes as well.

The mortality benefit persisted with subgroup analysis by age, serum cholesterol, and serum triglycerides. Importantly, this benefit also was seen in patients with impaired fasting glucose (≥100 mg/dL). The survival curves of niacin and placebo were identical until month 72, when divergence begins. The initial analysis of CDP did note the start of this separation, but there was inadequate follow-up at that time to have statistical significance. The separation of curves continued despite the cessation of niacin treatment. It remains unclear why was there a 6-year delay before niacin treatment manifested a mortality benefit and why did this benefit persisted despite lack of treatment. One possibility is that the progression of atherosclerosis was most effectively altered by niacin. Compared to the other treatment groups, niacin treatment resulted in the greatest reduction in serum cholesterol and triglycerides, −10.1 % and −26.9 %, respectively. The clinical benefit of this was initially manifested by a reduction in nonfatal MI seen in the niacin group starting about 2 years after randomization.

## Stockholm Ischemic Heart Disease Secondary Prevention Study

Performed in the "pre-statin" era, this open-label, secondary prevention trial enrolled 554 survivors of MI's and randomized them to either placebo or combination clofibrate/niacin for five years. The specific form of niacin used was a nicotinic acid ester called pentaerythrityl tetranicotinate or niceritrol, which has delayed release characteristics. Though insulin-dependent diabetic patients were excluded, the trial still enrolled a small cohort of diabetic subjects, 3.6 and 3.0 % in the control and treatment groups, respectively. There were no specific subgroup analyses of outcomes for patients with diabetes [66].

Most notably there was a 26 % reduction of all-cause mortality and a 36 % of CV death in patient's treatment with clofibrate/niacin vs. placebo ($p<0.01$). Patients in the treatment arm were observed to have a significant improvement in their lipid profile: serum triglycerides were reduced by 19 % and serum cholesterol decreased by 13 % ($p<0.001$ for both end points). HDL-C was not reported. Interestingly, the authors concluded that the CV mortality benefit correlated with reduction in serum triglycerides rather than serum cholesterol.

## Cholesterol-Lowering Atherosclerosis Study

This relatively small angiographic study was a randomized, placebo-controlled, selectively blinded trial which randomized 162 male post-CABG patients to either 30 g of colestipol hydrochloride plus niacin (titrated to 3–12 g/day) or placebo. Patients with diabetes, hypertension, or hypertriglyceridemia (>500 mg/dL) were excluded from the trial. The trial was designed to evaluate the change of coronary or peripheral arterial stenosis after two years of treatment using a semiquantitative measurement called the "Global Change Score." Based on this assessment, overall progression of disease was significantly reduced with colestipol–niacin treatment. Importantly, the lipid profile significantly improved in colestipol–niacin-treated patients compared to placebo: LDL-C levels decreased −43 % vs. −5 % ($p<0.001$), HDL-C increased 37 % vs. 2 % ($p<0.001$), and total cholesterol decreased −26 % vs. −4 % ($p<0.001$) [67].

## Familial Atherosclerosis Treatment Study

This small, randomized, doubled trial assessed the change in the severity of proximal coronary artery disease assessed by a semiquantitative analysis [68]. The trial population consisted of 146 men with angiographically proven CAD, as well as elevated ApoB levels (>125 mg/dL) and family history of CAD. Diabetic subjects were excluded from the trial. Participants were randomized to one of three treatment groups for 2½ years: lovastatin (20 mg twice a day) plus colestipol (10 g three times a day), niacin (1 g four times a day) plus colestipol (10 g three times a day), or conventional treatment (diet counseling and "placebo"). However, as per protocol, subjects could receive colestipol if LDL-C was above the 90th percentile for age. Thus, 43 % of patients in the placebo group received colestipol.

Participants underwent a baseline coronary angiogram and a 2½ year follow-up. In the conventional treatment group, 46 % had progression of at least one lesion at one of nine proximal coronary artery segments. By comparison, the incidence of progression of proximal stenosis was approximately half that observed in the conventional treatment group, 23 % ($p=0.005$). Since the trial was relatively small, there were few clinical events observed. However, the primary clinical composite end point (CV death, MI, or revascularization for worsening ischemic) was observed significantly more in the placebo group than in the active treatment group (11 vs. 5, $p=0.01$). In the conventional treatment group, LDL-C and HDL changed modestly: −7 % and +5 %, respectively. In contrast, the lipid profile was significantly improved in the niacin–colestipol group: LDL-C decreased 32 % and HDL-C increased 43 % ($p<0.001$). ApoB levels significantly decreased with both lovastatin–colestipol and niacin–colestipol treatment: −35 % and −28 %, respectively ($p<0.001$).

A few side effects were noted. Two patients in the niacin–colestipol group had to receive antidiabetic medications, and two other patients developed gout. Mean AST increased by about 20 % in both niacin–colestipol and lovastatin–colestipol groups, but no individual patient developed significant AST elevation greater than three times normal.

Multivariate stepwise analysis of mean change in proximal stenosis found %Δ HDL-C and %ΔLDL-C as independently predictive. Other variables also independently predictive were

ST-segment depression at peak exercise during baseline treadmill stress testing, %Δ ApoB, and %Δ systolic blood pressure during treatment. These results of Familial Atherosclerosis Treatment Study (FATS) suggested that significant improvements in CAD, assessed by angiographic and clinically metrics, could be observed with therapies that effectively raised HDL-C and lowered LDL-C.

## HDL-Atherosclerosis Treatment Study

This was a randomized, double-blind, placebo-controlled angiographic trial that used a two-by-two factorial design to evaluate the effects of combination simvastatin–niacin therapy and/or antioxidant therapy (vitamin E, C, β-carotene, and selenium) vs. placebo [69]. The primary end point was the mean change of stenosis caused by the most severe lesion in a proximal coronary artery segment using quantitative coronary angiography (QCA). The pre-specified primary clinical end point was the time to occurrence of cardiovascular death, non-fatal MI, CVA, or revascularization due to worsening ischemia.

The study population consisted of 160 patients; 55 % had prior MI and 49 % had undergone prior angioplasty. Sixteen percent had diabetes mellitus, although uncontrolled diabetic subjects were excluded from the trial. The patients were randomized to one of four groups: placebo ($n=44$), simvastatin–niacin ($n=33$), antioxidant vitamins ($n=39$), or simvastatin–niacin plus antioxidants ($n=40$). Of note, in an effort to maintain blinding, the placebo group received a small dose of immediate-release niacin (50 mg twice daily) to provoke flushing. Simvastatin–niacin-treated patients experienced a 42 % reduction of LDL-C and a 26 % increase in HDL-C levels. The addition of antioxidants to simvastatin–niacin blunted both the lipid-lowering effects and the capacity to raise HDL-C of simvastatin–niacin [70]. Coronary artery disease as measured by angiography worsened in patients assigned to placebo but regressed in the simvastatin–niacin group ($p<0.001$) [69].

## Atherothrombosis Intervention in Metabolic Syndrome with Low HDL/High Triglycerides: Impact on Global Health Outcomes (AIM-HIGH)

Despite aggressive pharmacologic therapies to reduce LDL-C to target levels, a large proportion of patients with CAD will continue to have CV events. In these patients, HDL-C levels have independent prognostic value. The AIM-HIGH investigators hoped to demonstrate that HDL-C raising and triglyceride lowering with Niaspan ER after aggressive LDL-C lowering with statins and ezetimibe (for some of the patients) would improve cardiovascular outcomes in patients with stable coronary artery disease [71, 72].

AIM-HIGH enrolled patients age 45 years or older who had established cardiovascular disease, defined as documented stable CAD, cerebrovascular disease, carotid artery disease, or peripheral arterial disease. At entry, patients had low baseline levels of HDL-C (<40 mg/dL for men, <50 mg/dL for women). LDL-C levels were required to be lower than 180 mg/dL. Compared to the placebo, the baseline mean LDL-C (mg/dL) was not significantly different in patients randomized to ERN plus simvastatin: 75.8 ± 24.3 vs. 76.2 ± 25.7, respectively. Mean HLD-C was nominally higher in the placebo group: 35.3 ± 5.9 vs. 34.8 ± 5.9 ($p=0.04$). The trial was multicenter and enrolled patients from the USA and Canada.

The trial's primary end point was the composite of CV death, nonfatal MI, ischemic CVA, hospitalization for an ACS, or cerebral revascularization. It was an event-driven trial expected to have 800 adjudicated events with a mean follow-up period of 4.6 years. The trial was proposed to have 85 % power to detect a 25 % relative risk reduction in the primary end point.

A total of 3,414 patients were randomized to ERN (1,500–2,000 mg/day) plus simvastatin or placebo plus simvastatin. It must be noted that the placebo group (like other trials) received niacin IR (50–100 mg twice a day) to mask treatment. Simvastatin was adjusted based upon a prespecified algorithm to maintain LDL in the range of 40–80 mg/dL. In addition, subjects in either group could receive an adjunctive daily dose of ezetimibe 10 mg/day to achieve the target LDL-C level of 70 mg/dL.

Patients with diabetes were included in the trial and were one of the six prespecified subgroups for analysis. Of subjects with a history of diabetes, 570 (33.6 %) were randomized to placebo plus simvastatin and 588 (34.2 %) were randomized to ERN plus simvastatin. The mean baseline HbA1c was similar: 6.68 ± 0.85 % and 6.70 ± 0.88, respectively. There was no significant difference in mean baseline glucose or serum insulin either.

AIM-HIGH was stopped early by the Data Safety Monitoring Board (DSMB) due to lack of efficacy and a trend towards a higher rate of ischemic strokes in the ERN-treated group: 556 patients had a primary end point event (282 [6.4 %] in the niacin group and 274 [16.2 %] in the placebo group, HR 1.02; $p = 0.80$). There was a trend towards a higher incidence of ischemic strokes in the niacin group: 27 patients (1.6 %) vs. 15 (0.9 %) and hazard ratio (HR) 1.61; $p = 0.11$. In subgroup analysis no benefit for niacin could be detected among subjects with diabetes.

The trial's results were very controversial and received considerable attention regarding its design, early termination, and negative findings. It was criticized for being underpowered to detect a clinical benefit since the between group difference of HDL-C was only 4 mg/dL. This resulted from a higher than expected increase in the HDL-C in the placebo group, which did receive a small dose of immediate-release niacin.

Other critiques focused on the possible differential effects of niacin on total cholesterol (HDL-C or LDL-C) vs. modulation of particle size (HDL-P or LDL-P). Niacin can cause discordant effects on total measured cholesterol (HDL-C or LDL-C) and particle size/number [73]. While combination therapy of ERN and simvastatin compared to atorvastatin monotherapy has been shown to favorably increase the number and size of HDL particle subclasses, the effect of ERN and simvastatin in the AIM-HIGH trial is still unknown pending results of the nuclear magnetic resonance substudy [74]. Thus, if Apo B or LDL-P levels have been lowered to very low values, then raising HDL-C without accompanying changes in HDL-P offers no additional incremental CV risk reduction benefit [75, 76].

### The Treatment of HDL to Reduce the Incidence of Vascular Events (HPS2-THRIVE)

The ongoing HPS2-THRIVE trial is by far the largest trial to evaluate the clinical benefits of niacin treatment (Clinicaltrials.gov: NCT0046-1630). This trial is a multicenter, randomized, double-blind, placebo-controlled trial which enrolled over 25,000 patients with CAD, cerebrovascular disease, peripheral arterial disease, and diabetes from the UK, Scandinavia, and China. More patients have been enrolled in this single trial than all previous randomized niacin trials combined. Furthermore, HPS2-THRIVE will enroll more than 7,000 patients with diabetes which will finally allow for a robust understanding of the beneficial or potentially deleterious effects of niacin in people with diabetes. The study is headed by the Clinical Trial Service Unit of the University of Oxford. The goal of the study is to evaluate the clinical benefits of adjunctive treatment with extended-release niacin 1 g/laropiprant (ERN/LPRT) in patients already treated with simvastatin 40 mg/day ± ezetimibe. ERN/LPRT (Tredaptive®; Merck & Co, Inc) was approved for use in the EU in 2008, but is not yet approved for use in the USA. LPRT is a selective prostaglandin D receptor antagonist that significantly reduces the frequency and intensity of niacin-induced flushing [77]. The primary end point will be time to first major vascular event: nonfatal MI, CV death, CVA, or revascularization. Patients will be followed for a mean of at least 4 years. Enrollment in HPS2-THRIVE was completed in June 2010, and preliminary results are anticipated in 2013.

## Non-invasive Imaging Trials

### Arterial Biology for the Investigation of the Treatment Effects of Reducing Cholesterol (ARBITER-2/ARBITER-3)

ARBITER-2 was a small, randomized trial that measured changes in carotid intima media thickness (CIMT) to compare ERN vs. placebo in patients already being treated with statin (>90 %

of patients used simvastatin) and low LDL-C (≈80 mg/dL) levels. The trial enrolled 167 subjects with known CAD and low HDL-C levels (mean 40 mg/dL). There was a high prevalence of insulin resistance (46 with type 2 diabetes mellitus and 85 with metabolic syndrome). After one year, there was a small progression of mean CIMT ($0.044 \pm 0.100$ mm, $p < 0.001$) in the statin plus placebo GROUP, but unchanged in the statin plus ERN group. The overall progression of mean CIMT was not significantly different between the placebo and ERN groups. Post hoc analysis of subjects with insulin resistance also showed no significant difference between placebo and niacin. However, when the subjects with insulin resistance were excluded from the analysis, a statistically significant difference was observed [78].

Building on these results, ARIBTER-3 continued niacin treatment in 130 subjects (36 with diabetes) for another 12 months in an open-label design. Patients who were initially randomized to placebo in ARBITER-2 crossed over to treatment with ERN. Sixty-nine subjects who had initially been treated with ERN were continued on ERN to complete 24 months of treatment. Both groups showed significant regression of mean CIMT, with the 24 month ERN group demonstrating the most regression ($p < 0.001$). Glucose values were not significantly different in the 24 month ERN group compared to baseline ($p = 0.20$). This was the first trial to show additional treatment benefit of niacin to a background of statin therapy. Despite the negative results of ARBITER-2 in patients with insulin resistance, these results from ARBITER-3 suggest a benefit of niacin to patients with diabetes and metabolic syndrome [79].

## ARBITER 6-HALTS

Again using CIMT as surrogate marker for atherosclerosis, the ARBITER 6-HALTS study compared two different adjunctive strategies for lipid modification in patients already being treated with statins [80]. Three hundred sixty-three subjects with known vascular disease or CAD risk equivalents were randomized to either ezetimibe (10 mg/day) or ERN (2,000 mg/day) in addition to long treatment with statins. Subjects had CIMT measured at baseline and at 14 months follow-up. Compared to ezetimibe, subjects treated with ERN had significantly larger regression of mean ($p = 0.001$) and maximal CIMT ($p \leq 0.001$). LDL-C and TG levels decreased significantly in niacin-treated patients, and mean HDL-C level increased 18.4 % in niacin-treated patients. Though the trial was not powered for clinical end points, it was unfortunately stopped early due to the CIMT results. This may have exaggerated the efficacy of niacin on CIMT compared to ezetimibe [81].

## Guidelines

While not specifically discussing diabetic patients, ATPIII NCEP guidelines suggest adding niacin or fibrate therapy to statins in high-risk patients with elevated triglycerides or low HDL-C levels [82]. In 2010, the American Diabetes Association (ADA) published the Standard of Medical Care in Diabetes. The recommended target levels for LDL-C in diabetic patients without CVD was <100 mg/dL and <70 mg/dL in patients with CVD. The ADA also recommended using statins as the primary agent to reduce LDL-C levels and reserved the use of niacin (along with fenofibrate, ezetimibe, and bile acid sequestrants) in patients who did not achieve LDL-C targets with statins or were intolerant to statins. Niacin was acknowledged as a potent agent that can raise HDL-C levels and improve the lipid profile of diabetic patients; however, the guidelines cautioned that there was sparse and insufficient data compared to statins regarding its clinical benefits [83]. The ADA and the American College of Cardiology (ACC) addressed lipoprotein management in patients with CMR in a consensus statement in 2008. The same LDL-C targets were recommended for patients with CMR as diabetic patients. If needed, niacin was recommended as the preferred adjuvant agent to statins in patients with low HDL-C and elevated TG levels [84].

## Conclusions

Niacin is the first pharmacologic agent known to reduce cholesterol levels in humans and the most effective to increase HDL-C levels, but much remains to be understood regarding the mechanisms of its action and clinical benefit. Niacin induces favorable changes across the spectrum of lipoproteins which may reduce atherogenic potential and CV risk. These effects may be of particularly benefit in patients with diabetes or CMR. There have been few studies of niacin's clinical benefits, and data regarding outcomes in patients with diabetes are even more scant. Although statins and LDL-C reduction are the cornerstones of modern antilipidemic therapy, there is clinical equipoise regarding niacin's benefits. Given this though, a significant role for niacin may still exist as adjuvant therapy for LDL-C or LDL-p lowering or in statin-intolerant patients. Further data from large studies such as HPS2-THRIVE are eagerly anticipated and hopefully should clarify the role and utility of niacin therapy.

## References


1. National Cholesterol Education Program (NCEP) Expert Panel on Detection, Evaluation, and Treatment of High Blood Cholesterol in Adults (Adult Treatment Panel III). Third report of the National Cholesterol Education Program (NCEP) Expert Panel on Detection, Evaluation, and Treatment of High Blood Cholesterol in Adults (Adult Treatment Panel III) final report. Circulation. 2002;106:3143–421.
2. Hegyi J, Schwartz RA, Hegyi V. Pellagra: dermatitis, dementia, and diarrhea. Int J Dermatol. 2004;43:1–5.
3. Hoffer A. Niacin and cholesterol: the history of a discovery. J Clin Lipidol. 2009;3:244–6.
4. Altschul R, Hoffer A, Stephen JD. Influence of nicotinic acid on serum cholesterol in man. Arch Biochem Biophys. 1955;54:558–9.
5. Altschul R. Effect of nicotine acid on the blood cholesterol level and experimental atherosclerosis. Z Kreislaufforsch. 1956;45:573–6.
6. Shepherd J, Packard CJ, Patsch JR, Gotto Jr AM, Taunton OD. Effects of nicotinic acid therapy on plasma high density lipoprotein subfraction distribution and composition and on apolipoprotein A metabolism. J Clin Invest. 1979;63:858–67.
7. Sakai T, Kamanna VS, Kashyap ML. Niacin, but not gemfibrozil, selectively increases LP-AI, a cardioprotective subfraction of HDL, in patients with low HDL cholesterol. Arterioscler Thromb Vasc Biol. 2001;21:1783–9.
8. Carlson LA, Hamsten A, Asplund A. Pronounced lowering of serum levels of lipoprotein Lp(a) in hyperlipidaemic subjects treated with nicotinic acid. J Intern Med. 1989;226:271–6.
9. Airan-Javia SL, Wolf RL, Wolfe ML, Tadesse M, Mohler E, Reilly MP. Atheroprotective lipoprotein effects of a niacin-simvastatin combination compared to low- and high-dose simvastatin monotherapy. Am Heart J. 2009;157:687.e1–8.
10. Jafri H, Alsheikh-Ali AA, Mooney P, Kimmelstiel CD, Karas RH, Kuvin JT. Extended-release niacin reduces LDL particle number without changing total LDL cholesterol in patients with stable CAD. J Clin Lipidol. 2009;3:45–50.
11. Knopp RH, Retzlaff BM, Fish B, et al. The SLIM Study: Slo-Niacin(R) and atorvastatin treatment of lipoproteins and inflammatory markers in combined hyperlipidemia. J Clin Lipidol. 2009;3:167–78.
12. Insull Jr W, Toth PP, Superko HR, et al. Combination of niacin extended-release and simvastatin results in a less atherogenic lipid profile than atorvastatin monotherapy. Vasc Health Risk Manag. 2010;6:1065–75.
13. Carlson LA, Oro L. The effect of nicotinic acid on the plasma free fatty acid; demonstration of a metabolic type of sympathicolysis. Acta Med Scand. 1962;172:641–5.
14. Vega GL, Cater NB, Meguro S, Grundy SM. Influence of extended-release nicotinic acid on nonesterified fatty acid flux in the metabolic syndrome with atherogenic dyslipidemia. Am J Cardiol. 2005;95:1309–13.
15. Aktories K, Schultz G, Jakobs KH. Regulation of adenylate cyclase activity in hamster adipocytes. Inhibition by prostaglandins, alpha-adrenergic agonists and nicotinic acid. Naunyn Schmiedebergs Arch Pharmacol. 1980;312:167–73.
16. Aktories K, Jakobs KH, Schultz G. Nicotinic acid inhibits adipocyte adenylate cyclase in a hormone-like manner. FEBS Lett. 1980;115:11–4.
17. Soga T, Kamohara M, Takasaki J, et al. Molecular identification of nicotinic acid receptor. Biochem Biophys Res Commun. 2003;303:364–9.
18. Tunaru S, Kero J, Schaub A, et al. PUMA-G and HM74 are receptors for nicotinic acid and mediate its anti-lipolytic effect. Nat Med. 2003;9:352–5.
19. Wise A, Foord SM, Fraser NJ, et al. Molecular identification of high and low affinity receptors for nicotinic acid. J Biol Chem. 2003;278:9869–74.
20. Zellner C, Pullinger CR, Aouizerat BE, et al. Variations in human HM74 (GPR109B) and HM74A (GPR109A) niacin receptors. Hum Mutat. 2005;25:18–21.
21. Offermanns S. The nicotinic acid receptor GPR109A (HM74A or PUMA-G) as a new therapeutic target. Trends Pharmacol Sci. 2006;27:384–90.
22. Linke A, Sonnabend M, Fasshauer M, et al. Effects of extended-release niacin on lipid profile and adipocyte biology in patients with impaired glucose tolerance. Atherosclerosis. 2009;205:207–13.

23. Nirogi R, Kandikere V, Komarneni P, et al. Quantification of methyllycaconitine, selective alpha(7) nicotinic receptor antagonist, in rodent plasma and brain tissue by liquid chromatography tandem mass spectrometry—application to neuro-pharmacokinetics of methyllycaconitine in rats. Biomed Chromatogr. 2011.
24. Ganji SH, Tavintharan S, Zhu D, Xing Y, Kamanna VS, Kashyap ML. Niacin noncompetitively inhibits DGAT2 but not DGAT1 activity in HepG2 cells. J Lipid Res. 2004;45:1835–45.
25. Lukasova M, Hanson J, Tunaru S, Offermanns S. Nicotinic acid (niacin): new lipid-independent mechanisms of action and therapeutic potentials. Trends Pharmacol Sci. 2011;32:700–7.
26. Kang I, Kim SW, Youn JH. Effects of nicotinic acid on gene expression: potential mechanisms and implications for wanted and unwanted effects of the lipid-lowering drug. J Clin Endocrinol Metab. 2011;96:3048–55.
27. Offermanns S. It ain't over 'til the fat lady sings. Sci Transl Med. 2012;4:148fs30.
28. Lauring B, Taggart AK, Tata JR, et al. Niacin lipid efficacy is independent of both the niacin receptor GPR109A and free fatty acid suppression. Sci Transl Med. 2012;4:148ra15.
29. Acton S, Rigotti A, Landschulz KT, Xu S, Hobbs HH, Krieger M. Identification of scavenger receptor SR-BI as a high density lipoprotein receptor. Science. 1996;271:518–20.
30. Steinberg D. A docking receptor for HDL cholesterol esters. Science. 1996;271:460–1.
31. Fidge NH. High density lipoprotein receptors, binding proteins, and ligands. J Lipid Res. 1999;40: 187–201.
32. Nieland TJ, Shaw JT, Jaipuri FA, et al. Identification of the molecular target of small molecule inhibitors of HDL receptor SR-BI activity. Biochemistry. 2008;47: 460–72.
33. Nieland TJ, Shaw JT, Jaipuri FA, et al. Influence of HDL-cholesterol-elevating drugs on the in vitro activity of the HDL receptor SR-BI. J Lipid Res. 2007;48: 1832–45.
34. Martinez LO, Jacquet S, Esteve JP, et al. Ectopic beta-chain of ATP synthase is an apolipoprotein A-I receptor in hepatic HDL endocytosis. Nature. 2003;421: 75–9.
35. Zhang LH, Kamanna VS, Zhang MC, Kashyap ML. Niacin inhibits surface expression of ATP synthase beta chain in HepG2 cells: implications for raising HDL. J Lipid Res. 2008;49:1195–201.
36. van der Hoorn JW, de Haan W, Berbee JF, et al. Niacin increases HDL by reducing hepatic expression and plasma levels of cholesteryl ester transfer protein in APOE*3Leiden.CETP mice. Arterioscler Thromb Vasc Biol. 2008;28:2016–22.
37. Digby JE, Lee JM, Choudhury RP. Nicotinic acid and the prevention of coronary artery disease. Curr Opin Lipidol. 2009;20:321–6.
38. Piepho RW. The pharmacokinetics and pharmacodynamics of agents proven to raise high-density lipoprotein cholesterol. Am J Cardiol. 2000;86:35L–40.
39. Stern RH, Freeman D, Spence JD. Differences in metabolism of time-release and unmodified nicotinic acid: explanation of the differences in hypolipidemic action? Metabolism. 1992;41:879–81.
40. McKenney JM, Proctor JD, Harris S, Chinchili VM. A comparison of the efficacy and toxic effects of sustained- vs immediate-release niacin in hypercholesterolemic patients. JAMA. 1994;271:672–7.
41. Physicians' desk reference: PDR. In: Oradell NJ (ed) Medical Economics Co.:v.
42. Garg A, Grundy SM. Nicotinic acid as therapy for dyslipidemia in non-insulin-dependent diabetes mellitus. JAMA. 1990;264:723–6.
43. Adler E, Paauw D. Medical myths involving diabetes. Prim Care. 2003;30:607–18.
44. Management of dyslipidemia in adults with diabetes. American Diabetes Association. Diabetes Care. 1998; 21:179–82.
45. Clofibrate and niacin in coronary heart disease. JAMA. 1975;231:360–81.
46. W.H.O. cooperative trial on primary prevention of ischaemic heart disease using clofibrate to lower serum cholesterol: mortality follow-up. Report of the Committee of Principal Investigators. Lancet. 1980;2:379–85.
47. Guyton JR, Bays HE. Safety considerations with niacin therapy. Am J Cardiol. 2007;99:22C–31.
48. Goldberg RB, Jacobson TA. Effects of niacin on glucose control in patients with dyslipidemia. Mayo Clin Proc. 2008;83:470–8.
49. Kelly JJ, Lawson JA, Campbell LV, et al. Effects of nicotinic acid on insulin sensitivity and blood pressure in healthy subjects. J Hum Hypertens. 2000;14:567–72.
50. Alvarsson M, Grill V. Impact of nicotinic acid treatment on insulin secretion and insulin sensitivity in low and high insulin responders. Scand J Clin Lab Invest. 1996;56:563–70.
51. Kahn SE, Beard JC, Schwartz MW, et al. Increased beta-cell secretory capacity as mechanism for islet adaptation to nicotinic acid-induced insulin resistance. Diabetes. 1989;38:562–8.
52. Canner PL, Furberg CD, Terrin ML, McGovern ME. Benefits of niacin by glycemic status in patients with healed myocardial infarction (from the Coronary Drug Project). Am J Cardiol. 2005;95:254–7.
53. Zhao XQ, Morse JS, Dowdy AA, et al. Safety and tolerability of simvastatin plus niacin in patients with coronary artery disease and low high-density lipoprotein cholesterol (The HDL Atherosclerosis Treatment Study). Am J Cardiol. 2004;93:307–12.
54. Bays HE, Shah A, Lin J, McCrary Sisk C, Paolini JF, Maccubbin D. Efficacy and tolerability of extended-release niacin/laropiprant in dyslipidemic patients with metabolic syndrome. J Clin Lipidol. 2010;4:515–21.
55. Elam MB, Hunninghake DB, Davis KB, et al. Effect of niacin on lipid and lipoprotein levels and glycemic control in patients with diabetes and peripheral arterial disease: the ADMIT study: a randomized trial. Arterial Disease Multiple Intervention Trial. JAMA. 2000;284:1263–70.
56. Grundy SM, Vega GL, McGovern ME, et al. Efficacy, safety, and tolerability of once-daily niacin for the

treatment of dyslipidemia associated with type 2 diabetes: results of the assessment of diabetes control and evaluation of the efficacy of niaspan trial. Arch Intern Med. 2002;162:1568–76.
57. Meyers CD, Carr MC, Park S, Brunzell JD. Varying cost and free nicotinic acid content in over-the-counter niacin preparations for dyslipidemia. Ann Intern Med. 2003;139:996–1002.
58. McKenney J. Niacin for dyslipidemia: considerations in product selection. Am J Health Syst Pharm. 2003;60:995–1005.
59. Jungnickel PW, Maloley PA, Vander Tuin EL, Peddicord TE, Campbell JR. Effect of two aspirin pretreatment regimens on niacin-induced cutaneous reactions. J Gen Intern Med. 1997;12:591–6.
60. Dunn RT, Ford MA, Rindone JP, Kwiecinski FA. Low-dose aspirin and ibuprofen reduce the cutaneous reactions following niacin administration. Am J Ther. 1995;2:478–80.
61. Davidson MH. Niacin use and cutaneous flushing: mechanisms and strategies for prevention. Am J Cardiol. 2008;101:14B–9.
62. Paolini JF, Bays HE, Ballantyne CM, et al. Extended-release niacin/laropiprant: reducing niacin-induced flushing to better realize the benefit of niacin in improving cardiovascular risk factors. Cardiol Clin. 2008;26:547–60.
63. Plaisance EP, Lukasova M, Offermanns S, Zhang Y, Cao G, Judd RL. Niacin stimulates adiponectin secretion through the GPR109A receptor. Am J Physiol Endocrinol Metab. 2009;296:E549–58.
64. Westphal S, Luley C. Preferential increase in high-molecular weight adiponectin after niacin. Atherosclerosis. 2008;198:179–83.
65. Digby JE, McNeill E, Dyar OJ, Lam V, Greaves DR, Choudhury RP. Anti-inflammatory effects of nicotinic acid in adipocytes demonstrated by suppression of fractalkine, RANTES, and MCP-1 and upregulation of adiponectin. Atherosclerosis. 2010;209:89–95.
66. Carlson LA, Rosenhamer G. Reduction of mortality in the Stockholm Ischaemic Heart Disease Secondary Prevention Study by combined treatment with clofibrate and nicotinic acid. Acta Med Scand. 1988;223:405–18.
67. Blankenhorn DH, Nessim SA, Johnson RL, Sanmarco ME, Azen SP, Cashin-Hemphill L. Beneficial effects of combined colestipol-niacin therapy on coronary atherosclerosis and coronary venous bypass grafts. JAMA. 1987;257:3233–40.
68. Brown G, Albers JJ, Fisher LD, et al. Regression of coronary-artery disease as a result of intensive lipid-lowering therapy in men with high-levels of apolipoprotein-B. N Engl J Med. 1990;323:1289–98.
69. Brown BG, Zhao XQ, Chait A, et al. Simvastatin and niacin, antioxidant vitamins, or the combination for the prevention of coronary disease. N Engl J Med. 2001;345:1583–92.
70. Cheung MC, Zhao XQ, Chait A, Albers JJ, Brown BG. Antioxidant supplements block the response of HDL to simvastatin-niacin therapy in patients with coronary artery disease and low HDL. Arterioscler Thromb Vasc Biol. 2001;21:1320–6.
71. The role of niacin in raising high-density lipoprotein cholesterol to reduce cardiovascular events in patients with atherosclerotic cardiovascular disease and optimally treated low-density lipoprotein cholesterol Rationale and study design. The Atherothrombosis Intervention in Metabolic syndrome with low HDL/high triglycerides: Impact on Global Health outcomes (AIM-HIGH). Am Heart J. 2011;161:471–7.e2.
72. Niacin in patients with low HDL cholesterol levels receiving intensive statin therapy. N Engl J Med. 2011.
73. Otvos JD. The surprising AIM-HIGH results are not surprising when viewed through a particle lens. J Clin Lipidol. 2011;5:368–70.
74. Toth PP, Thakker KM, Jiang P, Padley RJ. Niacin extended-release/simvastatin combination therapy produces larger favorable changes in high-density lipoprotein particles than atorvastatin monotherapy. Vasc Health Risk Manag. 2012;8:39–44.
75. Otvos JD, Collins D, Freedman DS, et al. Low-density lipoprotein and high-density lipoprotein particle subclasses predict coronary events and are favorably changed by gemfibrozil therapy in the Veterans Affairs High-Density Lipoprotein Intervention Trial. Circulation. 2006;113:1556–63.
76. Otvos JD, Mora S, Shalaurova I, Greenland P, Mackey RH, Goff Jr DC. Clinical implications of discordance between low-density lipoprotein cholesterol and particle number. J Clin Lipidol. 2011;5:105–13.
77. Paolini JF, Mitchel YB, Reyes R, et al. Effects of laropiprant on nicotinic acid-induced flushing in patients with dyslipidemia. Am J Cardiol. 2008;101:625–30.
78. Taylor AJ, Sullenberger LE, Lee HJ, Lee JK, Grace KA. Arterial Biology for the Investigation of the Treatment Effects of Reducing Cholesterol (ARBITER) 2: a double-blind, placebo-controlled study of extended-release niacin on atherosclerosis progression in secondary prevention patients treated with statins. Circulation. 2004;110:3512–7.
79. Taylor AJ, Lee HJ, Sullenberger LE. The effect of 24 months of combination statin and extended-release niacin on carotid intima-media thickness: ARBITER 3. Curr Med Res Opin. 2006;22:2243–50.
80. Taylor AJ, Villines TC, Stanek EJ, et al. Extended-release niacin or ezetimibe and carotid intima-media thickness. N Engl J Med. 2009;361:2113–22.
81. Blumenthal RS, Michos ED. The HALTS trial—halting atherosclerosis or halted too early? N Engl J Med. 2009;361:2178–80.
82. Grundy SM, Cleeman JI, Merz CN, et al. Implications of recent clinical trials for the National Cholesterol Education Program Adult Treatment Panel III guidelines. Circulation. 2004;110:227–39.
83. American Diabetes Association. Standards of medical care in diabetes—2010. Diabetes Care. 2010;33 Suppl 1:S11–61.
84. Brunzell JD, Davidson M, Furberg CD, et al. Lipoprotein management in patients with cardiometabolic risk: consensus statement from the American Diabetes Association and the American College of Cardiology Foundation. Diabetes Care. 2008;31: 811–22.

# Cholesterol Absorption Inhibitors (Ezetimibe) and Bile Acid Binding Resins (Colesevelam HCl) as Therapy for Dyslipidemia in Patients with Diabetes Mellitus

22

Harold Bays

## Introduction

Ezetimibe blocks the intestinal absorption of both biliary and dietary cholesterol by inhibiting intestinal sterol transporters. Therapeutically, ezetimibe alone and in combination with statins is primarily indicated to lower low-density lipoprotein (LDL) cholesterol levels. Additionally, ezetimibe lowers non-high-density lipoprotein (non-HDL) cholesterol, apolipoprotein B, triglycerides, and remnant-like particle cholesterol and modestly raises HDL cholesterol levels. When combined with statins, ezetimibe may also lower C-reactive protein levels. These lipid effects have particular application when treating the dyslipidemia often found in patients with type 2 diabetes mellitus (T2DM). Colesevelam HCl is another gastrointestinal-acting lipid-altering drug, which is classified as a bile acid sequestrant (BAS). Earlier, BAS were among the first drugs approved to lower cholesterol levels, and clinical outcomes trials supported their use in not only lowering cholesterol but also improving atherosclerotic coronary heart disease (CHD) outcomes. Unfortunately, the first marketed BAS (e.g., cholestyramine and colestipol) were poorly tolerated and had substantial potential for drug interactions which substantially limited their clinical use. Colesevelam HCl was approved in the year 2000 as a new generation of BAS that was specifically designed to be better tolerated, with less potential for drug interactions. Additionally, BAS were known for decades to not only reduce cholesterol levels but also reduce glucose levels. In 2008, colesevelam HCl received regulatory approval as an anti-diabetes mellitus agent, which was in addition to its established indication as a cholesterol-lowering agent. This chapter focuses on the use of ezetimibe and colesevelam HCl in the management of dyslipidemia in patients with T2DM.

## Diabetes Mellitus and Dyslipidemia

A dyslipidemia often described in association with metabolic syndrome and T2DM includes elevated levels of triglycerides (TG), very low-density lipoprotein (and other triglyceride rich lipoproteins (TRL) and their remnants), small dense low-density lipoproteins (LDL), and increased levels of apolipoprotein B, as well as decreased levels of high-density lipoprotein (HDL) and apolipoprotein A-1. Most studies suggest that when corrected for applicable demographics (age, gender, adiposity, etc.), LDL

H. Bays, M.D., F.T.O.S., F.A.C.E., F.N.L.A. (✉)
Louisville Metabolic and Atherosclerosis Research Center, 3288 Illinois Avenue, Louisville, KY 40213, USA
e-mail: hbaysmd@aol.com

A.J. Jenkins et al. (eds.), *Lipoproteins in Diabetes Mellitus*, Contemporary Diabetes,
DOI 10.1007/978-1-4614-7554-5_22, © Springer Science+Business Media New York 2014

cholesterol may not substantively differ between those with and without T2DM [1].

The cause of the dyslipidemia associated with T2DM is multifactorial. The most common modifiable lifestyle contributor to T2DM and its associated dyslipidemia involves the pathogenic endocrine and immune effects of excessive adipose tissue, termed "adiposopathy" (Fig. 22.1).

Adiposopathy [2] is caused by positive caloric and sedentary lifestyle in genetically and environmentally susceptible patients [3]. Anatomically, adiposopathy is manifest by adipocyte hypertrophy, as well as increased visceral, pericardial, perivascular, and other periorgan adiposity, growth of adipose tissue beyond its vascular supply, increased number of adipose tissue immune cells, and "ectopic fat deposition" in other body organs [4]. Pathophysiological manifestations of adiposopathy include impaired adipogenesis, adipocyte organelle dysfunction, increased circulating free fatty acid levels, and adverse adipocyte and adipose tissue endocrine and immune responses [5]. As importantly, the pathogenic potential of adipose tissue is highly dependent upon interactions or cross talk with other body organs. If such actions and interactions are pathogenic, then the potential clinical manifestations of adiposopathy include hyperglycemia, high blood pressure, dyslipidemia, metabolic syndrome, atherosclerosis, fatty liver, and increased risk of cancer [2].

Hormonal abnormalities associated with adiposopathy include hyperandrogenemia in women and hypoandrogenemia in men. Thus, fat weight gain resulting in adiposopathy may "approximate the genders," at least with respect to sex hormone status [6, 7]. Women may develop insulin resistance on the basis of inherited postreceptor defects in insulin signaling, irrespective of adiposity. Women who gain body fat may develop adiposopathic responses that also may contribute to insulin resistance. In either circumstance, the resultant compensatory hyperinsulinemia enhances ovarian androgen production and inhibits hepatic synthesis of sex hormone binding globulin (SHBG), which increases free testosterone. These mechanisms help account for the clinical presentations and common endocrinopathies associated with the polycystic ovarian syndrome (PCOS), which depending on the underlying pathophysiology, may occur with and without adiposity. The adverse clinical consequences of PCOS include infertility, increased risk of cardiovascular disease, and increased risk of T2DM [8]. Regarding men, adiposopathic responses may lead to hypoandrogenemia via various mechanisms [9]. Hyperinsulinemia may decrease SHBG, which decreases total circulating testosterone. Hyperleptinemia may suppress testicular androgen production. Increased adipose tissue aromatase activity may increase the conversion of testosterone to estradiol, which may decrease pulsatile luteinizing hormone secretion, which in turn, decreases testicular androgen production. The reduction in male androgens may promote even further adiposity, which may potentially worsen adiposopathy, creating a circular and interconnected pathologic process leading to a number of metabolic abnormalities. This is yet another example as to how adiposopathic responses lead to the clinical and laboratory findings described by the "metabolic syndrome," as well as an increased risk of atherosclerotic coronary heart disease and T2DM [10].

Conceptually, the origins of the dyslipidemia associated with T2DM are shown in Figs. 22.2, 22.3, and 22.4. If during positive caloric balance, adipose tissue responds with pathogenic endocrine and immune responses, and if adipose tissue is unable to adequately store free fatty acids, then these pathogenic responses and energy overflow are directed to other body organs. If non-adipose tissue body organs (such as the liver and muscle) are not sufficiently "flexible" in their capacity to manage the adverse metabolic onslaught, then such organs may become dysfunctional, contributing to metabolic disease (Fig. 22.2). An illustrative example most applicable to this discussion is shown in Figs. 22.3 and 22.4. If due to genetic or environmental limitations, the liver is unable to oxidize the excessive

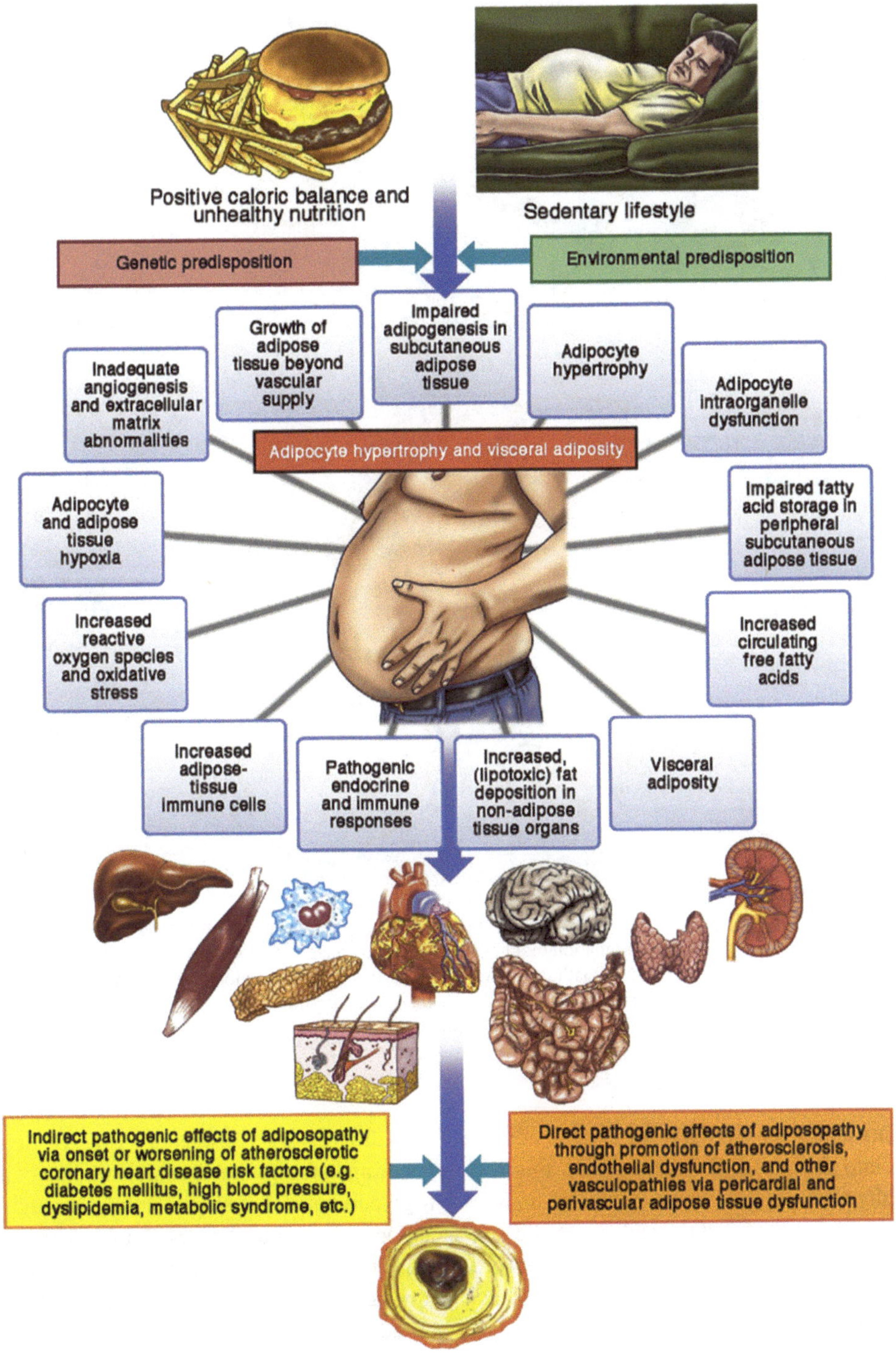


**Fig. 22.1** Title: Adiposopathy: Simplified relationship between pathogenic adipose tissue and cardiovascular disease [2]. Adiposopathy is promoted by unhealthy nutrition and a sedentary lifestyle in genetically and environmentally predisposed individuals. With impaired adipogenesis of peripheral, subcutaneous adipose tissue during positive caloric balance, existing fat cells may hypertrophy, circulating free fatty acids may increase, and lipids may be deposited in non-adipose tissue organs (e.g., liver, muscle, possibly pancreas) resulting in lipotoxicity. Adiposopathic endocrine and immune responses may be directly pathogenic to the cardiovascular system or otherwise interact with other body systems. If not mitigated by these other body organs, adiposopathy may indirectly cause or promote major atherosclerotic risk factors (type 2 diabetes mellitus, high blood pressure, or dyslipidemia)

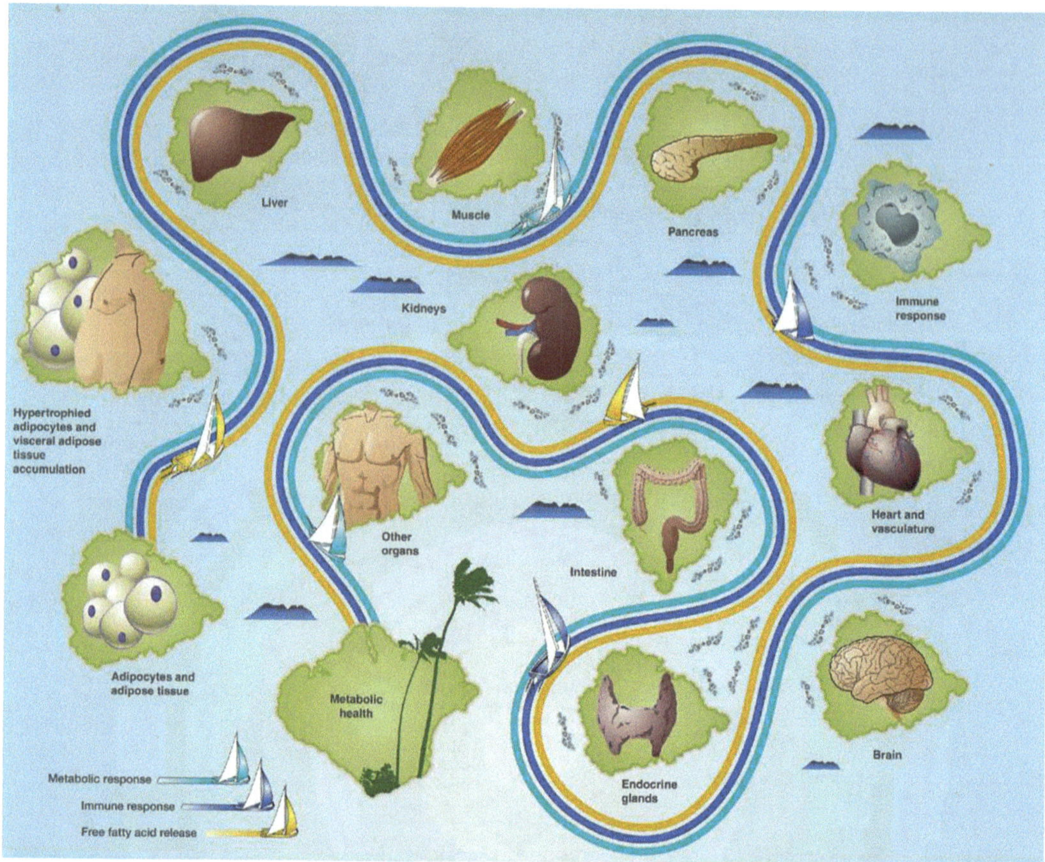


**Fig. 22.2** Navigating the pathogenic potential of adiposopathy. Fat cell enlargement and accumulation of adipose tissue in the visceral area often result in pathogenic adipose tissue metabolic and immune responses, including the net release of free fatty acids, which may be lipotoxic to peripheral organs. The potential of pathogenic adipose tissue to cause metabolic disease is largely dependent on cross talk and interactions with, as well as responses of other body tissues

free fatty acid load derived from visceral adipose tissue into the portal circulation, then this may clinically result in the common clinical findings among patients with T2DM and metabolic syndrome, such as fatty liver, increased VLDL secretion, as well as generation of small LDL and HDL particles, and increased triglyceride rich lipoprotein remnants [11].

In addition to the increased VLDL secretion, as shown in Fig. 22.4, one of the endocrinopathies associated with adiposopathy is a relative decrease in lipoprotein lipase activity [4]. Thus, in addition to increased secretion of VLDL, adiposopathy may also result in a reduced capacity to hydrolyze triglycerides in VLDL particles, all resulting in the common clinical finding of hypertriglyceridemia. Subsequently, through the actions of various lipases, VLDL particles are converted to remnant lipoproteins (incompletely digested VLDL particles), which are thought to be atherogenic. Triglycerides carried by VLDL particles may also undergo a 1:1 stoichiometric exchange with LDL and HDL particles via cholesteryl ester transfer protein (CETP). Triglyceride-enriched LDL and HDL particles are better substrates for lipase activity, which results in the formation of smaller and more dense particles.

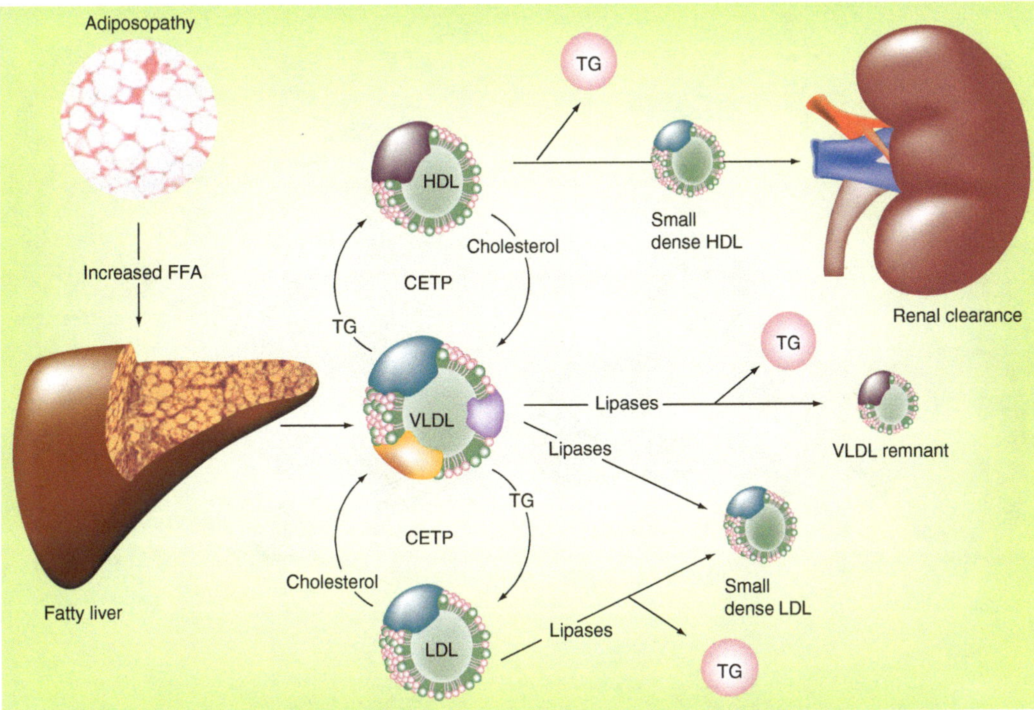


**Fig. 22.3** Adiposopathy and the dyslipidemia associated with the metabolic syndrome [6]. Relation between pathogenic adipose tissue and the characteristic lipid pattern described by the metabolic syndrome: hypertriglyceridemia, low high-density lipoprotein (HDL) cholesterol levels, and small, dense low-density lipoprotein (LDL) particles. *CETP* cholesterol ester transfer protein, *FFA* free fatty acid, *TG* triglyceride, *VLDL* very low-density lipoprotein

## Cholesterol Flux and the Importance of Intestinal Cholesterol

Irrespective of cause, dyslipidemia in patients with T2DM is a modifiable risk factor, which is especially important given that patients with T2DM are at high risk for CHD [11]. Statins are the first treatment of choice to lower cholesterol levels in T2DM patients. However, when statins are not tolerated or if statin therapy alone is not sufficient in achieving LDL cholesterol treatment goals, then ezetimibe is another lipid-altering drug treatment option.

In both peripheral tissues and the liver, the major precursor for cholesterol synthesis is acetyl coenzyme A (acetyl-CoA), which gives rise to hydroxy-methylglutaryl coenzyme A (HMG-CoA). HMG-CoA reductase is the rate-limiting enzyme in cholesterol biosynthesis. This enzyme converts HMG-CoA to mevalonic acid. Statins inhibit HMG-CoA reductase. Clinically, statins are the most commonly used drug to treat high cholesterol and were originally termed HMG-CoA reductase inhibitors, reflecting their mechanism of action, which was to inhibit the rate-limiting step of cholesterol production.

Textbook descriptions differ when describing the origin of bodily cholesterol production. Strictly speaking, primate studies suggest the greatest amount of cholesterol produced in the body is derived from non-hepatic tissues, such as skin, muscle, and intestine, with the greatest amount of cholesterol produced per gram of tissue being endocrine organs, such as the adrenal gland and sex organs [12] (Fig. 22.5). This is because cholesterol is required for cell membranes, cellular functions, and especially for

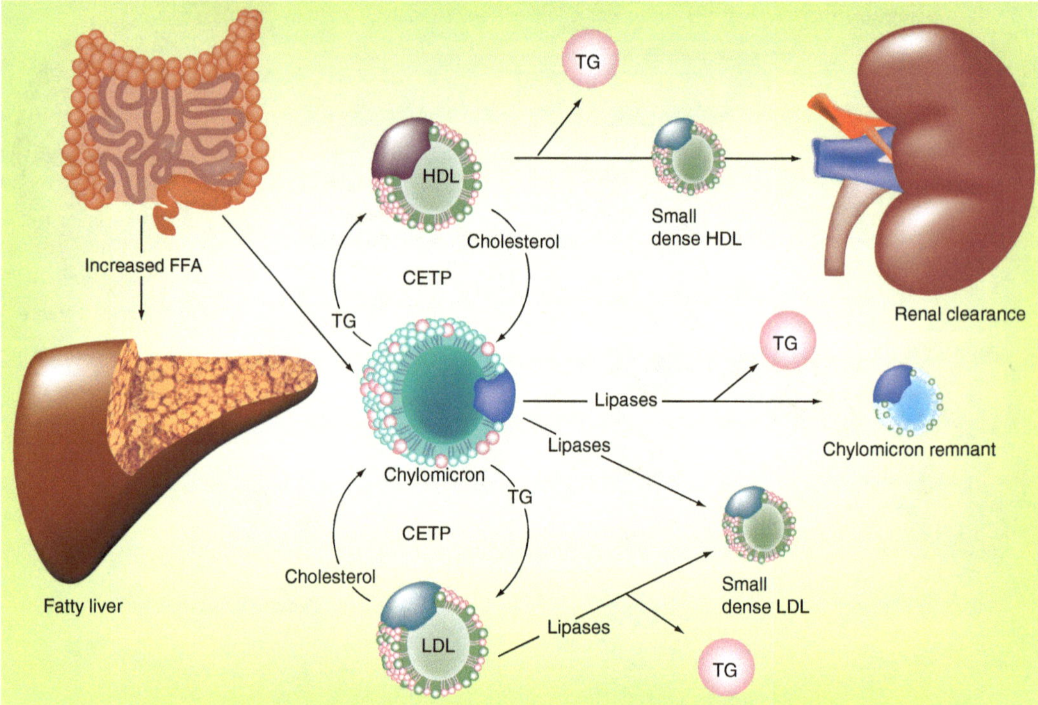


**Fig. 22.4** Postprandial contribution to the metabolic syndrome [6]. Adiposopathy may result in an inability of the adipose tissue organ to adequately clear postprandial FFA. This results in diversion (and potential lipotoxicity) of FFA to organs such as the liver. Such increases in FFA may also be lipotoxic to other organs, including muscle and pancreas (Fig. 22.2). The effect of excessive postprandial FFA upon lipid parameters is illustrated. *CETP* cholesteryl ester transfer protein, *FFA* free fatty acid, *HDL* high-density lipoprotein, *LDL* low-density lipoprotein, *TG* triglyceride

steroidogenesis. However, what is most clinically relevant regarding dyslipidemia and CHD is not where most total body cholesterol is produced but rather the origin of the cholesterol carried in the blood. Cholesterol is a waxy substance first described in gallstones. The Greek derivation of the term "cholesterol" refers to "chole" for bile and "stereos" for solid. Because cholesterol (a lipid) is insoluble in water, it must be packaged and carried in the blood by polar protein-containing biochemical particles, known as lipoproteins. Thus, most of the circulating cholesterol is hepatic/gastrointestinal in origin, in that most of the cholesterol carried by lipoproteins originates from the liver or intestine.

Once released in the blood, different lipoproteins may undergo enzymatic exchanges of cholesterol (for TG) with other lipoproteins (e.g., via cholesteryl ester transfer protein) [13]. Furthermore, LDL particles may transfer cholesterol to peripheral tissues. In most cases peripheral tissues have the capacity to synthesize their own cholesterol. Conversely, HDL particles may transfer free cholesterol from peripheral tissues back to the liver via peripheral cholesterol transport (Fig. 22.5). The fact that cellular production of cholesterol is sufficient for cellular function and that lipoprotein delivery of cholesterol is not required for peripheral tissue function is supported by the lack of widespread tissue and organ failure among patients with homozygous familial hypercholesterolemia, a genetic disorder wherein tissue LDL receptors are lacking. Even when patients with homozygous familial hypercholesterolemia (with lack of LDL receptors) undergo steroidogenesis stress testing, endocrine glands (i.e., body tissues dependent upon cholesterol for steroidogenesis, and thus among the most

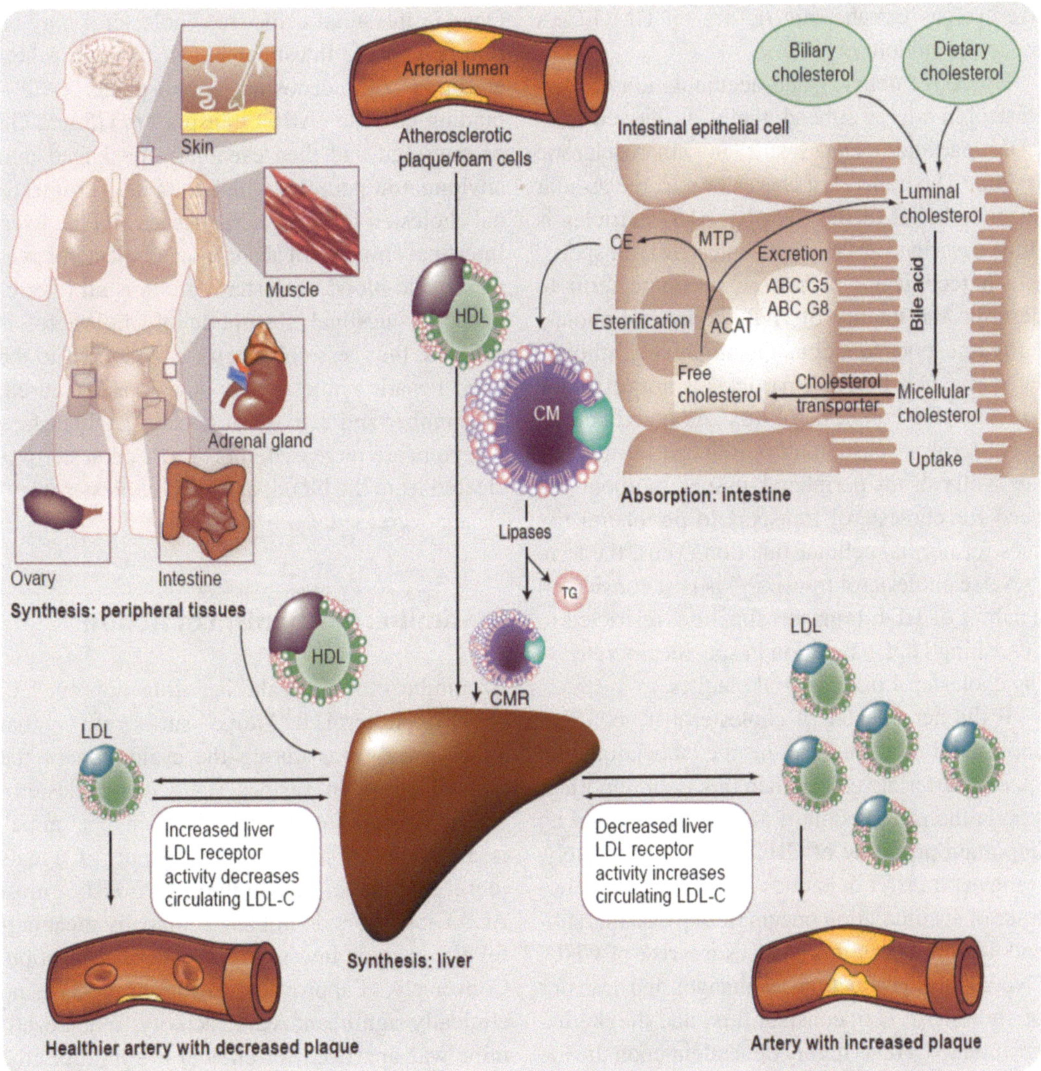


**Fig. 22.5** Simplified, global overview of major organs involved in lipoprotein metabolism and subsequent risk for CHD [13]. The liver normally serves as the main regulatory organ determining LDL-C blood levels. Impaired hepatic cholesterol synthesis (such as through administration of "statins") or impaired intestinal cholesterol delivery (such as through administration of cholesterol absorption inhibitors) result in increased hepatic LDL receptor activity with increased clearance of circulating LDL-C from the blood. Cholesterol from peripheral tissues, including macrophages associated with arterial cholesterol plaques, is transported to the liver via HDL particles. *ABC* adenosine triphosphate-binding cassette transporter, *ACAT* acyl-coenzyme A: cholesterol acyltransferase, *CE* cholesterol ester, *CM* chylomicron, *CMR* chylomicron remnant, *HDL* high-density lipoprotein, *LDL* low-density lipoprotein, *MTP* microsomal triglyceride transfer protein

potentially vulnerable to deficiency of cholesterol transport) hormone production is not diminished, again, due to sufficient intracellular cholesterol production. In fact, it is only after administration of statins in patients with homozygous familial hypercholesterolemia that minor, nonclinically significant reductions in steroidogenesis are observed [14]. The modest, if any clinical effect upon peripheral tissues with statins is likely because statin concentrations are effectually higher in the liver than peripheral tissues, with greater inhibition of cholesterol synthesis in the liver versus extrahepatic tissues by HMG-CoA reductace inhibitors [15].

Excessive delivery and accumulation of cholesterol in arterial subendothelia, as derived from LDL particles, can result in atherosclerotic lesions. The transfer of cholesterol from vascular subendothelial to the liver by HDL particles is often described as "reverse cholesterol transport," which technically, is not an adequate term to describe the totality of HDL peripheral cholesterol transport function. Quantitatively, cholesterol transport by HDL particles is not restricted to "reversing" cholesterol flux. As noted before, cholesterol is substantially produced from cellular synthesis in peripheral tissues, without the need for cholesterol transport to peripheral tissues for normal cellular function. Thus, the term "reverse cholesterol transport" is best considered a subset of HDL transport function, restricted to describing HDL's function in specifically retrieving cholesterol from arterial plaques.

If the net transfer of cholesterol is such that cholesterol accumulates in the subendothelial space of arterial vessels, then this is an important step in the progression of atherosclerosis and an important promoter of CHD events. Conversely, if the net transfer dynamics are such that no cholesterol accumulation occurs in the vascular subendothelium, then this reduces the risk of CHD. Overall, the production, exchange, and transfer of cholesterol is in constant flux, and the predisposition to CHD is highly dependent upon the net effect of this flux.

Beyond tissue production, another important contributor to the cholesterol pool, and thus contributor to cholesterol flux, is intestinal cholesterol. Dietary sterols may not substantially contribute to circulating cholesterol and other sterols, except during times of very high cholesterol consumption, because up to three-quarters of the cholesterol delivered to the intestine is derived from biliary cholesterol excretion from the liver, not dietary consumption [12]. Once in the intestinal lumen, both biliary and dietary cholesterol (and other lipids) interact with bile acids allowing for micelle formation, which enhances transport of cholesterol through the jejunal brush border membranes into intestinal epithelial cells. Once in intestinal cells, free cholesterol may be returned to the intestinal lumen through a heterodimer of adenosine triphosphate (ATP)-binding cassette (ABC) transporters G5 and G8 or esterified and then eventually packaged into chylomicron particles which then deliver intestinal cholesterol to peripheral tissues and the liver. Intestinal cholesterol absorption, cholesterol synthesis, and blood cholesterol are thus all interrelated. If intestinal absorption of cholesterol is reduced, then less cholesterol is delivered to the liver, hepatic cholesterol synthesis is increased, the number and activity of hepatic LDL surface receptors are increased, more LDL cholesterol is cleared from the blood, and LDL cholesterol levels are decreased.

## Ezetimibe: Mechanism of Action

Ezetimibe is a lipid-altering drug approved to lower cholesterol. Its "mibe" suffix reflects that its discovery was during the evaluation of the clinical utility of various acyl-CoA cholesterol acyltransferase (ACAT) inhibitors, in that "mibe" is a designated name for this group of agents (e.g., avasimibe, pactimibe). Curiously, most ACAT inhibitors do not have clinically meaningful effects upon intestinal cholesterol absorption. Conversely, at approved doses, ezetimibe has no clinically significant ACAT activity. When ezetimibe was approved for clinical use in 2002, the precise molecular target was unknown and was classified as a cholesterol absorption inhibitor. Subsequently, ezetimibe was found to competitively inhibit the sterol transporter, Niemann-Pick C1-like 1 protein (NPC1L1), located on the brush border membrane of intestinal epithelial cells (and at sites in the liver). However, ezetimibe is not classified as an intestinal transport inhibitor, but rather maintained in a class termed intestinal absorption inhibitor. Through inhibiting intestinal cholesterol transport, ezetimibe reduces cholesterol entering the enterocyte, reduces the cholesterol packaged into chylomicrons, decreases the amount of cholesterol delivered to the liver, promotes a compensatory upregulation of hepatic LDL receptors, enhances

LDL-C clearance from the circulation, and thus lowers LDL cholesterol blood levels.

This mechanism of action of ezetimibe is complementary to statins, with the combination sometimes described as representing "dual inhibition," referring to the inhibition of cholesterol production by statins and the inhibition of intestinal cholesterol absorption by ezetimibe. In some ways, both statins and ezetimibe share the same mechanism of action in that both increase hepatic LDL receptor activity resulting in enhance clearance of LDL particles, with a greater potential to reduce cholesterol blood levels, compared to either agent alone. Increased LDL receptor activity may also increase clearance of other apolipoprotein B containing lipoproteins, such as TRL (e.g., VLDL), helping to account for why both statins and ezetimibe lower TG levels.

## Ezetimibe: Effects Upon Dyslipidemia Associated with Diabetes Mellitus

Lowering LDL cholesterol remains the primary lipid treatment target for most patients with T2DM. While ezetimibe's main clinical use is lowering LDL cholesterol, ezetimibe has other effects applicable to the dyslipidemias so often found in patients with T2DM. This may be of clinical importance because CHD risk reduction may best be achieved by modification of multiple CHD risk factors.

### Non-HDL Cholesterol

Non-HDL cholesterol is the sum of cholesterol carried by all atherogenic lipoproteins such as LDL, very low-density lipoprotein (VLDL), intermediate density lipoprotein (IDL), remnant lipoprotein (RLP), lipoprotein(a) [Lp(a)], and chylomicrons. Non-HDL cholesterol is calculated as total cholesterol minus HDL cholesterol. Given that non-HDL cholesterol is more inclusive in assessing the cholesterol carried by atherogenic lipoproteins, it should not be surprising that clinical trial data suggests non-HDL cholesterol may be a better predictor of CHD risk than LDL-C levels [16]. In recognition of the clinical importance of non-HDL cholesterol, the National Cholesterol Education Program (NCEP) ATP III has recommended non-HDL-C treatment goals be set at levels 30 mg/dl above the respective LDL-C treatment goals, as a secondary target for high-risk patients with TG of more than 200 mg/dl [1]. Measurement of non-HDL-cholesterol in patients with metabolic syndrome and T2DM is particularly relevant, because many of these patients have increased levels of TRL, apolipoprotein B, and small, dense LDL particles which, while reflected in non-HDL cholesterol, may not be adequately reflected by measuring LDL cholesterol alone. In statin-treated patients, ezetimibe significantly reduces non-HDL cholesterol approximately 15–20 % in those with metabolic syndrome and reduces non-HDL cholesterol approximately 20–25 % in patients with T2DM [17, 18].

### Apolipoprotein B

As with non-HDL cholesterol, apolipoprotein B may be a better predictor of CHD risk than LDL cholesterol alone [19], and apolipoprotein B levels less than 90 mg/dl may be considered an alternative secondary target for patients at high CHD risk [20]. Unlike non-HDL cholesterol, apolipoprotein B provides a direct assessment of atherogenic particle number, which is thought to be an important determinant of atherogenic burden and CHD risk. Chylomicron particles contain one molecule of ApoB-48, while lipoprotein particles such as LDL, VLDL, IDL, and other TRL contain one molecule each of ApoB-100. Some assays may measure both apolipoprotein B 48 and 100. Many other apolipoprotein assays only assess apolipoprotein B100. Either way, apolipoprotein B blood levels represent the concentration of atherogenic lipoproteins, which is a measurement of atherogenic risk beyond measuring the cholesterol carried by LDL alone (as reflected by LDL cholesterol levels). This may be especially of clinical importance among metabolic syndrome and T2DM patients who have elevated TG levels, and thus elevated TRL. Adding ezetimibe to ongoing statin therapy significantly reduces ApoB levels approximately 13 % in patients with metabolic syndrome and approximately 18 % among those with T2DM [17].

## Triglycerides

Hypertriglyceridemia is generally considered a CHD risk factor. Elevated TG levels are often found in patients with metabolic syndrome and T2DM. If after LDL cholesterol goals are reached, and TG levels remain ≥200 mg/dl, then national guidelines suggest non-HDL cholesterol be assessed, with treatment to non-HDL-C treatment goals [1]. Although support via clinical trial outcome data is lacking among patients with T2DM, achieving a TG level of <150 mg/dl is considered desirable [21]. When added to statin therapy, ezetimibe significantly reduces TG levels in patients with metabolic syndrome by approximately 5–10 % and approximately 10 % in patients with T2DM [17, 18].

## HDL Cholesterol

Low levels of HDL cholesterol correlates with increased CHD risk. Although support via clinical trial outcome data is lacking, raising HDL cholesterol is recommended by some organizations in patients at higher risk for CHD [22]. Some suggest that among those with T2DM, achieving HDL cholesterol >40 mg/dl in men and HDL cholesterol >50 mg/dl in women is desirable [21]. When added to statin therapy, ezetimibe significantly increases HDL cholesterol levels in patients with metabolic syndrome and T2DM by approximately 3 % [17, 18].

## Remnant-Like Lipoproteins

Elevated levels TRL and their remnants are associated with an increased CHD risk [22, 23]. The cholesterol carried by remnant TRL is included in measurements of non-HDL-C levels, and the number of particles are reflected in measurements of apolipoprotein B. TRL (e.g., chylomicrons, IDL, and VLDL and their remnants) may undergo intravascular remodeling into metabolic by-products of smaller and more dense particles, which may have higher atherogenic potential than larger, more buoyant, particles. Ezetimibe reduces remnant lipoprotein cholesterol approximately 10–20 % [24].

## Lipoprotein Particle Size

Both metabolic syndrome and T2DM are often associated with a disproportionate baseline number of smaller LDL particles, which is often described as increasing CHD risk (Figs. 22.3 and 22.4). However, while baseline lipoprotein particle size may have some utility in predicting CHD risk, no evidence suggests that the assessment of lipoprotein particle size is useful in determining the efficacy of lipid-altering intervention. In fact, in some circumstances, post-treatment lipoprotein particle size analyses may be misleading [25].

Mechanistically, it is suggested that smaller, more dense LDL particles may (1) have decreased affinity for tissue and liver LDL receptors, thus prolonging LDL particle presence in the blood; (2) have increased permeability through the arterial endothelium with preferential retention in the arterial wall; and (3) be more readily oxidized, further increasing their atherogenic potential [25]. However, while the lipoprotein particle size effects of a lipid-altering intervention may be scientifically intriguing, the vast majority of scientific data supports LDL cholesterol reduction, non-HDL cholesterol reduction, and atherogenic lipoprotein particle number reduction (as reflected by a reduction in apolipoprotein B) as not only what is most clinically relevant but also what represents validated lipid treatment targets. A challenge to some clinicians arises when administration of cholesterol-lowering drugs (such as statins or ezetimibe) lowers LDL cholesterol, lowers non-HDL cholesterol, and reduces apolipoprotein B levels, but also results in an increase in the proportion of remaining LDL particles that are more small and dense [25].

While lipoprotein particle size may be helpful in assessing baseline CHD risk, no evidence that such measurements are helpful to assess efficacy of lipid-altering therapy [26].

Physiologically, reduced LDL clearance due to impaired LDL receptor binding is one of the proposed reasons why smaller, more dense LDL particles are potentially more atherogenic. It might therefore be expected that when hepatic LDL receptors are upregulated through therapies such as statins and/or ezetimibe, then the larger circulating LDL particles are preferentially cleared. This leaves a disproportionate amount of smaller, more dense LDL particles. But what is most clinically relevant is that both small and large LDL particles are atherogenic and that both statins and ezetimibe reduce the number of large and small LDL particles, both reduce apolipoprotein B, both reduce LDL cholesterol, and both reduce non-HDL cholesterol, which are the lipid parameters of most clinical relevance when assessing post-treatment lipid-altering efficacy [25].

## High-Sensitivity C-Reactive Protein

Atherosclerosis is promoted by inflammation. C-reactive protein is an acute phase reactant and biomarker of inflammation whose increase is associated with increased CHD risk. The reduced progression of CHD associated with intensive statin treatment somewhat correlates with reductions in hs-CRP levels [27]. While ezetimibe monotherapy may reduce hs-CRP compared to placebo, these modest differences are generally not statistically significant [28]. However, when ezetimibe is added to ongoing statin therapy, this is when hs-CRP is found to be most consistently and significantly reduced [28, 29].

## Ezetimibe: Clinical Trials in Patients with Diabetes Mellitus

In a post hoc assessment of metabolic syndrome or T2DM patients treated with ongoing statin therapy, adding ezetimibe significantly lowered LDL cholesterol, non-HDL cholesterol, total cholesterol, apolipoprotein B, and TG levels, irrespective of the presence of metabolic syndrome or T2DM [17]. In a pooled post hoc analysis of 27 clinical trials ($n=6{,}541$ with T2DM; $n=15{,}253$ without T2DM), ezetimibe combined with statin was more effective than statin monotherapy in improving LDL cholesterol, total cholesterol, HDL cholesterol, TGs, non-HDL-cholesterol, apolipoprotein B, and hs-CRP in the overall population, as well as both subgroups with and without T2DM. The safety profile was also similar between groups. This analysis also suggested that ezetimibe combined with statin may lower LDL cholesterol, total cholesterol, and non-HDL cholesterol more among those with T2DM, compared to those without T2DM [30]. In a study of 1,229 hypercholesterolemic T2DM patients comparing ezetimibe 10 mg/simvastatin 20 mg per day versus atorvastatin 10 or 20 mg per day or ezetimibe 10 mg/simvastatin 40 mg per day versus atorvastatin 40 mg per day, ezetimibe/simvastatin generally provided additional improvements over atorvastatin with regard to LDL cholesterol, total cholesterol, HDL cholesterol, non-HDL cholesterol, TG, and hs-CRP, although these findings were not statistically significant at all dose comparisons. Ezetimibe/simvastatin was also superior to atorvastatin in allowing T2DM patients to attain LDL cholesterol levels less than 70 mg/dl ($P<0.001$ for all dose comparisons) [31].

Ezetimibe can be prescribed as monotherapy or combined in a single pill with either simvastatin or atorvastatin. Compared to simvastatin alone, a subgroup analysis of three similarly designed, randomized, double-blind, placebo-controlled studies in patients with primary hypercholesterolemia revealed that ezetimibe plus simvastatin significantly reduced LDL cholesterol, non-HDL cholesterol, apolipoprotein B, TG, and C-reactive protein. These effects were similar among those with and without metabolic syndrome [32]. When compared to doubling of the atorvastatin dose in hypercholesterolemic patients at high CHD risk, T2DM, and metabolic syndrome, a post hoc analysis of a double-blind, parallel group trial of hypercholesterolemia at high CHD risk demonstrated that atorvastatin plus ezetimibe resulted in greater reductions in LDL cholesterol, TG, apolipoprotein B, non-HDL cholesterol, total cholesterol, and lipid ratios in the T2DM, metabolic syndrome, and neither groups [33]. When ezetimibe plus simvastatin was compared to atorvastatin or rosuvastatin in patients with metabolic syndrome or T2DM, subgroup analyses supported ezetimibe plus simvastatin as providing greater improvements than atorvastatin or rosuvastatin in LDL cholesterol, total cholesterol, HDL cholesterol (versus atorvastatin only), non-HDL cholesterol, LDL-C:HDL-C ratio, TC:HDL-C ratio, and apolipoprotein B in all subgroups. A greater percentage of patients receiving ezetimibe plus simvastatin attained their individual National Cholesterol Education Program Adult Treatment Panel III LDL cholesterol goals of <100 mg/dl or LDL-C <70 mg/dl [1, 34], as well as non-HDL cholesterol treatment goal, again, regardless of subgroup [35].

Because patients with metabolic syndrome and T2DM are at higher CHD risk, attainment of LDL cholesterol treatment goals may be especially challenging, because the LDL cholesterol targets are likely to be lower than among many of those without metabolic syndrome and T2DM. Greater LDL cholesterol reduction is usually required to achieve desired lipid targets among patients with metabolic syndrome and/or T2DM. In an analysis of a study of metabolic syndrome and T2DM patients wherein ezetimibe was added on to statin therapy, LDL cholesterol was significantly reduced by a placebo-corrected 23 % among those with metabolic syndrome and 25 % among those with T2DM. In both groups, approximately 70 % of patients receiving ezetimibe added to statins achieved LDL cholesterol goal versus about 20 % who had placebo added to statins [18].

In order to better achieve lipid treatment targets, multiple lipid-altering drugs are often required. In a long-term efficacy and safety subgroup analysis of a 64-week trial of 1,220 patients with metabolic syndrome, T2DM, or neither, who were administered ezetimibe plus simvastatin versus ezetimibe plus simvastatin and niacin, the triple combination was significantly better than either alone in lowering LDL cholesterol and raising HDL cholesterol compared to ezetimibe plus simvastatin. As expected, the niacin treated groups had greater flushing and increases in glucose levels with the greatest increases in new onset T2DM being among those with metabolic syndrome, and the greatest glucose rises among those with T2DM [36]. Mixed dyslipidemia is another clinical situation requiring multiple lipid-altering drug therapies, because statin monotherapy is frequently inadequate for normalizing simultaneous derangements in multiple lipid parameters. In a study of metabolic syndrome patients with mixed dyslipidemia, ezetimibe plus simvastatin, as well as ezetimibe plus simvastatin and fenofibrate significantly reduced LDL cholesterol better than fenofibrate alone, in patients with or without metabolic syndrome. Similarly, improvements in total cholesterol, TG, non-HDL cholesterol, apolipoprotein B, HDL cholesterol, apolipoprotein A-1, and hs-CRP were greater with ezetimibe plus simvastatin or ezetimibe plus simvastatin and fenofibrate compared to fenofibrate alone. These effects appeared to be consistent in patients with or without metabolic syndrome [37].

## Bile Acid Sequestrants

In addition to intestinal cholesterol absorption inhibitors such as ezetimibe, another class of gastrointestinal lipid-altering drug are bile acid sequestrants (BAS), sometimes referred to as "resins." The most direct mechanism of action of BAS (e.g., cholestyramine, colestipol, and colesevelam HCl) is the binding of bile acids in the intestine. Because this effect is restricted to the gastrointestinal (GI) tract, BAS are considered non-systemic agents, although they clearly have metabolic effects beyond the GI tract. BAS hold a special place in lipid-altering drug history in that they were among the first such drugs to be found to both reduce cholesterol and improve CHD outcomes (Table 22.1) [38]. In fact, in 1988 before statins and other therapies became more established, the initial Expert Panel of the

**Table 22.1** Examples of cardiovascular disease outcome trials of bile acid sequestrants

| Clinical trial (year published) | Demographics | Duration (years) | Intervention | Lipid effect[a] | Results |
|---|---|---|---|---|---|
| CHD outcome study | | | | | |
| LRC-CPPT (1984) [41] | 3806 men w/o CHD | 7.4 | Cholestyramine 24 g/day | LDL-C: −20.3 %<br>HDL-C: +1.6 % | 19 % reduction in fatal and nonfatal MI in treated group |
| Angiographic studies | | | | | |
| NHLBI (1984) [42] | 116 men and women with CHD | 5 | Cholestyramine 24 g/day | LDL-C: −26 %<br>HDL-C: +8 % | Significant decreased progression in coronary artery lesions >50 % stenosis at baseline |
| CLAS I (1987) [43] | 162 men with CABG | 2 | Colestipol 30 g/day and Niacin 4.3 g/day | LDL-C: −43 %<br>HDL-C: +37 % | Significant increased regression, and decreased progression in treated group than placebo group |
| CLAS II (1990) [44] | 103 men with CABG | 4 | Colestipol 30 g/day and Niacin 4.2 g/day | LDL-C: −40 %<br>HDL-C: +37 % | Significant increased regression and decreased progression in treated group than placebo group |
| FATS (1990) [45] | 38 men with coronary atherosclerosis and family history of CVD | 2.5 | Colestipol 30 g/day and Lovastatin 40 mg/day | LDL-C: −46 %<br>HDL-C: +15 % | Significant increased regression, decreased progression, and decreased CHD events compared to conventional therapy |
| FATS (1990) [45] | 36 men with coronary atherosclerosis and family history of CVD | 2.5 | Colestipol 30 g/day and Niacin 4 g/day | LDL-C: −32 %<br>HDL-C: +43 % | Significant increased regression, decreased progression, and decreased CHD events compared to conventional therapy |
| UCSF-SCOR (1990) [46] | 72 men and women with familial hypercholesterolemia | 2 | Colestipol, niacin, and lovastatin | LDL-C: −39 %<br>HDL-C: +26 % | Mean within-patient change in percent area stenosis was significantly greater in diet than drug intervention group with the treatment group demonstrating mean regression and the diet group demonstrating mean progression |
| STARS (1992) [47] | 90 men with CHD | 3 | Cholestyramine 16 g/day | LDL-C: −35.7 %<br>HDL-C: +4 % | Change in mean absolute width of the coronary segment (MAWS) was decreased with dietary and dietary + cholestyramine intervention compared to control group. The change in MAWS was independently and significantly correlated with LDL cholesterol levels. Both diet and diet + cholestyramine groups had significant increased regression, decreased progression, and decreased CHD events compared to "usual care" therapy |

Recreated from [40]

*CABG* coronary artery bypass graft, *CHD* atherosclerotic coronary heart disease, *CVD* cardiovascular disease, *CLAS* Cholesterol Lowering Atherosclerosis Study, *FATS* Familial Atherosclerosis Treatment Study, *HDL-C* high-density lipoprotein cholesterol, *LCAS* Lipoproteins in Coronary Atherosclerosis Study, *LDL-C* low-density lipoprotein cholesterol, *LRC-CPPT* Lipid Research Clinics Coronary Primary Prevention Trial, *MI* myocardial infarction, *NHLBI* National Heart and Lung Blood Institute, *STARS* St. Thomas Arteriosclerosis Regression Study, *UCSF-SCOR* University of California, San Francisco Specialized Center of Research

[a]Values Compared to Baseline

**Table 22.2** Examples of clinical trials evaluating the effects of bile acid sequestrants upon glucose levels

| Clinical trial | Demographics | Duration | Intervention | Lipid effect | Baseline HbA1c | Results at study end[a] |
|---|---|---|---|---|---|---|
| Garg and Grundy [50] | 20 men and 1 woman with T2DM | Crossover study; 6 weeks for each period | Cholestyramine 16 g a day | LDL-C = −28 %<br>HDL-C = No change<br>TG = +13.5 % | Not reported | FPG = −13 %<br>HbA1c = −0.5 % (NS) |
| Yamakawa et al. [51] | 70 men and women with T2DM | 3 months | Colestimide 6 g per day or pravastatin 10 mg per day | LDL-C = −23 %[b]<br>HDL-C = −0.06 % (NS)<br>TG = +14 %(NS) | 7.7 % | FPG = −8 %<br>HbA1c = −0.9 % |
| Zieve et al. (GLOWS trial) [52] | 65 men and women with T2DM | 12 weeks | Colesevelam 3.75 mg/day[c] | LDL-C: −11.7 %<br>HDL-C: −1.5 % (NS)<br>TG: +7.8 % (NS) | 7.9 % | HbA1c: −0.5 %<br>FPG: −14 mg/dl (NS)<br>PPG: −31.5 mg/dl |

Recreated from [40]

*CHD* atherosclerotic coronary heart disease, *FPG* fasting plasma glucose, *GLOWS* Glucose Lowering effects of WelChol Study, *HDL-C* high-density lipoprotein cholesterol, *LDL-C* low-density lipoprotein cholesterol, *NS* not a statistically significant change, *OAD* oral anti-diabetes drugs, *PPG* two-hour postprandial glucose, *T2DM* type 2 diabetes mellitus, *TG* triglycerides

[a]FPG values represent percent change in glucose levels; HbA1c values reduction in HbA1c percent

[b]Lipid and glucose values were colestimide-treated subjects compared to baseline

[c]In addition to other OAD

National Cholesterol Education Program listed BAS as a first treatment of choice for hypercholesterolemia (along with niacin), because BAS were generally safe with long-term use, and because studies that began in the 1970s supported BAS as reducing CHD risk [39]. One of the illustrative studies listed in Table 22.2 was the Lipid Research Clinics Coronary Primary Prevention Trial (LRC-CPPT), which was a primary prevention trial evaluating cholestyramine administered over 7 years in 3,806 men. In this study, cholestyramine reduced total cholesterol by 13 %, reduced LDL cholesterol by 20 %, and reduced CHD death or nonfatal myocardial infarction by 19 %. Unfortunately, 68 % of study participants experienced adverse gastrointestinal experiences, with the average cholestyramine dose actually taken being 14 g/day, although the study called for a dose of 24 g per day. The LRC-CPPT study was a landmark study in that it was one of the first CHD outcomes studies to support the "cholesterol hypothesis," in that not only was an elevated cholesterol level contributive to CHD, but the LRC-CPPT demonstrated that a reduction of cholesterol could reduce CHD events. However, in retrospect, the poor compliance during the study was predictive of the challenges of its future use in clinical practice. Due to their poor gastrointestinal tolerability (e.g., constipation and other GI adverse experiences), high potential for drug interactions, and predominant administration via multiple daily scoops of sandy-textured drug, once statins were introduced, the use of BAS declined, representing a small fraction of the drugs utilized for treatment of hypercholesterolemia.

## Colesevelam HCl

In the 1990s, colesevelam hydrochloride was developed as a BAS with a unique polymer structure specifically designed to maintain lipid efficacy, but improve BAS tolerability. Regarding efficacy and compared to placebo, early monotherapy trials demonstrated that six 625 mg colesevelam HCl tablets per day significantly reduced LDL cholesterol levels 15–21 %, increased HDL cholesterol levels 3–9 %, and increased TG levels 2–16 % [38]. Similarly, early statin combination trials likewise supported six 625 mg tablets/day of colesevelam HCl per day significantly reduced LDL-C 10–16 %, increased HDL-C 3–7 %, and increased TG levels 5–23 % compared with statin alone [38]. Regarding tolerability, in addition to the first-introduced tablet formulation, a subsequent "sugar free" (phenylalanine) colesevelam HCl powder was developed wherein, as opposed to multiple scoops of sandy-textured drug (as was typical of cholestyramine), colesevelam HCl powder could be administered via one small 3.75 g packet of drug, once a day. In a BAS acceptability trial, 71 % of study participants reported taste as being important for long-term compliance. In this controlled comparison study, those participating in the study found the colesevelam HCl powder tasted significantly better than generic cholestyramine [48].

## Colesevelam HCl: Cholesterol Lowering of Bile Acid Sequestration

While colesevelam HCl and ezetimibe are both gastrointestinal lipid-altering drugs, they do have important differences. Ezetimibe is administered as a single pill, while colesevelam HCl is administered as six pills per day or one packet of colesevelam HCl powder per day. Ezetimibe inhibits cholesterol transporters, while colesevelam HCl binds bile acids. Ezetimibe is technically a systemic drug, in that it undergoes enterohepatic circulation, while colesevelam HCl is non-systemic, in that the colesevelam HCl drug remains limited to the intestine, without systemic exposure. But while these two agents do have differences, much of the physiology of the GI tract in lipid metabolism previously described with ezetimibe are similar and applicable to colesevelam HCl. As seen in Fig. 22.5, cholesterol is converted into bile acids in the liver via the enzyme 7 alpha-hydroxylase. Bile acids are secreted into the biliary system, and then into the intestine, predominantly for the purpose of micelle formation and fat digestion. Over 95 % of bile acids are transported to the terminal ileum, where they are then returned to the liver via enterohepatic recirculation. Once these bile acids are bound by BAS such as colesevelam HCl, these bile acids are excreted in the feces and do not undergo enterohepatic recirculation. The decreased bile acid return to the liver upregulates enzymes that increase the cholesterol catabolism to bile acids, resulting in a compensatory increase in hepatic LDL receptor activity, clearing LDL from the circulation, and reducing LDL-C levels [38]. Thus, the increase in LDL receptor activity is a mechanism shared by colesevelam HCl, ezetimibe, and statins for that matter. Finally, another similarity to ezetimibe is that colesevelam HCl was the first BAS to report reductions in CRP when added to statins, which is an effect most consistently reported in well-controlled trials of combination lipid-altering drug trials with statins [49].

## Colesevelam HCl: Glucose Lowering of Bile Acid Sequestration

Another important difference between BAS such as colesevelam HCl and ezetimibe is that while ezetimibe has no effects upon blood glucose levels, colesevelam HCl is approved as a glucose-lowering agent for treatment of T2DM. In the years spanning the 1990s and 2000s, some smaller pilot studies consistently suggested BAS may lower glucose and HbA1c levels in patients with T2DM (Table 22.2).

Subsequently, colesevelam HCl underwent a robust development program for the intent of being the first BAS to obtain an approval and indicated use as an anti-diabetes mellitus agent. This development program involved three pivotal trials as summarized in Table 22.3. Each of these trials evaluated colesevelam HCl added to a specified anti-diabetes drug regimen, which included metformin, insulin, or sulfonylurea-based therapies, either alone, or in combination with other anti-diabetes mellitus drugs. These clinical trials demonstrated colesevelam HCl consistently reduced fasting glucose levels approximately 13–15 %, reduced HbA1c approximately 0.5–0.54 %, and reduced LDL-C 12–17 %. Regarding tolerability and safety, the only noteworthy differences in reported adverse experiences between placebo and colesevelam HCl were numerical increases in constipation and dyspepsia.

Although many potential mechanisms have been proposed (e.g., effects upon luminal bile acid composition, effects on cholecystokinin, effects on hepatocyte nuclear factor 4 alpha, and increases in incretins), the manner by which BAS reduce glucose levels is largely unknown [40].

**Table 22.3** Prospective phase III clinical trials investigating the effects of colesevelam upon glucose levels

| Clinical trial | Demographics of total study participants | Duration | Intervention | Lipid effect | Baseline HbA1c | Results at study end[a] |
|---|---|---|---|---|---|---|
| Bays et al. [53] (Metformin ± OAD) | 316 men and women with T2DM | 26 weeks | Colesevelam 3.75 mg/day[b] | LDL-C: −15.9 %<br>HDL-C: +0.9<br>TG: +4.7 % (NS) | 8.1 % | HbA1c: −0.54 %<br>FPG: −13.9 mg/dl |
| Goldberg et al. [54] (Insulin ± OAD) | 287 men and women with T2DM | 16 weeks | Colesevelam 3.75 mg/day[c] | LDL-C: −12.8 %<br>HDL-C: −0.9 % (NS)<br>TG: +21.5 % | 8.2 % | HbA1c: −0.50 %<br>FPG: −14.6 mg/dl (NS) |
| Fonseca et al. [55] (Sulfonylurea ± OAD) | 461 men and women with T2DM | 26 weeks | Colesevelam 3.75 mg/day[d] | LDL-C: −16.7 %<br>HDL-C: +0.1 % (NS)<br>TG: +17.7 % | 8.3 % | HbA1c: −0.54 %<br>FPG: −13.5 mg/dl |

Recreated from [40]

*FPG* fasting plasma glucose, *NS* not a statistically significant change, *OAD* oral anti-diabetes drugs, *PPG* two-hour postprandial glucose, *T2DM* type 2 diabetes mellitus

[a]FPG values represent percent change in glucose levels; HbA1c values reduction in HbA1c percent

[b]Study medication mean percent compliance was 93.3 % in the colesevelam HCl group and 91.9 % in the placebo

[c]Study medication mean percent compliance was 92.7 % in the colesevelam HCl group and 94.5 % in the placebo group

[d]Study medication mean percent compliance was 92.7 % in the colesevelam HCl group and 90.8 % in the placebo group

One might imagine that the most likely mechanism is related to the direct action of these agents, which is the binding of bile acids. Bile acids are the natural ligand for farnesoid X receptors associated with enterocytes. If a lack of intestinally active bile acid availability (due to bile acid sequestration) reduces farnesoid X receptor activity, then this "deactivation" may lead to increased liver X receptor (LXR) activity. LXR is considered a glucose sensor whose increased activity may increase pancreatic insulin secretion, increase adipogenesis and adipose tissue functionality, and thus improve glucose disposal. Increased hepatic LXR activity may also downregulate enzymes relative to hepatic insulin resistance, glucose intolerance, and hepatic gluconeogenesis with a net effect of improved glucose utilization and glucose uptake. Interestingly, investigational LXR agonists are known to lower glucose, lower LDL-C, and raise HDL cholesterol levels, but have experienced limitations in their development as therapeutic agents, at least partially because they also raise triglyceride levels. BAS such as colesevelam HCl have similar glucose and lipid effects as LXR agonists [40]. Irrespective of whether the increase in triglyceride levels are due to increased LXR activity or other mechanisms resulting in increased VLDL secretion, BAS should be used with caution in patients with triglyceride levels >300 mg/dl and contraindicated in patients with triglyceride levels >500 mg/dl.

## Ezetimibe and Colesevelam HCl

One of the challenges for clinicians in achieving acceptable lipid treatment targets involves the care of patients with statin intolerance, with the most common reported statin intolerance being myalgias defined as muscle pain with or without elevated muscle enzymes [56]. In most clinical trials, statin-induced myalgias are reported in only about 5 % of study participants. However, in other trials and clinical practice surveys, the reports of myalgias are widely variable, ranging between 0.3 and 33 % [56]. Thus, having non-statin lipid-altering drug options is often useful in clinical practice.

In a multicenter, randomized, double-blind, parallel group study of patients with primary hypercholesterolemia, the colesevelam HCl plus ezetimibe combination (i.e., without statins) significantly reduced LDL-C levels by 32.3 %. This was in contrast to a reduction of 21.4 % with ezetimibe alone. Also compared to ezetimibe monotherapy, colesevelam HCl plus ezetimibe significantly reduced total cholesterol, non-HDL cholesterol, and apolipoprotein B, and increased apolipoprotein A-1 levels. Neither treatment regimen significantly increased median triglyceride levels compared with baseline, and both regimens were safe and generally well-tolerated. The conclusion was that colesevelam HCl plus ezetimibe combination therapy significantly improved important lipid parameters compared to ezetimibe alone. According to the authors, combining colesevelam HCl with ezetimibe may be a therapeutic option in hypercholesterolemic patients, such as those in whom statins are contraindicated and/or who may have intolerances to statin therapy [57].

## Conclusion

- Diabetes mellitus and/or metabolic syndrome is often associated with elevated triglyceride, very low-density lipoprotein (and other triglyceride rich lipoproteins (TRL) and their remnants), small dense low-density lipoproteins (LDL), and increased apolipoprotein B, as well as decreased levels of high-density lipoprotein (HDL) and apolipoprotein A-1 levels.
- The mechanisms contributing to this common dyslipidemia may be substantially due to the adverse consequences of adiposopathy, which is the most common reversible cause of the most common metabolic diseases encountered in clinical practice, such as elevated glucose levels, high blood pressure, and dyslipidemia.
- Ezetimibe is a cholesterol absorption inhibitor, that primarily lowers LDL-C levels, which is the primary lipid treatment target to reduce CHD risk.
- Colesevelam HCl is a BAS that not only lowers LDL-C levels but also reduces glucose levels.

## References

1. Expert Panel on Detection E. Treatment of high blood cholesterol in A. Executive summary of the third report of The National Cholesterol Education Program (NCEP) Expert Panel on Detection, Evaluation, and Treatment of High Blood Cholesterol in Adults (Adult Treatment Panel III). JAMA 2001;285:2486–97.
2. Bays HE. Adiposopathy is "sick fat" a cardiovascular disease? J Am Coll Cardiol. 2011;57:2461–73.
3. Bays H, Abate N, Chandalia M. Adiposopathy: sick fat causes high blood sugar, high blood pressure and dyslipidemia. Future Cardiol. 2005;1:39–59.
4. Bays HE, Gonzalez-Campoy JM, Bray GA, et al. Pathogenic potential of adipose tissue and metabolic consequences of adipocyte hypertrophy and increased visceral adiposity. Expert Rev Cardiovasc Ther. 2008;6:343–68.
5. Bays HE, Gonzalez-Campoy JM, Henry RR, et al. Is adiposopathy (sick fat) an endocrine disease? Int J Clin Pract. 2008;62:1474–83.
6. Bays HBC. Adiposopathy: why do adiposity and obesity cause metabolic disease? Future Lipidol. 2006;1:389–420.
7. Bays HE, Gonzalez-Campoy JM, Schorr AB. What men should know about metabolic syndrome, adiposopathy and "sick fat". Int J Clin Pract. 2010;64:1735–9.
8. Goodarzi MO, Dumesic DA, Chazenbalk G, Azziz R. Polycystic ovary syndrome: etiology, pathogenesis and diagnosis. Nat Rev Endocrinol. 2011;7:219–31.
9. Mammi C, Calanchini M, Antelmi A, et al. Androgens and adipose tissue in males: a complex and reciprocal interplay. Int J Endocrinol. 2012;2012:789653.
10. Gould DC, Kirby RS, Amoroso P. Hypoandrogen-metabolic syndrome: a potentially common and underdiagnosed condition in men. Int J Clin Pract. 2007;61:341–4.
11. Bays HE. "Sick fat," metabolic disease, and atherosclerosis. Am J Med. 2009;122:S26–37.
12. Bays H. Ezetimibe. Expert Opin Investig Drugs. 2002;11:1587–604.
13. Bays H, McKenney J, Davidson M. Torcetrapib/atorvastatin combination therapy. Expert Rev Cardiovasc Ther. 2005;3:789–820.
14. Laue L, Hoeg JM, Barnes K, Loriaux DL, Chrousos GP. The effect of mevinolin on steroidogenesis in patients with defects in the low density lipoprotein receptor pathway. J Clin Endocrinol Metab. 1987;64:531–5.
15. Parker RA, Clark RW, Sit SY, Lanier TL, Grosso RA, Wright JJ. Selective inhibition of cholesterol synthesis in liver versus extrahepatic tissues by HMG-CoA reductase inhibitors. J Lipid Res. 1990;31:1271–82.
16. Xydakis AM, Ballantyne CM. Role of non-high-density lipoprotein cholesterol in prevention of cardiovascular disease: updated evidence from clinical trials. Curr Opin Cardiol. 2003;18:503–9.
17. Simons L, Tonkon M, Masana L, et al. Effects of ezetimibe added to on-going statin therapy on the lipid profile of hypercholesterolemic patients with diabetes mellitus or metabolic syndrome. Curr Med Res Opin. 2004;20:1437–45.
18. Denke M, Pearson T, McBride P, Gazzara RA, Brady WE, Tershakovec AM. Ezetimibe added to ongoing statin therapy improves LDL-C goal attainment and lipid profile in patients with diabetes or metabolic syndrome. Diab Vasc Dis Res. 2006;3:93–102.
19. Sniderman AD. Apolipoprotein B, versus non-high-density lipoprotein cholesterol: and the winner is. Circulation. 2005;112:3366–7.

20. Genest J, Frohlich J, Fodor G, McPherson R, Working Group on H, Other D. Recommendations for the management of dyslipidemia and the prevention of cardiovascular disease: summary of the 2003 update. CMAJ 2003;169:921–4
21. American Diabetes Association. Executive summary: standards of medical care in diabetes—2011. Diabetes Care 2011;34 Suppl 1:S4–10.
22. Grundy SM, Cleeman JI, Daniels SR, et al. Diagnosis and management of the metabolic syndrome: an American Heart Association/National Heart, Lung, and Blood Institute scientific statement. Curr Opin Cardiol. 2006;21:1–6.
23. Twickler TB, Dallinga-Thie GM, Cohn JS, Chapman MJ. Elevated remnant-like particle cholesterol concentration: a characteristic feature of the atherogenic lipoprotein phenotype. Circulation. 2004;109:1918–25.
24. Bays HE, Ose L, Fraser N, et al. A multicenter, randomized, double-blind, placebo-controlled, factorial design study to evaluate the lipid-altering efficacy and safety profile of the ezetimibe/simvastatin tablet compared with ezetimibe and simvastatin monotherapy in patients with primary hypercholesterolemia. Clin Ther. 2004;26:1758–73.
25. Bays H, Conard S, Leiter LA, et al. Are post-treatment low-density lipoprotein subclass pattern analyses potentially misleading? Lipids Health Dis. 2010;9:136.
26. Davidson MH, Ballantyne CM, Jacobson TA, et al. Clinical utility of inflammatory markers and advanced lipoprotein testing: advice from an expert panel of lipid specialists. J Clin Lipidol. 2011;5:338–67.
27. Ridker PM, Cannon CP, Morrow D, et al. C-reactive protein levels and outcomes after statin therapy. N Eng J Med. 2005;352:20–8.
28. Bays HE, Neff D, Tomassini JE, Tershakovec AM. Ezetimibe: cholesterol lowering and beyond. Expert Rev Cardiovasc Ther. 2008;6:447–70.
29. Gagne C, Bays HE, Weiss SR, et al. Efficacy and safety of ezetimibe added to ongoing statin therapy for treatment of patients with primary hypercholesterolemia. Am J Cardiol. 2002;90:1084–91.
30. Leiter LA, Betteridge DJ, Farnier M, et al. Lipid-altering efficacy and safety profile of combination therapy with ezetimibe/statin vs. statin monotherapy in patients with and without diabetes: an analysis of pooled data from 27 clinical trials. Diabetes Obes Metab. 2011;13:615–28.
31. Goldberg RB, Guyton JR, Mazzone T, et al. Ezetimibe/simvastatin vs. atorvastatin in patients with type 2 diabetes mellitus and hypercholesterolemia: the VYTAL study. Mayo Clin Proc. 2006;81:1579–88.
32. Feldman T, Ose L, Shah A, et al. Efficacy and safety of ezetimibe/simvastatin versus simvastatin monotherapy in hypercholesterolemic patients with metabolic syndrome. Metab Syndr Relat Disord. 2007;5:13–21.
33. Conard S, Bays H, Leiter LA, et al. Ezetimibe added to atorvastatin compared with doubling the atorvastatin dose in patients at high risk for coronary heart disease with diabetes mellitus, metabolic syndrome or neither. Diabetes Obes Metab. 2010;12:210–8.
34. Grundy SM, Cleeman JI, Merz CN, et al. Implications of recent clinical trials for the National Cholesterol Education Program Adult Treatment Panel III guidelines. Circulation. 2004;110:227–39.
35. Abate N, Catapano AL, Ballantyne CM, et al. Effect of ezetimibe/simvastatin versus atorvastatin or rosuvastatin on modifying lipid profiles in patients with diabetes, metabolic syndrome, or neither: results of two subgroup analyses. J Clin Lipidol. 2008;2:91–105.
36. Fazio S, Guyton JR, Lin J, Tomassini JE, Shah A, Tershakovec AM. Long-term efficacy and safety of ezetimibe/simvastatin coadministered with extended-release niacin in hyperlipidaemic patients with diabetes or metabolic syndrome. Diabetes Obes Metab. 2010;12:983–93.
37. Gil-Extremera B, Mendez G, Zakson M, et al. Efficacy and safety of ezetimibe/simvastatin co- administered with fenofibrate in mixed hyperlipidemic patients with metabolic syndrome. Metab Syndr Relat Disord. 2007;5:305–14.
38. Bays H, Dujovne C. Colesevelam HCl: a non-systemic lipid-altering drug. Expert Opin Pharmacother. 2003;4:779–90.
39. The Expert Panel. Report of the National Cholesterol Education Program Expert Panel on Detection, Evaluation, and Treatment of High Blood Cholesterol in Adults. Arch Intern Med 1988;148:36–69.
40. Bays HE, Goldberg RB. The "forgotten" bile acid sequestrants: is now a good time to remember? Am J Ther. 2007;14:567–80.
41. The lipid research clinics coronary primary prevention trial results. I. Reduction in incidence of coronary heart disease. JAMA 1984;251:351–64.
42. Brensike JF, Levy RI, Kelsey SF, et al. Effects of therapy with cholestyramine on progression of coronary arteriosclerosis: results of the NHLBI Type II Coronary Intervention Study. Circulation. 1984;69:313–24.
43. Blankenhorn DH, Nessim SA, Johnson RL, Sanmarco ME, Azen SP, Cashin-Hemphill L. Beneficial effects of combined colestipol-niacin therapy on coronary atherosclerosis and coronary venous bypass grafts. JAMA. 1987;257:3233–40.
44. Cashin-Hemphill L, Mack WJ, Pogoda JM, Sanmarco ME, Azen SP, Blankenhorn DH. Beneficial effects of colestipol-niacin on coronary atherosclerosis. A 4-year follow-up. JAMA. 1990;264:3013–7.
45. Brown G, Albers JJ, Fisher LD, et al. Regression of coronary artery disease as a result of intensive lipid-lowering therapy in men with high levels of apolipoprotein B. N Eng J Med. 1990;323:1289–98.
46. Kane JP, Malloy MJ, Ports TA, Phillips NR, Diehl JC, Havel RJ. Regression of coronary atherosclerosis during treatment of familial hypercholesterolemia with combined drug regimens. JAMA. 1990;264:3007–12.
47. Watts GF, Lewis B, Brunt JN, et al. Effects on coronary artery disease of lipid-lowering diet, or diet plus cholestyramine, in the St Thomas' Atherosclerosis Regression Study (STARS). Lancet. 1992;339:563–9.

48. Bays HE, Maki KC, Schmitz K. Colesevelam hydrochloride powder for oral suspension versus cholestyramine powder for oral suspension: comparison of acceptability and tolerability. Endocr Pract. 2011;17: 218–25.
49. Bays HE, Davidson M, Jones MR, Abby SL. Effects of colesevelam hydrochloride on low-density lipoprotein cholesterol and high-sensitivity C-reactive protein when added to statins in patients with hypercholesterolemia. Am J Cardiol. 2006;97: 1198–205.
50. Garg A, Grundy SM. Cholestyramine therapy for dyslipidemia in non-insulin-dependent diabetes mellitus. A short-term, double-blind, crossover trial. Ann Intern Med. 1994;121:416–22.
51. Yamakawa T, Takano T, Utsunomiya H, Kadonosono K, Okamura A. Effect of colestimide therapy for glycemic control in type 2 diabetes mellitus with hypercholesterolemia. Endocr J. 2007;54:53–8.
52. Zieve FJ, Kalin MF, Schwartz SL, Jones MR, Bailey WL. Results of the glucose-lowering effect of WelChol study (GLOWS): a randomized, double-blind, placebo-controlled pilot study evaluating the effect of colesevelam hydrochloride on glycemic control in subjects with type 2 diabetes. Clin Ther. 2007;29:74–83.
53. Bays HE, Goldberg RB, Truitt KE, Jones MR. Colesevelam hydrochloride therapy in patients with type 2 diabetes mellitus treated with metformin: glucose and lipid effects. Arch Intern Med. 2008;168: 1975–83.
54. Goldberg RB, Fonseca VA, Truitt KE, Jones MR. Efficacy and safety of colesevelam in patients with type 2 diabetes mellitus and inadequate glycemic control receiving insulin-based therapy. Arch Intern Med. 2008;168:1531–40.
55. Fonseca VA, Rosenstock J, Wang AC, Truitt KE, Jones MR. Colesevelam HCl improves glycemic control and reduces LDL cholesterol in patients with inadequately controlled type 2 diabetes on sulfonylurea-based therapy. Diabetes Care. 2008;31: 1479–84.
56. Bays H. Statin safety: an overview and assessment of the data—2005. Am J Cardiol. 2006;97:6C–26C.
57. Bays H, Rhyne J, Abby S, Lai YL, Jones M. Lipid-lowering effects of colesevelam HCl in combination with ezetimibe. Curr Med Res Opin. 2006;22: 2191–200.

# 23 Emerging Lipoprotein-Related Therapeutics for Patients with Diabetes

Peter J. Little, Alan Chait, Andrzej S. Januszewski, Alex Bobik, David O'Neal, and Alicia J. Jenkins

## Introduction

Dyslipidemia is a major risk factor for atherosclerosis in both diabetic and nondiabetic subjects, which is a common cause of morbidity and premature mortality. Based on and supported by favorable outcomes of clinical trials, drugs targeting lipoprotein metabolism are widely used, particularly in developed countries. Drugs to improve lipid levels, in particular to lower low-density lipoprotein (LDL) cholesterol (LDL-C), are commonly used for the primary and secondary prevention of cardiovascular disease. Of the LDL-C-lowering drugs, HMG-CoA reductase inhibitors ("statins") are particularly effective at reducing cardiovascular disease, both in people with and without diabetes mellitus [1, 2], with more intensive LDL-C lowering being more effective than less intensive LDL-C lowering [3–12]. Statins are effective cardioprotective agents in both type 1 and type 2 diabetes patients [2].

PPARα agonists (fibrates) also have a small (≈10 %) effect in reducing cardiovascular events [13, 14], and as shown by the FIELD [15, 16] and ACCORD-Lipid [17] studies, fenofibrate is also effective in reducing cardiovascular disease in people with type 2 diabetes and dyslipidemia (high fasting triglyceride levels and low high-density lipoprotein cholesterol (HDL-C) levels. Fenofibrate can also reduce lower-limb amputations (predominantly those due to small vessel disease) [18], as demonstrated by the FIELD study and as shown by both the FIELD and ACCORD-Lipid studies, the retinal and renal complications of type 2 diabetes [19–22]. These (predominantly triglyceride-lowering) fibrate drugs are also useful for the prevention of acute pancreatitis in people with severe hypertriglyceridemia [23, 24], which is often related to an

P.J. Little, B.Pharm., Ph.D. (✉)
Department of Pharmacy, RMIT University, Plenty Road, P.O. Box 71, Bundoora, VIC 3083, Australia

Monash University, Melbourne, VIC, Australia
e-mail: peter.little@rmit.edu.au

A. Chait
Division of Metabolism, Endocrinology and Nutrition, University of Washington School of Medicine, Seattle, WA, USA

A. Bobik
Vascular Biology and Atherosclerosis, BakerIDI Heart and Diabetes Insitute, Melbourne, VIC, Australia

A.S. Januszewski
Department of Medicine, The University of Melbourne, St. Vincent's Hospital, Melbourne, VIC, Australia

NHMRC Clinical Trials Centre, University of Sydney, Sydney, NSW, Australia

D. O'Neal
University of Melbourne, Department of Medicine, St. Vincent's Hospital, Fitzroy, 3065, Melbourne, VIC, Australia

A.J. Jenkins, M.D., F.R.A.C.P.
Section of Endocrinology and Diabetes, University of Oklahoma Health Sciences Center, 941 Stanton L. Young Blvd., BSEB 302F, Oklahoma City, OK, USA

University of Sydney, NHMRC Clinical Trials Centre, Camperdown, Sydney, NSW, Australia

A.J. Jenkins et al. (eds.), *Lipoproteins in Diabetes Mellitus*, Contemporary Diabetes,
DOI 10.1007/978-1-4614-7554-5_23, © Springer Science+Business Media New York 2014

**Table 23.1** Current lipid-modifying treatments used in clinical practice for people with diabetes

| |
|---|
| Lifestyle |
| Optimize glycemic control in people with diabetes |
| Weight loss if overweight or obese |
| Physical exercise |
| Nonsmoking |
| Healthy diet |
| Plant sterol-supplemented foods |
| Predominantly LDL-lowering treatments |
| HMG-CoA reductase inhibitors |
| e.g., rosuvastatin, lovastatin, pravastatin, fluvastatin, simvastatin |
| Cholesterol absorption inhibitors |
| Bile acid-binding resins |
| e.g., cholestyramine, colestipol |
| Ezetimibe |
| LDL (and Lp(a)) apheresis |
| Predominantly triglyceride-lowering agents |
| Fibrates |
| e.g., fenofibrate, gemfibrozil |
| Nicotinic acid |
| Fish oils |
| Combination tablets |
| Simvastatin and ezetimibe |
| Pravastatin and nicotinic acid |

underlying genetic defect in lipoprotein metabolism compounded by acquired conditions such as poorly controlled diabetes, alcohol excess, pregnancy, or drugs.

Diabetes care guidelines, such as by the American Diabetes Association, usually recommend the regular measurement of lipid levels and aggressive lipid targets [25]. Lifestyle treatments and approved lipid drug classes which are currently available for clinical use to achieve these lipid treatment goals are listed in Table 23.1 and are discussed in more detail in other chapters in this book. The general drug classes are predominantly LDL-C lowering, "statins," and cholesterol absorption inhibitors, such as bile acid-binding resins and ezetimibe, and the predominantly triglyceride-lowering agents fibrates, fish oils, and nicotinic acid. Nicotinic acid is one of the few drugs in clinical practice which can also lower levels of lipoprotein(a) (Lp(a)), but unfortunately it is often poorly tolerated, but some novel agents (discussed below) can also lower Lp(a).

**Table 23.2** Potential pleiotropic effects of lipid drugs

| |
|---|
| Improve endothelial function |
| e.g., statins and fibrates induce NOS |
| Stabilize atherosclerotic plaques |
| Antioxidant |
| Anti-inflammatory |
| Antithrombotic effects |
| Antiplatelet effects |
| Angiogenesis related |
| e.g., statins may have pro-angiogenic effects, and fibrates are anti-angiogenic in the eye |
| Cell signaling effects |
| e.g., fibrates activate PPARα and AMP kinase and suppress Wnt signaling pathways |
| Neuroprotective effects (e.g., of fibrates) |
| Protection against telomere shortening (e.g., of statins) |
| Skin protective effects (of fibrates via keratinocyte differentiation and epidermal effects) |

Clinical benefits of lipid-targeting drugs may be related to both improvements in the lipid profile and also an array of potential pleiotropic effects [26–28], summarized in Table 23.2. Additional as yet unknown pleiotropic effects may also exist. The relative importance and dose relatedness of the pleiotropic effects of these drug classes are not fully elucidated in either diabetic or nondiabetic subjects. Some of the novel agents in development are targeting lipid levels and also have pleiotropic effect(s), and it remains to be seen if this approach provides additional vasoprotection. Greater knowledge of the beneficial pleiotropic effects of lipid drugs on hemostasis, inflammation, vasoreactivity, and on the cardiovascular, retinal, renal, and neural systems and their mechanisms may facilitate the development of new drug classes to ameliorate the chronic complications of diabetes.

While many people with type 2 diabetes and with type 1 diabetes are prescribed lipid drugs, in particular a statin, some have contraindications to their use, for example, severe renal or liver disease, some do not meet the desired lipid goal even when at maximum tolerated drug dose, some are intolerant of the prescribed medication, and some are reluctant to or cannot afford to take them. Even in this era of evidence-based medi-

**Table 23.3** Emerging lipid therapeutic agents

| |
|---|
| Combination lipid drugs |
| New "statins" |
| New "fibrates" |
| New fish oil-like agents |
| New LDL-lowering agents |
| Inhibitors of proprotein convertase subtilin kexin 9 (PCSK9) |
| Thyromimetic agents |
| Inhibitors of ApoB-containing lipoproteins: antisense oligonucleotides and siRNAs inhibitors of (early and late) glycation |
| HDL-elevating drugs |
| ApoA1 mimetics |
| Modulators of lipoprotein-related enzymes, e.g., CETP inhibitors |
| Triglyceride-lowering drugs |
| Modulators of lipoprotein-related enzymes, e.g., inhibitors of CETP, DGAT2, ACAT, and MTP |
| ApoC-III ASO |
| Miscellaneous |
| Inhibitors of lipoprotein glycation and AGE modification |
| Inhibitors of lipoprotein immune complex formation |
| Inhibitors of lipoprotein and matrix interactions |
| Inhibitors of foam cell formation |
| Antioxidants |
| Anti-inflammatory agents |

cine, not all available lipid drugs and lipid drug combinations have been tested in major vascular end-point clinical trials in people with diabetes, especially those with type 1 diabetes and younger type 2 diabetes patients. The latter group, which is becoming more common [29], often includes obese youth from high-risk ethnic groups [29–31] and is of major concern, as they often have dyslipidemia and are at particularly high risk of vascular disease [31, 32]. Indeed their vascular complication rates are higher than that of young people with type 1 diabetes [32]. As we also now recognize that atheroma begins in childhood, particularly in those on a western diet, and in those who are obese, dyslipidemic, or dysglycemic [33, 34], the safety and efficacy of lipoprotein treatments in youth must be assessed.

In this chapter we will discuss emerging treatments closely related to approved lipid drugs and lipid treatments in development, relating them to their primary lipid target, such as LDL lowering, triglyceride lowering, and HDL elevating. These categories are summarized in Table 23.3. Some of the agents are in or have been in clinical trials, while others are in earlier phases of development.

## Strategies Aimed at Lowering LDL

*New Statins*. Since the advent of statins over 20 years ago, this class of drugs has been the mainstay of lipid-lowering therapy. While early studies with relatively weaker statins showed modest effects, more recent studies using powerful statins in very high-risk individuals indicate that a reduction of 30–40 % in relative risk might be expected from statin monotherapy [1–12]. With the statins in use today, doubling their daily dose only results in only about 6 % further reduction in LDL-C levels and a greater risk of side effects such as myalgia/myositis [35]. The development and trials of even more potent statins are in progress. One such novel statin, which is licensed for use in some countries is *pitavastatin* [36–38]. As shown by large phases 3 and 4 studies, pitavastatin can lower LDL-C levels by 40–65 % and lower triglyceride levels by about 20 % and has more marked HDL-C-elevating effects (up to 14 %) than current commonly used statins [36–38]. In vitro studies demonstrate potent stimulation of ApoA1 production by hepatocyte-like cells [39]. Pitavastatin has minimal metabolism via cytochrome P450 (CYP) enzymes, which may benefit patients requiring multiple drugs, as is common in people with type 2 diabetes [40]. About 10 % of subjects experienced adverse events of a similar nature to that of other statins. In a large ($n \sim 20{,}000$) Japanese long-term prospective post-marketing surveillance LIVALO Effectiveness and Safety (LIVES) study, 2-year pitavastatin use was associated with 29 % lower LDL-C levels and 5.9 % higher HDL-C levels, with a 24.6 % HDL-C rise in those with low (<40 mg/dL) HDL-C levels at baseline [41]. In a LIVES substudy, HDL-C levels rose in subjects changing from other statins to pitavastatin [42]. This potent statin has shown longer-term safety and efficacy in acute myocardial infarction patients, including diabetes subjects [43], can improve insulin resistance, and has shown no deleterious effects on glycemia in people with diabetes [44]. As shown by the Japanese Assessment of Pitavastatin and Atorvastatin in Acute Coronary Syndrome (JAPAN-ACS) study [45] and other longitudinal trials with intermediate coronary and carotid vascular end points [46–48], pitavastatin significantly improves atheroma volume and quality.

Interestingly in animal studies, including diabetic rodents [49, 50], and in some human studies, this new statin improves renal function in chronic renal disease subjects [51], including lowering albuminuria in type 2 diabetic patients [52]. The results of long-term studies with mortality and clinical cardiovascular, renal, and retinal end points in diabetes are awaited with interest.

Another statin in development is NCX6560 (NicOx, Sophia-Antipolis, France), which combines a statin with a nitric oxide (NO) donor to enhance vasodilatory effects [53]. As diabetes is associated with impaired vascular endothelial function and reduced NO bioavailability [54], this is of particular interest in diabetes.

*Combination Therapies.* As greater LDL lowering is associated with greater risk reduction [1, 2] and statin monotherapy alone leaves many patients with LDL-C levels above target, in which case combination therapy is often recommended. As well as increased efficacy in improving the lipid profile and reducing vascular events combination tablets are often helpful in increasing adherence and reducing drug costs to individuals.

Statins can be used in combination with *bile acid-binding resins* to achieve additional ≈10 % LDL-C lowering, but gastrointestinal side effects are common. Resins bind bile acids in the gut and induce secondary upregulation of hepatic LDL receptors, thus lowering LDL-C levels. Resins do not significantly alter HDL-C levels and can elevate serum triglyceride levels (via effects on the liver X receptor (LXR) [55, 56]. Bile acid sequestrants can also lower blood glucose levels via a farnesoid-X-receptor action, and colesevelam is approved for both lipid- and glucose-improving effects [57–59].

A better tolerated (than resins) combination is that of a statin with the cholesterol absorption inhibitor [60], *ezetimibe*, which acts by inhibiting the intestinal cholesterol transporter, NPC1-L1 and usually lowers LDL-C by an additional 20 % [60–62]. There are ongoing trials of statins plus ezetimibe, with the recently reported SHARP study finding benefit of 20 mg simvastatin plus 10 mg ezetimibe vs. placebo in a RCT of 9,270 chronic kidney disease patients, including approximately 20 % with diabetes, with a 17 % reduction in risk of a first major atherosclerotic event over a 4.9-year follow-up [63].

The combination of a statin with *fish oils* can address the combined dyslipidemia that is common in type 2 diabetes. In the COMBination of Omega-3 preparation with Simvastatin (COMBOS) study, 4 g daily prescription omega-3 fatty acids or placebo was added to simvastatin 40 mg daily in 254 patients with hypertriglyceridemia. Relative to the placebo group, the fish oil group demonstrated significantly lower triglycerides (29.5 vs. 6.3 %) and higher HDL-C (3.4 vs. −1.2 %), which was well tolerated and sustained for 2 years [64–66]. There are no clinical endpoint trials in diabetes yet.

The effects of most of these combination therapies have not been tested in major clinical endpoint outcome trials with large numbers of people with diabetes. In the future additional combination therapies may also become available. Diabetes-specific trials or adequately sized subgroups of patients with diabetes and with macrovascular and microvascular end points are desirable.

*Preprotein convertase subtilin kexin 9* (PCSK-9) is a secreted protein that degrades the LDL receptor in hepatocytes and increases LDL-C levels [67, 68]. Genetic mutations in PCSK-9 cause FH, and loss of function mutations of this protein is associated with modest reductions in LDL-C levels, yet considerable protection from cardiovascular disease [69, 70]. The extent of protection is much greater than that seen with comparable degrees of LDL lowering in clinical trials [71, 72]. In human populations, PCSK-9 levels in blood are usually correlated with BMI and lipid levels (triglycerides, total and LDL-C) and are affected by sex hormones and growth hormone [73]. Some of the LDL-C-lowering effects of fibrates are thought to be mediated by PCSK-9 [74]. In several prospective studies in statin-treated type 2 diabetic patients, fenofibrate effects on PCSK-9 levels are divergent, with some finding lowering effects of fenofibrate [75] and others finding elevated PCSK-9 levels [76]. PCSK-9 is upregulated by statins [72, 77], thus potentially limiting the full potential of statins to lower LDL-C levels. Ezetimibe intervention is also associated with increased circulating PCSK-9 levels [77]. Thus, the combination of a statin and/or ezetimibe with a PSCK-9 inhibitor might prove to be particularly effective at lowering LDL-C levels and vascular events. The challenge is how best to inhibit PSCK9 in vivo. At present, the most promising response appears to be by the administration of antibodies, although these would need to be administered parenterally. Human monoclonal antibodies to PCSK-9 (e.g., RGEN-727 (Regeneron, Tarrytown, NY)) given parenterally have lowered LDL-C levels in statin-treated heterozygous FH patients and in nonfamilial hyperlipidemic subjects [78].

*Thyromimetic Agents.* D-Thyroxine was evaluated in the Coronary Drug Project many years ago but resulted in cardiac arrhythmias and in increased mortality [79, 80], an effect that has been attributed to contamination of the medications used with small amounts of L-thyroxine. Thyroid hormone administration can lower LDL-C levels by increasing hepatic LDL receptor expression via activation of thyroid hormone receptor, but has adverse effects on the heart and bone via activation of thyroid hormone receptor [81, 82]. These effects are highly undesirable in people with diabetes who are at higher risk of osteopenia and osteoporosis [83] and for those with type 1 diabetes who are also at increased risk of (autoimmune) thyroid disease [84]. With the development of selective activators of thyroid hormone receptor-β, there has been renewed interest in the use of selective thyromimetics for lowering LDL levels without having an adverse effect on the heart and bones. Selective thyroid hormone receptor-β agonists appear to deplete hepatocytes of cholesterol in addition to activating LDL receptors directly [85, 86], so they may have a somewhat different mechanism of action to statins. Unlike statins, thyromimetics can also lower Lp(a) levels [87]. They have been shown to reduce atherosclerosis in an animal model [88] and are beginning to be tested for their lipid-lowering effects in human subjects. Studies in people with diabetes will be of interest.

## Antisense Oligonucleotides (ASOs) and Small Interfering RNA

ASO and siRNA constructs that target ApoB are in development and may, with time, prove useful in the management of certain patients with increased LDL levels and/or some forms of hypertriglyceridemia. ASOs are single-stranded RNA that bind to mRNA, whereas siRNAs are short duplexes of RNA that contain a sequence identical to that in the target RNA. Both lead to destruction of the mRNA target and inhibition of protein synthesis [88]. A downside of both is that they need to be administered by injection, which to date has been associated with marked injections site reactions and also with hepatic steatosis, so they are likely to only be useful for very specific patients in whom adequate LDL lowering cannot be readily achieved by other means. The most well developed of these agents is the ASO Mipomersen (Isis, Carlsbad, CA) which targets ApoB and is in phase 3 trials in FH [89]. An additional potential advantage of these agents is that they may also reduce Lp(a) levels, although there currently is no information as to whether or not that would be beneficial for cardiovascular disease prevention [87].

*Other Drugs.* Several other drug classes that lower LDL-C levels by modulating lipoprotein metabolism are being investigated but have been limited by adverse effects. *Squalene synthase inhibitors*, such as lapaquistat (Takeda, Osaka, Japan), act in the endoplasmic reticulum to limit synthesis of cholesterol, but not of geranyl pyrophosphate-derived compounds (such as coenzyme Q10). LDL-C reductions were relatively small (about

15 %), and there were hepatic side effects [90]. Similarly *microsomal transfer protein (MTP) inhibitors*, such as lomitapide (Aegerion Pharmaceuticals, Cambridge, MA) which lower LDL-C by up to 80 % and triglycerides by 40 %, also caused hepatic dysfunction (fatty liver and elevated transaminases) [91, 92]. *Acyl-cholesterol acyltransferase (ACAT) inhibitors* which block lipoprotein synthesis and foam cell formation have reached clinical trials [93–95] but did not reduce coronary atheroma burden in IVUS studies [93, 94] or slow carotid IMT increase in familial hypercholesterolemia (FH) patients [95].

## Addressing Residual Risk Beyond Statin-Mediated LDL Lowering

Despite the success with statin therapy in all types of high-risk individuals, a considerable residual risk nonetheless exists in many individuals even after appropriate statin therapy. Some of this residual might be reduced by even more aggressive LDL-C lowering, which potentially could be achieved by using even more powerful statins, by the use of the combination therapies, or by using some of the newer strategies that are undergoing clinical testing and are not yet available for routine use (described above).

Much of the residual cardiovascular risk in both the nondiabetic and diabetic population appears to be related to low HDL cholesterol (HDL-C) and hypertriglyceridemia [97, 98], which often is associated with the metabolic syndrome and with type 2 diabetes [99]. Much less data is available regarding specific approaches to lower triglycerides and increase HDL-C levels than is available for LDL-C lowering. Also, much less is known concerning mechanism of atherosclerosis with these lipoproteins than for LDL. For example, although triglyceride-rich lipoproteins and their remnants can bind to and be retained by vascular proteoglycans [100–103], triglycerides do not accumulate to any major extent in atherosclerotic lesions, and it is not clear whether triglyceride-rich lipoproteins are directly atherogenic, or whether their effect is indirect, or both [104–106]. Hypertriglyceridemia is often accompanied by low HDL levels, an accumulation of remnant lipoproteins, and the presence of small, dense LDL particles, which appear to be particularly atherogenic [107, 108]. HDL is believed to exert its atheroprotective effect largely by facilitating reverse cholesterol transport. However, HDL also has anti-inflammatory, antioxidant, and antithrombotic properties and vasodilatory effects [109–113], all of which may play a role in reducing atherosclerosis risk and potentially also diabetic retinopathy and nephropathy [114].

## HDL Raising and TG Lowering as Targets

### Approaches to Lowering Triglycerides and Raising HDL

High triglycerides and low HDL levels are amenable to therapeutic approaches other than statins. Although statins in general result in modest elevations of HDL-C and modest reductions in triglycerides, other drugs more specifically target HDL and triglycerides. The two most widely used classes of drugs that target both hypertriglyceridemia and low HDL-C levels are fibrates and niacin [115–120]. However, clinical trials with fibrates, discussed in other chapters in this book, have yielded mixed and sometimes disappointing results with regard to cardiovascular disease [13–15, 17]. Fibrates and specifically fenofibrate have shown cardiovascular benefit in type 2 diabetes patients with high triglyceride and low HDL-C levels [15–17, 120] and microvascular benefit [18–22]. As yet there are no known clinical end-point trials of fibrates in type 1 diabetes, and there is also a paucity of data concerning the vascular effects of niacin in diabetes. New versions of both fibrates and niacin are undergoing investigation.

*Fibrates and Other PPAR Agonists*. The PPARα agonists such as fenofibrate lower VLDL and increase HDL by increasing expression of lipoprotein lipase and apoA1 and apoA2 and also have pleiotropic effects including related to blood clotting and inflammation (Table 23.2). Fibrates have shown clinical benefit in RCTs in type 2 diabetes patients [15–22], but many of these favorable responses do not correlate strongly with the changes in lipid levels [18–22]. While fenofibrate was well tolerated in the large FIELD and ACCORD-Lipid studies [15–22] and is used in clinical practice for hypertriglyceridemia, more specific PPARα agonists have not progressed due to side effects such as muscle toxicity. Agonists to other PPAR ligands may also be of interest in the management of lipids in diabetes.

PPARγ agonists (such as the thiazolidinediones) also lower triglycerides and increase HDL as do PPARα agonists, and they also improve glycemia, lowering HbA1c levels up to 1 % [121]. While they reached clinical practice, they caused excessive fluid retention and increased the risk of bone fractures and in some cases (rosiglitazone) of myocardial infarction [122] and concerns about bladder cancer (pioglitazone) [123]. In clinical trials the combined PPARα and PPARγ agonists such as muraglitazar and ragaglitazar also had serious adverse effects related to bladder cancer and excess cardiovascular events [124, 125]. Of this class aleglitazar, which improves the lipid profile and HbA1c levels in type 2 diabetes patients, is still undergoing assessment in clinical trials. The phase 2 SYNCHRONY trial demonstrated adverse effects such as fluid retention with high-dose (600 μg) aleglitazar [126], and using this dose, the SESTA R trial demonstrated a reversible 19 % reduction in eGFR levels in type 2 diabetes patients [127]. The ALECARDIO phase 3 study of cardiovascular outcomes in 6,000 type 2 diabetes patients with acute coronary syndromes is in progress (as of 2012) [128].

PPARγ and PPARδ co-agonists and PPARα and PPARγ co-agonist drugs are also undergoing testing [129].

*Niacin-Related.* Like the fibrates, nicotinic acid (niacin)-related drugs also effectively lower triglyceride levels [130, 131], whereas niacin is more effective in raising HDL-C levels than fibrates [132, 133]. As well as reducing LDL-C levels to a modest extent, niacin is the most effective drug currently clinically available for reducing Lp(a) levels [134]. In the old Coronary Drug Project, niacin monotherapy was associated with risk reduction [135] and reduced mortality several years after the conclusion of the study [136]. Niacin has been available for many years, but its widespread use has been limited by nuisance side effects, particularly flushing, which is believed to be due to niacin-induced production of prostaglandin D2 and other prostaglandins in skin immune cells [137], by hepatotoxicity and impaired glucose tolerance [138, 139]. Since the advent of relatively effective slow-release forms of niacin and the approval in some countries of niacin combined with a prostaglandin D2 type 1 receptor inhibitor, laropiprant, that reduces flushing by up to 80 % [140], there has been a renewed interest in this old drug. In a 64-week study of 949 hyperlipidemic subjects on simvastatin and ezetimibe, the addition of slow-release niacin increased blood glucose levels and new-onset diabetes which often improved or remitted without specific treatment [141]. Although use of niacin plus a statin led to lesion regression and improved clinical outcomes in small angiographic studies [142], the large AIM-HIGH study of 3,414 patients with low HDL-C levels on intensive statin therapy, including about one third with type 1 or type 2 diabetes, the clinical cardiovascular benefit of added slow-release niacin (1,500–2,000 μg daily) was tested, but the trial was stopped after 3 years due to lack of clinical efficacy [143]. The HPS2/THRIVE study is also testing the clinical vascular effects of niacin/laropiprant [144]. Other non-flushing niacin variants have been developed and at least one has reached clinical trial phase.

## Newer Targets for Increasing HDL

Several new targets to raise HDL are being tested. These include the CETP inhibitors and apoA mimetic peptides.

## CETP Inhibitors

The initial enthusiasm for CETP inhibitors has been dampened considerably by the negative experience with torcetrapib, trials of which led to a predicted increase in blood pressure, an unpredicted increase in cardiovascular events, cancer deaths, and deaths due to infections [145, 146]. These events occurred despite very favorable changes in plasma lipid and lipoproteins, i.e., a marked increase (up to 150 %) in HDL-C levels, a respectable 25 % decrease in LDL-C levels, and a highly favorable change in the LDL-C/HDL-C ratio [147]. In lipoprotein kinetic studies, torcetrapib did not improve cholesterol efflux to fecal sterols [148]. Therefore, the relationship between HDL and cardiovascular disease appears to be a lot more complex than is apparent from the epidemiology.

It has been suggested that the increase in cardiovascular disease was due to an off-target effect of torcetrapib to increase blood pressure by increasing aldosterone levels [149, 150]. However, concern has been raised that the adverse effect of these inhibitors on cardiovascular outcomes might be related to their ability to block part of the reverse cholesterol pathway [145]. Moreover, the increase in cancer and infective deaths raises concern that CETP inhibitors might be interfering with HDL's role in innate immunity. Other CETP inhibitors that do not have this effect on the renin-angiotensin system are currently being tested in large outcome studies.

Dalcetrapib, which increases HDL-C by 33 %, including levels of pre-beta HDL does increase fecal sterol excretion and does not cause hypertension [151]. In intermediate end-point studies, dalcetrapib did not improve endothelial function [152] or plaque composition (DAL-PLAQUE study) [153], and recently (May 2012) due to lack of efficacy, but not safety concerns, the company ceased its clinical end-point studies (DAL-ACUTE and DAL-OUTCOMES).

Another CETP inhibitor in clinical trial phase is anacetrapib. Anacetrapib is structurally closer to torcetrapib than to dalcetrapib and unlike dalcetrapib decreases pre-beta HDL-1. In the 3-month DEFINE study of coronary heart disease (CHD) or CHD-risk equivalents on a statin background, 100 mg anacetrapib increased HDL levels by 138 %, decreased LDL by 40 %, and also decreased Lp(a) levels, with no effects on blood pressure or the renin-angiotensin-aldosterone system [154]. Anacetrapib is, as of 2012, in a large 4-year atorvastatin background placebo-controlled clinical trial ($n \approx 30{,}0000$ subjects, including people with diabetes) (REVEAL) with a primary end point of cardiac death, myocardial infarction, or coronary revascularization [155].

If they too have adverse effects similar to what was observed with torcetrapib or lack clinical efficacy as with dalcetrapib, this might severely dampen enthusiasm for developing drugs that increase HDL levels. The torcetrapib experience also points out the need to differentiate HDL levels from HDL functionality and points out the need to develop relatively simple, widely applicable, and reproducible assays of HDL function that can be correlated with outcomes in clinical trials.

## ApoA-I Mimetic Agents

Many of the beneficial effects of HDL, particularly its role in reverse cholesterol transport, are likely to be largely due to the major apolipoprotein in HDL, apoA-I. Since apoA-I has to be administered by intravenous injection, attempts have been made to create small peptides that mimic the effect of the intact apolipoprotein. Several small apoA-I mimetic agents have been shown to have anti-inflammatory and antioxidant effects in vitro [156–158] and anti-atherogenic effects in animal studies [159, 160]. More recently they have begun to be tested in human subjects.

Many of the beneficial effects of apoA-I have been attributed to the ability of the class A amphipathic helices of this apolipoprotein to bind oxidized lipids, particularly oxidized phospholipids [161]. These mimetic peptides were designed to contain class A amphipathic helices and have been shown to have high affinity for oxidized phospholipids [161]. They are believed to work by tightly binding these toxic lipids, thereby preventing them from having adverse effects on vascular cells. While intact apoA-I has to be administered by intravenous infusion and has a relatively short half-life, an advantage of some of these smaller apoA-I mimetic peptides is that they can be administered orally. Future studies will determine whether they will have a role to play in the prevention and treatment of atherosclerosis, including in people with diabetes.

An ideal approach to raising HDL would be to stimulate the synthesis of endogenous apoA-I in a more potent manner than fibrates. Indeed, initial testing on one such small molecule that stimulates apoA-I synthesis has been reported [162]. Further studies using this approach are awaited with interest.

*Apheresis*. Both plasmapheresis and LDL apheresis, which involve weekly or biweekly invasive and costly procedures, substantially lower both LDL-C and Lp(a) levels with only slight HDL-C increases. Such treatments prolong life in homozygous FH patients and are now used in children and pregnant women with FH and increasingly for heterozygous FH subjects and other patients with aggressive coronary artery disease on or intolerant of maximal lipid drug therapy [163]. Apheresis can also be used to selectively remove ApoA1-containing HDL particles, which can then be delipidated and reinfused. This has shown promise in reducing atheroma in nonhuman primates [164] and (IVUS determined) carotid plaque in acute coronary syndrome patients [165]. In the future these types of apheresis therapies may be of clinical benefit to a limited subset of people with diabetes.

## Newer Targets for Triglyceride Lowering

Similar to the situation with increasing HDL levels by pharmacologic means, there are no data that definitely show that lowering triglyceride levels leads to a reduction in clinical events. As noted earlier, many of the fibrate trials have been handicapped by the fact that they were not performed in hypertriglyceridemic subjects. In the FIELD study, many of the vascular benefits, such as the retinopathy benefit [20], did not correlate with reduction in the standard lipid measures. Even if the ongoing niacin trials are positive, they are unlikely to show a definitive role for triglyceride lowering because of the multiple other effects of niacin. Nonetheless, there have been considerable efforts over the past several years to develop hypotriglyceridemic drugs that work by reducing hepatic triglyceride production. These include inhibitors of DGAT2, ACAT, and MTP, discussed above, which lower both VLDL and LDL levels. None have been very successful to date, with lipid accumulation in the liver, skin, and other tissues being the biggest problems with these agents.

## Fish Oils

High doses of fish oils, which contain docosahexaenoic acid (DHA) and eicosapentaenoic acid (EPA), greater than that usually achievable by the regular consumption of oily fish meals, are effective at lowering triglyceride levels, usually by 10–30 %, in a dose-dependent manner. Other effects such as antiplatelet, antiarrhythmic, and anti-inflammatory effects may also contribute to clinical benefit. The wide range of fish oil capsules available in the supermarkets, health food stores, and in pharmacies (without a prescription) attest to the public interest in the use of fish oil supplements. In a recent analysis of 20 fish oil trials of at least 1 year between 1982 and 2012 including 68,860 subjects, there was no statistically significant association between all deaths, cardiac-related deaths, sudden deaths, heart attacks, and strokes among people taking the supplements [166].

In the GISSI-Prevenzione study (using DHA and EPA) [166] and the Japan EPA Lipid Intervention Study (JELIS) (using 1.8 g EPA daily) in statin-treated postmenopausal women and men [168], a prescribed fish oil supplement significantly reduced cardiovascular events in people, including subjects with diabetes, though did not specifically enrol hypertriglyceridemic subjects. Unfortunately in the recent ORIGIN trial of dysglycemic people with or at high risk of type 2 diabetes, 1 g of n-3 fatty acids daily for a median of 6.2 years reduced triglyceride levels (0.16 mmol/L) but did not demonstrate any clinical benefit re cardiovascular or arrhythmia-related death or cardiovascular event reduction [169].

AMR101, a purified fish oil EPA, is in human clinical trials. In the 12-week ANCHOR study (on a statin background) [170] and in the MARINE study [171] of high cardiovascular disease risk subjects with hypertriglyceridemia, 2–4 g a day of AMR101 was well tolerated and was associated with lower triglycerides (up to 21 %), VLDL-C, total cholesterol, ApoB, lipoprotein-associated phospholipase A(2), and CRP levels. LDL-C levels did not change significantly.

A large 6-year clinical end-point study of AMR101 in 8,000 patients with hypertriglyceridemia—the Reduction of Cardiovascular Events with EPA-Intervention Trial (REDUCE-IT)—is in progress.

Other drugs in development may target the recently identified omega-3 receptor which mediates lipid, anti-inflammatory, and insulin-sensitizing effects [172].

## Apo C-III ASO

ApoC-III, an apolipoprotein that is transported on both VLDL and HDL, is an inhibitor of lipoprotein lipase [173, 174]. High circulating levels of apoC-III associate with hypertriglyceridemia and increased risk of cardiovascular disease. Recently it was shown that a null mutation in the apoC-III gene was associated with reduced triglyceride levels, a favorable lipid profile, and reduced risk of cardiovascular disease [175]. This has prompted a renewed search for approaches to lower apoC-III levels. One specific approach that might have promise in special circumstances is the use of an ASO directed specifically at apoC-III. Since ASOs need to be administered parenterally, this would obviously not have widespread use and is unlikely to be tested in a large outcomes study. Nonetheless, it demonstrates the potential use of a novel molecular approach based on molecular epidemiological findings.

## Other Novel Agents

As well as quantitative changes, qualitative changes in lipoproteins are also implicated in the lipoprotein-mediated vascular complications of diabetes. Such changes, including lipoprotein glycation, oxidation, immune complex formation, and matrix-binding effects, have been discussed in other chapters in this book. Novel therapies that ameliorate these processes and vascular responses to native and modified lipoproteins could also contribute to reducing vascular damage and improving clinical outcomes in people with diabetes.

## Drugs to Reduce Common Lipid Drug Side Effects

A common clinical problem in general practice and in specialist lipid clinics is that people with dyslipidemia are appropriately prescribed lipid-modifying drugs and they cannot tolerate them due to side effects. Myalgia related to statins is one such example. Sometimes these problems can be overcome by finding and (where possible) treating the alternate cause of the problematic symptom (such as a myopathy, hypothyroidism, low vitamin D levels, or drug interactions causing muscle-related problems [176]), by dosage reduction and slow up-titration of the lipid drug, or by changing to an alternate lipid drug. Other agents that are often suggested to reduce statin-related muscle symptoms, thought to be related to mitochondrial effects in muscle, include vitamin D, coenzyme Q10, and magnesium supplements [176, 177]. Randomized controlled placebo-controlled trials are desirable.

Nicotinic acid is another lipid drug whose side effects, including glucose intolerance and flushing, can limit its tolerability and clinical usefulness. Attempts to ameliorate these problems include the development of slow-release preparations and coadministration with aspirin and with laropiprant (discussed above). Similar challenges may also occur with the emerging treatments.

## Conclusions

Dyslipoproteinemia contributes to the macrovascular and microvascular complications of diabetes. Improving lipid levels with oral agents such as statins and fibrates has improved cardiovascular outcomes in the general population and also in people with diabetes. Some lipid drugs can also protect the microvasculature in people with type 2 diabetes, but as yet this is an off-label effect (of fenofibrate). These important clinical benefits may relate to the direct effects of the improved lipid profile or to pleiotropic effects. Emerging lipid agents include more potent agents of the currently available lipid drug classes, combinations thereof (which may increase patient adherence and reduce cost), and more novel modulators of genes and enzymes related to lipoprotein metabolism, such as antisense therapeutics and enzyme inhibitors or activators. Drugs that safely alter lipoprotein interactions with matrix and cells or relevant cell signaling pathways may also prove useful, as could agents that mimic and amplify the pleiotropic effects of lipid drugs.

The development and testing of even more effective lipoprotein-targeted therapies will be a costly endeavor, but there are many millions of people with diabetes, and also people without diabetes, who may benefit by reduced rates of vascular damage and by improved quality and quantity of life. Avoidance of costly clinical events by primary or secondary prevention may also be cost-effective for those agencies that fund the treatments. This major and costly pharmaceutical and academic endeavor should also be complemented by clinical research to identify who requires such treatment(s), when they should take them, and for how long. Post-marketing surveillance and oversight by regulatory bodies will help ensure the safety of these new treatments as their use spreads beyond randomized controlled trials. Treatment algorithms, health economics analyses, and health-care policy should ensure translation of this evolving area of research into optimal clinical practice.

## References

1. Cholesterol Treatment Trialists' (CTT) Collaboration; Baigent C, Blackwell L, Emberson J, Holland LE, Reith C, Bhala N, Peto R, Barnes EH, Keech A, Simes J, Collins R. Efficacy and safety of more intensive lowering of LDL cholesterol: a meta-analysis of data from 170,000 participants in 26 randomised trials. Lancet 2010;376(9753): 1670–1681.
2. Cholesterol Treatment Trialists' Collaborators, Kearney PM, Blackwell L, Collins R, Keech A, Simes J, Peto R, Armitage J, Baigent C. Efficacy of cholesterol-lowering therapy in 18,686 people with diabetes in 14 randomised trials of statins: a meta-analysis. Lancet. 2008;371:117–25.
3. Study of the Effectiveness of Additional Reductions in Cholesterol and Homocysteine (SEARCH) Collaborative Group, Armitage J, Bowman L, Wallendszus K,Bulbulia R, Rahimi K, Haynes R, Parish S, Peto R, Collins R. Intensive lowering of LDL cholesterol with 80 mg versus 20 mg simvastatin daily in 12,064 survivors of myocardial infarction: a double-blind randomised trial. Lancet. 2010;376(9753):1658–69.
4. Chan DK, O'Rourke F, Shen Q, Mak JC, Hung WT. Meta-analysis of the cardiovascular benefits of intensive lipid lowering with statins. Acta Neurol Scand. 2011;124(3):188–95.
5. Murphy SA, Cannon CP, Wiviott SD, McCabe CH, Braunwald E. Reduction in recurrent cardiovascular events with intensive lipid-lowering statin therapy compared with moderate lipid-lowering statin therapy after acute coronary syndromes from the PROVE IT-TIMI 22 (Pravastatin or Atorvastatin Evaluation and Infection Therapy-Thrombolysis In Myocardial Infarction 22) trial. J Am Coll Cardiol. 2009;54(25): 2358–62.
6. LaRosa JC, Deedwania PC, Shepherd J, Wenger NK, Greten H, DeMicco DA, Breazna A. TNT investigators. Comparison of 80 versus 10 mg of atorvastatin on occurrence of cardiovascular events after the first event (from the Treating to New Targets [TNT] trial). Am J Cardiol. 2010;105(3):283–7.
7. Tikkanen MJ, Szarek M, Fayyad R, Holme I, Cater NB, Faergeman O, Kastelein JJ, Olsson AG, Larsen ML, Lindahl C, Pedersen TR. IDEAL investigators. Total cardiovascular disease burden: comparing intensive with moderate statin therapy insights from the IDEAL (Incremental Decrease in End Points Through Aggressive Lipid Lowering) trial. J Am Coll Cardiol. 2009;54(25):2353–7.
8. Josan K, Majumdar SR, McAlister FA. The efficacy and safety of intensive statin therapy: a meta-analysis of randomized trials. CMAJ. 2008;178(5):576–84.
9. Deedwania P, Stone PH, Bairey Merz CN, Cosin-Aguilar J, Koylan N, Luo D, Ouyang P, Piotrowicz R, Schenck-Gustafsson K, Sellier P, Stein JH, Thompson PL, Tzivoni D. Effects of intensive versus moderate lipid-lowering therapy on myocardial ischemia in older patients with coronary heart disease: results of the Study Assessing Goals in the Elderly (SAGE). Circulation. 2007;115(6):700–7.
10. Rouleau J. Improved outcome after acute coronary syndromes with an intensive versus standard lipid-lowering regimen: results from the Pravastatin or Atorvastatin Evaluation and Infection Therapy-Thrombolysis in Myocardial Infarction 22 (PROVE IT-TIMI 22) trial. Am J Med. 2005;118(Suppl 12A): 28–35.

11. Nissen SE. Halting the progression of atherosclerosis with intensive lipid lowering: results from the Reversal of Atherosclerosis with Aggressive Lipid Lowering (REVERSAL) trial. Am J Med. 2005;118(Suppl 12A):22–7.
12. LaRosa JC, Grundy SM, Waters DD, Shear C, Barter P, Fruchart JC, Gotto AM, Greten H, Kastelein JJ, Shepherd J. Wenger NK; Treating to New Targets (TNT) Investigators. Intensive lipid lowering with atorvastatin in patients with stable coronary disease. N Engl J Med. 2005;352(14):1425–35.
13. Lee M, Saver JL, Towfighi A, Chow J, Ovbiagele B. Efficacy of fibrates for cardiovascular risk reduction in persons with atherogenic dyslipidemia: a meta-analysis. Atherosclerosis. 2011;217(2):492–8.
14. Jun M, Foote C, Lv J, Neal B, Patel A, Nicholls SJ, Grobbee DE, Cass A, Chalmers J, Perkovic V. Effects of fibrates on cardiovascular outcomes: a systematic review and meta-analysis. Lancet. 2010;375(9729):1875–84.
15. Keech A, Simes RJ, Barter P, Best J, Scott R, Taskinen MR, Forder P, Pillai A, Davis T, Glasziou P, Drury P, Kesaniemi YA, Sullivan D, Hunt D, Colman P, d'Emden M, Whiting M, Ehnholm C. Effects of long-term fenofibrate therapy on cardiovascular events in 9,795 people with type 2 diabetes mellitus (the FIELD study): randomised controlled trial. Lancet. 2005;366(9500):1849–61.
16. Scott R, O''Brien R, Fulcher G, Pardy C, d'Emden M, Tse D, Taskinen MR, Ehnholm C, Keech A, on behalf of the FIELD Study Investigators. The effects of fenofibrate treatment on cardiovascular disease risk in 9,795 people with type 2 diabetes and various components of the metabolic syndrome: the FIELD study. Diabetes Care. 2009;32(3):493–8.
17. ACCORD Study Group, Ginsberg HN, Elam MB, Lovato LC, Crouse 3rd JR, Leiter LA, Linz P, Friedewald WT, Buse JB, Gerstein HC, Probstfield J, Grimm RH, Ismail-Beigi F, Bigger JT, Goff Jr DC, Cushman WC, Simons-Morton DG, Byington RP. Effects of combination lipid therapy in type 2 diabetes mellitus. N Engl J Med. 2010;362(17):1563–74.
18. Rajamani K, Colman PG, Li LP, Best JD, Voysey M, D'Emden MC, Laakso M, Baker JR, Keech AC, on behalf of the FIELD Study Investigators. Effect of fenofibrate on amputation events in people with type 2 diabetes mellitus (FIELD study): a prespecified analysis of a randomised controlled trial. Lancet. 2009;373(9677):1780–8.
19. ACCORD Study Group; ACCORD Eye Study Group, Chew EY, Ambrosius WT, Davis MD, Danis RP, Gangaputra S, Greven CM, Hubbard L, Esser BA, Lovato JF, Perdue LH, Goff Jr DC, Cushman WC, Ginsberg HN, Elam MB, Genuth S, Gerstein HC, Schubart U, Fine LJ. Effects of medical therapies on retinopathy progression in type 2diabetes. N Engl J Med. 2010;363(3):233–44.
20. Keech AC, Mitchell P, Summanen PA, O'Day J, Davis TM, Moffitt MS, Taskinen MR, Simes RJ, Tse D, Williamson E, Merrifield A, Laatikainen LT, d'Emden MC, Crimet DC, O'Connell RL, Colman PG. FIELD study investigators. Effect of fenofibrate on the need for laser treatment for diabetic retinopathy (FIELD study): a randomised controlled trial. Lancet. 2007;370(9600):1687–97.
21. Davis TM, Ting R, Best JD, Donoghoe MW, Drury PL, Sullivan DR, Jenkins AJ, O'Connell RL, Whiting MJ, Glasziou PP, Simes RJ, Kesäniemi YA, Gebski VJ, Scott RS, Keech AC, on behalf of the FIELD Study Investigators. Effects of fenofibrate on renal function in patients with type 2 diabetes mellitus: the Fenofibrate Intervention and Event Lowering in Diabetes (FIELD) Study. Diabetologia. 2011;54(20): 280–90.
22. Ting RD, Keech AC, Drury PL, Donoghoe MW, Hedley J, Jenkins AJ, Davis TM, Lehto S, Celermajer D, Simes RJ, Rajamani K, Stanton K, FIELD Study Investigators. Benefits and safety of long-term fenofibrate therapy in people with type 2 diabetes and renal impairment: the FIELD Study. Diabetes Care. 2012;35(2):218–25.
23. Sandhu S, Al-Sarraf A, Taraboanta C, Frohlich J, Francis GA. Incidence of pancreatitis, secondary causes, and treatment of patients referred to a specialty lipid clinic with severe hypertriglyceridemia: a retrospective cohort study. Lipids Health Dis. 2011;10:157.
24. Viljoen A, Wierzbicki AS. Diagnosis and treatment of severe hypertriglyceridemia. Expert Rev Cardiovasc Ther. 2012;10(4):505–14.
25. American Diabetes Association Clinical Practice Guidelines. VI. Prevention, management of complications. Diabetes Care. 2011;34 Suppl 1:S29.
26. Mihos CG, Salas MJ, Santana O. The pleiotropic effects of the hydroxy-methyl-glutaryl-CoA reductase inhibitors in cardiovascular disease: a comprehensive review. Cardiol Rev. 2010;18(6):298–304.
27. Florentin M, Liberopoulos EN, Kei A, Mikhailidis DP, Elisaf MS. Pleiotropic effects of nicotinic acid: beyond high density lipoprotein cholesterol elevation. Curr Vasc Pharmacol. 2011;9(4):385–400.
28. Tsimihodimos V, Liberopoulos E, Elisaf M. Pleiotropic effects of fenofibrate. Curr Pharm Des. 2009;15(5):517–28.
29. D'Adamo E, Caprio S. Type 2 diabetes in youth: epidemiology and pathophysiology. Diabetes Care. 2011;34 Suppl 2:S161–5.
30. Azzopardi P, Brown AD, Zimmet P, Fahy RE, Dent GA, Kelly MJ, Kranzusch K, Maple-Brown LJ, Nossar V, Silink M, Sinha AK, Stone ML, Wren SJ. Type 2 diabetes in young Indigenous Australians in rural and remote areas: diagnosis, screening, management and prevention. Med J Aust. 2012;197(1):32–6.
31. Pavkov ME, Bennett PH, Knowler WC, Krakoff J, Sievers ML, Nelson RG. Effect of youth-onset type 2 diabetes mellitus on incidence of end-stage renal disease and mortality in young and middle-aged Pima Indians. JAMA. 2006;296(4):421–6.
32. Eppens MC, Craig ME, Cusumano J, Hing S, Chan AK, Howard NJ, Silink M, Donaghue KC. Prevalence of diabetes complications in adolescents

with type 2 compared with type 1 diabetes. Diabetes Care. 2006;29(6):1300–6.

33. McGill Jr HC, McMahan CA, Herderick EE, Malcom GT, Tracy RE, Strong JP. Origin of atherosclerosis in childhood and adolescence. Am J Clin Nutr. 2000;72 Suppl 5:1307S–15S.
34. Strong JP, Malcom GT, Newman 3rd WP, Oalmann MC. Early lesions of atherosclerosis in childhood and youth: natural history and risk factors. J Am Coll Nutr. 1992;11(Suppl):51S–4S.
35. Illingworth DR. Management of hypercholesterolemia. Med Clin North Am. 2000;84(1):23–42.
36. Chapman MJ. Pitavastatin: novel effects on lipid parameters. Atheroscler Suppl. 2011;12(3):277–84.
37. Betteridge J. Pitavastatin - results from phase III & IV. Atheroscler Suppl. 2010;11(3):8–14.
38. Teramoto T. The clinical impact of pitavastatin: comparative studies with other statins on LDL-C and HDL-C. Expert Opin Pharmacother. 2012;13(6): 859–65.
39. Yamashita S, Tsubakio-Yamamoto K, Ohama T, Nakagawa-Toyama Y, Nishida M. Molecular mechanisms of HDL-cholesterol elevation by statins and its effects on HDL functions. J Atheroscler Thromb. 2010;17(5):436–51.
40. Catapano AL. Statin-induced myotoxicity: pharmacokinetic differences among statins and the risk of rhabdomyolysis, with particular reference to pitavastatin. Curr Vasc Pharmacol. 2012;10(2):257–67.
41. Teramoto T. Pitavastatin: clinical effects from the LIVES Study. Atheroscler Suppl. 2011;12(3):285–8.
42. Yokote K, Shimano H, Urashima M, Teramoto T. Efficacy and safety of pitavastatin in Japanese patients with hypercholesterolemia: LIVES study and subanalysis. Expert Rev Cardiovasc Ther. 2011;9(5):555–62.
43. Suh SY, Rha SW, Ahn TH, Shin EK, Choi CU, Oh DJ, Bae JH, Hur SH, Yun KH, Oh SK, Kim JH, Kim SW, Chae IH, Kim KS, Hong YJ, Jeong MH, LAMIS investigators. Long-term safety and efficacy of Pitavastatin in patients with acute myocardial infarction (from the Livalo Acute Myocardial Infarction Study [LAMIS]). Am J Cardiol. 2011;108(11): 1530–5.
44. Matsubara T, Naruse K, Arakawa T, Nakao M, Yokoi K, Oguri M, Marui N, Amano T,Ichimiya S, Ohashi T, Imai K, Sakai S, Sugiyama S, Ishii H, Murohara T. Impact of pitavastatin on high-sensitivity C-reactive protein and adiponectin in hypercholesterolemic patients with the metabolic syndrome: The PREMIUM Study. J Cardiol. 2012. [Epub ahead of print] PubMed PMID: 22884685.
45. Hibi K, Kimura T, Kimura K, Morimoto T, Hiro T, Miyauchi K, Nakagawa Y, Yamagishi M, Ozaki Y, Saito S, Yamaguchi T, Daida H, Matsuzaki M, JAPAN-ACS Investigators. Clinically evident polyvascular disease and regression of coronary atherosclerosis after intensive statin therapy in patients with acute coronary syndrome: serial intravascular ultrasound from the Japanese assessment of pitavastatin and atorvastatin in acute coronary syndrome (JAPAN-ACS) trial. Atherosclerosis. 2011;219(2):743–9.
46. Nozue T, Yamamoto S, Tohyama S, Umezawa S, Kunishima T, Sato A, Miyake S, Takeyama Y, Morino Y, Yamauchi T, Muramatsu T, Hibi K, Sozu T, Terashima M, Michishita I. Statin treatment for coronary artery plaque composition based on intravascular ultrasound radiofrequency data analysis. Am Heart J 2012;163(2):191–9.e1.
47. Ikeda K, Takahashi T, Yamada H, Matsui K, Sawada T, Nakamura T, Matsubara H. Effect of intensive statin therapy on regression of carotid intima-media thickness in patients with subclinical carotid atherosclerosis (a prospective, randomized trial: PEACE (Pitavastatin Evaluation of Atherosclerosis Regression by Intensive Cholesterol-lowering Therapy) study). Eur J Prev Cardiol 2012. [Epub ahead of print] PubMed PMID: 22689416.
48. Hong YJ, Jeong MH, Ahn Y, Kim SW, Bae JH, Hur SH, Ahn TH, Rha SW, Kim KS,Chae IH, Kim JH, Yun KH, Oh SK; Other LAMIS investigators. Effect of pitavastatin treatment on changes of plaque volume and composition according to the reduction of high-sensitivity C-reactive protein levels. J Cardiol. 2012;60(4):277–82. doi:10.1016/j.jjcc.2012.04.003.
49. Mori Y, Hirano T. Ezetimibe alone or in combination with pitavastatin prevents kidney dysfunction in 5/6 nephrectomized rats fed high-cholesterol. Metabolism. 2012;61(3):379–88.
50. Tamura Y, Murayama T, Minami M, Yokode M, Arai H. Differential effect of statins on diabetic nephropathy in db/db mice. Int J Mol Med. 2011;28(5):683–7.
51. Kakuda H, Kanasaki K, Koya D, Takekoshi N. The administration of pitavastatin augments creatinine clearance associated with reduction in oxidative stress parameters: acute and early effects. Clin Exp Nephrol. 2012 Sep 5. [Epub ahead of print] PubMed PMID: 22948417.
52. Kimura S, Inoguchi T, Yokomizo H, Maeda Y, Sonoda N, Takayanagi R. Randomized comparison of pitavastatin and pravastatin treatment on the reduction of urinary albumin in patients with type 2 diabetic nephropathy. Diabetes Obes Metab. 2012;14(7):666–9.
53. Dijan JP, Maucci R, Guilmin L, Ferreirira T, Prister P. NCS a6560, a novel nitric oxide donating atorvastatin with a promising safety and efficacy profile: a randomised double blind placebo and active control study. Circulation. 2010;122 Suppl 21:A14267.
54. Masha A, Dinatale S, Allasia S, Martina V. Role of the decreased nitric oxide bioavailability in the vascular complications of diabetes mellitus. Curr Pharm Biotechnol. 2011;12(9):1354–63.
55. Out C, Groen AK, Brufau G. Bile acid sequestrants: more than simple resins. Curr Opin Lipidol. 2012;23(1):43–55.
56. Prawitt J, Staels B. Bile acid sequestrants: glucose-lowering mechanisms. Metab Syndr Relat Disord 2010;8(Suppl 1):S3–8. Epub 2010 Oct 26.

57. Zema MJ. Colesevelam hydrochloride: evidence for its use in the treatment of hypercholesterolemia and type 2 diabetes mellitus with insights into mechanism of action. Core Evid. 2012;7:61–75.
58. Bays HE. Long-term (52–78 weeks) treatment with colesevelam HCl added to metformin therapy in type 2 diabetes mellitus patients. Diabetes Metab Syndr Obes. 2012;5:125–34.
59. Younk LM, Davis SN. Evaluation of colesevelam hydrochloride for the treatment of type 2 diabetes. Expert Opin Drug Metab Toxicol. 2012;8(4): 515–25.
60. Descamps OS, De Sutter J, Guillaume M, Missault L. Where does the interplay between cholesterol absorption and synthesis in the context of statin and/or ezetimibe treatment stand today? Atherosclerosis. 2011;217(2):308–21.
61. Gupta EK, Ito MK. Ezetimibe: the first in a novel class of selective cholesterol-absorption inhibitors. Heart Dis. 2002;4(6):399–409.
62. Bays H. Ezetimibe. Expert Opin Investig Drugs. 2002;11(11):1587–604.
63. Baigent C, Landray MJ, Reith C, Emberson J, Wheeler DC, Tomson C, Wanner C, Krane V, Cass A, Craig J, Neal B, Jiang L, Hooi LS, Levin A, Agodoa L, Gaziano M, Kasiske B, Walker R, Massy ZA, Feldt-Rasmussen B, Krairittichai U, Ophascharoensuk V, Fellström B, Holdaas H, Tesar V, Wiecek A, Grobbee D, de Zeeuw D, Grönhagen-Riska C, Dasgupta T, Lewis D, Herrington W, Mafham M, Majoni W, Wallendszus K, Grimm R, Pedersen T, Tobert J, Armitage J, Baxter A, Bray C, Chen Y, Chen Z, Hill M, Knott C, Parish S, Simpson D, Sleight P, Young A, Collins R, SHARP Investigators. The effects of lowering LDL cholesterol with simvastatin plus ezetimibe in patients with chronic kidney disease (Study of Heart and Renal Protection): a randomised placebo-controlled trial. Lancet. 2011;377(9784):2181–92.
64. Davidson MH, Stein EA, Bays HE, Maki KC, Doyle RT, Shalwitz RA, Ballantyne CM, Ginsberg HN. COMBination of prescription Omega-3 with Simvastatin (COMBOS)Investigators. Efficacy and tolerability of adding prescription omega-3 fatty acids 4 g/d to simvastatin 40 mg/d in hypertriglyceridemic patients: an 8-week,randomized, double-blind, placebo-controlled study. Clin Ther. 2007; 29(7):1354–67.
65. Maki KC, Dicklin MR, Davidson MH, Doyle RT, Ballantyne CM. COMBination of prescription Omega-3 with Simvastatin (COMBOS) Investigators. Baseline lipoprotein lipids and low-density lipoprotein cholesterol response to prescription omega-3 acid ethyl ester added to Simvastatin therapy. Am J Cardiol. 2010;105(10):1409–12.
66. Bays HE, Maki KC, McKenney J, Snipes R, Meadowcroft A, Schroyer R, Doyle RT, Stein E. Long-term up to 24-month efficacy and safety of concomitant prescription omega-3-acid ethyl esters and simvastatin in ypertriglyceridemic patients. Curr Med Res Opin. 2010;26(4):907–15.
67. Mousavi SA, Berge KE, Leren TP. The unique role of proprotein convertase subtilisin/kexin 9 in cholesterol homeostasis. J Intern Med. 2009;266(6):507–19.
68. Lambert G, Charlton F, Rye KA, Piper DE. Molecular basis of PCSK9 function. Atherosclerosis. 2009;203(1):1–7.
69. Humphries SE, Neely RD, Whittall RA, Troutt JS, Konrad RJ, Scartezini M, Li KW, Cooper JA, Acharya J, Neil A. Healthy individuals carrying the PCSK9 p.R46L variant and familial hypercholesterolemia patients carrying PCSK9 p.D374Y exhibit lower plasma concentrations of PCSK9. Clin Chem. 2009;55(12):2153–61.
70. Abifadel M, Rabès JP, Devillers M, Munnich A, Erlich D, Junien C, Varret M, Boileau C. Mutations and polymorphisms in the proprotein convertase subtilisin kexin 9 (PCSK9) gene in cholesterol metabolism and disease. Hum Mutat. 2009;30(4):520–9.
71. Zhao Z, Tuakli-Wosornu Y, Lagace TA, Kinch L, Grishin NV, Horton JD, Cohen JC, Hobbs HH. Molecular characterization of loss-of-function mutations in PCSK9 and identification of a compound heterozygote. Am J Hum Genet. 2006;79(3):514–23.
72. Awan Z, Seidah NG, MacFadyen JG, Benjannet S, Chasman DI, Ridker PM, Genest J. Rosuvastatin, proprotein convertase subtilisin/kexin type 9 concentrations, and LDL cholesterol response: the JUPITER trial. Clin Chem. 2012;58(1):183–9.
73. Baass A, Dubuc G, Tremblay M, Delvin EE, O'Loughlin J, Levy E, Davignon J, Lambert M. Plasma PCSK9 is associated with age, sex, and multiple metabolic markers in a population-based sample of children and adolescents. Clin Chem. 2009;55(9):1637–45.
74. Lambert G, Ancellin N, Charlton F, Comas D, Pilot J, Keech A, Patel S, Sullivan DR, Cohn JS, Rye KA, Barter PJ. Plasma PCSK9 concentrations correlate with LDL and total cholesterol in diabetic patients and are decreased by fenofibrate treatment. Clin Chem. 2008;54(6):1038–45.
75. Chan DC, Hamilton SJ, Rye KA, Chew GT, Jenkins AJ, Lambert G, Watts GF. Fenofibrate concomitantly decreases serum proprotein convertase subtilisin/kexin type 9 and very-low-density lipoprotein particle concentrations in statin-treated type 2 diabetic patients. Diabetes Obes Metab. 2010;12(9): 752–6.
76. Costet P, Hoffmann MM, Cariou B, Guyomarc'h Delasalle B, Konrad T, Winkler K. Plasma PCSK9 is increased by fenofibrate and atorvastatin in a non-additive fashion in diabetic patients. Atherosclerosis. 2010;212(1):246–51.
77. Davignon J, Dubuc G. Statins and ezetimibe modulate plasma proprotein convertase subtilisin kexin-9 (PCSK9) levels. Trans Am Clin Climatol Assoc. 2009;120:163–73.
78. Stein EA, Mellis S, Yancopoulos GD, Stahl N, Logan D, Smith WB, Lisbon E, Gutierrez M, Webb C, Wu R, Du Y, Kranz T, Gasparino E, Swergold GD. Effect of a monoclonal antibody to PCSK9 on LDL cholesterol. N Engl J Med. 2012;366(12): 1108–18.

79. Stamler J. The coronary drug project-findings with regard to estrogen, dextrothyroxine, clofibrate and niacin. Adv Exp Med Biol. 1977;82:52–75.
80. The coronary drug project. Findings leading to further modifications of its protocol with respect to dextrothyroxine. The coronary drug project research group. JAMA. 1972;220(7):996–1008.
81. Medici M, Rivadeneira F, van der Deure WM, Hofman A, van Meurs JB, Styrkársdottir U, van Duijn CM, Spector T, Kiel DP, GEFOS Consortium, Uitterlinden AG, Visser TJ, Peeters RP. A large-scale population-based analysis of common genetic variation in the thyroid hormone receptor alpha locus and bone. Thyroid. 2012, 22(2):223–4
82. Goumidi L, Gauthier K, Legry V, Mayi TH, Houzet A, Cottel D, Montaye M, Proust C, Kee F, Ferrières J, Arveiler D, Ducimetière P, Staels B, Dallongeville J, Chinetti G, Flamant F, Amouyel P, Meirhaeghe A. Association between a thyroid hormone receptor-α gene polymorphism and blood pressure but not with coronary heart disease risk. Am J Hypertens. 2011;24(9):1027–34.
83. Mazziotti G, Canalis E, Giustina A. Drug-induced osteoporosis: mechanisms and clinical implications. Am J Med. 2010;123(10):877–84.
84. Moriguchi M, Noso S, Kawabata Y, Yamauchi T, Harada T, Komaki K, Babaya N, Hiromine Y, Ito H, Yamagata S, Murata K, Higashimoto T, Park C, Yamamoto A, Ohno Y, Ikegami H. Clinical and genetic characteristics of patients with autoimmune thyroid disease with anti-islet autoimmunity. Metabolism. 2011;60(6):761–6.
85. Kowalik MA, Perra A, Pibiri M, Cocco MT, Samarut J, Plateroti M, Ledda-Columbano GM, Columbano A. TRbeta is the critical thyroid hormone receptor isoform in T3-induced proliferation of hepatocytes and pancreatic acinar cells. J Hepatol. 2010;53(4):686–92.
86. Tancevski I, Demetz E, Eller P. Sobetirome: a selective thyromimetic for the treatment of dyslipidemia. Recent Pat Cardiovasc Drug Discov. 2011;6(1):16–9.
87. Parhofer KG. Lipoprotein(a): medical treatment options for an elusive molecule. Curr Pharm Des. 2011;17(9):871–6.
88. Shiohara H, Nakamura T, Kikuchi N, Ozawa T, Nagano R, Matsuzawa A, Ohnota H, Miyamoto T, Ichikawa K, Hashizume K. Discovery of novel indane derivatives as liver-selective thyroid hormone receptor β (TRβ) agonists for the treatment of dyslipidemia. Bioorg Med Chem. 2012;20(11):3622–34.
89. Merki E, Graham MJ, Mullick AE, Miller ER, Crooke RM, Pitas RE, Witztum JL, Tsimikas S. Antisense oligonucleotide directed to human apolipoprotein B-100 reduces lipoprotein(a) levels and oxidized phospholipids on human apolipoprotein B-100 particles in lipoprotein(a) transgenic mice. Circulation. 2008;118(7):743–53.
90. Visser ME, Wagener G, Baker BF, Geary RS, Donovan JM, Beuers UH, Nederveen AJ, Verheij J, Trip MD, Basart DC, Kastelein JJ, Stroes ES. Mipomersen, an apolipoprotein B synthesis inhibitor, lowers low-density lipoprotein cholesterol in high-risk statin-intolerant patients: a randomized, double-blind, placebo-controlled trial. Eur Heart J. 2012;33(9):1142–9.
91. Stein EA, Bays H, O'Brien D, Pedicano J, Piper E, Spezzi A. Lapaquistat acetate: development of a squalene synthase inhibitor for the treatment of hypercholesterolemia. Circulation. 2011;123(18):1974–85.
92. Wierzbicki AS, Hardman T, Prince WT. Future challenges for microsomal transport protein inhibitors. Curr Vasc Pharmacol. 2009;7(3):277–86.
93. Samaha FF, McKenney J, Bloedon LT, Sasiela WJ, Rader DJ. Inhibition of microsomal triglyceride transfer protein alone or with ezetimibe in patients with moderate hypercholesterolemia. Nat Clin Pract Cardiovasc. 2008;5(8):497–505.
94. Tardif JC, Grégoire J, L'Allier PL, Anderson TJ, Bertrand O, Reeves F, Title LM, Alfonso F, Schampaert E, Hassan A, McLain R, Pressler ML, Ibrahim R, Lespérance J, Blue J, Heinonen T, Rodés-Cabau J, Avasimibe and Progression of Lesions on UltraSound (A-PLUS) Investigators. Effects of the acyl coenzyme A: cholesterol acyltransferase inhibitor avasimibe on human atherosclerotic lesions. Circulation. 2004;110(21):3372–7.
95. Nissen SE, Tuzcu EM, Brewer HB, Sipahi I, Nicholls SJ, Ganz P, Schoenhagen P, Waters DD, Pepine CJ, Crowe TD, Davidson MH, Deanfield JE, Wisniewski LM, Hanyok JJ, Kassalow LM, ACAT Intravascular Atherosclerosis Treatment Evaluation (ACTIVATE) Investigators. Effect of ACAT inhibition on the progression of coronary atherosclerosis. N Engl J Med. 2006;354(12):1253–63.
96. Meuwese MC, de Groot E, Duivenvoorden R, Trip MD, Ose L, Maritz FJ, Basart DC, Kastelein JJ, Habib R, Davidson MH, Zwinderman AH, Schwocho LR, Stein EA, CAPTIVATE Investigators. ACAT inhibition and progression of carotid atherosclerosis in patients with familial hypercholesterolemia: the CAPTIVATE randomized trial. JAMA. 2009;301(11):1131–9.
97. Arsenault BJ, Boekholdt SM, Kastelein JJ. Lipid parameters for measuring risk of cardiovascular disease. Nat Rev Cardiol. 2011;8(4):197–206.
98. Mangalmurti SS, Davidson MH. The incremental value of lipids and inflammatory biomarkers in determining residual cardiovascular risk. Curr Atheroscler Rep. 2011;13(5):373–80.
99. Jenkins AJ, Best JD, Klein RL, Lyons TJ. Lipoproteins, glycoxidation and diabetic angiopathy. Diabetes Metab Res Rev. 2004;20(5):349–68.
100. Mahley RW, Huang Y. Atherogenic remnant lipoproteins: role for proteoglycans in trapping, transferring, and internalizing. J Clin Invest. 2007;117(1):94–8.
101. Mulder M, Lombardi P, Jansen H, van Berkel TJ, Frants RR, Havekes LM. Low density lipoprotein receptor internalizes low density and very low den-

sity lipoproteins that are bound to heparan sulfate proteoglycans via lipoprotein lipase. J Biol Chem. 1993;268(13):9369–75.

102. de Beer F, Hendriks WL, van Vark LC, Kamerling SW, van Dijk KW, Hofker MH, Smelt AH, Havekes LM. Binding of beta-VLDL to heparan sulfate proteoglycans requires lipoprotein lipase, whereas ApoE only modulates binding affinity. Arterioscler Thromb Vasc Biol. 1999;19(3):633–7. PubMed PMID: 10073967.
103. Anber V, Millar JS, McConnell M, Shepherd J, Packard CJ. Interaction of very-low-density, intermediate-density, and low-density lipoproteins with human arterial wall proteoglycans. Arterioscler Thromb Vasc Biol. 1997;17(11):2507–14. PubMed PMID: 9409221.
104. Kohli P, Cannon CP. Triglycerides: how much credit do they deserve? Med Clin North Am. 2012;96(1): 39–55.
105. Wierzbicki AS, Clarke RE, Viljoen A, Mikhailidis DP. Triglycerides: a case for treatment? Curr Opin Cardiol. 2012;27(4):398–404. PubMed PMID: 22565137.
106. Talayero BG, Sacks FM. The role of triglycerides in atherosclerosis. Curr Cardiol Rep. 2011;13(6):544–52.
107. Dallinga-Thie GM, Franssen R, Mooij HL, Visser ME, Hassing HC, Peelman F, Kastelein JJ, Péterfy M, Nieuwdorp M. The metabolism of triglyceride-rich lipoproteins revisited: new players, new insight. Atherosclerosis. 2010;211(1):1–8.
108. Austin MA. Refining and expanding the role of small, dense low-density lipoproteins. Atherosclerosis. 2009;207(2):350–1.
109. Barter P. HDL-C: role as a risk modifier. Atheroscler Suppl. 2011;12(3):267–70.
110. Tabet F, Rye KA. High-density lipoproteins, inflammation and oxidative stress. Clin Sci (Lond). 2009;116(2):87–98.
111. Rye KA, Bursill CA, Lambert G, Tabet F, Barter PJ. The metabolism and anti-atherogenic properties of HDL. J Lipid Res. 2009;50(Suppl):S195–200.
112. Barter PJ, Puranik R, Rye KA. New insights into the role of HDL as an anti-inflammatory agent in the prevention of cardiovascular disease. Curr Cardiol Rep. 2007;9(6):493–8.
113. Barter PJ, Baker PW, Rye KA. Effect of high-density lipoproteins on the expression of adhesion molecules in endothelial cells. Curr Opin Lipidol. 2002;13(3):285–8.
114. Jenkins AJ, Rowley KG, Lyons TJ, Best JD, Hill MA, Klein RL. Lipoproteins and diabetic microvascular complications. Curr Pharm Des. 2004;10(27): 3395–418.
115. Watts GF, Karpe F. Why, when and how should hypertriglyceridemia be treated in the high-risk cardiovascular patient? Expert Rev Cardiovasc Ther. 2011;9(8):987–97.
116. Mehra S, Movahed H, Movahed A. Emerging therapies for residual risk. Rev Cardiovasc Med. 2012;13(1):e24–31.
117. Judge EP, Phelan D, O'Shea D. Beyond statin therapy: a review of the management of residual risk in diabetes mellitus. J R Soc Med. 2010;103(9): 357–62.
118. Wanner C, Krane V. Recent advances in the treatment of atherogenic dyslipidemia in type 2 diabetes mellitus. Kidney Blood Press Res. 2011;34(4):209–17.
119. Kumar A, Singh V. Atherogenic dyslipidemia and diabetes mellitus: what's new in the management arena? Vasc Health Risk Manag. 2010;6:665–9.
120. Bruckert E, Labreuche J, Deplanque D, Touboul PJ, Amarenco P. Fibrates effect on cardiovascular risk is greater in patients with high triglyceride levels or atherogenic dyslipidemia profile: a systematic review and meta-analysis. J Cardiovasc Pharmacol. 2011;57(2):267–72. Review. PubMed PMID: 21052016.
121. Stumvoll M, Häring HU. Glitazones: clinical effects and molecular mechanisms. Ann Med. 2002;34(3): 217–24.
122. Singh S, Loke YK, Furberg CD. Long-term risk of cardiovascular events with rosiglitazone: a meta-analysis. JAMA. 2007;298(10):1189–95.
123. Piccinni C, Motola D, Marchesini G, Poluzzi E. Assessing the association of pioglitazone use and bladder cancer through drug adverse event reporting. Diabetes Care. 2011;34(6):1369–71.
124. Nissen SE, Wolski K, Topol EJ. Effect of muraglitazar on death and major adverse cardiovascular events in patients with type 2 diabetes mellitus. JAMA. 2005;294(20):2581–6.
125. Kendall DM, Rubin CJ, Mohideen P, Ledeine JM, Belder R, Gross J, Norwood P, O'Mahony M, Sall K, Sloan G, Roberts A, Fiedorek FT, DeFronzo RA. Improvement of glycemic control, triglycerides, and HDL cholesterol levels with muraglitazar, a dual (alpha/gamma) peroxisome proliferator-activated receptor activator, in patients with type 2 diabetes inadequately controlled with metformin monotherapy: A double-blind, randomized, pioglitazone-comparative study. Diabetes Care. 2006;29(5):1016–23.
126. Henry RR, Lincoff AM, Mudaliar S, Rabbia M, Chognot C, Herz M. Effect of the dual peroxisome proliferator-activated receptor-alpha/gamma agonist aleglitazar on risk of cardiovascular disease in patients with type 2 diabetes (SYNCHRONY): a phase II, randomised, dose-ranging study. Lancet. 2009;374(9684):126–35.
127. Herz M, Gaspari F, Perico N, Viberti G, Urbanowska T, Rabbia M, Wieczorek Kirk D. Effects of high dose aleglitazar on renal function in patients with type 2 diabetes. Int J Cardiol. 2011;151(2):136–42.
128. Wilding JP. PPAR agonists for the treatment of cardiovascular disease in patients with diabetes. Diabetes Obes Metab. 2012;14(11):973–82. doi:10.1111/j.1463-1326.2012.
129. Cariou B, Zaïr Y, Staels B, Bruckert E. Effects of the new dual PPAR α/δ agonist GFT505 on lipid and glucose homeostasis in abdominally obese patients with combined dyslipidemia or impaired glucose metabolism. Diabetes Care. 2011;34(9):2008–14.

130. Crouse 3rd JR. New developments in the use of niacin for treatment of hyperlipidemia: new considerations in the use of an old drug. Coron Artery Dis. 1996;7(4):321–6.
131. Faergeman O. Hypertriglyceridemia and the fibrate trials. Curr Opin Lipidol. 2000;11(6):609–14.
132. Niacin, fenofibrates increase benefits for statin users. These HDL- raising, triglyceride-lowering drugs beat out the use of additional LDL-lowering drugs. Duke Med Health News. 2010;16(8):1–2.
133. Nichols GA, Koro CE, Chan W, Bowlin SJ, Sprecher DL. The association between fibrate use, change in high-density lipoprotein cholesterol, and the risk of cardiovascular disease: a retrospective chart review involving up to 8 years of follow-up. Clin Ther. 2006;28(2):243–50.
134. Helmbold AF, Slim JN, Morgan J, Castillo-Rojas LM, Shry EA, Slim AM. The effects of extended release niacin in combination with omega 3 fatty acid supplements in the treatment of elevated lipoprotein (a). Cholesterol. 2010;2010:306147.
135. Canner PL, Halperin M. Implications of findings in the coronary drug project for secondary prevention trials in coronary heart disease. The coronary; drug project research group. Circulation. 1981;63(6):1342–50.
136. Schlant RC, Forman S, Stamler J, Canner PL. The natural history of coronary heart disease: prognostic factors after recovery from myocardial infarction in 2,789 men. The 5-year findings of the coronary drug project. Circulation. 1982;66(2):401–14.
137. Song WL, Stubbe J, Ricciotti E, Alamuddin N, Ibrahim S, Crichton I, Prempeh M, Lawson JA, Wilensky RL, Rasmussen LM, Puré E, FitzGerald GA. Niacin and biosynthesis of $PGD_2$ by platelet COX-1 in mice and humans. J Clin Invest. 2012;122(4):1459–68.
138. Stern RH. The role of nicotinic acid metabolites in flushing and hepatotoxicity. J Clin Lipidol. 2007;1(3):191–3.
139. Cooper-DeHoff RM, Pacanowski MA, Pepine CJ. Cardiovascular therapies and associated glucose homeostasis: implications across the dysglycemia continuum. J Am Coll Cardiol. 2009;53 Suppl 5:S28–34.
140. Maccubbin DL, Chen F, Anderson JW, Sirah W, McCrary Sisk C, Kher U, Olsson AG, Bays HE, Mitchel YB. Effectiveness and safety of laropiprant on niacin-induced flushing. Am J Cardiol. 2012;110(6):817–22.
141. Guyton JR, Fazio S, Adewale AJ, Jensen E, Tomassini JE, Shah A, Tershakovec AM. Effect of extended-release niacin on new-onset diabetes among hyperlipidemic patients treated with ezetimibe/simvastatin in a randomized controlled trial. Diabetes Care. 2012;35(4):857–60.
142. Brown BG, Zhao XQ, Chait A, Fisher LD, Cheung MC, Morse JS, Dowdy AA, Marino EK, Bolson EL, Alaupovic P, Frohlich J, Albers JJ. Simvastatin and niacin, antioxidant vitamins, or the combination for the prevention of coronary disease. N Engl J Med. 2001;345(22):1583–92.
143. Michos ED, Sibley CT, Baer JT, Blaha MJ, Blumenthal RS. Niacin and statin combination therapy for atherosclerosis regression and prevention of cardiovascular disease events: reconciling the AIM-HIGH (Atherothrombosis Intervention in Metabolic Syndrome With Low HDL/High Triglycerides: Impact on Global Health Outcomes) trial with previous surrogate endpoint trials. J Am Coll Cardiol. 2012;59(23):2058–64.
144. HPS2/THRIVE Clinical Trials.gov. http://www.thrivestudy.org/ (as accessed June 2013).
145. Johns DG, Duffy J, Fisher T, Hubbard BK, Forrest MJ. On- and off-target pharmacology of torcetrapib: current understanding and implications for the structure activity relationships (SAR), discovery and development of cholesteryl ester-transfer protein (CETP) inhibitors. Drugs. 2012;72(4):491–507.
146. Shear C, Beltangady M, Ports W, Duggan W, Barter P. Torcetrapib: predictors of increased clinical risk in the ILLUMINATE study. Circulation 2008;118: S_370–S_371. Abstract 1694
147. Yvan-Charvet L, Matsuura F, Wang N, Bamberger MJ, Nguyen T, Rinninger F, Jiang XC, Shear CL, Tall AR. Inhibition of cholesteryl ester transfer protein by torcetrapib modestly increases macrophage cholesterol efflux to HDL. Arterioscler Thromb Vasc Biol. 2007;27:1132–8.
148. Brousseau ME, Diffenderfer MR, Millar JS, Nartsupha C, Asztalos BF, Welty FK, Wolfe ML, Rudling M, Björkhem I, Angelin B, Mancuso JP, Digenio AG, Rader DJ, Schaefer EJ. Effects of cholesteryl ester transfer protein inhibition on high-density lipoprotein subspecies, apolipoprotein A-I metabolism, and fecal sterol excretion. Arterioscler Thromb Vasc Biol. 2005;25(5):1057–64.
149. Hu X, Dietz JD, Xia C, Knight DR, Loging WT, Smith AH, Yuan H, Perry DA, Keiser J. Torcetrapib induces aldosterone and cortisol production by an intracellular calcium-mediated mechanism independently of cholesteryl ester transfer protein inhibition. Endocrinology. 2009;150:2211–9.
150. Forrest MJ, Bloomfield D, Briscoe RJ, Brown PN, Cumiskey AM, Ehrhart J, Hershey JC, Keller WJ, Ma X, McPherson HE, et al. Torcetrapib-induced blood pressure elevation is independent of CETP inhibition and is accompanied by increased circulating levels of aldosterone. Br J Pharmacol. 2008;154:1465–73.
151. Stein EA, Roth EM, Rhyne JM, Burgess T, Kallend D, Robinson JG. Safety and tolerability of dalcetrapib (RO4607381/JTT-705): results from a 48-week trial. Eur Heart J. 2010;31(4):480–8.
152. Lüscher TF, Taddei S, Kaski JC, Jukema JW, Kallend D, Münzel T, Kastelein JJ, Deanfield JE, dal-VESSEL Investigators. Vascular effects and safety of dalcetrapib in patients with or at risk of coronary heart disease: the dal-VESSEL randomized clinical trial. Eur Heart J. 2012;33(7):857–65.
153. Fayad ZA, Mani V, Woodward M, et al. Safety and efficacy of dalcetrapib on atherosclerotic disease using novel non-invasive multimodality imaging

(dal-PLAQUE): a randomised clinical trial. Lancet. 2011;378(9802):1547–59.

154. Cannon CP, Dansky HM, Davidson M, Gotto AM Jr, Brinton EA, Gould AL,Stepanavage M, Liu SX, Shah S, Rubino J, Gibbons P, Hermanowski-Vosatka A,Binkowitz B, Mitchel Y, Barter P, DEFINE Investigators. Design of the DEFINE trial: determining the EFficacy and tolerability of CETP INhibition with AnacEtrapib. Am Heart J 2009;158(4): 513–519.e3.
155. REVEAL trial. Clinicaltrials.gov. http://clinicaltrials.gov/show/NCT01252953. (as accessed June 2013).
156. White CR, Datta G, Mochon P, Zhang Z, Kelly O, Curcio C, Parks D, Palgunachari M, Handattu S, Gupta H, Garber DW, Anantharamaiah GM. Vasculoprotective effects of apolipoprotein mimetic peptides: an evolving paradigm in Hdl therapy. Vasc Dis Prev. 2009;6:122–30.
157. Bucci M, Cigliano L, Vellecco V, D'Andrea LD, Ziaco B, Rossi A, Sautebin L, Carlucci A, Abrescia P, Pedone C, Ianaro A, Cirino G. Apolipoprotein A-I (ApoA-I) mimetic peptide P2a by restoring cholesterol esterification unmasks ApoA-I anti-inflammatory endogenous activity in vivo. J Pharmacol Exp Ther. 2012;340(3):716–22.
158. Di Bartolo BA, Vanags LZ, Tan JT, Bao S, Rye KA, Barter PJ, Bursill CA. The apolipoprotein A-I mimetic peptide, ETC-642, reduces chronic vascular inflammation in the rabbit. Lipids Health Dis. 2011;10:224.
159. Imaizumi S, Navab M, Morgantini C, Charles-Schoeman C, Su F, Gao F, Kwon M, Ganapathy E, Meriwether D, Farias-Eisner R, Fogelman AM, Reddy ST. Dysfunctional high-density lipoprotein and the potential of apolipoprotein A-1 mimetic peptides to normalize the composition and function of lipoproteins. Circ J. 2011;75(7):1533–8.
160. Vecoli C, Cao J, Neglia D, Inoue K, Sodhi K, Vanella L, Gabrielson KK, Bedja D, Paolocci N, L'abbate A, Abraham NG. Apolipoprotein A-I mimetic peptide L-4F prevents myocardial and coronary dysfunction in diabetic mice. J Cell Biochem. 2011;112(9): 2616–26.
161. Datta G, Epand RF, Epand RM, Chaddha M, Kirksey MA, Garber DW, Lund-Katz S, Phillips MC, Hama S, Navab M, Fogelman AM, Palgunachari MN, Segrest JP, Anantharamaiah GM. Aromatic residue position on the nonpolar face of class a amphipathic helical peptides determines biological activity. J Biol Chem. 2004;279(25):26509–17.
162. Carballo-Jane E, Chen Z, O'Neill E, Wang J, Burton C, Chang CH, Chen X, Eveland S, Frantz-Wattley B, Gagen K, Hubbard B, Ichetovkin M, Luell S, Meurer R, Song X, Strack A, Langella A, Cianetti S, Rech F, Capitò E, Bufali S, Veneziano M, Verdirame M, Bonelli F, Monteagudo E, Pessi A, Ingenito R, Bianchi E. ApoA-I mimetic peptides promote pre-β HDL formation in vivo causing remodeling of HDL and triglyceride accumulation at higher dose. Bioorg Med Chem. 2010;18(24):8669–78.
163. Thompson GR, HEART-UK LDL Apheresis Working Group. Recommendations for the use of LDL apheresis. Atherosclerosis. 2008;198(2):247–55.
164. Sacks FM, Rudel LL, Conner A, et al. Selective delipidation of plasma HDL enhances reverse cholesterol transport in vivo. J Lipid Res. 2009;50(5): 894–907.
165. Waksman R, Torguson R, Kent KM, et al. A first in-man, randomized, placebo-controlled study to evaluate the safety and feasibility of autologous delipidated high-density lipoprotein plasma infusions in patients with acute coronary syndrome. J Am Coll Cardiol. 2010;55(24):2727–35.
166. Rizos EC, Ntzani EE, Bika E, Kostapanos MS, Elisaf MS. Association between omega-3 fatty acid supplementation and risk of major cardiovascular disease events: a systematic review and meta-analysis. JAMA. 2012;308(10):1024–33.
167. Gruppo Italiano per lo Studio della Sopravvivenza nell'Infarto miocardico. Dietary supplementation with n-3 polyunsaturated fatty acids and vitamin E after myocardial infarction: results of the GISSIPrevenzione trial. Lancet 1999;354(9177):447–55.
168. Yokoyama M, Origasa H, Matsuzaki M, Matsuzawa Y, Saito Y, Ishikawa Y, Oikawa S, Sasaki J, Hishida H, Itakura H, Kita T, Kitabatake A, Nakaya N, Sakata T, Shimada K, Shirato K, Japan EPA. lipid intervention study (JELIS) Investigators. Effects of eicosapentaenoic acid on major coronary events in hypercholesterolaemic patients (JELIS): a randomised open-label, blinded endpoint analysis. Lancet. 2007;369(9567):1090–8.
169. ORIGIN Trial Investigators, Bosch J, Gerstein HC, Dagenais GR, Díaz R, Dyal L, Jung H, Maggiono AP, Probstfield J, Ramachandran A, Riddle MC, Rydén LE, Yusuf S. n-3 fatty acids and cardiovascular outcomes in patients with dysglycemia. N Engl J Med. 2012;367(4):309–18.
170. Ballantyne CM, Bays HE, Kastelein JJ, Stein E, Isaacsohn JL, Braeckman RA, Soni PN. Efficacy and safety of eicosapentaenoic acid ethyl ester (AMR101) therapy in statin-treated patients with persistent high triglycerides (from the ANCHOR study). Am J Cardiol. 2012;110(7):984–92.
171. Bays HE, Ballantyne CM, Kastelein JJ, Isaacsohn JL, Braeckman RA, Soni PN. Eicosapentaenoic acid ethyl ester (AMR101) therapy in patients with very high triglyceride levels (from the multi-center, plAcebo-controlled, randomized, double-blINd, 12-week study with an open-label extension [MARINE] trial). Am J Cardiol. 2011;108(5):682–90.
172. Oh DY, Talukdar S, Bae EJ, Imamura T, Morinaga H, Fan W, Li P, Lu WJ, Watkins SM, Olefsky JM. GPR120 is an omega-3 fatty acid receptor mediating potent anti-inflammatory and insulin-sensitizing effects. Cell. 2010;142(5):687–98.
173. Gerritsen G, Rensen PC, Kypreos KE, Zannis VI, Havekes LM, Willems van Dijk K. ApoC-III deficiency prevents hyperlipidemia induced by apoE overexpression. J Lipid Res. 2005;46(7):1466–73.

174. Yamamoto M, Morita SY, Kumon M, Kawabe M, Nishitsuji K, Saito H, Vertut-Doï A, Nakano M, Handa T. Effects of plasma apolipoproteins on lipoprotein lipase-mediated lipolysis of small and large lipid emulsions. Biochim Biophys Acta. 2003; 1632(1–3):31–9.
175. Pollin TI, Damcott CM, Shen H, Ott SH, Shelton J, Horenstein RB, Post W, McLenithan JC, Bielak LF, Peyser PA, Mitchell BD, Miller M, O'Connell JR, Shuldiner AR. A null mutation in human APOC3 confers a favorable plasma lipid profile and apparent cardioprotection. Science. 2008;322(5908):1702–5.
176. Glueck CJ, Budhani SB, Masineni SS, Abuchaibe C, Khan N, Wang P, Goldenberg N. Vitamin D deficiency, myositis-myalgia, and reversible statin intolerance. Curr Med Res Opin. 2011;27(9): 1683–90.
177. Mas E, Mori TA. Coenzyme Q(10) and statin myalgia: what is the evidence? Curr Atheroscler Rep. 2010;12(6):407–13.

# Index



A.J. Jenkins et al. (eds.), *Lipoproteins in Diabetes Mellitus*, Contemporary Diabetes,
DOI 10.1007/978-1-4614-7554-5, © Springer Science+Business Media New York 2014

## M

**R**

FSC
www.fsc.org
MIX
Papier | Fördert gute Waldnutzung
FSC® C083411

Kolibri 360 GmbH
Ferdinand-Jühlke-Straße 7
99095 Erfurt, Deutschland
produktsicherheit@kolibri360.de